# Medical, Psychosocial, and Vocational Aspects of Disability

Edited by

**Martin G. Brodwin, Ph.D., C.R.C.**
Coordinator of the Rehabilitation Counselor Education Program
California State University, Los Angeles
Los Angeles, California

**Fernando A. Tellez, M.D.**
Chief Medical Consultant
State of California, Department of Rehabilitation
Sacramento, California

and

**Sandra K. Brodwin, M.S., C.R.C.**
Rehabilitation Counselor and Consultant
Image Development
Los Angeles, California

# Medical, Psychosocial, and Vocational Aspects of Disability

Edited by

*Martin G. Brodwin, Ph.D., C.R.C.,*

*Fernando A. Tellez, M.D.*

*and*

*Sandra K. Brodwin, M.S., C.R.C.*

ISBN #0-945019-34-3
© Copyright Martin G. Brodwin, 1993

Published and Marketed by:

Elliott & Fitzpatrick, Inc.
P.O. Box 1945
Athens, GA 30603
1-706-548-8161

# PREFACE

The recent enactment of the Americans with Disabilities Act signaled a new era in America for persons with disabilities. These individuals, often excluded from mainstream society, will now be able to participate in all phases of life to a far greater extent. Rehabilitation counselors, as well as educators, nurses, counselors in other settings, work evaluators, and vocational experts have the responsibility to facilitate increasing progression into independent living, education, employment, and leisure-time activities for persons with disabilities. The Americans with Disabilities Act defines a "person with a disability" as someone who: "(1) has a physical or mental impairment that substantially limits one or more major life activities; (2) has a record of such an impairment; or (3) is regarded as having such an impairment."

Rehabilitation involves counseling a person with a disability to assist that individual to acquire skills necessary for maximum functioning and independence. The professional who has an understanding of medical aspects of disabling conditions and its relationship to employment is unique within the counseling profession. Counselors need to read, understand, and interpret medical reports and other medical information regarding the client. Knowledge of medical aspects of disability is crucial for counselors working with persons with disabilities. With comprehension of this information, the counselor will be able to determine the person's functional limitations and potential for rehabilitation.

Knowledge of functional limitations allows the counselor and the individual with a disability to obtain information necessary for developing positive directions for rehabilitation. Rehabilitation may include job modification, reasonable accommodation, educational pursuit, training or on-the-job training, supported employment, job placement, and independent living. The purpose of any rehabilitation counseling goal is to empower the individual with a disability to successfully participate in all phases of life.

This book is a textbook for students and a reference book for practicing counselors. Its intended audience includes rehabilitation counselors in both public and private sectors, rehabilitation educators and their students (undergraduate and graduate programs), vocational experts, work evaluators, and counselors in a variety of settings. It also can be used by allied health professionals in various related disciplines.

The reader is encouraged to have a medical dictionary available when reading this book. A glossary was not included as the writers have found glossaries to be inadequate, both in providing sufficient explanations and in defining most of the required vocabulary. Many words are provided with a short definition in parentheses within the text.

## Overview of the Contents

The book contains thirty-three chapters encompassing the common disabilities. Many of the chapters have case studies to help stimulate thinking and discussion about the particular topic. All the cases are hypothetical and do not relate to any particular individual. Section I includes "Rehabilitation: A Case Study Approach", "Medical Terminology", and "The Medical Examination", all of which help establish a foundation for subsequent chapters. Chapter 1 contains two case studies; one has appropriate responses to the questions, while the questions on the second case study are left open for discussion. Other topics found in Section I include: drug abuse, alcoholism, sexuality and disability, and the acquired immunodeficiency syndrome.

Section II contains information regarding coping with a physical disability, plastic and reconstructive surgery, image of people with disabilities, psychiatric disabilities, mental retardation, and chronic pain syndromes.

Section III focuses on hearing and visual disabilities.

Section IV discusses the disabilities of cancer, hemophilia, sickle cell disease, diabetes mellitus, respiratory dysfunction, and cardiovascular disease.

In Section V are found the topics of back and neck pain in industrial injuries, rheumatic diseases, paraplegia and quadriplegia, evaluating hand function and impairment, and orthotics and prosthetics.

Section VI includes chapters on neurological conditions, epilepsy, multiple sclerosis, acquired traumatic brain injury, learning disabilities, cerebrovascular accidents, and cerebral palsy.

## *Acknowledgements*

The editors did their utmost to maintain the meaning and philosophy of each author and, at the same time, to have the chapters conform to a similar style. We sincerely appreciate each author's time and patience during the difficult editing process.

Our sincere appreciation to all of the authors of the chapters in this book. They each spent many hours writing and revising their manuscripts; we believe that through their efforts this text will provide the reader with an excellent resource of medical aspects of disabling conditions and their relationship to employment issues.

We wish to thank many individuals for their thoughtful reviews, helpful comments, and suggestions: Kathy Casey, Rosemary Hendrix, Sallye Kaproff, Kris Kohler, Robert Liebman, Rebecca Macrory, Leo Orange, Julie Seguin, Carol St. John, Barbara Woodall, among others.

A special thanks to Joyce Brendle, Hearing Office Manager, and the staff of the Office of Hearings and Appeals, Social Security Administration, Pasadena, California for their constant encouragement and support; Lynn Willmott for her review and editing of many of the chapters; and Linda Marubayashi, for the typing and re-typing of seemingly endless manuscript drafts.

# FOREWORD

Rehabilitationists have an acknowledged need to synthesize a vast array of information about their clients from a multitude of sources, including physicians, psychologists, occupational and physical therapists, vocational evaluators, and social workers. All this information must be condensed into a comprehensive analysis, the result being a complete plan of rehabilitation services. The development of a current, comprehensive, and useable resource to enable rehabilitationists to complete these tasks has been a long-standing need for both students and practitioners.

Medical, psychosocial, and vocational aspects of disability are at the very core of rehabilitation counseling. To attempt to cover these three areas in a coherent and substantial manner was indeed a bold challenge. When Dr. Brodwin first shared his plans with me, we discussed the difficulties in achieving such a task. Yet, Dr. Brodwin, Dr. Tellez, and Ms. Brodwin have achieved all that they set out to do. Those of us who have taught medical and psychosocial aspects of disability have long desired a book that would address these issues in a working manner. Professionals involved in rehabilitation and other forms of counseling have also wanted such a book because of the necessity to forage through numerous references when seeking an answer to a question involving disability.

The editors have accomplished what this writer considers to be a major achievement in that they have brought up to date and greatly supplemented the information contained in standard textbooks and references in the field. This book has a consistent chapter organization and uses a functional holistic approach, as well as incorporating new topics to enable the rehabilitationist to more effectively use the information. One topic finally addressed in a comprehensive manner is sexuality and disability, a point usually either glossed over or ignored in other texts of disability. A feature that makes this book more valuable is the consistent use of case studies to demonstrate the material presented.

**Medical, Psychosocial, and Vocational Aspects of Disability** is intended to be both a textbook and a reference. It suits both purposes well. The up-to-date and comprehensive nature of the information will make it the viable resource on these crucial disability issues for the foreseeable future.

Joseph E. Havranek, Ed.D., C.R.C.
Assistant Professor of Rehabilitation Counseling
Bowling Green State University
Bowling Green, Ohio

# TABLE OF CONTENTS

## Medical, Psychosocial, and Vocational Aspects of Disability

# Chapter 1

# REHABILITATION: A CASE STUDY APPROACH

by
*Martin G. Brodwin, Ph.D., C.R.C.*
*and*
*Sandra K. Brodwin, M.S., C.R.C.*

## INTRODUCTION

Rehabilitation professionals (counselors, rehabilitation providers, and job placement specialists) need expertise in the area of medical aspects of disabling conditions to work effectively with persons who have disabilities. It is the function of the rehabilitation professional to apply this expertise when developing vocational plans and when determining the functional limitations and rehabilitation potential of clients. Knowledge of medical aspects of disability is a significant component in the development of appropriate rehabilitation interventions. The "vocational profile" case study approach is one method of evaluating a client from the aspects of age, education, work history, occupationally significant characteristics of work, and transferability of work skills.

Development of vocational and educational rehabilitation plans and programs relies heavily on the expertise of the rehabilitation professional. A realistic objective for a vocational or educational plan is one that is within the client's physical, intellectual, and emotional capacities. To establish a realistic objective, the rehabilitation professional applies knowledge of the client's vocational profile, medical aspects of the particular disability, the client's interaction with the environment, and the effort and persistence the client demonstrates at a task in the face of obstacles. Another issue often disregarded is the counselor's efforts and persistence at providing rehabilitation services.

This chapter addresses the functions of the rehabilitation professional who provides services within the parameters of a variety of rehabilitation systems. The authors believe the use of the "vocational profile" will assist in client case analysis and improve the chances for a successful return to employment. This chapter focuses on the importance of the "holistic approach" for successful rehabilitation. Maximizing the "self-efficacy" of the client is the final component of this chapter.

## VOCATIONAL PROFILE

The "vocational profile" is a term used to describe certain characteristics of a person. Vocational Experts (VEs) for the Social Security Administration's (SSA) Office of Hearings and Appeals, use the vocational profile when testifying on disability and related issues. We are using the SSA vocational profile model as it is part of a nationally-mandated program that is uniform throughout the country. The vocational profile includes the categories of age, education, and work history as they relate to a client, as well as occupationally significant characteristics and transferability of work skills. The following categories - **age** (SSA Section # 404.1563), **education** (SSA Section # 404.1564), and **work experience** (SSA Section #s 404.1565, 404.1567, and 404.1568) - are taken from the guidelines of the Social Security Administration (U.S. Department of Health & Human Services, 1988).

## Age Category

Age is important in evaluating the total person. As an individual ages, it becomes more difficult to adapt to new and unfamiliar work situations. Age becomes more crucial when an individual has had only physically demanding jobs and has developed few, if any, work skills. The following categories are taken from the guidelines of the Social Security Administration (U.S. Department of Health & Human Services, 1988).

**Younger person.** An individual is in this category if under the age of 50. Generally, age in this category will not affect the person's ability to adapt to a new work situation.

**Person approaching advanced age.** An individual between 50-54 years of age is considered a "person approaching advanced age." This age category, along with a severe impairment and limited work experience, may seriously affect the ability to adjust to a significant number of jobs in the national economy.

**Person of advanced age.** This category is appropriate if a person is between 55-59 years of age. With advancing age, it becomes more difficult to obtain employment, especially when the individual has an unskilled work background, a history of physically arduous work, and a minimal education. Skills a person possesses that can be transferred to other similar jobs and work activity (often less physically demanding) become very important as an individual ages.

**Close to retirement age.** When individuals are 60 years of age or older, they are considered to be "close to retirement age." Skills at this age need to be highly transferable and are pivotal to an individual's success in the rehabilitation process.

The rehabilitation professional needs to consider age as a factor. All aspects of the vocational profile will affect the determination of the importance of age to the total rehabilitation potential of the individual. However, age should never be cited as a reason for denying rehabilitation services. Also, it is discriminatory for a potential employer to make hiring decisions based on a person's age.

## Educational Level

Educational level is the amount of formal schooling a person achieves. Although a specific grade level is important, it is only one means of assessment. When evaluating rehabilitation potential, the counselor needs to consider how long ago a person attended school, the quality of the educational experience, additional informal or formal education, and other training.

**Illiteracy.** Illiteracy means the inability to read or write. People are placed in this category if they cannot read or write simple messages, such as instructions or inventory lists.

**Marginal education.** Generally, this indicates a formal education at the 6th grade level or less. The person who has a "marginal education" has only a basic ability in reasoning, arithmetic, and language.

**Limited education.** A person of "limited education" has a formal education between the 7th and 11th grades (without having attained a high school diploma or its equivalence).

**High school education and above.** "High school education and above" means the person has a high school diploma or the equivalence. Persons with additional education beyond high school are also classified within this category. The individual in this category has obtained abilities in reasoning, arithmetic, and language skills to do more complex work activity.

## Work History

This section will be subdivided into the following categories: specific vocational preparation, skill requirements, physical exertion, occupationally significant characteristics, vocational skills, and transferability of skills.

**Specific vocational preparation (training time).** This represents the amount of time required to learn the techniques, acquire information, and develop the facility needed for average performance in a specific job situation. One may acquire the training in a school, work, military, or institutional setting. It does not include orientation training required of a fully qualified worker to become accustomed to the special conditions of a job. Specific vocational preparation includes training given in any of the following circumstances:

1. Vocational education (such as high school and that part of college training organized around a specific vocational objective).

2. Apprentice training (for apprenticeship jobs only).

3. In-plant training (given by an employer in an organized classroom situation).

4. On-the-job training (training on the actual job under the instruction of a qualified worker).

5. Essential experience in other jobs (serving in less responsible jobs which lead to the higher grade job or serving in other jobs that provide skills that are transferable).

The following identify the various levels of specific vocational preparation.

| Level | Time |
|---|---|
| 1 | Short demonstration |
| 2 | Anything beyond short demonstration up to and including 30 days |
| 3 | Over 30 days up to and including 3 months |
| 4 | Over 3 months up to and including 6 months |
| 5 | Over 6 months up to and including one year |
| 6 | Over one year up to and including 2 years |
| 7 | Over 2 years up to and including 4 years |
| 8 | Over 4 years up to and including 10 years |
| 9 | Over 10 years |

In terms of skill levels, we typically find unskilled work to have a specific vocational preparation (SVP) of levels 1 or 2 (occasionally at level 3). Semiskilled work usually has an SVP level of 3, 4, 5, or 6. Skilled work typically has an SVP classification level of 7, 8, or 9. These categories are only general guidelines; each job must be evaluated individually. For example, a job with an SVP level of 3 may be unskilled or semiskilled, depending on whether there are specific skills learned on the job. This decision is made by an individual experienced in the analysis of jobs and job-related skills.

**Skill requirements.**

*Unskilled work* - Work is in this category if it requires little or no judgement to do simple duties and if it can be learned on the job in a short time. A person can learn to do unskilled jobs in 30 days or less. These jobs frequently require considerable strength. For example, jobs are unskilled if the primary work duties involve stock or material handling, machine feeding, sorting, simple assembling, or machine tending. Work in this category requires little specific vocational preparation and judgement. **A person does not gain work skills by doing unskilled jobs.**

*Semiskilled work* - Semiskilled work requires some skills but not complex work activity. These jobs may involve alertness and close attention to observing machine processes or inspecting, testing, or quality control. Other aspects of semiskilled work include guarding equipment, materials, or persons against damage, loss, or injury. This category consists of other types of activities which are similarly less complex than skilled work but more complex than unskilled work, and can involve dexterity such as working with tools, equipment, and measuring devices. Typically, semiskilled work activity requires training over 30 days up to a maximum of 2 years.

*Skilled work* - This category of work requires an individual to use judgement to determine fairly complex machine and manual operations to be performed to obtain proper form, quality, and quantity of materials produced. Skilled work may require laying out work, estimating quality, determining suitability and needed quantities of material, making precise measurements, reading blueprints or other specifications, or making necessary complex computations or mechanical adjustments to control or regulate the work. Other skilled jobs involve dealing with people, facts, or figures, or abstract ideas at a high level of complexity. This work activity typically requires more than 2 years to learn.

**Physical exertion requirements.** In reviewing a client's past relevant work experience, the counselor evaluates the physical exertion requirements of the person's work duties. Physical exertion requirements are summarized in the following categories. If medical reports regarding the client's disability indicate return to work at one exertion level, the counselor and client need to investigate work situations requiring equal or lessor physical exertion requirements.

*Sedentary work* - Work in this category involves lifting a maximum of 10 pounds at a time and frequently lifting or carrying articles weighing 5 pounds or less, such as clerical materials, charts, books, small tools, and instruments. The work activity performed is primarily in a seated position, although occasional standing and walking may be required.

*Light work* - This involves lifting a maximum of 20 pounds at a time with frequent lifting or carrying of objects weighing up to 10 pounds. A job is in the light category if there is frequent standing and walking, even if it requires substantially less lifting and carrying (such as in sedentary work). If a job involves primarily sitting, with pushing and pulling of arm or leg controls, it may also be in this category.

*Medium work* - This category requires lifting a maximum of 50 pounds at a time with frequent lifting or carrying of up to 25 pounds.

*4*

*Heavy work* - Lifting a maximum of 100 pounds at a time with frequent lifting or carrying of up to 50 pounds defines heavy work.

*Very heavy work* - This involves lifting more than 100 pounds at a time with frequent lifting or carrying of 50 pounds or more.

The following table summarizes the above exertional categories of work in terms of lifting and carrying.

## Table 1
## EXERTIONAL CATEGORIES OF WORK

| Category | Lifting/Carrying | |
|---|---|---|
| | Frequent | Maximum (occasional) |
| Sedentary | 2-5 pounds | 10 pounds |
| Light | 10 pounds | 20 pounds |
| Medium | 25 pounds | 50 pounds |
| Heavy | 50 pounds | 100 pounds |
| Very Heavy | 50 pounds or more | More than 100 pounds |

**Occupationally significant characteristics.** These are distinctive elements that are part of the job, the work environment, or work functions that are normally present for all persons employed in a particular vocational position. They **do not involve skills or characteristics of a person.** The occupational characteristics are present, no matter who does the job. These characteristics can be modified if the need arises. Examples of occupationally significant characteristics include: eye-hand-foot coordination, visual perception, working with other people, exertional level of work (sedentary, light, medium, heavy, or very heavy), inside work, routine and repetitive work, work requiring occasional bending and stooping, work involving fumes and irritants, among others.

An individual who has worked as a secretary may have some or all (depending on the particular job) of the following occupationally significant characteristics: indoor work, eye-hand coordination, sedentary work activity, work with other people, use of office equipment, clerical work, and work with information. In contrast, the work of a truck driver may include characteristics such as: manual dexterity, eye-hand-foot coordination, work in the transportation industry, medium work, work alone, and work in a variety of environmental conditions. **As can be seen from these examples, occupationally significant characteristics do not involve acquisition or use of skills.**

**Vocational skills and transferability of skills.** Skills involve abilities that are learned while a person is working on a job. They are distinct from occupationally significant characteristics in that they require work experience and the acquisition of abilities. Skills involve expertise or knowledge specific to work functions. They may involve the ability to use personal judgement, to work with specific tools and equipment, to operate complex machinery, to work with people or ideas at a high level of intricacy, among others.

The skills of a rehabilitation counselor may include: the ability to counsel persons regarding personal concerns, career development, and vocational pursuits; skills involved in helping individuals secure employment; capabilities in management and supervision; organizational skills; knowledge of medical aspects of disability, medical terminology, and medical treatment; and ability to work with troubled and distraught individuals with serious problems. On the other hand, the skills of a secretary may involve: clerical skills; ability to effectively operate various office machines; capability to type, file, compile letters, and answer business telephones; ability to use a word processor or computer; and organizational skills in terms of maintaining the clerical flow of an office.

Field and Weed (1988) thoroughly discussed transferability of job skills. They explain in detail how the **Dictionary of Occupational Titles (D.O.T.)** (U.S. Department of Labor, 1991) and other resources can be used effectively in transferring skills from one job to another. Only skilled and semiskilled work have transferable skills. Unskilled work, by definition, does not involve skills and, therefore, transferability of skills is not relevant. Skills found in skilled and semiskilled work can be transferred to a position of equal or lessor skill requirements, but not to a position of greater skill requirements.

An example of transferability involving a skilled position can be illustrated by the occupation of a rehabilitation counselor. The duties of this job can transfer to other skilled or semiskilled positions. Skilled positions include manager of a human resource department, college counselor, rehabilitation director, academic advisor, supervisor, teacher, mental health clinician, parole or probation officer, or work evaluator. The skills also transfer to semiskilled work activity such as personnel interviewer, job analyst, research assistant, or work evaluation technician. A semiskilled occupation, such as secretary, has transferable skills to other semiskilled work such as office clerk, receptionist, file clerk, general office worker, or word processor. Since the work is semiskilled, there is no transferability to skilled work.

In analyzing rehabilitation cases, care must be given to evaluate all job possibilities. Initial exploration includes determining the skill requirements of the jobs held by the client in order to define possible transferable skills. The counselor can identify other jobs within the same industry that use these skills. Next, the research process expands to jobs within related industries using transferability of work skills. Finally, if no positions exist within the client's physical exertional (or emotional) restrictions using transferable skills, the counselor then investigates alternative rehabilitation plans. In determining transferability of skills, the counselor needs to assess how long ago the job was last performed and whether the skills are outdated or forgotten. The length of time the individual held the job is an additional factor to consider.

If the client's skills are not immediately transferable to jobs within the current labor market (using direct job placement), the rehabilitation professional may consider on-the-job training, vocational training, or educational programs. The rehabilitationist uses a variety of criteria for deciding on the type of plan best suited to assist the client.

The rehabilitation professional in a provider system applies expertise in medical aspects of disabilities to develop vocational and educational plans with practical, realistic, and obtainable objectives. The basis for the rehabilitation objective includes analysis of the client's age, education, work history, occupationally significant characteristics, transferability of skills, and the client's functional limitations.

# FUNCTIONAL LIMITATIONS

A functional limitation is the inability to perform an action or a set of actions, either physical or mental, because of a physical or emotional restriction (often referred to as a disability). A clearly specified limitation of function can help the counselor understand the actual limitation(s) of the client. The case can be analyzed with clear understanding when medical conditions are stated in functional terms to describe the disability.

## *Examples*

1. An individual has a below the knee (BK) amputation of the left lower extremity. In functional terms, this person may be limited to maximum ambulation of one hour during an 8-hour work day, no ambulation on rough or uneven surfaces, and no stair climbing.

2. A client has a low back injury and a problem with lifting and carrying. Functionally, the individual has limitations of lifting a maximum of 20 pounds on an occasional basis with repetitive lifting and carrying not to exceed 10 pounds.

3. This person has a psychiatric diagnosis involving moderate depression and anxiety. In functional terms, this individual needs low stress work with an understanding female supervisor (because of a problem with dominant male authority figures).

4. The individual has a diagnosis of schizophrenia, chronic undifferentiated type. In functional terms, this person needs work that involves simple, routine, and repetitive activity with minimal personal interaction and a structured work environment.

Medical conditions described in functional terms enable the counselor to readily understand the client's limitations. First, the rehabilitation professional evaluates the client's vocational profile. The second step is to review the client's medical file to insure the limitations are understood in functional terms. The rehabilitationist can then determine the client's potential for vocational rehabilitation.

# REHABILITATION POTENTIAL

Rehabilitation potential consists of three characteristics: (1) attaining increased functioning in the direction of maximizing physical and emotional growth; (2) having a sense of well-being; and (3) facilitating development of a personally satisfying level of independence. Different rehabilitation systems (workers' compensation, long-term disability, Social Security, state vocational rehabilitation, independent living) define a client's rehabilitation potential within their particular parameters. A person may have rehabilitation potential within an independent living program but not with a State Department of Rehabilitation program. Another individual may be considered to have rehabilitation potential within a public agency but not in certain private agencies (such as workers' compensation or long-term disability). A third individual may be considered too disabled to benefit from vocational rehabilitation under workers' compensation, but not sufficiently disabled to receive Social Security disability benefits.

The counselor needs to be cognizant of the distinct requirements of the particular rehabilitation system(s) providing the services. Each system has its own advantages and limitations. Once the counselor determines the client's rehabilitation potential within the specific system, reasons must be presented to support the decision as to whether or not rehabilitation services will be provided. The counselor needs to clarify if the medical conditions appear to be temporary or permanent, and whether they may be expected to improve, remain the same, or deteriorate.

Also, one needs to assess whether the particular rehabilitation system providing services influenced this determination (e.g., eligibility criteria). The counselor should inform the client of the decision and the basis for that decision. If denying services, the counselor may be able to refer the client to another system where appropriate and applicable services or benefits can be provided. Each rehabilitation system evaluates a client's rehabilitation potential, including length of time typically provided for rehabilitation services, medical costs, rehabilitation costs, and the likelihood of the client returning to gainful employment.

# REHABILITATION INTERVENTION

Rehabilitation intervention attempts to modify the environment for a person with a disability to empower that person to succeed in a beneficial activity. Modifications of the environment include accommodation, job modification, and restructuring of job sites (Wright, 1980).

## *Job Analysis*

The purpose of a job analysis is to analyze the work-related measures of a specific employment position. This analysis will assist the rehabilitation professional in identifying occupationally significant characteristics, skills, and potential transferable skills of the position. Information from medical reports and a detailed job analysis help determine a client's rehabilitation potential. Possible accommodations, modifications, and restructuring of work situations may result from an accurate job analysis.

Job analysis information serves the rehabilitationist, client, and employer. This data can help identify characteristics of the job that are important when providing reasonable accommodation, to allow the client to continue or return to work. The job analysis identifies primary (essential) and secondary (nonessential) aspects of the job. The counselor may identify and suggest modifications of the nonessential aspects of the job to accommodate the employee who has a disability. Job analysis can enable a current employer to continue to benefit from a worker's knowledge, abilities, and loyalty, and can identify skills for work with other employers.

Ideally, the job analysis needs to be completed at the work site. It is essential all parties involved in the job, including the client, supervisor, foreman, human resources department, and employer provide input. Identifying these parties requires contact with the employer before conducting the job analysis, to ensure the person providing the on-site information is the most knowledgeable regarding the position.

A thorough job analysis requires time and detail. The rehabilitationist completes research on the medical status of the client and attempts to have a general knowledge of the industry before the on-site appointment. This information prepares the job analyst to ask questions pertinent to the client's functional limitations, rehabilitation potential, and possibilities for reasonable accommodation.

## *Job Accommodation, Modification, and Restructuring*

"Reasonable accommodation" is a logical adjustment made to a job or the work environment that enables a qualified person with a disability to perform the duties of the position (Berkeley Planning Associates, 1982). Reasonable accommodation recommendations must be considered on an individual basis for each employee and employer.

Section 503 of the Federal Rehabilitation Act of 1973 and the Americans with Disabilities Act (ADA) of 1990 mandate reasonable accommodation (Berkeley Planning Associates, 1982; Greenwood & Johnson, 1985; King & Backer, 1989; West, 1991). Employers now have an obligation to make reasonable accommodation for physical and mental limitations, unless the accommodation imposes an "undue hardship" on the employer. Undue hardship depends on several factors including cost; financial resources of the company; overall size of the employer; employer's operation, including composition and structure of the workplace; and the nature and cost of the proposed accommodation.

The Americans with Disabilities Act states that modifications necessary under the "reasonable accommodation" provisions include (West, 1991):

1. Modifying the physical layout of a job facility to make it accessible to individuals who use wheelchairs or who have other impairments that make access difficult.

2. Restructuring a job to enable the person with a disability to perform the essential functions of the job.

3. Establishing a part-time or modified work schedule (for example, accommodating people with disabilities who have medical treatment appointments or fatigue problems).

4. Reassigning a person with a disability to a vacant job.

5. Acquiring or modifying equipment or devices (for example, buying a hearing telephone amplifier for a person with a hearing impairment).

6. Adjusting or modifying exams, training materials, or policies (for example, giving an application examination orally to a person with dyslexia, or modifying a policy against dogs in the workplace for a person with a service dog).

7. Providing qualified readers or interpreters for people with vision or hearing impairments.

Reasonable accommodation rarely involves considerable cost. Berkeley Planning Associates (1982) conducted a study for the U.S. Department of Labor on accommodation in private sector employment and noted the following results:

1. About 50% of the reasonable accommodations surveyed cost nothing.

2. Thirty percent cost less than $500.00.

3. Ten percent cost between $500.00-$2,000.00.

4. Ten percent cost in excess of $2,000.00.

The Department of Labor study concluded that, based on the above figures, reasonable accommodation is "no big deal." This study reported the most expensive and extensive accommodations tended to be provided to the blind and to those persons who use wheelchairs. Frequently, the reasonable accommodations that are expensive and extensive are provided by employers to current employees to maintain their ability to continue work.

The public perceives accommodation efforts as helping persons with disabilities become employed or remain successful on the job. There appears to be no significant relationship between accommodation and upward mobility, either in providing an advantage to a specific employee or in limiting job potential. Highly skilled workers more often receive environmental adaptations of the work place or special equipment, while lower skilled workers receive job redesign, retraining, or selective placement.

Large firms are most likely to hire and accommodate persons with disabilities for the following reasons (Berkeley Planning Associates, 1982):

1. The existence of affirmative action mechanisms in larger firms.

2. The likelihood of encountering persons with disabilities because of the sheer numbers of workers employed.

3. The much greater diversity of job types in larger firms that leads to more possibilities of hiring and greater flexibility in job assignments.

**Types of Reasonable Accommodation**

I. Physical access accommodation

    A. A change or modification of the physical structure

    B. Examples - Accessibility/ambulation solutions

        1. Situate job on first floor

        2. Situate job near employee parking lot

        3. Situate job near restroom

II. Resource accessibility accommodation

    A. Providing assistive persons to enable the individual to do the job duties

    B. Examples

        1. Hearing impairment - Provide note taker or sign language interpreter

        2. Visual impairment - Provide reader or note taker

        3. Developmental disability (mental retardation) - Provide a job coach

III. Adaptive equipment accommodation

    A. The provision of "low tech" and "high tech" assistive devices

    B. Examples

        1. Person with arthritis or carpal tunnel syndrome - Provide special pen/pencil holders

        2. Orthopedic problems

            a. Provide desk or chair modifications

            b. Provide speaker and earphone on telephone

        3. Reaching problems

            a. Provide a turntable on a desk

            b. Provide a special desk that has easy accessibility

        4. Neck problems - Provide a slant board on a desk

        5. Visual impairment - Provide a talking calculator or talking computer

        6. Hearing impairment

            a. Provide a telephone amplifier

            b. Provide a speaker telephone

7. Quadriplegia - Provide a computer with specialized keyboard and an electronic wheelchair with assistive devices

## IV. Job Modification

A. Modifying the performance of job duties while maintaining the same job duties

B. Examples

1. Energy or ambulation problems - Salesperson can do more telephone sales and decrease field appointments

2. Energy problem - Design drafter can work part-time and receive less pay

3. Orthopedic problems

a. Parking-lot attendant can use a chair for sitting instead of standing throughout the day

b. Warehouse worker can lift and carry lesser weights by making more frequent trips with lighter weights

4. Scheduling - Secretary can leave early for physical therapy appointments by coming to work earlier

## V. Job restructuring

A. Changing some of the actual job duties performed (maintain, eliminate, or replace job duties)

B. Examples

1. Ambulation problem - Rehabilitation counselor can be assigned more office work (labor market surveys, job development, job placement, initial interviews) and less field work activity (on-site job analyses, school visits, employer visits)

2. Emotional stress

a. Social worker can be assigned more case file analysis and paperwork and less interviewing and field visits

b. Attorney can be assigned more research, case preparation, and legal briefs and less time litigating in court

3. Lower extremity problems - Shipping and receiving clerk can be assigned more clerical work (typing reports, bills of lading, and expediting) and less lifting, carrying, standing, walking, and forklift driving

Job Accommodation Network (JAN) is a resource available for additional information on employer accommodations. They have an 800 toll-free telephone number. This telephone service is provided at no cost and allows the counselor, employer, and consumer access to information on restructuring possibilities and costs. There are consultants available Monday through Friday.

Before calling this resource, it is necessary to have specific medical restrictions regarding the client, job duties which are precluded as a result of the restrictions, and general information about the industry in which the job is located. The JAN consultant will provide information at the time of the telephone call. Additional information will be mailed. There are also referrals to companies which provide restructuring and accommodation materials for specific costs.

# A HOLISTIC APPROACH TO REHABILITATION

An individual, with or without disability, cannot be perceived as an isolated entity. There is continuous interaction between the individual and the environment. Interventions in one area of the individual's environment will have an influence on the other areas. The five areas are the person's disability, psychological status, vocational experiences, educational background, and social issues (see Figure 1). The disability can be expressed in terms of functional limitations. Psychological status involves any emotional factors that may impede rehabilitation planning. The more extensive the vocational experiences and educational background, the more opportunities for a successful outcome. Lastly, the social functioning of the person, involving interaction with family, friends, and associates is an important factor that must not be overlooked. The rehabilitation professional needs to look at rehabilitation from a holistic perspective.

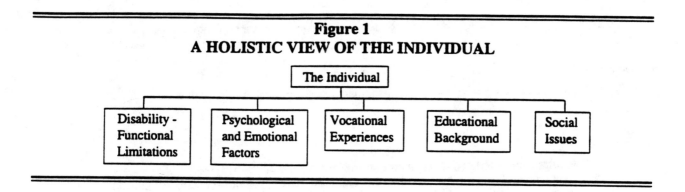

**Figure 1**
**A HOLISTIC VIEW OF THE INDIVIDUAL**

# SELF-EFFICACY AND REHABILITATION COUNSELING

Self-efficacy theory is concerned with the personal self-judgements which influence the environments that people choose, the activities in which they engage, and the effort and persistence they demonstrate at a task in the face of obstacles (Bandura, 1982). The theory of self-efficacy has application to rehabilitation within the parameters of any of the rehabilitation systems, but especially for systems that involve litigation (i.e., workers' compensation). The theory provides an overall framework for why some clients are successful in rehabilitation and others are not. It also addresses how counselors can most effectively help clients maximize rehabilitation potential.

## *What is Self-Efficacy?*

A rapidly growing body of research (Bandura, 1982, 1989; Betz & Hackett, 1981) supports the hypothesis that "self-efficacy beliefs" are cognitive mediators of assured, purposeful, and persistent behavior. These are behaviors that need to be developed and increased in clients with disabilities if they are to receive maximum benefit from the various rehabilitation systems.

**Efficacy expectations and outcome expectations.** Self-efficacy beliefs consist of these two components.

1. **Efficacy expectations** concern a person's beliefs about his or her ability to undertake a given task, and can be high or low.

2. **Outcome expectations** involve a person's beliefs about whether the outcomes of effort will be beneficial or not. Both efficacy and outcome expectations can be high or low, but must be high for persons to attempt and succeed at difficult tasks. Self-efficacy includes four essential elements:

   1. In a given situation, an individual knows what to do and how to do it.

   2. The individual has confidence he or she can succeed in the activity.

   3. The individual believes that what he or she does will have an impact on the end result.

   4. The outcome is of sufficient importance for the individual to want what the outcome will provide.

When the levels of these four components are high, the client will demonstrate goal-oriented, self-assured, and persistent behavior. The higher the self-efficacy of the rehabilitation client, the greater the chances of a successful rehabilitation outcome.

**Self-efficacy and disability.** Applying these four elements of self-efficacy systematically to persons with disabilities (especially those involved in workers' compensation and similar rehabilitation systems), we see the following (Mitchell, Brodwin, & Benoit, 1990):

1. The client often does not know what to do once in the disability system. Conflicting or contradictory advice received from physicians and counselors exacerbates this problem. For example, treating physicians may have said little about the disability, minimized it, or not clarified their remarks in easy-to-understand terminology. An applicant's attorney, if there is one, may see the case from the standpoint of maximizing disability. From a legal standpoint, the longer the person is unable to return to work, the larger the potential financial settlement. An insurance company wants to see minimal expenses in rehabilitation and an early return to work (case closure). The rehabilitation counselor focuses on vocational feasibility, vocational enhancement, and early return to work. Counselors encourage the client to focus not on the disability but on the abilities that remain or those that can be developed. This often conflicting state may be extremely confusing for clients.

2. A client may lack confidence in his or her ability to succeed in the rehabilitation system. This is especially true when the client needs to learn a new job or return to school. The individual may perceive further education or training as overwhelming and want to avoid it. To do this, one may attempt to remain on disability longer than necessary.

3. Even when the client demonstrates ability, knowledge, and confidence, he or she still may not believe that the effort will produce the desired outcome (e.g., succeeding in a return to gainful employment). The client may be of the opinion that no matter what effort is made, the result will be unsuccessful.

4. A client may not believe that, even if successful, rehabilitation will result in adequate salary, status, or benefits needed. The outcome is not perceived as having sufficient importance to put forth the effort and strive to achieve.

Figure 2 is modified from Bandura (1982); it presents a useful grid for exploring self-efficacy configurations and patterns of behavior. This figure presents the possible combinations of high (+) and low (-) efficacy and outcome expectations.

# Figure 2
## INTERACTIVE EFFECTS OF EFFICACY RATINGS
## AND OUTCOME EXPECTATIONS
(adapted from Bandura, 1982)

|  | OUTCOME EXPECTATIONS | |
|---|---|---|
|  | (+) | (-) |
| EFFICACY EXPECTATIONS (+) | **A**<br>Feel Capable (+)<br>Feel Confident (+)<br>Know what to do (+)<br>Belief in the rehabilitation system (+) | **B**<br>Feel Capable (+)<br>Feel Confident (+)<br>Unaware of what to do (-)<br>Disbelief in the rehabilitation system (-) |
| EFFICACY EXPECTATIONS (-) | **C**<br>Do not feel capable (-)<br>Have no self-confidence (-)<br>Know what to do (+)<br>Belief in the rehabilitation system (+) | **D**<br>Do not feel capable (-)<br>Have no self-confidence (-)<br>Unaware of what to do (-)<br>Disbelief in the rehabilitation system (-) |

## *Methods for Self-Efficacy Enhancement*

**Element #1.** In a given situation, the person knows what to do and how to do it. This element can be enhanced by insuring that the rehabilitation counselor not only explains to the client what needs to be done, but how to accomplish the task.

**Element #2.** The individual has confidence he or she can accomplish the task. Insuring that this second element exists is where the counselor needs assistance from the other members of the rehabilitation team. The client is more likely to succeed if all parties involved in the case (physicians, attorney, client's family and friends) have instilled confidence in the client's abilities.

It is also crucial for the counselor to build and reinforce confidence in the client periodically throughout the process. If an individual will not act, or has ceased to act, given adequate incentives and outcome expectancies, this loss of confidence is most likely attributable to the perception of excessive task difficulty. The counselor must be skilled at aiding the client with dividing seemingly impossible tasks into easily achievable units. This process effectively builds an individual's level of confidence step-by-step.

**Element #3.** The third element of self-efficacy is that the individual believes that what he or she does will have an impact on how things turn out. It is very important for the counselor to stress the functional relationship between the career search process and success in rehabilitation. Client involvement in early stages of rehabilitation will help facilitate this. Rehabilitation planning should be a shared responsibility between counselor and client. The client needs sufficient information to have an impact on the decision-making process regarding the selection of a rehabilitation plan.

Client involvement in test review, conducting labor market surveys for potential programs, and job placement activities are ways to enhance self-efficacy. The client becomes an active participant in determining rehabilitation outcome. "Locus of control" is then within the client, not the counselor, physician, attorney, insurance company, or rehabilitation system.

**Element #4.** The fourth element of self-efficacy is that the individual wants what the outcome will provide. This element also points out the importance of client choice in rehabilitation planning. The client assumes some of the decision-making responsibility in choosing an appropriate plan. The eventual goal, of course, needs to be a joint decision between counselor and client with approval of all concerned parties. If the plan is not what the client wants, efforts to succeed may be less than optimal.

# CASE STUDIES - A VOCATIONAL PROFILE APPROACH

The following case studies are examples of those which are found in most of the remaining chapters in this book. Each case study describes a person with presenting disabilities. After each case study is a series of questions. Case #1 includes answers to the questions to illustrate how one analyzes the case studies found in this book. The second case study, as well as all other case studies found in subsequent chapters, has questions which are to be answered by the reader.

## Case #1

Mr. Samuel Williams is 60 years of age and is currently married with three grown children. He has a Bachelor of Arts Degree in Fine Arts, completed a real estate course, and holds a current real estate license. For the past seven years, he has been active and successful in residential real estate sales. Previous to this, he was both a salesperson and an assistant manager in a men's specialty clothing store for 21 years.

This client has hypertension (high blood pressure) and a heart condition. Six months ago, he suffered a myocardial infarction (heart attack). The treating physician reported that Mr. Williams had coronary artery disease and restricted him to a maximum of light work that does not involve excessive emotional stress. It was also recommended that he consider sedentary work, as it would be less physically demanding. No surgery is contemplated at this time.

The position of real estate sales agent, **Dictionary of Occupational Titles #250.357-018** (U.S. Department of Labor, 1991), involves renting, buying, and selling real estate property for clients. An agent is paid on a commission basis only and does not earn a salary. Real estate sales agents are familiar with all state and local regulations relating to the purchase and sale of property. They review trade journals and other publications to keep current in the field and to be informed about marketing conditions and property values. A real estate sales agent must hold a current license issued by the state. Agents interview perspective clients to solicit listings. They accompany potential clients to property sites, show properties, quote purchase prices, and describe features and conditions of sale or terms of lease. Agents draw up real estate contracts, such as deeds, leases, and mortgages, and negotiate loans on properties. Real estate agents are typically paid on a commission-only basis.

In addition to these functions, Mr. Williams served as an office manager, supervising clerical personnel in the real estate office. This was on a part-time basis for which he was paid a salary.

## Questions

1. Describe the client's vocational profile, including age, educational level, work history (skill and exertional levels), occupationally significant characteristics, and job skills.

2. How do the occupationally significant characteristics of the job impact the client's disability?

3. What, if any, reasonable accommodations can be made for the client to return to his usual and customary occupation as a real estate sales agent?

4. What is the client's rehabilitation potential? Your rehabilitation supervisor is of the opinion this client may be too old for the provision of rehabilitation services.

5. What jobs can the client perform using transferable skills?

## Answers

1. The vocational profile for this client is as follows:

**Age:** 60 years of age - **Close to retirement age.**

**Education:** Bachelor of Arts Degree and real estate license training
**High school education and above.**

**Work History:** 1985-1992: Real Estate Sales Agent
**Skilled. Light exertion.**
1989-1992: Real Estate Sales Office Manager
(part-time)
**Skilled. Light exertion.**
1964-1985:Retail Sales and Assistant Manager
(men's clothing store)
**Semiskilled. Light exertion.**

**Occupationally Significant Characteristics:** Manual dexterity; eye-hand-foot coordination; attention to detail; visual perception and acuity; capacity to work with others; inside, as well as outside work; varying work tasks; clerical work activity; light work involving frequent standing and walking; work involving emotional stress.

**Transferable Skills:** An ability to rent, buy, and sell property for clients on a commission basis; knowledge of property listings and ability to study real estate listings; capability to review trade journals to keep current on market conditions and property values; skills in interviewing clients; an ability to show property; the capability to draw up real estate contracts; ability to negotiate loans on property; current real estate license issued by the state; ability to calculate costs, taxes, discounts, and other charges; arithmetic abilities as applied to retail sales; capability to work with finances and financial matters; capacity to present property in a positive light; ability to persuade, convince, and finalize sales; a facility with words to clearly describe the advantages of a particular product; and the capacity to use diplomacy and tact when dealing with people.

2. The work of a real estate agent and a salesperson involve physical exertion at the light level. This is within Mr. Williams' physical limitations, although the physician recommends that Mr. Williams consider sedentary work, as it would be less physically demanding. The work of a real estate agent is emotionally

demanding, although the work of an office manager (real estate) or salesperson (not in real estate) are less emotionally demanding.

3. Mr. Williams can be assigned more office work, involving less standing and walking, and less emotional stress. Working in the office and assuming office management duties, the employer may be willing to pay him a greater salary. Salaried work is typically less stressful than commission only work. This client's perception of emotional stress as it relates to prior work activities must be explored.

4. This client has good rehabilitation potential. He has a medical condition that is apparently under control with clearly specified functional limitations. There is at least a 28 year consistent work history at the skilled and semiskilled levels. During these 28 years, he has developed a variety of transferable skills. Age, in and of itself, cannot be used to deny provision of rehabilitation services.

5. The following jobs use this client's transferable skills to light and sedentary jobs that are considered to involve low emotional stress.

Light:
Salesperson (furniture, appliances, among other areas)
Counter clerk (clerical)
Sales representative (retail trade; wholesale trade)
File clerk (clerical; real estate)
Office clerk (clerical; real estate)

Sedentary:
Real estate clerk (clerical)
Real estate assistant (real estate)
Receptionist (real estate)
Credit-reference clerk (clerical)
Credit clerk (clerical)
Cashier (clerical)
Credit-card clerk (retail trade)
Check cashier (business services)
Information clerk/assistant (real estate)

## Case #2

Ms. Patricia Duvall is 56 years of age, not married, and has no dependent children. This worker had a low back injury and is restricted to light work activity. The treating physician recommends alternate sitting and standing/walking throughout the work shift. She has work experience as a registered nurse and a medical laboratory technician, and has an Associate of Science degree. Between 1984-1991, Ms. Duvall worked as a medical-laboratory technician (medical services) **D.O.T. #: 078.381-014**, a position that is classified as semiskilled, light. Previous to this, she worked for many years as a registered nurse (medical services), **D.O.T. #: 075- 364.010.** This hospital job was skilled, and medium in exertion.

The **Dictionary of Occupational Titles** (U.S. Department of Labor, 1991) describes Medical-Laboratory Technician as follows: Performs routine tests in medical laboratory to provide data for use in diagnosis and treatment of disease: Conducts quantitative and qualitative chemical analysis of body fluids, such as blood, urine, and spinal fluid, under supervision of a medical technologist. Performs blood counts, using microscope. Conducts blood tests for transfusion purposes. May draw blood from patient's finger, ear lobe, or vein, observing principles of asepsis to obtain blood samples. May specialize in hematology, blood bank, cytology, histology, or chemistry.

The **D.O.T.** (U.S. Department of Labor, 1991) notes the following job description for Nurse, General Duty: Provides general nursing care to patients in hospitals, nursing homes, infirmaries, or similar health-care facilities: Administers prescribed medications and treatment in accordance with approved nursing techniques. Prepares equipment and aids physician during treatment and examination of patients. Observes patient, records significant conditions and reactions, and notifies supervisor or physician of patient's condition and reaction to drugs, treatment, and significant incidents. Takes temperature, pulse, blood pressure, and other vital signs to detect deviations from normal and assesses condition of patient.

## *Questions*

1. What is this client's vocational profile, including age, educational level, work history (skill and exertional levels), occupationally significant characteristics, and job skills?

2. Identify the client's transferable skills?

3. What jobs could be found in the economy for this client if she could only return to a semiskilled, low stress job in the light or sedentary categories?

4. List the functional limitations for this client if her physician restricted her to a) no "light work," b) no "medium work," or c) no "heavy work" (describe each category).

5. The client is interested in returning to her usual and customary occupation. Her employer is willing to have her return, if she can function within the job description. What reasonable accommodations can you suggest for successful return to employment?

6. The client has stated interest in the following areas for return to gainful employment, as alternatives to returning to her current employer: teacher at a community college, hospital administrator, rehabilitation counselor, and Medicare analyst (determines if money is available for a hospital to continue the person as an in-patient). Describe your role, as the counselor, in addressing these areas of interest.

# REFERENCES

Bandura, A. (1982). Self-efficacy mechanism in human agency. **American Psychologist, 37,** 122-147.

Bandura, A. (1989). Human agency in social cognitive theory. **American Psychologist, 44,** 1175-1183.

Berkeley Planning Associates (1982). **A study of recommendations provided to handicapped employees by federal contractors** (Contract No. J-9-E-1-009). Berkeley, CA: Author.

Betz, N.E., & Hackett, G. (1981). The relationship of career-related self-efficacy expectations to perceived career options in college women and men. **Journal of Counseling Psychology, 28,** 399-410.

Field, T.F., & Weed, R.O. (1988). **Transferable work skills.** Athens, GA: Elliott and Fitzpatrick.

Greenwood, R., & Johnson, V.A. (1985). **Employer concerns regarding workers with disabilities.** Hot Springs, AR: Arkansas Research and Training Center in Vocational Rehabilitation.

King, R.B., & Backer, T.E. (1989). **Overcoming challenges: A guide to selective job placement of workers with disabilities.** Los Angeles, CA: National Medical Enterprises.

Mitchell, L.K., Brodwin, M.G., & Benoit, B.R. (1990). Strengthening the workers' compensation system by increasing client efficacy. **Journal of Applied Rehabilitation Counseling, 21,** 22-26.

U.S. Department of Labor (1991). **Dictionary of occupational titles** (4th ed., revised). Washington, DC: Author.

U.S. Department of Health & Human Services. (1988). **Social security handbook** (10th ed.). Washington, D.C.: Author.

West, J. (Ed.). (1991). **The Americans with Disabilities Act: From policy to practice.** New York, N.Y.: Milbank Memorial Fund.

Wright, G.N. (1980). **Total rehabilitation.** Boston: Little, Brown.

## About the Authors:

Martin G. Brodwin, Ph.D., C.R.C., is an Assistant Professor and Coordinator of the Rehabilitation Counselor Education Programs at California State University, Los Angeles, in Los Angeles, California. He is a vocational expert for the Office of Hearings and Appeals, Social Security Administration, providing testimony on disability-related issues. As a counselor and co-owner of Image Development, located in Los Angeles, he provides consultation on workers' compensation and long-term disability.

Sandra K. Brodwin, M.S., C.R.C., is a counselor at Pasadena Community College, in Pasadena, California in the Center for Students with Learning Disabilities. She is a member of the Panel of Vocational Experts for the Office of Hearings and Appeals, Social Security Administration. As a counselor and co-owner of Image Development, she provides counseling and administrative services for workers' compensation and long-term disability cases.

# Chapter 2

# MEDICAL TERMINOLOGY

by
*Jean Spencer Felton, M.D.*

The principle objective in understanding medical terminology is to have physicians' reports become meaningful without having to resort to a dictionary for the definition of every technical word. The rehabilitation counselor, however, needs a medical dictionary available for quick and easy reference (Cohen, 1989; Dorland, 1988; Glanze, Anderson, & Anderson, 1990; Miller & Keane, 1987; Stedman, 1990; Thomas, 1989). In verbal discussions with health care professionals, there will be no need to paraphrase, translate each word, or convert to the use of lay terms. Many physicians have difficulty expressing themselves in lay terms and rely on technical words, phrases, and sentences. When speaking with an individual who understands the nomenclature, the physician will speak more readily and more completely, to the advantage of the counselor who needs an understanding of the client's medical condition (Berkow, 1987).

## MEDICAL TERMS

It is an easier task to bring this new terminology into one's vocabulary if the counselor makes an effort to learn the meanings of the parts of words (the combining forms) that make up the whole word. For example, at first reading, the terms **sternocleidomastoid** or **hypertrophic pulmonary osteoarthropathy** can be awesome to the uninformed; they can become understandable and useful when divided into their parts. In the first example, the prefix **stern** refers to the sternum or breast bone; **cleid** indicates the clavicle; and **mastoid** means the bony process behind the ear. (The "o"s are connectors.) The word itself is the name of the muscle that attaches to the three bony structures included in the full term.

The second lengthy and possibly frightening technical term is the scientific name for "clubbing of the fingers." **Hyper** translates as "in excess or more than normal"; **trophic** refers to nutrition; the whole word denotes the enlargement or overgrowth of a body part. **Pulmonary** pertains to the lungs (from the Latin for lung, **pulmo**). **Osteo** is the combining form signifying a relationship to a bone or the bones (from the Greek **osteon** or bone), while **arthr(o)** denotes a relationship to a joint or joints (the Greek word for joint is **arthron**). The ending **-pathy** (from the Greek **pathos** for disease) signifies a morbid condition or disease; the full word means any disease of the joints and bones. When the words are in sequence, they denote a disease overgrowth of the bones and joints (in this instance the terminal phalanges), secondary to a lung disorder.

These examples exemplify the manner in which medical terms, usually for clinical disorders or diseases, become clear through a knowledge of the parts or combining forms they comprise. Medical nomenclature, like the language of any science, profession, or technology, provides precision, speed, and economy in communication.

## Medical Terminology and the Counselor

Since most of the clients receiving services from rehabilitation counselors will have an impairment or disability, it is necessary for the counselor to understand the language of medicine and health care. The counselor, in evaluating clients and developing rehabilitation programs, has access to various reports from medical specialists. There is both a basic medical language and a specialized terminology that counselors need to comprehend.

Much of the rehabilitation effort involves physical restoration, medical control of chronic disease, and possible restitution of emotional stability. The rehabilitationist is in constant contact with representatives of many disciplines composing the health care team: physicians, nurses, physical therapists, occupational therapists, orthotists, prosthetists, psychologists, and social workers, among others. Each care provider uses a specialized nomenclature in formal interchange and a unique jargon (or medical shorthand) in informal conversation (Tyrrell, 1989). This will differ not only among professions, but also among professionals in the same field of specialization. It is necessary for the counselor to understand this language to help facilitate the rehabilitation process.

The counselor who has attained this new fluency should not indulge in overuse or inappropriate usage of technical terms in order to impress others. In discussing health problems with a client, the counselor should not use technical terms unless the client clearly understands the meanings. Many patients will not ask for an explanation due to embarrassment and confusion; to use a technical vocabulary in an interview only confuses the exchange of information. In short, the client may understand **heart murmur**, but will become confused if the condition is called **mitral stenosis**.

## Analysis of Terms

Like many specialized vocabularies, medical terminology is built upon recurring components (Barrow, 1960; Haubrich, 1984; Jaeger, 1978; Pepper 1949). The more familiar the counselor is with these verbal building blocks, the more readily new terms will be understood. In the division of words, as in the examples cited previously, one identifies the components: there is the core of the word, its **root** or **stem**, plus the modifying terms which precede (**prefixes**) or follow (**suffixes**) the root. As an example, in the word **dysmenorrhea**, the root is -**men**-, for month. The prefix **dys**- means difficult or painful, and the suffix, -**rrhea**, denotes flow. With a knowledge of the components, the meaning of **dysmenorrhea** is understood as painful menstruation.

The lexicon of medicine is essentially a way of organizing medical information (Lorenzini, 1989). It is the organization of a constantly changing and growing body of knowledge and is not always as clear and predictable as one might like. There are ambiguities and inconsistencies, duplications and contradictions. Medical terminology still embodies archaic terms generated by theories no longer valid; it also contains clever concepts from "Madison Avenue". The current direction in terminology is toward order and understanding. The hazards of language confusion can be partially overcome if one is familiar with the origins of medical terms (Jaeger, 1978; Pepper, 1949).

## Origins of Medical Terms

Most of the terms encountered today have their origin in Greek or Latin words and, infrequently, in a combination of these two sources. Most of the familiar terms for body parts are of Anglo-Saxon origin: eye (**eage**), heart (**heorte**), skull (**skulle** [a bowl]), hip (**hype**), and kidney (**kidenei**), for example. From French have come such terms as jaundice (**jaune** [yellow]), malaise, gout, curette, grand mal, and gavage. German contributed **anlage**, Dutch gave us **sprue**, and from Italian, we derived **influenza** and **petechia**. **Agar** (initially agar agar) was Singalese in origin, as was **beriberi**. Japan added **tsutsugamuchi** fever, and from the Amazon Indians came **ipecac**. **Alkali**, **alcohol**, and **bezoar** descended from Arabic, while a few terms are given different beginnings such as **dengue**, which is attributed to Spanish by one source and Swahili by a second.

Several word roots occur in both Latin and Greek, but have considerably different meanings. Perhaps the most frequently encountered pair is the root **ped(o)-**, which in Latin means **foot** (**pedicle, pedicure**), but in Greek means **child** (**pediatrics**). Other word roots might prove confusing because they sound alike, but have different meaning: **hydr(o)** - for water (as in **hydrarthrosis**) and **hidr(o)** - for sweat (as in **anhidrosis**). Other difficulties arise when both Latin and Greek forms are inserted into contemporary language. For example, numbers derived from Latin and Greek are used in prefixes, yet each system is different. From Latin, **one** (1) provides the prefix **uni-**, as in **unilateral** (affecting one side only) or **unidirectional** (flowing in one direction only). **One** in Greek provides the prefix **mono-**, as in **monochromatic** (existing in or having only one color) or **monocyte** (a leukocyte [white blood cell] having only one nucleus). Also, iron compounds usually carry the prefix **ferr(o)**, from the Latin **ferrum**, meaning iron, as in **ferrous** gluconate or **ferric** oxide. Still, there are many words that use the Greek **sider(o)**, from **sideros** (iron), as in **siderosis** (a lung disorder resulting from the inhalation of iron particles), or **sideropenia** (an iron deficiency in the body).

One must be careful not to confuse a current definition of the word with its origin. As an example, the term **mastoid** is the rounded prominence of the temporal bone behind the ear. In pre-antibiotic days it was subject to inflammation and corrective surgery. It was believed to resemble a female breast, so the name was drawn from the Greek **mastos** (breast) and **eidos** (like). The anatomic designation should not be misinterpreted as being similar to such terms as **mastitis** or **mastectomy**.

Not all medical terms emerge purely from language roots. There are **eponyms** which are names based on a person, usually the individual who first described the clinical entity or advanced a theory concerning the disorder. Many diseases have such name origins, e.g., **Alzheimer's disease, Hansen's disease, Hodgkin's disease,** and **Paget's disease**. Eponyms are also used for reactions or tests in clinical medicine, such as **Arthus' reaction, Mantoux' test,** and **Rubin's test.** Operative procedures carry the originators' names as in **Matas' operation** or **Potts' operation.** Eponyms appear in the names of body parts such as **Hesselbach's triangle** and instruments such as **galvanometer** and **voltmeter.** Occasionally, a disease will derive its name from a geographic location such as **Bornholm disease** or **Lyme disease.**

The method in which medical terms are derived is changing and as more is learned of an old perplexing disorder or as a new disease is identified, more descriptive names of the process are given. **Bornholm disease,** just mentioned, is also currently called **epidemic pleurodynia**; others, like **tularemia** (Tulare, California) continue to be identified by the old designation.

There are certain disorders bearing the designation **syndrome,** which is a set of symptoms occurring together that results in specific or probable outcomes. Examples are **acute radiation syndrome, Cushing's syndrome,** and **Horner's syndrome.** Physicians naming disorders may be from any one of many countries, adding more to the international flavor of medical nomenclature. From literature are the **"Alice in Wonderland" syndrome,** a delusional state, and the **Münchhausen syndrome,** a chronic factitious disorder with physical symptoms. The former comes, of course, from Lewis Carroll's (Charles Dodgson's) wonderful story, while the latter is from the eighteenth century baron, the teller of tall tales.

Acronyms are formed from the initials of lengthy names. **ACTH** (adrenocorticotropic hormone), **HIV** (human immunodeficiency virus), **LASER** (light amplification by stimulated emission or radiation), and **MRI** (magnetic resonance imaging) are examples.

Names of pharmaceuticals are derived in a variety of ways. Some are given acronyms from abbreviations of their chemical names. Others are derived from random computer trials; occasionally, designations are selected that are easy to remember or can be used readily in promotional activities and sales.

Certain words are derived from an entity or action by a vocal imitation of the sound associated with it (onomatopoeic), as heard in **buzz** or **hiss.** Examples in medical terminology include **hiccup, tympany** (the sound produced by percussion over a cavity containing air), and **belch. Rale** (from the French **râle** meaning rattle) indicates an abnormal sound heard when listening to respiration with the stethoscope.

It is not within the scope of this chapter to provide a comprehensive glossary of medical terms. Medical dictionaries and other reference works cited at the end of this chapter will be useful in the counselor's library. Medical terminology can be understood by analysis of the prefixes and suffixes added to words. A list of the important components of medical terms needed by rehabilitation counselors follows below. These will appear repeatedly in written medical reports and during counselors' discussions with physicians.

# MASTERING MEDICAL TERMINOLOGY

## *Prefixes*

Word roots can be modified by prefixes that denote:

1. Position in time or space

    **Ab-** means **away from**
        **abnormal** - away from normal
        **abduction** - drawing away from the mid-line of the body by the arm or leg
    **Circum-** means **around**
        **circumcision** - a cutting around of the prepuce
        **circumarticular** - around a joint

2. Quantitative information

    **A-** or **an-** means **without**
        **anorexia** - without appetite
        **anoxia** - without enough oxygen
    **Hemi-** means **half**
        **hemiplegia** - paralysis of one lateral half of the body
        **heminephrectomy** - removal of a portion of a kidney
    **Diplo-** means **double**
        **diplopia** - double vision
        **diploscope** - an apparatus for the study of binocular vision
    **Quint-** means **fifth**
        **quintipara** - a woman who has five pregnancies continued beyond the 20th week of gestation
        **quintuplet** - one of five offspring produced in one gestation period

3. Qualitative information

    **Mal-** means **bad** or **ill**
        **malfunction** - defective function
        **malocclusion** - faulty positioning of the upper or lower teeth in relation to the other

Eu- means **good** or healthy

    **euphoria** - sense of well-being or condition of good health

    **euthanasia** - easy or painless death

4. Sameness and difference

    Hetero- means **different**

        **heterogeneous** - differing in kinds or nature

        **heterosexual** - sexual orientation directed to the opposite sex

    Homo- means **same**

        **homogeneous** - of the same kind

        **homosexual** - sexual orientation directed to the same sex

5. Physical attributes (size, shape, color)

    Micro- means **small**

        **microcephalia** - abnormal smallness of the head

        **micromelia** - abnormal smallness or shortness of the extremities

    Brachy- means **short**

        **brachycephalia** - having a short head

        **brachydactylia** - having abnormally short fingers and toes

    Oxy- means **pointed** or **sharp**

        **oxycephaly** - having a high and pointed head

    Albo- means **white**

        **albinism** - absence of pigmentation

## *Suffixes*

Suffixes and significant word endings characteristically function in compound words to:

1. Form adjectives

    -al means **pertaining to**

        peritoneal - pertaining to the peritoneum

        arterial - pertaining to an artery

    -ible, or -able means **ability**

        digestible - capable of being digested

        operable - subject to being operated

2. Express diminutive size - a number of suffixes serve this purpose, including -cule, -icle, -ium, -ole, -ule, and variations

    diverticulum means a small outpocketing from a hollow organ

    arteriole means a small artery

    granule means a small grain

3. Indicate a surgical procedure

> **-ectomy** means **removal** of an organ or part
>> **appendectomy** - removal of the appendix
>
> **-lysis** means **loosening**, usually of adhesions
>> **cardiolysis** - freeing of the heart of pericardial adhesions
>
> **-ostomy** means an operation in which an **artificial opening** is formed between two hollow organs or between one or more such viscera and the abdominal wall for discharge of intestinal content or urine
>> **colostomy** - the surgical creation of an opening between the colon and the exterior of the body
>
> **-pexy** means **fixation**
>> **nephropexy** - the surgical attachment of a floating kidney
>
> **-plasty** means **plastic surgery**
>> **blepharoplasty** - plastic surgery of the eyelids
>
> **-rrhaphy** means **suture** or **operative repair**
>> **tenorrhaphy** - the suturing of a tendon
>
> **-scopy** means **viewing** or **examining**, usually with an instrument
>> **endoscopy** - visual inspection of any body cavity by means of an endoscope
>
> **-tomy** means **cutting** or **incision**
>> **laparotomy** - the surgical opening of the abdomen
>
> **-tripsy** means the **intentional surgical crushing** of a structure
>> **lithotripsy** - the disintegration of a kidney stone by a high-energy shockwave

4. Express conditions or changes related to pathological processes

> **-mania** means excessive excitement or obsessive preoccupation
>> **pyromania** - an irrational compulsion to set fires
>
> **-sis** means an action, process, or condition
>> **silicosis** - a fibrotic disorder of the lungs following inhalation of dust containing silicon dioxide
>>
>> **thoracentesis** - surgical puncture of the chest wall for removal of fluid
>>
>> **moniliosis** - an infection caused by **Monilia**
>
> **-itis** means inflammation
>> **appendicitis** - an inflammation of the appendix

Besides these loosely formulated classes of suffixes, there are a number of miscellaneous word endings, the most significant of which is included in the vocabulary that follows. These are also important to the rehabilitation counselor.

## Basic Terms

The following list of prefixes and suffixes will aid in the understanding of medical terminology. This list will familiarize the reader with the flexibility of nomenclature. As new terms are encountered, the counselor can more readily recognize the components from which they are made.

| Prefix/Suffix | Definition | Example |
|---|---|---|
| -algia | pain | neuralgia |
| angio- | blood vessel | angiogram |
| ante- | before | antecubital |
| arth- | joint | arthroscopy |
| blephar- | eyelid | blepharospasm |
| cardi- | heart | electrocardiography |
| cele- | 1) a swelling | |
| | 2) a hernia | varicocele, rectocele |
| cerebro- | cerebrum | cerebral |
| chole- | gall or bile | cholecystectomy |
| chondr- | cartilage | chondrocostal |
| contra- | opposed to | contraception |
| cost- | rib | intercostal |
| cysto- | bladder | cystitis |
| -desis | fusion | arthrodesis |
| derm- | skin | dermatology |
| dys- | difficult, abnormal | dyspnea |
| ect- | outside | ectomorph |
| -ectomy | removal | splenectomy |
| -emia | condition of the blood | polycythemia |
| enceph- | brain | encephalitis |
| end- | within | endocrine |
| enter- | intestine | enterostomy |
| epi- | upon, above | epithelium |
| genic- | giving rise to | psychogenic |
| glyco- | sugar | glycosuria |
| hemi- | half | hemiplegia |
| hepat- | liver | hepatitis |
| hyper- | in excess | hypertension |
| hyster- | uterus | hysterectomy |
| -iosis | a pathologic condition | amebiosis |
| -itis | inflammation | tonsillitis |
| leuk- | white | leukocyte |
| lip- | fat | hyperlipemia |
| -lith | stone | nephrolithiasis |
| -megaly | a state of largeness | hepatomegaly |
| myel- | 1) bone marrow | myelocyte |
| | 2) spinal cord | poliomyelitis |
| myo- | muscle | myocardium |
| neph- | kidney | nephrosis |
| -oid | resembling | thyroid |

| -oma | tumor or swelling | carcinoma |
| -oscopy | visual examination | laparoscopy |
| -osis | disease process or condition | necrosis |
| osteo- | bone | osteoarthritis |
| -ostomy | creation of an artificial opening in an organ | tracheostomy |
| -otomy | incision | craniotomy |
| para- | near, alongside, beyond, outside | paravertebral |
| -pathy | disease of | cardiomyopathy |
| -penia | lack of | leukopenia |
| -plasty | reparative or reconstructive surgery | rhinoplasty |
| pneumo- | air | pneumothorax |
| pre- | before | precancerous |
| pro- | in front of, before | prognathism |
| proct- | rectum or anus | proctology |
| -ptosis | lowering of an organ or part | nephroptosis |
| pyel- | pelvis | pyelogram |
| pyo- | pus | pyorrhea |
| spondyl- | vertebra | spondylolysis |
| sub- | under | submandibular |
| super- | above, excessive | supersensitivity |
| supra- | above | supraventricular |
| syn- | together | synarthrosis |
| trans- | across | transurethral |
| tri- | three | triceps |

## Landmarks

To understand medical information, one should be familiar not only with the names of anatomic structures and pathological conditions, but also with the "landmark" terms that designate relative position and direction. They are described in relation to a patient who is standing in the erect position looking forward with arms to the side of the body and hands with palms forward (see Figure 1). The most commonly used are the following:

**lateral -** to the side (used in contradistinction to medial)
**medial -** to the center
**superior -** above (used in contradistinction to inferior)
**inferior -** below
**anterior -** before or in front (used in contradistinction to posterior)
**posterior -** behind or in back
**proximal -** nearest to the point of attachment or center of the body (used in contradistinction to distal)
**distal -** farthest from the center
**prone -** lying face downward (used in contradistinction to supine)
**supine -** lying face upward
**volar -** pertaining to the sole of the foot or the palm of the hand

| | |
|---|---|
| **dorsal -** | pertaining to the back (used in contradistinction to ventral) |
| **ventral -** | pertaining to the front or abdominal surface |
| **palmar -** | pertaining to the palm of the hand |
| **plantar -** | pertaining to the sole of the foot |

---

### Figure 1
## ANATOMICAL POSITION OF THE HUMAN BODY
## FOR DESCRIPTIVE PURPOSES

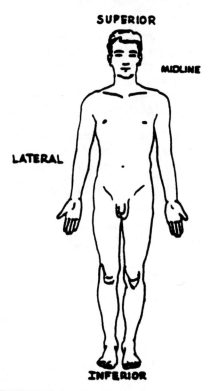

---

## Body Areas

Specific sites of illness or injury are usually designated by terms derived from the adjacent anatomic structure. Among the commonly used terms to indicate body areas are the following:

| | |
|---|---|
| **abdominal -** | pertaining to the stomach and intestinal area |
| **carpal -** | pertaining to the wrist |
| **cervical -** | pertaining to the seven vertebrae in the neck |
| **costal -** | pertaining to the ribs |
| **cranial -** | pertaining to the skull |
| **femoral -** | pertaining to the thigh |

| | |
|---|---|
| **frontal** - | pertaining to the forehead |
| **lumbar** - | pertaining to the five vertebrae in the lower portion of the back |
| **pelvic** - | pertaining to the pelvic girdle |
| **renal** - | pertaining to the kidney area |
| **sacral** - | pertaining to the four vertebrae in the lowest portion of the back |
| **sternal** - | pertaining to the sternum or breastbone |
| **thoracic** - | pertaining to the twelve vertebrae in the upper portion of the back |

## *Medical Abbreviations*

Understanding verbal and written communication with physicians involves knowledge of the terms used and a familiarity with the abbreviations in widespread use within the profession. This nomenclature changes with medical developments and, to some extent, may vary in different regions of the country. While some abbreviations may be used by all practitioners, there are others which are unique to the particular physician and may be puzzling. One physician consistently wrote H.A. to mean "headache." Abbreviations, incorrectly used, can be as different as NP for "neuropsychiatric" or for "new patient" or AA meaning "Alcoholics Anonymous," "achievement age," or "arteries."

Abbreviations denote instructions that are included in prescriptions for medications; some signify symptoms as reported by patients and some refer to anatomic parts or body systems. A few examples are noted:

| | |
|---|---|
| a.c. - | before meals (ante cibum) |
| b.i.d. - | twice daily (bis in die) |
| B.P. - | blood pressure |
| C-1, C-2, C-3 - | cervical vertebrae by number |
| CBC - | complete blood count |
| C.C. - | chief complaint |
| C.N. - | cranial nerve |
| C.N.S. - | central nervous system |
| CPR - | cardiopulmonary resuscitation |
| CT - | computed tomography |
| CVA - | cerebrovascular accident |
| dB - | decibel |
| DX - | diagnosis |
| ESR - | erythrocyte sedimentation rate |
| F.H. - | family history |
| FX - | fracture |
| GI - | gastrointestinal |
| Hg - | hemoglobin |
| GU - | genitourinary |
| HBV - | hepatitis B virus |
| HDL - | high density lipoprotein |
| Hg - | mercury |
| h.s. - | at bedtime (hora somni) |
| H & P - | history and physical examination |
| HX - | history |
| L-1, L-2, L-3 - | lumbar vertebrae by number |
| L.L.Q. - | left lower quadrant |
| L.M.P. - | last menstrual period |

| L.U.Q. - | left upper quadrant |
| MRI - | magnetic resonance imaging |
| OA - | osteoarthritis |
| O.D. - | right eye (oculus dexter) |
| O.S. - | left eye (oculus sinister) |
| p.c. - | after meals (post cibum) |
| P.H. - | past history |
| P.I. - | present illness |
| p.r.n. - | as needed (pro re nata) |
| q.i.d. - | four times daily (quater in die) |
| RA - | rheumatoid arthritis |
| R.B.C. - | red blood count |
| R.L.Q. - | right lower quadrant |
| R/O - | rule out |
| R.U.Q. - | right upper quadrant |
| RX - | treatment |
| S-1, S-2, S-3 - | sacral vertebrae by number |
| SOAP - | subjective findings, objective findings, assessment, plan |
| T-1, T-2, T-3 - | thoracic vertebrae by number |
| t.i.d. - | three times daily (ter in die) |
| W.B.C. - | white blood count |

The abbreviations cited are examples of the hundreds, perhaps thousands in use. New chemicals are named and given acronyms or abbreviations. A recent example is the abbreviation, AIDS, for acquired immunodeficiency syndrome. Unlike medical nomenclature, abbreviations cannot be divided logically into components, nor is it feasible to try to memorize a list of abbreviations. With experience, one becomes increasingly competent in interpreting this medical shorthand. Care must also be used when writing abbreviations. CA, for example, may mean cancer, carcinoma, chemical abstracts, and the like. When it is written Ca, it means calcium; the ca form might stand for circa. Available sources such as those noted in the reference section of this chapter must be used.

One other precaution is suggested. Professional journals ordinarily write out a long medical title when it is first introduced in an article. Following the name, the initials are given in parentheses. The initials or acronym will be used thereafter without the actual name. This use of abbreviations makes reading difficult because the full medical term is not readily recalled. The custom is universal in scholarly journals and may confuse persons new to medical terminology.


# INCONSISTENCIES, CONTRADICTIONS, AND TRENDS


## Inconsistencies and Contradictions


In all fairness, the newcomer to medical terminology should be informed of some of the problems that exist. Certain words within the medical lexicon have multiple meanings. The word **sinus**, for instance, can be used in several contexts, according to the specific meaning intended. The reader needs to be sensitive to the context in which it is used to determine which of the several meanings is intended. Conversely, several names may apply to a single medical entity without necessarily conveying different meaning. **Brucellosis**, for example, is sometimes called undulant fever, sometimes Bruce's septicemia, and sometimes by a geographic name, Malta fever. Some disorders still carry names originally given to workers that were affected by the disease. Some examples follow: arc-welder lung (siderosis), brown lung (byssinosis), white lung (asbestosis), and metal fume fever (whose colloquial names have included brassfounders' ague, braziers' disease, smelter shakes, brass chills, zinc chills, Monday fever, and the smothers). Although these old "shop" terms are not in use, they may appear in medical histories or infrequently be used by health care personnel unaware of the designations of contemporary occupational illnesses.

## Trends in Medical Nomenclature

Medical terminology has come down through an impressive span of time, but the vocabulary of medicine, like the science itself, is not without change. A counselor must be alert to shifts in usage and be aware of additions being made. For example, the trend is away from the use of eponyms, for such designations provide little information about the nature of the disease or the body organ system which is affected. Accordingly, they are felt to lack precision as a basis for nomenclature. Another recent trend is to use generic names rather than the brand or trademark name in specifying medication or in describing clinical use in a medical report. For example, the generic name for Valium (an anti-anxiety and sedative drug) is diazepam.

Technological changes generate new words for new processes and equipment; these innovations find a place within medical terminology, as did LASER when the device first appeared. When this book is published and is being read, other new terms will have been developed and accepted. Keeping current with medical terminology is a continuing assignment for both the physician and the rehabilitation counselor. It is imperative that the counselor have a medical dictionary close by whenever reviewing medical reports.

# REFERENCES

Barrow, D.J. (1960). **Dictionary of word roots and combining forms**. Palo Alto, CA: N-P Publications.

Berkow, R. (1987). **The Merck manual** (15th ed.). Rahway, NJ:Merck, Sharp, and Dohme.

Cohen, B.J. (1989). **Medical terminology: An illustrated guide.**Philadelphia, PA: J.B. Lippincott.

**Dorland's illustrated medical dictionary** (1988). (27th ed.).Philadelphia, PA: W.B. Saunders.

Glanze, W.D., Anderson, K.N., & Anderson, L.E. (Eds.). (1990). **Mosby's medical, nursing and allied health dictionary** (3rd ed.). St. Louis, MO: C.V. Mosby.

Haubrich, W.S. (1984). **Medical meanings - a glossary of word origins**. New York: Harcourt Brace Jovanovich.

Jaeger, E.C. (1978). **A source book of biological names and terms** (3rd ed.). Springfield, IL: Charles C Thomas.

Lorenzini, J.A. (Ed.). (1989). **Medical phrase index: A one-step reference to the terminology of medicine** (2nd ed.). Oradell, NJ: Medical Economics Books.

Miller, B.F., & Keane, C.B. (1987). **Encyclopedia and dictionary of medicine, nursing, and allied health** (4th ed.). Philadelphia, PA: W.B. Saunders.

Pepper, O.H.P. (1949). **Medical etymology**. Philadelphia, PA: W.B. Saunders.

**Stedman's medical dictionary** (1990). (25th ed.). Baltimore, MD: Williams and Wilkins.

Thomas, C.L. (Ed.). (1989). **Taber's cyclopedic medical dictionary** (16th ed.). Philadephia, PA: F.A. Davis.

Tyrrell, W.B. (1989). **Medical terminology for medical students** (2nd ed.). Springfield, IL: Charles C Thomas.

*About the Author:*

Jean Spencer Felton, M.D., is a Clinical Professor of Community and Environmental Medicine at the University of California, Irvine, California and a Clinical Professor (Emeritus) of Preventive Medicine, University of Southern California, Los Angeles, California. Dr. Felton is a member of the President's Committee on Employment of People with Disabilities.

# Chapter 3

# THE PHYSICAL EXAMINATION

by
*Jean Spencer Felton, M.D.*

Medical reports and records constitute the continuing bond between the rehabilitation counselor and the physician. Through practice and use of a good medical dictionary (Dorland, 1988; Glanze, Anderson, & Anderson, 1990; Thomas, 1989), the counselor can become reasonably adept at interpreting and comprehending these documents. To understand them properly, the counselor should be familiar with the physical examination, a procedure by which the physician obtains information concerning the patient's medical history and elicits findings. The physician will enter the data obtained into the medical record; it is from this record that medical reports are derived (Coy, 1990; Krupp, Tierney, Jawetz, Roe, & Camargo, 1985).

## CONTEMPORARY MEDICAL PRACTICE

The contemporary practice in diagnosing any disease or disabling disorder involves obtaining (a) a complete medical history and (b) conducting a comprehensive physical examination (Clayman, 1989; Williams, Warwick, Dyson, & Bannister, 1989). It must be pointed out that the words, "the physical examination," are employed universally. Many practitioners prefer the designation, "the health examination," when the individual presumably is well and the evaluation is being performed on a periodic basis for purposes of disease prevention. In some settings, at the time of hire in business or industry, the term "medical examination" is applied to the process for it may include more than just the physical examination. There may be a psychological evaluation as part of the requirement, a step which is outside the realm of a pure "physical" review. As used here, "physical examination" will be the preferred term; determinations of mental health status will be performed by other professionals engaged in the evaluation of the client.

### Objectives of the Physical Examination

To understand the objectives of a physical examination, it is necessary to understand the various components. Examples used in this chapter involve the evaluation of a patient being seen by a family physician or internist for the first time. If referred by a rehabilitation counselor or State Department of Rehabilitation, the findings resulting from such an examination may be entered on a form provided by the referral source. Most agencies forward such printed forms to be used for the general medical report. In addition, some agencies have special forms for the reporting of certain disabilities such as visual or hearing impairments, dental problems, cardiac disease, or psychiatric disorders. The counselor also may request the physician to determine work tolerances and functional limitations. Most specialty examinations are reported in a narrative form.

The thorough physician will enter both positive and negative findings in accurate detail in the medical record. Frequently, preprinted schematic or outline drawings of various body parts or organ systems are used to enhance or clarify the written description (see Figure 1 for an example). All physicians use abbreviations in the record documents; this chapter will provide many of the abbreviated entries that represent the recordings of findings on examination. To illustrate this usage, hypothetical medical records of two patients have been reproduced. The examples will be paired. The one on the reader's left represents a record (or report) with many common abbreviations; on the right is the translation of the report with all the words spelled out. As will be apparent in the exhibits used, no two physicians follow an identical style in examining patients and recording information.

## The Issue of Rapport

The written medical evaluation reflects the communication established between physician and patient; the quality of reporting depends so much on this relationship. Rapport between physician and patient at the initial meeting is crucial; the patient often has mixed emotions when seeing a physician for the initial appointment. These emotions may include anxiety, depression, fear, anger, hostility, guilt, and shame. These feelings may obscure or alter what the patient hears the physician say. To a considerable extent, these intangible barriers can be removed only when the physician has successfully established a good relationship with the patient. The physician, like the counselor, must build rapport slowly and patiently, partially through positive attitudes and behavior.

As the modes of health care are undergoing change, it is particularly important that the physician retain humanistic qualities. These qualities have been defined by the American Board of Internal Medicine and encompass integrity, respect, and compassion:

"The expression of sincere concern, the willingness to take the time to explain all aspects of the patient's illness, and an attitude of being nonjudgmental with patients who have lifestyles, attitudes, and values which are different from the physician's own and which he or she in some instances may even find repugnant. . . " (Braunwald et al., 1987, p. 82).

These qualities of a physician can help a patient maintain a positive outlook and thereby aid in the future success of a rehabilitation effort. The attitudes of the reporting physician can also be seen in written medical reports.

**Figure 1**

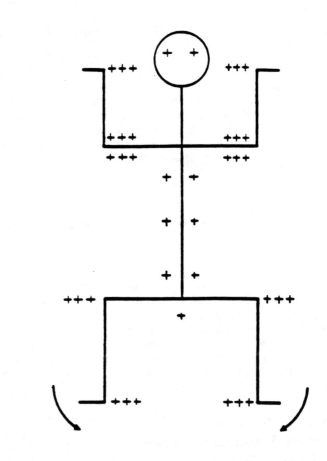

*Schematic representation of the results of testing the deep tendon reflexes, conducted as part of the physical examination.*

# THE MEDICAL HISTORY

Apart from the patient's current presenting problem, the medical history should include all factual material of a medical nature relating to the patient's life (Andreoli, Carpenter, Plum, & Smith, 1990; Conn & Conn, 1985; Schroeder, 1990; Wyngaarden & Smith, 1988). The history is composed of what the patient states and what the physician may imply from what is not said. Nonverbal behavior, such as mannerisms, facial expressions, personal hygiene, posture, and gait, can be extremely meaningful. With careful listening, the physician will begin to detect the nature of the disease entity and learn about the patient as a human being.

Not all histories are readily compiled for some patients are not sufficiently verbal to articulate clearly the symptoms or events leading to illness. Some patients have difficulty reporting a reasonable chronological history of events leading up to the presenting problem. When a physician claims certain patients are poor historians, the physician may not have taken the time necessary to obtain the significant information. A detailed medical history is essential and, as much as possible, the historical data should be in the patient's own words, in quotes.

## Chief Complaint

The starting point in taking the medical history is noting the patient's chief complaint and recording it exactly as expressed by the patient, including its duration.

**Record Segment With Abbreviations**
**Patient A**
c.c.    "Weak and tired" - 3 weeks duration

**Record Segment in Full Form**

Chief Complaint - "Weak and tired" - 3 weeks duration.

**Patient B**
c.c.    SOB, severe - 4 days.

Chief Complaint - Shortness of breath, severe - 4 days.

Additional complaints will be noted in descending order of importance.

## Present Illness

The physician will ask about the onset and duration of the present illness and obtain a full description of the symptoms. This description should include the location, the duration, and the intensity of the symptoms. The circumstances under which symptoms become more acute or subside need to be noted; effects of medication taken should be specified. It is important to ask if any other family members have this or related conditions. There may be barriers to obtaining a fully detailed clinical history. Differences in socio-economic level, a patient's limited language skills, organic changes due to disease or injury, and cultural differences may make it difficult to obtain a complete picture. The physician should discuss the issues of confidentiality with the patient.

**Record Segment With Abbreviations**

**Record Segment in Full Form**

*Patient A*

C.C.

P.I. Three weeks ago, this 40 y/o w/m ♀ homemaker had a cold with ass'd mild cough & temp. elev. which lasted 2 days. At this time, there was a loss of appetite and food intake was ↓.

After the cough & temp. elev. subsided, pt. noted ↑ weakness and general malaise. Exercise which was tolerated well ā the URI now tires her considerably.

One week ago she noticed thirst & a feeling of nausea. She had n & v yesterday (date) and was advised to seek medical attention.

There has been a 25-35 lb. weight loss during the past year.

**Chief Complaint**

Present Illness - Three weeks ago, this 40-year-old white married female homemaker had a cold with associated mild cough and temperature elevation which lasted two days. At this time, there was a loss of appetite and food intake was decreased.

After the cough and temperature elevation subsided, the patient noted increased weakness and general malaise. Exercise which was tolerated well before the upper respiratory infection now tires her considerably.

One week ago she noticed thirst and a feeling of nausea. She had nausea and vomiting yesterday (date) and was advised to seek medical attention.

There has been a 25-35 pound weight loss during the past year.

*Patient B*

C.C.

P.I. This 60 y/o w/m ♂ welder was N & W until approx. 4d ago. Noted onset of SOB c̄ sl. exertion which w/in 4-6h became SOB even at rest. This has ↑ in the last 3d. Past 2 nights, pt. has had to sit up in chair while sleeping, c̄ no prev. HX of orthopnea or PND. Denies any prev. HX of heart disease, hypertension; re lungs, pt. states he has had "cough c̄ lots of phlegm" qd for last 3-4 yrs; otherwise, denies lung disease.

**Chief Complaint**

Present Illness - This 60-year-old white married male welder was normal and well until approximately 4 days ago. Noted onset of shortness of breath with slight exertion which within 4-6 hours became shortness of breath even at rest. This has increased in the last 3 days. The past 2 nights, the patient has had to sit up in a chair while sleeping, with no previous history of orthopnea or paroxysmal nocturnal dyspnea. Denies any previous history of heart disease or hypertension; regarding the lungs, patient states he has had "cough with lots of phlegm" each day for the last 3-4 years; otherwise, denies lung disease.

Following a thorough discussion of the health problem or problems, the physician evaluates the patient in relationship to a full range of hereditary and environmental (work, home, and leisure) factors.

## Family History

The physician will take a family history concerning medical events in the lives of relatives, including information about parents, grandparents, siblings, spouse, and children. Familial diseases can provide significant clues, as can the cause of death of any deceased relatives. In certain diseases that may involve multiple family members, the physician may actively intervene to prevent the onset of symptoms before the actual development of apparent disease. This is particularly important when working with hereditary factors that may predispose an individual to certain diseases.

Many patients do not know the cause of death of close relatives. If a parent died of cancer, the patient often cannot identify the type or primary site of the growth. When multiple cancer deaths are reported in a family constellation, the patient often shows little concern that the disease may have a hereditary link.

| Record Segment With Abbreviations | Record Segment in Full Form |
|---|---|
| *Patient A* | |
| C.C. | Chief Complaint |
| P.I. | Present Illness |
| F.H.  Mother A & W age 67. Father died age 55 of "heart trouble." An aunt (maternal) has diabetes. Fourth of 5 sibs - 2♀, 3♂. Mother of 3 children, 1♀, 2♂. | Family History - Mother alive and well, aged 67. Father died age 55 of "heart trouble." An aunt (maternal) has diabetes. Patient is the fourth of 5 siblings, 2 female, 3 male. Mother of 3 children, 1 daughter, 2 sons. |

## Past [Medical] History

The next step involves obtaining extensive information concerning the patient's past medical history. Inquiries will be made about diseases that occurred in childhood, serious adult illnesses, injuries, surgical procedures, and hospitalizations. If the patient is a female, she will be asked about pregnancies, both those carried to term and those interrupted. The individual's diet; smoking habits (if any); consumption of coffee, tea, alcohol, non-prescription drugs, prescribed medications, and self-medications; and hours of sleep will be recorded.

To obtain a total personal profile of the patient, data will be sought about the social history, marital status, educational background, present and past occupations, and possible exposure to hazardous substances.

| Record Segment With Abbreviations | Record Segment in Full Form |
|---|---|
| *Patient A* | |
| C.C. | Chief Complaint |
| P.I. | Present Illness |
| F.H. | Family History |
| P.H.  UCHD. Pneumonia age 31, no sequelae. Appendectomy, age 24 (date), Everytown General Hospital, Everytown, (State), A.B. Doe, M.D. Grava. IV, Para III, ab. I @ 2 mo. | Past History - Usual childhood diseases. Pneumonia at age 31, no sequelae (no complications following the pneumonia). Appendectomy at age 24 (date), Everytown General Hospital, Everytown, (State), A.B. Doe, M.D. Four pregnancies, 3 completed and 1 aborted in the second month. |
| S.H.  Born in Tulare, CA, 1943. High school education. Congenial family life. Habits: Smokes 1 - 1½ pks/ day (30 - 45 pk yrs). Denies use of alcohol, drugs, $R_x$ medications. | Social History - Born in Tulare, CA, 1943. High school education. Congenial family life. Habits: Smokes 1 - 1½ packs of cigarettes daily for a total of 30 - 45 pack years [1 x 30 years - 1½ x 30 years]. Denies use of alcohol, drugs, or prescribed medications. |
| O.H.  Has been homemaker all of working life. | Occupational History - Has been a homemaker all of her working life. |

| Record Segment With Abbreviations | Record Segment in Full Form |
|---|---|
| **Patient B** | |
| C.C. | **Chief Complaint** |
| P.I. | **Present Illness** |
| F.H. | **Family History** |
| P.H. NKA. Surgery - rt. inguinal herniorrhaphy approx. 30 yrs ago (place?); tonsillectomy in childhood (date?). Hospitalization - only for surg. above. Meds-none req. except ASA for H/A. Med illness-pneumonia p̄ flu, 1946 - not hosp. Frequent "chest colds" - chr. cough. | Past History - Allergies - none. Surgery - right inguinal herniorrhaphy approximately 30 years ago, place unknown; tonsillectomy in childhood, date unknown. Hospitalization - only for surgical procedures above. Medication - none regularly except aspirin [acetylsalicyclic acid] for headaches. Medical illness - pneumonia following the flu in 1946 - not hospitalized. Frequent "chest colds" - chronic cough. |
| S.H. Married, owns home, suburbs. Smokes 1-2 pks/day (45-60 pk yrs). Drinks "occas. cocktail," no beer, prob. mod. drinker at most. | Social History - Married, owns home in the suburbs. Smokes 1 - 2 packs of cigarettes daily for a total of 45 - 60 pack years [1 x 30 years - 2 x 30 years]. Drinks "occasional cocktail", but no beer. Probably a moderate drinker at most. |
| O.H. Linotype operator, local newspaper, 16 years, until tech. change and retirement. Prev. worked in small job shops around Midwest as compositor. Never any Pb exposure studies. U.S. Army 1950-1952. Clerk, never overseas. | Occupational History - Linotype operator, local newspaper, 16 years, until technology change and retirement. Previously worked in small job shops around the Midwest as compositor. Never any lead exposure studies. U.S. Army 1950-1952 - clerk, but never served overseas. |

## *Review of Systems*

To complete the medical history, the physician will review present and past disorders with the patient, as disclosed through questions involving all bodily organs or systems. These include: head, eyes, nose, throat, mouth, respiratory tract, cardiovascular system, gastrointestinal system, genitourinary system, menstrual cycle, metabolism, neurologic system, musculoskeletal system, and emotional status (psychiatric state). Such an orderly review may produce either a series of negative responses or will elicit coexisting symptoms or difficulties forgotten because of the current clinical problem.

| Record Segment With Abbreviations | Record Segment in Full Form |
|---|---|
| **Patient A** | |
| C.C. | Chief Complaint |
| P.I. | Present Illness |
| F.H. | Family History |
| P.H. | Past History |
| S.H. | Social History |
| O.H. | Occupational History |
| R.O.S. | Review of Systems |

HEENT: Frequent dull headaches of 2 weeks duration. Ears - No PRT. No disch. Eyes - NSA; wears glasses. Nose - NSA. Throat - NSA.

Neck: NSA

Resp.: Dyspnea on sl. exertion.

C.V.: Palpitation on exertion.

G.I.  See P.I.

G.U.  Frequency & nocturia, 4x. No hematuria. V.D.: Denies. Menses: Menarche 13, $\bar{q}$ 28-30 x 5 mod. heavy flow.

N.S.: Excessive drowsiness past 2-3 weeks. Has had PP drowsiness past 1-2 years.

M.S.: Vague pains thighs and calves. Infrequent leg cramps @ h.s. [hora somni].

Endocrine: See above for weakness, excessive thirst, wt. ↓, nocturia, dyspnea, tachycardia, etc.

*Patient B*

C.C.

P.I.

F.H.

P.H.

S.H.

O.H.

R.O.S.

HEENT: Occas. nosebleeds in last 8 mos; also headaches occas. in A.M.

Neck: NSA

Resp.: No hemoptysis.

C.V.: See P.I. Also has occas. ankle swelling, polyuria $\bar{c}$ nocturia x 2-3. No chest pain.

G.I.: No Hematemesis, no melena; has had occas. trouble $\bar{c}$ hemorrhoids - $\bar{o}$ recently.

G.U.: Denies V.D. Some recent trouble starting stream and dribbling. See C.V.

N.S.: NSA.

Head, Eyes, Ears, Nose, Throat: Frequent dull headaches of 2 weeks duration. Ears - No previous trouble. No discharge. Eyes - No significant abnormalities; wears glasses. Nose - No significant abnormalities. Throat - No significant abnormalities.

Neck: No significant abnormalities

Respiratory Tract: Difficulty in breathing on slight exertion.

Cardiovascular System: Palpitation on exertion.

Gastrointestinal System: See Present Illness.

Genitourinary System: Frequency of urination at night, 4 times. No blood in urine. Denies venereal disease. Menstrual cycle: Onset of menstruation at age 13, with periods of 5 days duration of moderately heavy flow, every 28-30 days.

Nervous System: Excessive drowsiness past 2-3 weeks. Has had drowsiness after meals for the past 1-2 years.

Musculoskeletal System: Vague pains in muscles of thighs and calves. Infrequent leg cramps at bedtime.

Endocrine System: See above for weakness, excessive thirst, weight loss, nocturia, dyspnea, rapid heart beat, etc.

Chief Complaint

Present Illness

Family History

Past History

Social History

Occupational History

Review of Systems

Head, Eyes, Ears, Nose, Throat: Occasional nosebleeds in the last 8 months; also headaches occasionally in the morning.

Neck: No significant abnormality.

Respiratory Tract: No expectoration of blood.

Cardiovascular System: See Present Illness. Also has occasional ankle swelling, frequent urination with nocturia, 2-3 times each night. No chest pain.

Gastrointestinal System: No vomiting of blood, no blood in bowel movements (black stools). Has had occasional trouble with hemorrhoids, but none recently.

Genitourinary System: Denies venereal disease. Some recent trouble with starting stream and dribbling. See Cardiovascular System.

Nervous System: No significant abnormality.

M.S.: Neg.  Musculoskeletal System: Negative.
Endocrine: Neg.  Endocrine System: Negative.

At this point in the interview, the physician may have reached a working diagnosis of the illness based on the data derived from the patient's responses. The diagnosis will be differentiated more precisely on completion of the physical examination, receipt of the results of subsequent clinical laboratory tests, and possible x-ray examinations.

# THE PHYSICAL EXAMINATION OF BODY SYSTEMS

The findings of the physical examination add to the content of the history; the physician may detect objective signs of disease that are verifiable either by another examiner or by clinical laboratory tests. Techniques used in the physical examination include inspection, palpation (feeling), percussion (sounding out), and auscultation (listening). The physician uses sensory instruments to look, feel, and listen, including visual illumination, magnification, and aural amplification. Most often, the examination is conducted from the external covering (the skin or integument) of the body internally through the various orifices and from the top (head) downward (to the toes).

The sequence of the medical evaluation is usually maintained and rarely deviates from the accustomed progression. More time will be spent by the physician in assuring that a certain finding truly represents a disease change in an organ or tissue. While some components of the examination may be carried out quickly, the amount of time spent represents the acquired and practiced systematic technique of an experienced observer. Important problem areas will frequently be given a second, more thorough examination.

It is good medical practice to record the findings as quickly as possible after completion of the examination. The physician should inform the patient of the findings, including the severity of the condition, in clear and understandable language.

## General Impression

On initial assessment, the physician will provide a general impression of the patient, including: the apparent state of health and nutrition, posture, muscular development, any abnormal body configuration, general level of intelligence, and evidence of any emotional reaction to physical illness.

**Record Segment with Abbreviation**
*Patient A*
P.E.: Wt. 108 T-97.4 P-136 R-32 B.P. 104/64. Age 40.

General Appearance: Pt. is FWD, PN, WF appearing both acutely and chronically ill. Respirations are rapid and pt. is restless.

**Record Segment in Full Form**

Physical Examination: Weight 108 pounds, temperature 97.4 F, Pulse 136, Respiration 32, Blood Pressure 104/64. Age 40.
General Appearance: Patient is a fairly well developed, poorly nourished, white female appearing both acutely and chronically ill. Respirations are rapid and patient is restless.

**Patient B**

P.E.: Pt. is a 60 y.o. Cauc., WD, WN, sl. obese, alert and coop., in some sl. resp. distress, well-oriented as to time, place, and person.

Physical Examination: Patient is a 60-year-old Caucasian, well developed, well nourished, slightly obese, alert and cooperative, in some slight respiratory distress, well-oriented as to time, place, and person.

V.S.: B.P. 185/105 R.A.S. P-104 and reg. 180/105 L.A.S. R-24 and labored. Afebrile.

Vital Signs: Blood Pressure 185/105, right arm, sitting. Pulse 104 and regular. B.P. 180/105, left arm, sitting. Respiration 24 and labored. Afebrile (no fever).

## Skin

Since many disabilities affect changes readily visible, the skin will be inspected for a variety of characteristics. The individual's general complexion, including cyanosis or jaundice, will be noted. Texture, abnormalities of turgor or pigmentation, folds, eruptions, moisture, hair quality, and distribution and elasticity will be evaluated. The physician will also note the presence of any traumatic or incisional scars, tumors, evidence of weight loss, occupational callouses, or similar changes.

**Record Segment with Abbreviation**
*Patient A*

Skin: Dry. Poor turgor (skin texture). Some areas of vitiligo (white patchy areas) on back of neck and forearms.

**Record Segment in Full Form**

Skin: (Same entry)

*Patient B*

Skin: Skin clear, moist, with some occupational soiling of hands and nails. Few keratoses on dorsa of hands.

Skin: (Same Entry)

## Head

In examination of the head, any dermatologic disorders of the scalp, texture of scalp hair, abnormal sensitivities, or evidence of old nasal fractures will be described.

**Record Segment with Abbreviation**
*Patient A*

Head: There are some dry, desquamating (scaly) elevated areas of reddening at the hairlines of the scalp and at the eyebrows. No tenderness to pressure over sinuses or mastoid areas.

**Record Segment in Full Form**

Head: (Same entry)

*Patient B*

Head: Normocephalic. There are some small xanthomatous (yellow) elevations over both upper lids. Transillumination of sinuses normal.

Head: (Same Entry)

## Eyes and Ears

The gross examination of the eyes identifies their alignment and functional coordination. The pupils are checked for their size, shape, equality, and reaction to light and accommodation. The physician notes the state of the sclerae in regard to possible jaundice, hemorrhage, or infection of the vessels. The corneas are examined for the possible presence of scarring, cloudiness, or ulceration. The reflected conjunctival lining of the lids are inspected for inflammatory change. Finger pressure over the eyeball establishes the tension of the fluid within the eyeball or globe.

The ophthalmoscope enables the physician to examine the background or fundus of the eye by means of a lens system and a beam of light (funduscopic examination). The state of the blood vessels of the retina in the back of the eye provides important diagnostic information, not only concerning the eyes but the possible presence of systemic disease. This location is one of the rare sites where blood vessels can be viewed directly.

External examination of the ears will establish their size, form, shape, and any evidence of infection. Using an otoscope, the physician is able to look into the ear canal for the presence of obstruction, excessive cerumen (wax), or infection. The state of the eardrum or tympanic membrane can be examined. Hearing acuity is tested by means of an audiometer, an electronic precision instrument.

**Record Segment with Abbreviation**
*Patient A*

Eyes and Ears: EOM intact. PERLA. Fundi Neg. TMs intact.

**Record Segment in Full Form**

Eyes and Ears: Extra-ocular movements intact. Pupils equal, round, and react to light and accommodation. Fundi are negative. Tympanic membranes (ear drums) are intact.

*Patient B*

Eyes and Ears: EOM Normal. Pupils R & E, and react to L & A. Fundi: some AV nicking bilat. A:V-1:3; no papilledema or hemorrhages. T.M.s both clear, with normal landmarks and good LR.

Eyes and Ears: Extra-ocular movements are normal. Pupils are round and equal, and react to light and accommodation. Fundi show some arteriovenous nicking bilaterally. Ratio of diameter of arteries to veins 1:3. There is no papilledema and there are no hemorrhages. Tympanic membranes are both clear, with normal landmarks and good light reflex.

## Nose, Mouth, Throat, and Neck

In examining the nose by means of a speculum, the physician looks for evidence of impairment to breathing, assesses the condition of the nasal septum, and inspects the mucous membrane.

The mouth is examined for changes or tumors of the lips. The mucous membrane lining the oral cavity and the gums are checked. Likewise, the teeth are inspected; those missing are noted. Changes are noted, as are the state of restoration and the presence of partial or full dentures; the general level of oral hygiene is indicated. Changes in the surface of the tongue can reveal the presence of various systemic disorders, and the inability of the patient to protrude the tongue in the midline has neurological significance. The soft palate and the pharynx are checked for the presence and condition of the tonsils, and for inflammation or tumors. A comment may be made about the patient's voice quality.

The neck is palpated to detect enlargement of the thyroid gland; the lymph nodes in the neck and under the arms will be checked. The position of the trachea is noted and the condition of the blood vessels is checked for abnormal pulsations.

**Record Segment with Abbreviation**
*Patient A*

Nose: Septum R, with some impairment of breathing space. No discharge. MM dry.

Mouth: Tongue red. Odor of acetone on breath. Edentulous.

Neck: Supple. Thyroid not palpable. Trachea in midline.

Lymphatics: NSA

*Patient B*

Nose: Septum in midline. Turbinates enlarged bilaterally, with considerable thick mucoid discharge.

Mouth: Tonsils sugically absent. Pharynx granular. Uvula deviated L. Tongue coated. Partial upper denture and moderate caries.

Neck: Trachea in midline, thyroid not enlarged, but palpable. No nodes felt. Jugular veins prominent, even c̄ pt. sitting up.

**Record Segment in Full Form**

Nose: Septum deviated to the right, with some impairment of breathing space. No discharge. Mucous membrane is dry.

Mouth: Tongue is red. There is an odor of acetone on the breath. No teeth are present.

Neck: (Same entry).

Lymphatics: No significant abnormality.

Nose: (Same entry).

Mouth: Tonsils surgically absent. Pharynx granular. Uvula deviated to the left. Tongue coated. Partial upper denture and moderate caries.

Neck: Trachea in midline, thyroid not enlarged, but palpable. No nodes felt. Jugular veins prominent, even with patient sitting up.

## *Chest*

The examination of the chest reveals the condition and level of functioning of the heart and lungs. In observing the movement of the chest as the patient breathes, the physician notes if respiratory movement is normal. Observation of the chest will reveal any asymmetry, flatness, or barrel configuration, evidence of possible abnormality, or disease process. The sounds evoked by percussing and the sensation of movement or vibration detected by the palpating hand of the physician convey information concerning the size and position of the organs and the presence of fluid, air, or solid structures.

Auscultation (listening to) of the lungs, through use of a stethoscope, provides information concerning the character and intensity of the breath sounds, the relative duration of inspiration and expiration, and the presence of abnormal lung sounds. Auscultation of the heart reveals the intensity of the heart sounds, the nature of the cardiac rhythm, and the presence and location of murmurs (abnormal heart sounds). Some physicians will take and record the blood pressure reading at this point, using a sphygmomanometer; others take the pressure at the beginning of the evaluation.

**Record Segment with Abbreviation**
*Patient A*

Chest: Symmetrical. Resp. rapid.
Lungs: Clear to P & A.

**Record Segment in Full Form**

Chest: Symmetrical. Respirations rapid.
Lungs: Clear to percussion and auscultation.

Heart: PMI in 5th LICS. Area of cardiac dullness normal. Rate 136/min, reg. R, A2>P2. No m s.

Heart: Point of maximum impulse in 5th left intercoastal space. Area of cardiac dullness normal. Rate 136/minute, regular rhythm, aortic second sound greater than pulmonic second sound. No murmurs.

## Patient B

Chest: ↑ A-P diam - secondary resp. muscles hypertrophied. Barrel-chested. Def. hyperres. on percussion. Decreased B.S. bilat. c̄ mod. number of rales (wet), both bases posteriorly, occas. rhonchus, no wheezes. Poor expan. bilat.

Chest: Increased anterior-posterior diameter-secondary respiratory muscles hypertrophied (enlarged). Barrel-chested. Definite hyperresonance on percussion. Decreased breath sounds bilaterally with a moderate number of rales (rattle-like sounds) at both bases posteriorly, with occasional rhonchus, no wheezes. Poor expansion bilaterally.

C.V.: Rate 96-108, reg. Heart sounds distant. Grade ii/vi syst. m aortic area c̄ minimal radiation (diamond-shaped); no other m detected, no T. Good pulses - radial, D.P., post tib. Positive hepatojugular reflex.

Cardiovascular system: Rate 96-108 and regular. Heart sounds are distant. There is a grade ii/vi systolic murmur at the aortic area with minimal radiation (diamond-shaped); no other murmur detected and there is no thrill. Good radial, dorsalis pedis and posterior tibial pulses (names of arteries). Positive hepatojugular reflex.

## Breasts, Abdomen, and Genitalia

With the patient lying in the supine position, the physician will palpate the abdomen, seeking signs of tenderness or the presence of masses. Also, it will be determined if there is any enlargement of the liver, spleen, or kidneys; the patient will be checked for the presence of hernia. The groin will be palpated to determine the size of the lymph nodes at that site.

If the patient is a woman, the breasts will be palpated for masses, and the nipples will be checked for possible ulceration, inversion, or secretion. The external genitalia will be examined; if the patient is female, a pelvic examination will be conducted.

**Record Segment with Abbreviation**
*Patient A*

Breasts: NSA.
Abd: Flat. LKS not palp. B.S. normal. 10 cm lower abd. healed incisional scar, RPM.

Pelvic: NSA.

**Record Segment in Full Form**

Breasts: No significant abnormality.
Abdomen: Flat. Liver, kidneys, and spleen are not palpable. Bowel sounds normal. There is a 10-centimeter lower abdominal healed incisional scar, right paramedian.
Pelvic Examination: No significant abnormality.

## Patient B

Abd: Sl. protub., minimal & questionable fluid wave. Liver edge felt 1-2 cm below RCM, sl. tenderness. No other masses or tenderness. Old 4 cm oblique RLQ healed surg. scar.

Abdomen: Slightly protuberant, with minimal and questionable fluid wave. Liver edge is felt 1-2 centimeters below the right coastal margin, and is slightly tender. No other masses or tenderness. There is an old 4-centimeter oblique right lower quadrant healed surgical scar.

GU: Testes ↓↓ and normal. No hernia detected. Normal external genitalia.

Genitourinary System: Both testes are descended and normal. No hernia detected. Normal external genitalia.

## Extremities, Rectum, Musculoskeletal System, and Nervous System

The upper and lower extremities are checked for swelling, deformity of the joints, and range of motion of the joints. In addition, the upper extremities examination includes a notation concerning the color and degree of moisture of the palms and the status of the fingernails. In the lower extremities, the physician looks for varicose veins, fungus infection of the feet and nails, edema of the feet and ankles, and the state of the arterial pulsations.

The digital examination of the rectum will reveal the tone of the sphincter and the presence of hemorrhoids or new growths. In men, the rectal examination provides a means to palpate the prostate gland, which is checked for size, consistency, and shape.

Unless there are specific indications such as symptoms or other pertinent findings, the initial neurological examination is usually limited to checking the biceps, triceps, and deep tendon reflexes. These findings may be entered in the record in the schematic manner shown in Figure 1.

To conclude the examination, the physician will observe the patient's gait and check the range of motion of the spine, including flexion, extension, lateral bending, and rotation.

### Record Segment with Abbreviation
*Patient A*
Ext:   No edema, trophic changes, or ulcerations.
Rectal: NSA.
Neuro: DTR physiologic.

B & J:  Full ROM. No HRST of joints.

*Patient B*
Ext:   No deformities, good pulses 2+ pitting edema, both ankles.
Rectal: Normal sphincter. Prostate grade ii-iii, firm throughout, no nodules. Feces on glove brown. Guaiac neg.

N.M.: Normal ROM all 4 ext. DTRs - 1+ - 2+ bilat. Cranial nerves, II-XII, intact. No sensory defects noted. No Babinski, Chaddock, Hoffmann. Gait and station WNL (within normal limits). Neg. cerebellar signs.

### Record Segment in Full Form

Extremities: (Same entry)
Rectal: No significant abnormality.
Neurologic Examination: Deep tendon reflexes are physiologic [physiologically normal].
Bones and Joints: Full range of motion. No heat, reddening, swelling, or tenderness of the joints.

Extremities: No deformities, good pulses 2+ [in range of 1-4], pitting edema (swelling) of both ankles.
Rectal Examination: Normal sphincter. Prostate gland grade ii-iii [in size, range of 1 - 4], firm throughout without nodules. Feces on examination glove are brown and Guaiac test for blood is negative.
Neuromuscular System: Normal range of motion of all 4 extremeties. Deep tendon reflexes are 1+-2+ [in an intensity range of 1-3] bilaterally. Cranial nerves II-XII are intact - I [one] was not tested. No sensory defects were noted. No Babinski, Chaddock, or Hoffmann reflex elicited. Gait and station are normal. There are no signs of cerebellar disease.

# DIAGNOSIS

## Diagnostic Impressions

On completion of the physical examination, the physician will record a diagnostic impression. Additional and further clarifying data studies will be needed for confirmation, since it is only an "impression" which is reached thus far. A diagnosis, or diagnoses, is made when conclusive evidence is obtained. In the cases of the two patients whose physical examinations have been presented here, the physician records a preliminary impression, subject to further studies.

## Patient A Impression

Diabetes mellitus, uncontrolled, complicated by acidosis.

## Patient B Impression

1. Congestive heart failure, acute.

2. Hypertension of unknown etiology (cause), probable cause of #1.

3. Chronic obstructive pulmonary disease, moderately advanced, also probably contributory cause of #1.

4. Bronchitis, chronic.

5. Prostatic hyperplasia (enlargement), probably benign.

## Further Diagnostic Studies

It is customary for most physicians to conduct further studies, the nature and extent of which will depend on the findings derived from the physical examination. Irrespective of findings, there probably will be a complete blood count, urinalysis, blood chemistry panel, and resting electrocardiogram. In the case of Patient B, a chest x-ray is warranted. Other test procedures, or repeated tests, will be conducted as indicated for fine tuning of the diagnosis or for determination of effectiveness of treatment.

## An Alternative Recording System

Some physicians employ a different framework for recording a patient's medical history data and physical examination findings. The "problem-oriented approach" uses the acronym SOAP: S standing for Subjective Findings, O meaning Objective Findings, A indicating Assessment, and P standing for Plan. Subjective Findings (S) encompasses the symptoms noted by the patient, along with pertinent historical data. Objective Findings (O) indicates the findings encountered by the physician through the physical examination. Assessment (A) comprises diagnostic impressions usually listed as problems. Plan (P) may include additional studies; the beginning of specific medication(s); counsel regarding diet, smoking, and exercise; and certain periodic follow-up visits or repeated clinical laboratory test procedures. Some physicians combine the formats using abbreviations (CC, PI, PH) and part of the problem-oriented approach (Assessment and Plan). In either case, records must be complete and legible.

In rare cases, records will be encountered in which recommendations will be made by the physician for procedures that will either not be wanted or flatly refused by the patient. In such cases, notes will appear in the record that recommendations were made but were refused by the patient. The patient will be asked to sign such an entry and the signature will be witnessed, in writing, by a member of the medical facility staff. Notes will be appended indicating what the patient was told about the examination findings, their significance, and the plan aimed at counteracting the disease process.

# REFERENCES

Andreoli, T.E., Carpenter, C.C.J., Plum, F., & Smith, L.H., Jr. (1990). **Cecil essential of medicine** (2nd ed.). Philadelphia, PA: Harcourt Brace Jovanovich.

Braunwald, E., Isselbacker, K.J., Petersdorf, R.G., Wilson, J.D., Martin, J.B., & Sauci, A.S. (Eds.). (1987). **Harrison's principles of internal medicine** (11th ed.). New York: McGraw Hill.

Clayman, C.B. (Ed.). (1989). **The American Medical Association encyclopedia of medicine.** New York: Random House.

Conn, H.F., & Conn, R.B., Jr. (Eds.). (1985). **Current diagnosis - 7.** Philadelphia, PA: W.B. Saunders.

Coy, J. (Ed.). (1990). **Physician's current procedural terminology.** Chicago, IL: American Medical Association.

**Dorland's illustrated medical dictionary** (27th ed.). (1988). Philadelphia, PA: W.B. Saunders.

Glanze, W.D., Anderson, K.N., & Anderson, L.E. (Eds.). (1990). **Mosby's medical, nursing, and allied health dictionary** (3rd ed.). St. Louis, MO: C.V. Mosby.

Krupp, M.A., Tierney, L.M., Jr., Jawetz, E., Roe, R.L., & Camargo, C.A. (Eds.). (1985). **Physician's handbook** (21st ed.). Los Altos, CA: Lange Medical Publications.

Schroeder, S.A., Krupp, M.A., Tierney, L.M., Jr., & McPhee, S.J. (1990). **Current medical diagnosis and treatment.** Norwalk, CT: Appleton and Lange.

Thomas, C.L. (Ed.). (1989). **Taber's cyclopedic medical dictionary** (16th ed.). Philadelphia, PA: F.A. Davis.

Williams, P.L., Warwick R., Dyson, M., & Bannister, L.H. (Eds.). (1989). **Gray's anatomy** (37th ed.). New York: Churchill Livingstone.

Wilson, J.D., Isselbacker, K.J., Petersdorf, R.G., Martin, J.B., Fanci, A.S., & Root, R.K., (Eds.). (1991). **Harrison's principles of internal medicine** (12th ed.). New York: McGraw Hill.

Wyngaarden, J.B., & Smith, L.H., Jr. (Eds.). (1988). **Cecil textbook of medicine** (18th ed.). Philadelphia, PA: W.B. Saunders.

## About the Author:

Jean Spencer Felton, M.D., is a Clinical Professor of Community and Environmental Medicine, at the University of California, Irvine, California and a Clinical Professor (Emeritus) of Preventive Medicine, at the University of Southern California, Los Angeles, California. Dr. Felton is also a member of the President's Committee on Employment of People with Disabilities.

# Chapter 4

# DRUG ABUSE

by
*E. W. (Bud) Stude, Ed.D., C.R.C., N.C.C.*

## INTRODUCTION

Substance abuse has become a major problem facing our society today. As such, it is a disability that will become even more prevalent in vocational rehabilitation caseloads, either as a primary or a secondary disability. The purpose of this chapter is to help the reader understand drug abuse in terms of basic concepts concerning use and abuse, incidence in our society and within rehabilitation counseling, pharmacological aspects, major treatment approaches, and vocational implications.

## BASIC CONCEPTS OF DRUG ABUSE

Drug abuse is a generic term which implies that an individual is taking substances (e.g., drugs) into the body in a continued, harmful, and compulsive manner that eventually damages or harms the body. Drug abuse produces a psychological dependence for relief of discomfort of a physical addiction that results in negative physical symptoms upon withdrawal. While psychological dependence on drugs may be mild or severe, physical addiction results in actual changes in the body causing the individual difficulty in functioning normally without the drug. Continual use of the drug results in abnormal behavior. In either case, the resulting behavior is counterproductive to effective functioning and results in disability to the individual and negative consequences for society.

### Major Effects

Common to all drugs that are abused is the affect they have on the central nervous system. This affect most often occurs at the synaptic junction in the brain where the drug blocks neural transmission. The result of this blocking produces pathological effects at the tissue level. The alteration of neuron function by influencing a receptor site between two neurons results in a S-shaped dose response. Low doses of the drug are accompanied initially by a slow appearance of drug effect that increases rapidly with intermediate doses followed by a gradual leveling-off of drug effect with higher doses (see Figure 1) (Westermeyer, 1986). To understand the major effects of drugs that are commonly abused, one must understand the concepts of tolerance, dependence, withdrawal, and addiction.

**Tolerance.** Tolerance is the progressive decrease in effectiveness of a drug. When a person uses a drug repeatedly and the effect of the drug plateaus or decreases, tolerance has been reached. An individual needs larger doses of the drug to obtain the same or an increased effect. To understand this phenomenon, one must be aware of the half-life of a drug. Half-life refers to the time it takes for a drug to decrease concentration in the body by 50%. If an individual takes a drug in intervals that are less than the half-life, the drug will accumulate in the body (Arif & Westermeyer, 1988). The lower the half-life of the drug, the sooner it is excreted and the greater the need for another dose to obtain the desired effects.

When a residual of the drug builds up in the body, the person will need larger doses to overcome the tolerance the body has built-up to the drug. In addition, many drugs (e.g., alcohol and barbiturates) have cross-tolerance. This refers to tolerance to one drug building up tolerance to another. Thus, higher doses of the second drug will be needed to obtain the desired effect (Westermeyer, 1986).

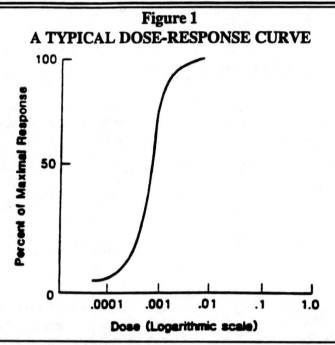

### Figure 1
### A TYPICAL DOSE-RESPONSE CURVE

Reprinted with permission of Greenwood Publishing Group, Inc., Westport, CT, from J. Westermeyer (1986). A clinical guide to alcohol and drug problems. New York: Praeger, P. 34.

**Dependence and withdrawal.** As mentioned earlier, the concept of dependence in relation to drug use has physical and psychological implications. Physical dependence is an altered physiological state because of repeated drug use. Withdrawal occurs with abstinence of the drug. The discomfort of withdrawal symptoms leads to continued drug use to prevent further withdrawal symptoms and sets up a vicious cycle of drug use leading to chronic drug abuse (Arif & Westermeyer, 1988; Westermeyer, 1986). Besides physical dependence, a psychological dependence may develop with chronic drug abuse, which is even more powerful in terms of its effects than physical dependence. The drug state may temporarily fulfill feelings of insecurity, the need to belong, striving for perfection, or need for power. This creates a strong drive to continue the use of drugs. Cessation of drug use creates psychological withdrawal symptoms if the individual does not find more appropriate ways of fulfilling these needs.

**Addiction.** The term addiction is associated with drug abuse. According to Benshoff and Riggar (1990), drug addiction includes the following three components: "(a) compulsive, repetitive use; (b) tolerance (the need to consume increasing amounts of the drug); and (c) withdrawal, generally of a marked physical nature" (p. 22). The definitions of tolerance, physical and psychological dependence, and withdrawal suggest that an individual who abuses drugs becomes unable to give up the habit of use because cessation causes severe trauma.

The resulting addiction has physical, psychological, and social aspects. Physically, the body may crave the drug. Psychologically, the individual may long for the euphoric feeling or mood induced by the drug. There are also social implications to drug addiction. Besides the social relationships that often accompany drug use and abuse, the individual expends tremendous physical and emotional energy and financial resources in obtaining drugs. This expenditure of energy is so all consuming that the welfare of those around have little meaning for the individual who is abusing drugs. This includes family members and significant others. It may also include people whose homes and businesses the abuser may burglarize to obtain necessary funds for drug purchases.

# OCCURRENCE OF SUBSTANCE ABUSE

Greer, Roberts, May, and Jenkins (1988) estimated the incidence of substance abuse in the general population to be as high as 35-40%. One in 10 individuals in the United States, who drinks, is prone to alcoholism, and there are 9-10 million adults who are alcoholics or problem drinkers (Taricone, Bordieri, & Scalia, 1989). Thirteen percent of men and 29% of women in this country use some form of psychotropic (mind altering) drug (Greer, 1986). There is additional data (Greer et al., 1988) that suggest individuals abusing one substance often concurrently or in the future will abuse other substances. The estimated annual cost of worker drug abuse to employers is $60 billion when taking into account health care costs, lost productivity, absenteeism, and job-related accidents (Backer, 1988).

The incidence of substance abuse among persons with disabilities approximates that of the general population (Dudek, 1984; Greer et al., 1988). Greer (1986) reported studies indicating 60% of 273 clients in a vocational rehabilitation facility experienced alcohol-related problems, while 30% were alcoholic. Forty-one of 47 spinal cord injured clients had problematic alcohol and drug use. Twenty-five percent of workers at a workshop for the blind had alcohol problems. Thirty-three percent of patients in the psychiatric service at a Veterans' Administration Hospital had problems with alcohol, while 4.6% abused drugs. Lett (1988) indicated that often the primary diagnosis of alcoholism is viewed as a secondary problem or is undetected in persons with severe psychiatric disorders. As many as 40% of persons with psychiatric diagnoses also abuse alcohol and should be considered as having a dual diagnosis of psychiatric disorder and substance abuse.

Keller and Green (1981), in a study of clients referred for psychological evaluation, found 44% were taking medications prescribed by at least two different physicians who were not in communication with one another. Of these, over 50% were not aware of the dangers involved in taking combinations of drugs, both prescribed and illegal. These studies indicated that besides substance abuse, the combination of substance abuse with physical, mental, and emotional problems has the potential for increasing the difficulty of providing effective medical treatment and rehabilitation.

# PHARMACOLOGY

Drugs that are most often abused include alcohol, hallucinogens, marijuana, nicotine, opiates, sedatives, stimulants, and inhalants (Wright, 1980). In addition, cocaine has become a major abused substance in the last decade. The following section will review the pharmacological factors associated with each drug, including the source and forms of the drug, effects, tolerance, dependence, and the withdrawal/abstinence syndromes. This discussion will be confined to abused substances other than alcohol, as alcohol is discussed in another chapter in this book.

## Hallucinogens

The common factor among hallucinogens is that they produce perceptual and cognitive changes. These drugs include the indole alkylamines such as lysergic acid diethylamide (LSD), psilocybin, phenylalkylamine derivatives such as mescaline (peyote cactus), and phencyclidine hydrochloride (PCP). Of these drugs, LSD and PCP ("angel dust") are the most commonly used. LSD reached popularity during the late 1960s. It produces perceptual and cognitive changes including delusions (a false belief despite overwhelming proof to the contrary), hallucinations (a sense of perception without the existence of a real source), and psychoses. It is most often taken orally and produces an effect in 30-40 minutes. The effects may result in somatic, perceptual, and psychic symptoms. Somatically, the individual may experience such symptoms as dizziness, weakness, tremors, nausea, and drowsiness. In terms of perceptual effects, the user may see alterations in shapes and colors (psychedelic) and have difficulty in concentration.

Psychiatric symptoms may include lability in mood, disorientation in time relationships, depersonalization, paranoid ideation, and hallucinations. While there are few physiological changes, somatic and perceptual changes occur before psychic effects. The latter may last up to 12 hours after a single dose. While a significant degree of tolerance develops to LSD after only a few doses, withdrawal effects do not occur and the user's baseline level of function usually returns rapidly after a somewhat brief, drug-free interval. However, persistent psychological impairment **can** occur with LSD use.

PCP ("angel dust"), as it is frequently called on the street, was originally used by veterinarians as a general anesthetic. It is very easy to produce in a simple laboratory. PCP can be taken by injection, but is most often sprinkled onto smoking material such as tobacco or marijuana. Its effects are many and varied. Neurologically, the user often experiences ataxia, dysarthria, tremors, muscular hypertonicity, and hyperflexion. Both systolic and diastolic blood pressures are often elevated, though, at higher doses, the drug acts as a myocardial depressant. While euphoria usually follows ingestion of lower doses, those periods of exaggerated well-being are often followed by heightened anxiety, unexplained and frequent mood changes, and hostility. Homicide has occurred following use in unusual cases.

The effect of PCP has often been compared to states of sensory deprivation. Higher doses may cause myoclonus (muscle twitching or spasm), continuous seizures, coma, and psychosis. Sometimes, an analgesic or anesthetic effect may lead to an indifferent reaction to painful stimuli resulting in self-injury. Animal experiments have demonstrated tolerance to the drug, and some human users may abuse the drug daily, unlike most of the other hallucinogens.

Psilocybin is found in certain mushrooms and has only 1% the potency of LSD. Phenylalkylamine derivatives such as mescaline and peyote, found in Mexican cactus, are approximately 1/1000 as potent as LSD. Native American Indians use peyote legally in religious rituals on Indian reservations (Arif & Westermeyer, 1988; Westermeyer, 1986).

## Cannabis

Cannabis comes from the resinous substance of the plant, **Cannabis sativa L.**, which contains psychoactive and intoxicating ingredients. Although beverages, soups, cakes, and other foods can be used, the most popular method of ingestion is by smoking the dried flower tops and leaves as marijuana or hashish (a more potent form of the drug). The psychoactive effects of the drug are primarily due to delta-9-tetrahydrocannabinol (THC). Although ingesting the drug through smoking results in only about half the available THC reaching the lungs, effects occur rapidly after inhalation; the effects of one marijuana cigarette last for about 3 hours.

While most smokers of marijuana and hashish seek relaxation and a sense of well-being from using the drug, THC produces changes in mood, sense of time, memory, and brain functions. It impairs short-term memory. Also, it interferes with coordination, balance, and stance, although simple motor tasks are not initially impaired. Inhibition of concentration and ability to converse meaningfully occur. Minutes may seem like hours with laughter and silliness prevalent. Acute effects include a dry mouth and throat, increased hunger, and tachycardia (abnormally rapid heart beat). Higher doses and chronic use may result in severe cognitive brain impairment, thought disruption, hallucination, delusions, mood changes, and paranoia. Diminished testosterone levels in males also have been reported. The tar produced by marijuana smoke is carcinogenic; frequent users often report a chronic cough.

Physical dependence on THC does occur in humans. Storage of THC in fatty tissues results in a physiological dependence, which may last for several days to several weeks following cessation of use. Tolerance occurs in both animals and humans. Withdrawal leads to adaptational decrease in heart rate, skin temperature, and pressure within the eyes (Arif & Westermeyer, 1988; Westermeyer, 1986).

## Opioids

Opiates are those drugs that, whether natural or synthetic, have specific morphine-like pharmacological properties. Opiates are naturally-occurring products derived from the opium poppy (papaver somniferum) and include morphine, codeine, and thebaine. Semisynthetic opiates, produced by chemical manipulation of these phenanthrene alkaloids of opium include heroin and oxycodone. Opioids which are entirely synthetic (produced in the laboratory) include methadone hydrochloride, meperidine hydrochloride, fentanyl, and propoxyphene hydrochloride. The preferred method of ingestion is through intravenous injection.

All the opioids have the beneficial effect of relieving pain, insomnia, anxiety, cough, visceral problems, and diarrhea. These actions are mediated via the depression or stimulation of various sites within the central nervous system. Larger doses may have more negative effects including respiratory depression, peripheral vasodilatation that may cause hypotension increasing the release of antidiuretic hormone, and inhibition of adrenocorticotropin and gonadotropin release. The latter has a direct affect on the testicular cells and may lead to diminished sexual interest.

Tolerance often develops with the first dose. While the user initially seeks the effects of the drug itself, eventually the discomfort of withdrawal symptoms also may lead to recurrent use. A key problem presented by increased tolerance is that the lethal dose does not change. The addicted person is not aware of the decreased margin between an effective maintenance dose and a lethal one. When the person who has developed dependence on an opioid stops taking the drug, withdrawal symptoms may occur within 4-25 hours. The symptoms worsen from 24-72 hours, with acute symptoms ending within 4-10 days. Although the ordinary dose of morphine is 15-30 milligrams, highly tolerant users of opioids may take up to 1000 milligrams per dose. This and the severity of withdrawal symptoms may lead to repeated detoxification to obtain the same effect from lower doses of the drug (Arif & Westermeyer, 1988; Westermeyer, 1986).

## Cocaine

Cocaine is extracted from the coca leaf as active alkaloid. Its anesthetic properties led to its use as a legal ingredient in wine, tonics, and soft drinks until the early twentieth century. The most common form of cocaine is the hydrochloride salt which is a white crystalline powder formed by processing coca paste, and it is usually consumed by insufflation (snorting). In recent years, smoking the alkaloid itself (free base or "crack" cocaine) has become popular. Free base is smoked in cigarette form or by using a water pipe and it produces an immediate, intense feeling of euphoria and well being. Its effect is brief, lasting only a few minutes. The preparation process which involves the use of a highly flammable solvent (ether), can result in explosion and severe burns.

Cocaine stimulates the central nervous system, producing euphoria, alertness, increased self-esteem, disinhibition, relief from fatigue, and psychomotor excitement. The euphoric effect disappears rapidly; larger doses may result in marked agitation, insomnia, loss of appetite, convulsions, paranoia, and acute psychosis. Physical consequences of chronic cocaine use may include constriction of blood vessels, degeneration of the nasal septum, pulmonary dysfunction, blood pressure problems, tachyarrhythmias (irregular and rapid heartbeat), and a variety of infections. Crack users may experience severe depression and suicidal ideation following cessation of use.

The World Health Organization has recognized cocaine as the most reinforcing and thus potentially addicting drug known. Animals and humans become compulsive users and both may use cocaine until death occurs because of its effects. Cocaine-dependent people often prefer cocaine intoxication to all other activities. This habit often results in behavior they previously thought unacceptable. As mentioned earlier, cessation of cocaine use leads to withdrawal characterized by severe depression. This may lead to self-treatment with cocaine to relieve the depression. While the depression is often not relieved, compulsive cocaine use recurs. Consequently, relapse is a high risk for cocaine users (Arif & Westermeyer, 1988; Benshoff & Riggar, 1990; Westermeyer, 1986).

## Sedatives

Besides sedatives, this broad category of drugs includes hypnotics and anxiolytics. Specific drugs include alcohol, barbiturates, benzodiazepines, ethchlorvynol, glutethimide, methaqualone hydrochloride, meprobamate, chloral hydrate, and paraldehyde. These drugs all tend to alleviate anxiety and induce sleep.

Barbiturates are derivatives of malonylurea and can be either short-acting or long-acting in their effect. Drug abusers prefer short-acting barbiturates, although long-acting barbiturates (e.g., phenobarbital) may pose fewer problems during withdrawal. Glutethimide has a longer duration of effect than barbiturates, and overdose can often result in prolonged coma and death. Ethchlorvynol is shorter acting and has some therapeutic properties, while methaqualone is popular among sedative abusers because it reduces cardiovascular activity and depresses respiration. It is important to note that respiratory depression and depressed cardiovascular activity are seen **less frequently** with methaqualone than with the other sedative-hypnotics. Chloral hydrate and meprobamate resemble barbiturates in relation to sedation tolerance and dependence. The benzodiazepines (which include valium, librium, xanax, and others) have been used medically since the 1960s for their antianxiety, sedative, anticonvulsant, and muscle-relaxing properties. Still, abuse of these drugs can lead to tolerance, dependence, dose escalation, and withdrawal symptoms.

The major physiological effects of this class of drugs is to inhibit or impair transmission of nervous impulses and increase the onset and duration of sleep. Suppression of rapid eye movement (REM) sleep often results in excessive dreaming with occasional vivid nightmares. Suppression of the central nervous system can be so complete as to cause respiratory cessation and death. Also occurring is suppression of cardiovascular function. These agents are often implicated in suicidal deaths.

The therapeutic effect of these drugs is usually short; tolerance can develop with a single dose. The chronic user needs continually larger doses to achieve the desired effect. Ataxia, dysarthria, and slowness in thought and movement may result. Withdrawal symptoms can include delirium tremens (DTs), convulsions, tachycardia, hallucinations, and delusions (Arif & Westermeyer, 1988; Westermeyer, 1986).

## Amphetamines

Amphetamine and amphetamine analogues may be taken orally or injected intravenously. By either method, they stimulate the central nervous system, producing increases in multiple aspects of the body's metabolic rate. They have been popular ingredients in diet pills for many years and, as with all substances that are abused, cause untoward physical and behavioral effects.

The effect of amphetamines on the central nervous system often results in increased blood pressure. Larger doses result in tachycardias (increased heart rate) and tachyarrhythmias (irregular heart beat). They increase the metabolic rate, relax bronchial muscles, and increase body temperature. Behaviorally, amphetamines result in increased alertness and wakefulness, elevated mood accompanied by increased self-confidence, and a hyperactive psychomotor response. These actions lead to an inability to rest or sleep. One also sees anorexia (decreased appetite).

Tolerance to amphetamines occurs in relation to its anorexiant effect, mood elevation, and euphoric effects. Both physical and psychological dependence occur and various withdrawal symptoms can be seen upon discontinuation of the drug. While these effects vary considerably with the individual, they may include profound fatigue, lack of energy, depression, nervousness, agitation, tremor, insomnia, confusion, delirium or panic states, and paranoid ideation. Two types of psychosis may result from amphetamine use: toxic psychosis, which usually improves within a few days of termination of drug use; and psychosis with schizophreniform, affective, or paranoid features. The latter usually persists beyond intoxication and resists improvement with supportive treatment alone. Individuals with a diagnosis and history of schizophrenia are very sensitive to even small doses of amphetamines (Arif & Westermeyer, 1988; Westermeyer, 1986).

## Volatile Solvents-Inhalants

There are several substances around the home and the workplace that contain psychoactive substances, which when inhaled as gases or vapors, result in intoxication. These substances include aromatic hydrocarbons found in benzene from coal and petroleum; aliphatic hydrocarbons or paraffins; amyl nitrites used in smelling salts in crushable glass ampules; halogenated solvents and propellants found in freon; trichlorinated solvents, chloroform, found in cleaning solvents and degreasers; and inhalational anesthetic drugs such as ether and nitrous oxide.

The effects of these solvents and inhalants are similar to alcohol in terms of their intoxication and resulting central nervous system depression. Euphoria and disinhibition also may result. Severe systemic changes leading to death may occur and include cardiac arrhythmias; chronic nervous system damage in the cerebral cortex, cerebellum, spinal cord, and peripheral nerves; hepatic necrosis; nephropathy; hypertension; dizziness; and tachycardia. Amyl nitrites also have properties that delay sexual climax. As such, a person may use the substance to enhance sexual pleasure by delaying orgasm, which can result in habituation as an adjunct to sexual activity. They are thought to contribute to the spread of acquired immune deficiency syndrome (AIDS) by lessening one's inhibition for casual sex and suppressing or damaging the immune system (Arif & Westermeyer, 1988; Westermeyer, 1986).

## Tobacco/Nicotine

Although tobacco is not a controlled substance, nicotine (the primary psychoactive substance in tobacco) and its many other active ingredients, can result in aversive effects on the body. Consequently, it is appropriate to discuss it in this chapter on drug abuse.

Tobacco and tobacco products may be ingested by smoking, chewing, or sniffing. Because of its toxic effect, nicotine is occasionally used as a pesticide. It can be fatal to a small child who accidentally eats one cigarette containing 20 milligrams of nicotine. Its initial effect is as a stimulant. Yet, its later effects are just the opposite, serving as a depressant. Small doses of nicotine appear to stimulate the autonomic nervous system and muscles, while larger doses inhibit or paralyze the autonomic ganglia and neuromuscular synaptic sites. Nicotine is a central nervous system stimulant, and in large oral doses, may result in convulsions. The drug inhibits gastric contractions, slowing down gastrointestinal emptying. A major side effect is vasoconstriction, which can pose serious vascular problems, especially in persons who already have compromised circulation due to such conditions as arteriosclerosis or diabetes mellitus.

Tolerance develops because of the depressant effects of nicotine after a few doses. This may result in physical dependence, although this issue is still controversial. Yet, psychological dependence also may occur in relation to the social situations in which one uses it (e.g., relaxing after a meal, dealing with the stress of making new acquaintances, taking a break during working hours). The withdrawal syndrome includes a craving for tobacco, irritability, restlessness, headaches, and impairment of concentration (Arif & Westermeyer, 1988; Westermeyer, 1986).

## Caffeine

Another very common drug used and potentially abused by a large part of the population is caffeine. Occurring in a variety of plants, alkaloid caffeine is most often found in coffee, cola beverages, tea, and other substances such as analgesic preparations, stimulants, and anorexiants. While some soft drinks contain no caffeine, others contain about 50 milligrams per 12-ounce serving; ground coffee has 80-180 milligrams per 5-ounce serving. Interestingly, decaffeinated coffee contains 3 milligrams of caffeine per 5-ounce serving.

The effects of caffeine may include diminished fatigue, enhanced mental abilities for some tasks, tachycardia, increased force of cardiac contraction, increased gastric acidity secretions, relaxation of smooth muscle, and a diuretic effect. Larger doses may result in increased excitement, anxiety, and insomnia.

While tolerance to caffeine may develop to a mild extent in individuals who consume small quantities daily, dependence and tolerance may occur in individuals who consume high doses (600 milligrams or more) daily. Abstinence may result in irritability, headaches, restlessness, lethargy, and excessive yawning. Individuals who consume high doses of caffeine can experience a syndrome characterized by headaches, irritability, agitation, anxiety, trembling, and insomnia (Arif & Westermeyer, 1988; Westermeyer, 1986).

# TREATMENT

For the past 20 years, three major types of treatment approaches to drug abuse have been used. These are (1) the outpatient program approach using methadone; (2) the residential program approach utilizing the therapeutic community; and, (3) the drug-free, outpatient program approach which does not use drugs. Each of these programs are discussed briefly in relation to their emphasis and approach in achieving and promoting drug independence. In addition, the conflict between professionals and paraprofessionals as suitable service providers in drug abuse treatment programs is addressed.

## Outpatient Methadone Treatment

Treatment programs using methadone came into prominence during the 1960s in treating heroin addiction. A daily dose of the drug methadone replaces the desire for heroin, leaving the individual able to function in a more normal manner than with heroin. More specifically, the U.S. Department of Health and Human Services (Hubbard et al., 1989) define this treatment as: "The continued administering or dispensing of methadone, in conjunction with provision of appropriate social and medical services, at a relatively stable dosage level for a period in excess of 21 days as an oral substitute for heroin or other morphine-like drugs for an individual dependent on heroin" (p. 44).

Treatment occurs on an outpatient basis where the heroin-dependent individual comes into a clinic for daily administration of methadone. Simultaneously, the clinic provides the individual with supportive social, psychotherapeutic, educational, vocational, and other assistive services. This treatment program encourages the addicted individual to substitute heroin addiction with a drug that allows normal functioning and helps the individual reach a drug-free state. Some individuals will need methadone for an extended period. This has led to controversy in that a methadone habit can be as difficult, if not more so, to "kick" than heroin itself.

**Two models of treatment.** Because of this controversy, two models of methadone treatment have evolved. One model views drug abuse as a specific physical defect with biochemical and metabolic properties. One satisfies opioid drug addiction by the administration of the drug methadone. Total drug abstinence or independence is not a goal of this treatment program. This approach sees supportive services as adjunctive aspects of treatment with the development of a person's vocational skills and a return to work, while continuing methadone maintenance. The second approach views drug abuse as a symptom of an emotional disorder or psychiatric condition. This model uses methadone as an adjunct to psychotherapy. The goal is eventual abstinence from all drugs, including methadone, resulting in drug-free living and resocialization in a productive lifestyle. These models are further contrasted in that the physical model approach administers high levels of methadone, while the psychotherapeutic model uses very low levels of the drug. Currently, the psychotherapeutic model or abstinence-based methadone programs are becoming increasingly popular.

**Self-administration.** In either treatment approach, the development and adherence to a treatment plan is very important. Eligibility for federal funds dictates development of such a plan with the cooperation and knowledge of the client, accompanied by periodic updating and adjustment of the plan. Another controversial aspect of methadone treatment is urine testing. Federal regulations require weekly urinalysis for the first 3 months of a program and monthly random urinalyses thereafter, to determine whether the client is using heroin. There is concern over communication of a negative message to the client in terms of the ability to be trusted and having control over one's life. There is also controversy over programs that allow clients to take their doses of methadone home for self-administration. This usually occurs after a 3-12 month demonstration of commitment to the treatment program. The concern is that the person will not take the methadone and will end up selling it "on the street." In spite of this controversy, home treatment is a frequent part of methadone maintenance programs.

**Services provided.** Counseling, primarily individual, is a service required by federal regulation in methadone treatment programs. A minimum of one counseling session per month is usually required. Although counseling sessions include discussion of drug use issues and psychotherapeutic counseling on life problems, practical problem-solving is a strong focus. Other services include education, vocational rehabilitation, job placement, family services, and legal services. The clinic's financial ability to provide these services dictates the extensiveness of services offered (Hubbard et al., 1989).

## Residential Therapeutic Community Treatment

**Synanon.** Residential therapeutic community treatment programs for drug abuse can be traced back to Synanon, begun by Charles Dederick in 1958. Based on the Alcoholics Anonymous (AA) approach, the Synanon program emphasized permanent participation in its program. In addition, Synanon rejected life outside the therapeutic community. While therapeutic community treatment programs developed after Synanon adopted many principles of that program, return to society and independence from drugs are the major goals.

**Self-reliance.** According to the therapeutic community treatment philosophy, one can only put addiction into remission, not cure, by reliance on help from other addicted individuals and a complete change in lifestyle. The goal of return to society is most likely to be achieved because of a change of lifestyle that includes abstinence from drugs, elimination of antisocial behavior, increased self-esteem, and return to work. Central to this treatment approach is eventual reliance on oneself. To break the cycle of drug abuse, it is necessary to undergo residential, 24-hour a day treatment within a therapeutic setting.

**Self-help.** The individual accomplishes the goal of changing dysfunctional behavior into a productive lifestyle by a long-term intensive communal experience, extensive use of paraprofessionals in therapeutic treatment, and a commitment to return to society by way of the therapeutic community subculture. Therapeutic communities strongly emphasize self-help. These helpers are usually graduates of the program and function as role models. The programs are very structured, with residents progressing through a series of stages that are initially very restrictive, with more responsibility added and freedom granted with the attainment of each additional stage. Openness, honesty, and direct confrontation by residents and staff, is very important in the treatment process. Each resident has a work assignment according to a level of responsibility as determined by members of the therapeutic community. These assignments increase in responsibility and requirements until more advanced residents become employed or involved in training programs outside the therapeutic community. Use of privileges and peer pressure are the primary means of motivating appropriate behavior. Counseling sessions are primarily group counseling, including encounter groups.

**Three phases of treatment.** Treatment is in three phases. The first consists of living in residence. This occurs only after careful screening to decide if an individual is ready to become a member of a therapeutic community. The next phase is gradual re-entry into society while remaining a resident of the therapeutic community. Lastly, a period of aftercare and follow-up occurs, once an individual has returned to society and no longer resides in the therapeutic community (Hubbard et al., 1989).

## Drug-Free Outpatient Treatment Programs

**Non-medication approach.** In contrast to outpatient drug treatment programs that use methadone, several outpatient programs do not use medication as a major part of the treatment process. These programs originally began as community-based clinics that provided services to drug abusers who were in crises. After the crisis subsided or was resolved, the individual continued residence in the community. These crisis clinics gradually evolved into longer-term treatment programs of two types. One type attempts to help individuals change through complete resocialization, resulting in a drug-free residence in the community. The other type considers resocialization to be an unrealistic goal and, therefore, helps individuals adapt to their unique situations and achieve existences free of substance abuse.

These programs emphasize the use of counseling modalities in place of medication and are often affiliated with or housed in mental health clinics or community centers. When the programs were mainly crisis clinics, former addicted individuals primarily staffed them. Today, educated, experienced, and professionally trained individuals make up the staffs of these facilities.

**Resocialization and independence.** As might be expected, outpatient drug-free programs vary in terms of their focus on complete resocialization. Change-oriented programs have a goal of complete resocialization. They provide services that attempt to help the individual move in that direction. Adaptive programs consider complete resocialization to be unrealistic, and provide services designed to help the recovering drug abuser cope with society in a more positive and independent manner. The latter seems the predominate approach among outpatient drug-free programs today. While counseling is the key ingredient in treatment, they provide other services including crisis intervention, day care, assistance with housing, employment opportunities, and legal intervention (Hubbard et al., 1989).

## Comparison of the Three Treatment Programs

In reviewing these various approaches for drug abuse treatment, one might wonder about the effectiveness of one approach over the other. While each treatment team involved feels they have an edge over the others, it appears that individuals who abuse drugs are as different as one individual is from another. These individual differences, and the complexities of the substance abuse problems in relation to society and its subcultures, result in the need for many different treatment approaches. Consequently, there is need for a variety of treatment approaches, each contributing to the elimination of drug abuse and the conditions that relate to the consequences of this abuse.

## Paraprofessional Versus Professional Providers

A final issue in drug abuse treatment involves identification of the most appropriate and effective provider of services, the paraprofessional (recovering substance abuser) or the professional (Nelson, 1986; Valle, 1979). The self-help emphasis in the treatment of drug abuse came about because professionals had neither interest nor training to deal with this problem. Consequently, the traditional approach to drug abuse counseling had been to rely upon individuals who were recovering substance abusers themselves in the belief that peers would facilitate change more effectively than those who had never experienced the problem (Wright, 1980).

Alcoholics Anonymous (AA) is the most popular treatment approach using this principle. Dudek (1984) indicated that "attending AA meetings has consistently been the most effective activity for alcoholics" (p. 20). Clifford (1986) reported a study in which AA membership was the strongest predictor for maintaining sober behavior. As mentioned earlier, the therapeutic community, as exemplified by Synanon, has long been a predominant approach in drug abuse treatment. The use of confrontation by peers is one foundation of this approach. Early employee assistance programs in business and industry almost exclusively used the recovering substance abuser as a key person in identifying and dealing with substance abuse problems among employees. Dickman and Phillips (1983) reported studies indicating that early intervention by employee assistance programs resulted in the recovery of 7 out of 10 employees, without the use of hospitalization.

Only since the adoption of the Hughes Act of 1970, establishing the National Institute on Alcohol Abuse and Alcoholism, have professionals made a concerted effort toward recognition and treatment of alcoholism (Valle, 1979). Paraprofessionals believe that the professional's reliance on theories and treatment procedures instead of a personal relationship with clients is not humanistic. Professionals view paraprofessionals as demonstrating lack of expertise, low standards, and facilitating maintenance instead of treatment (Bokos, Lipscomb, & Schwartzman, 1984).

At the center of this controversy is whether the degreed professional with a thorough understanding of behavioral sciences, or the nondegreed paraprofessional with natural ability because of personal experience, is the most qualified individual to provide substance abuse counseling (Valle, 1979). In addition, as certification and licensure increase the professionalization of counseling, it is becoming increasingly difficult for paraprofessionals to qualify for third-party payments. As a result, substance abuse treatment programs hire professional counselors for basic financing reasons. The resolution of this controversy is important if the substance abuser is to be given the best quality treatment leading to successful rehabilitation.

# VOCATIONAL FACTORS

Besides detoxification, strengthening of the ego, increasing self-esteem, and developing a constructive support system, the recovering drug abuser needs to be able to return to living in a healthy environment. A healthy environment is one that facilitates independence, minimizes the need for dependence, and reinforces non-enabling behaviors. When many drug abusers enter treatment, they have lost employment, friends, and family. An important aspect of their rehabilitation is return to work in an atmosphere that will allow self-support in an environment which is less susceptible to the influences that originally contributed to drug abuse. Recovery from long-term drug abuse requires more than a change in the motivation to take drugs. Social-vocational status is correlated with physical dependence on drugs. Treatment that offers the opportunity for social-vocational change enhances the long-term functioning of persons who abuse drugs (Baker & Cannon, 1988).

Hall, Sorensen, and Loeb (1988) reported that paid employment is very important for clients in drug treatment rehabilitation and is a replicable correlate of continued abstinence. Work is a crucial component in maintaining long-term abstinence in substance abuse; the type of work environment is also a critical factor. Newton, Elliott, and Meyer (1988) indicated that a structured work environment, one that is "non-enabling" in that it discourages substance abuse-related behaviors, can help the abstinence program. Work environments with minimum structure can be "enabling" in that they promote substance abuse and are not effective in establishing abstinence and minimizing relapse. It is unrealistic to expect a newly recovering drug abuser to make the change from treatment to employment without the benefit of professional assistance and support (Beale, 1988). Job seeking skills groups can provide such support as suggested by Hall, Sorensen, and Loeb (1988) and Beale (1988).

It is clear from the above discussion that vocational rehabilitation is an important part of drug abuse treatment. As pointed out by Buxbaum (1988), while substance abuse counselors are familiar with the treatment of drug addiction, they are usually unfamiliar with the psychological and social aspects of disability and its affect on vocational development. Counselors need expertise in dealing with persons with disabilities in a way that will result in their returning to productive work situations that will reinforce non-drug abusing behavior. While the rehabilitation counselor's expertise is in helping persons with disabilities return to work, they often do not understand the dependency needs that result in relapse of substance abuse. The rehabilitation counselor needs to comprehend the importance of attitudes toward drug abuse (their own as well as society's) to be effective in helping drug abusers achieve successful vocational rehabilitation.

## Attitudes in Drug Abuse Treatment

Allen, Peterson, and Keating (1982) found the attitudes of most mental health providers and rehabilitation counselors toward substance abusers were significantly lower than their attitudes toward gays, public offenders, mentally retarded, physically disabled, and mentally ill. Dudek (1984) indicated that the most important factor in successful intervention with substance abusers is not technique, but attitude. Counselors who do not have experience in working with substance abusers often feel uncomfortable in dealing with them as clients due to reservations concerning the success of rehabilitation efforts. To be effective in substance abuse counseling, rehabilitation counselors need to adopt positive attitudes toward the treatability of persons who abuse substances in three areas. These are (1) awareness of substance abuse as a problem, (2) the place of relapse in achieving vocational rehabilitation goals, and (3) substance abuse as a legitimate concern in workers' compensation rehabilitation systems.

**Awareness.** Lett (1988) suggested rehabilitation counselors without experience in working with persons abusing substances may not recognize significant signs in their client's history. A study of intake counselors (trained to be aware of alcohol and drug abuse) in a community-based counseling program, demonstrated the trained counselors identified alcohol or drug-related problems at a significantly higher rate (60.8%) than untrained counselors (6.1%) (Dalhauser, Dickman, Emener & Lewis, 1984). Even when aware of substance abuse as a problem, rehabilitation counselors are often reluctant to discuss it with their clients, feeling it is too personal or sensitive.

When counselors ignore this problem, they are participating in what Greer (1986) referred to as "enabling" behavior. The counselor's avoidance of the client's substance abuse reinforces the behavior. This avoidance behavior by many rehabilitation counselors contrasts with findings reported by Dickman and Phillips (1983), which suggested substance abuse is one of the most treatable disabilities. While substance abuse is often fatal when left untreated, successful diagnosis and treatment can result in complete recovery. To be successful in substance abuse counseling, the attitudes of rehabilitation counselors must reflect this reality.

**Relapse.** Traditional vocational rehabilitation has emphasized the one-stop approach. It was expected that diagnosis, treatment, evaluation, training, and placement would result in successful case closure. Failure at any point in the process often led to termination of the counseling relationship. Nelson (1986) suggested that substance abuse is often characterized by taking two steps backward for every three steps forward. The process of recovery is a lifelong effort in which a continuing support system is crucial to success (Dickman & Phillips, 1983).

The rehabilitation counselor can be an important part of this support system. Yet, to function effectively in this role, the counselor must realize clients will relapse, assist them to recover again, and proceed from there. A return to substance abuse behavior does not necessarily mean a client is not motivated for vocational rehabilitation. It may be a sign that the individual is making progress toward the goal of being able to deal successfully with substance abuse. Hunter and Salomone (1987) suggested there were even symptoms of behavior change (e.g., "dry drunks") that signal when a relapse is about to occur. They suggested substance abusers are at greatest risk of relapse in the first 3 months of recovery, "with a 50% to 75% rate of relapse within a 6 to 18 month follow-up period" (p. 23). Rehabilitation counselors, if they are aware of and sensitive to the symptoms that signal imminent relapse, can help recovering substance abusers by preventing the relapse or dealing constructively with the event.

## Workers' Compensation

A final comment on the importance of attitudes in successful substance abuse counseling relates to substance abuse as a legitimate concern in workers' compensation rehabilitation systems. There is a prevailing attitude in the insurance industry within this system that substance abuse should be ignored if it is not the disability that resulted directly from the industrial injury. Substance abuse, which often predates the industrial injury, is not considered the responsibility of the employer's insurance company. Consequently, insurance companies do not want to hear about the problem, especially in view of their fear of stress as related to employment issues that are difficult to define and deal with from their perspective.

Many rehabilitation counselors are faced with the dilemma of ignoring a problem that, though it may be secondary to the industrial accident, has the potential of becoming a greater barrier to employment. As a result, the counselor either does not deal with the substance abuse problem or helps the client deal with it informally, while not reporting it to the insurance company. In either case, the underlying message is "don't be sensitive to substance abuse." This negative attitude is counterproductive to substance abuse counseling and successful rehabilitation. Substance abuse awareness and treatment as an integral part of the rehabilitation plan must become a legitimate part of the workers' compensation rehabilitation system if counselors are to assist these clients to achieve successful vocational rehabilitation (Stude, 1990).

Besides constructive attitudes of service providers, there are several other vocational implications that must be considered by the rehabilitation counselor. Low self-esteem, lack of confidence, and fear of socialization outside a therapeutic community may result in feelings of discomfort in a training or work setting. Recovering substance abusers may be attempting to establish relationships with family members by focusing on caring for others rather than themselves. Concern that the job will meet financial needs may result from this rediscovered responsibility to others. Support groups and focusing on the development of problem-solving skills will be needed to help reach the goal of successful vocational rehabilitation (Zavolta & Rogoff, 1990).

Clients who are recovering from drug abuse may exhibit problems in motivation. The road to recovery is a difficult one. In the past, they may have relied on manipulation and exhibited immature behavior in dealing with problems. The rehabilitation counselor can help clients recognize this behavior as inappropriate and assist them in learning acceptable behavior. The problem of motivation may be further complicated by a past that included making somewhat large sums of money either legally or illegally to support a drug habit. Entry-level wages may not seem appealing. The counselor will need to stress the opportunity that will be afforded clients to increase income with continued drug abstinence and increased job experience.

These clients may have lost work personality characteristics such as good grooming, personal hygiene, appropriate relationships with co-workers and supervisors, the ability to delay need gratification, acceptance of criticism, and dealing effectively with frustration. The counselor must exercise patience, yet be willing to interact with clients in assisting them to relearn ways of interacting with others that will be appropriate at work.

Whether to volunteer information about one's drug abuse history in a work setting may become a problem for the recovering substance abuser. The honest, open, and direct confrontational techniques associated with treatment of substance abuse can be overpowering in the workplace. Whether to disclose previous drug abuse behavior will need to be evaluated by the counselor and client with careful consideration given to avoiding evasiveness, defensiveness, and falsifying information (Knowles, 1981).

Finally, it is important to remember that each person's drug abuse history is unique. Individual treatment with follow-up after the client has obtained employment will give the recovering person the greatest opportunity to reach full potential as an independent and responsible individual in society.

# CASE STUDY

Mr. Robert Johnson is a 35 year old, divorced male who is responsible for the child support of three children under the ages of 15, who live with his former wife. Upon graduation from high school, Mr. Johnson began driving delivery trucks, and for the past 15 years, has driven cross-country for various trucking firms hauling different types of freight. The **Dictionary of Occupational Titles** (1977) and **Selected Characteristics of Occupations Defined in the Dictionary of Occupational Titles** (1981) classifies the job of Truck Driver, Heavy (any industry), **D.O.T. #** 905.663-014, as medium exertion, semiskilled work.

Mr. Johnson first started using and abusing substances while he was a senior in high school, smoking marijuana and drinking alcohol. His drug use did not interfere with his vocational or social life until he began using cocaine when he was 25 years of age. Within two years, he lost his job, his marriage ended in divorce, and he was subsequently arrested and convicted for burglary. Robert served three years in prison as a result of trying to support a $300 per day cocaine habit. After he was released from prison, he was treated in an outpatient program for a period of six months. He subsequently returned to truck driving, which eventually led to him resuming the use of cocaine. Robert has just completed a year in a residential treatment program and has been referred by the director of the program for vocational rehabilitation, with a strong suggestion that he not return to truck driving.

## *Questions*

1.  Assign this individual a vocational profile, including age category, educational level, work history (including skill and exertional level), occupationally significant characteristics, and work skills (if any) obtained from work experience.

2.  What is Mr. Johnson's prognosis for continued substance abuse?

3.  What is the prognosis for him returning to work?

4.  What kind of support system would be most helpful for Robert in achieving a vocational objective?

5.  Should his family be involved in his vocational rehabilitation and, if so, in what manner?

6.  Why did the program director recommend Mr. Johnson not return to truck driving?

7.  Given his work history and disability, what type of work might be more suitable and why?

8.  How would you explain Robert's disability to a prospective employer?

# REFERENCES

Allen, H.A., Peterson, J.S., & Keating, G. (1982). Attitudes of counselors toward the alcoholic. **Rehabilitation Counseling Bulletin, 25**(3), 162-164.

Arif, A., & Westermeyer, J. (Eds.). (1988). **Manual of drug and alcohol abuse: Guidelines for teaching in medical and health institutions**. New York: Plenum Medical Books.

Baker, T.B., & Cannon, D.S. (1988). **Assessment and treatment of addictive disorders**. New York: Praeger.

Backer, T.E. (1988). The future of rehabilitation in the workplace: Drug abuse, aids, and disability management. **Journal of Applied Rehabilitation Counseling, 19**(2), 38-41.

Beale, A.V. (1988). A replicable program for teaching job interview skills to recovering substance abusers. **Journal of Applied Rehabilitation Counseling, 19**(1), 47-49.

Benshoff, J.J., & Riggar, T.F. (1990). Cocaine: A primer for rehabilitation counselors. **Journal of Applied Rehabilitation Counseling, 21**(3), 21-24.

Bokos, P.J., Lipscomb, S.T., & Schwartzman, J. (1984). Macrosystemic approaches to drug treatment. **The Personnel and Guidance Journal, 62**(10), 583-584.

Buxbaum, J. (1988). Helping the disabled alcohol-dependent client: A training program for rehabilitation counselors. **Rehabilitation Education, 2**(2), 113-119.

Clifford J.S. (1986). Neuropsychology: Implications for the treatment of alcoholism. **Journal of Counseling and Development, 65**(1), 31-34.

Dahlhauser, H.P., Dickman, F., Emener, W.G., & Lewis, B.Y. (1984). Alcohol and drug abuse awareness: Implications for intake interviewing. **Journal of Applied Rehabilitation Counseling, 15**(4), 31-34.

Dickman, F., & Phillips, E.A. (1983). Alcoholism: A pervasive rehabilitation counseling issue. **Journal of Applied Rehabilitation Counseling, 14**(3), 40-45.

Dudek, F.A. (1984). Rehabilitation counseling with alcoholics. **Journal of Applied Rehabilitation Counseling, 15**(2), 16-21.

Greer, B.G. (1986). Substance abuse among people with disabilities: A problem of too much accessibility. **Journal of Rehabilitation, 52**(1), 34-38.

Greer, B.G., Roberts, R., May, G., & Jenkins, W.M. (1988). Identification of substance abuse in a vocational evaluation setting. **Journal of Rehabilitation, 54**(3), 42-45.

Hall, S.M., Sorensen, J.L., & Loeb, P.C. (1988). Development and diffusion of a skills training intervention. In T.B. Baker & D.S. Cannon (Eds.), **Assessment and treatment of addictive disorders**, (pp. 180-204). New York: Praeger.

Hubbard, R.L., Marsden, M.E., Rachal, J., Harwood, H.J., Cavanaugh, E.R., & Ginzburg, H.M. (1989). **Drug abuse treatment: A national study of effectiveness**. Chapel Hill, NC: University of North Carolina.

Hunter, T.A., & Salomone, P.R. (1987). Dry drunk symptoms and alcoholic relapse. **Journal of Applied Rehabilitation Counseling, 18**(1), 22-25.

Keller, M.J., & Green, M.A. (1981). Multiple prescription drug use among rehabilitation clients referred for psychological evaluation. **Rehabilitation Counseling Bulletin, 25**(1), 26-29.

Knowles, R.R. (1981). Drug abuse. In W.C. Stolov & M.R. Clowers (Eds.), **Handbook of severe disability: A text for rehabilitation counselors, other vocational practitioners, and allied health professionals** (pp. 241-252). Washington, DC: U.S. Department of Education, Rehabilitation Service Administration.

Lett, P. (1988). Dual diagnosis: Psychiatric disorder and substance abuse. **Journal of Applied Rehabilitation Counseling, 19**(2), 16-20.

Nelson, S.J. (1986). Alcohol and other drugs: Facing reality and cynicism. **Journal of Counseling and Development, 66**(1), 4-5.

Newton, R.M., Elliott, T.A., & Meyer, A.A. (1988). The roll of structured work in alcoholism rehabilitation. **Journal of Rehabilitation, 54**(4), 63-67.

Stude, E.W. (1990). Professionalization of substance abuse counseling. **Journal of Applied Rehabilitation Counseling,** 21(3), 11-15.

Taricone, P.F., Bordieri, J.E., & Scalia, V.A. (1989). Assessing rehabilitation needs of clients in treatment for alcohol abuse. **Rehabilitation Counseling Bulletin, 32**(4), 324-332.

U.S. Department of Labor (1977). **Dictionary of occupational titles** (4th ed.). Washington, DC: Author.

U.S. Department of Labor (1981). **Selected characteristics of occupations defined in the dictionary of occupational titles.** Washington, DC: Author.

Valle, S.K. (1979). **Alcoholism counseling.** Springfield, IL: Charles C Thomas.

Westermeyer, J. (1986). **A clinical guide to alcohol and drug problems.**New York: Praeger.

Wright, G.N. (1980). **Total rehabilitation.** Boston, MA: Little, Brown.

Zavolta, H., & Rogoff, S. (1990). An overview of the vocational rehabilitation process in a long-term drug rehabilitation program. **Journal of Applied Rehabilitation Counseling, 21**(3), 40-44.

## *About the Author*

E.W. (Bud) Stude, Ed.D., C.R.C., N.C.C., is Professor and Coordinator, Master of Science Degree Program in Rehabilitation Counseling, California State University, Fresno, California. He is President of the National Council on Rehabilitation Education (NCRE) and has taught medical aspects of disability classes for the past 20 years.

# Chapter 5

# ALCOHOLISM

by
*Eugene H. Rogolsky, M.D.*
*and*
*Jack Little, Ph.D.*

## INTRODUCTION

Reports of the drinking of alcoholic beverages and the aberrant behavior associated with intoxication can be found in some of the earliest written accounts of human behavior. Consumption of alcohol is an integral part of the history of the world. The ingenuity demonstrated in the brewing, distilling, and fermenting of various fruits, vegetables, and grains to produce intoxicants is amazing. Virtually every civilized and many primitive societies have produced some form of intoxicant, with the majority of them containing alcohol. The use of alcohol, at all levels of society, was especially common in Europe. The New World saw no change in drinking customs. The colonists produced and consumed large quantities of spirits. There were almost no restrictions on either production or use of alcoholic beverages; taverns and public houses were a part of every community.

The consumption of alcohol has been commonplace for centuries, however, drunkenness or alcohol abuse, seldom has been tolerated. Drunkenness has been viewed historically as a matter of personal weakness or sin. It was assumed that one who was frequently or chronically inebriated was lacking in will, or was displaying a lack of morals. The consumption of alcohol has been discouraged or prohibited by some societies on either religious or moral grounds, while being institutionalized in others. It is only recently, since the 1950s, that alcoholism has been accepted as a disease. Prior to acceptance of the disease model, medical treatment was often unavailable. Treatment was frequently limited to the physical complications associated with the advanced condition.

### Definitions

**Alcoholism** is defined by the National Council on Alcoholism and the American Medical Society on Alcoholism as "a chronic, progressive and potentially fatal disease characterized by: tolerance, physical dependency, and/or pathological organ changes, all of which are the direct or indirect consequences of the alcohol ingested."

The American Psychiatric Association (**DSM-III-R**, 1987) defines **alcohol abuse** as synonymous with alcoholism. Contained within this definition are three elements:

1.  pathological use of alcohol, including need for daily use to maintain adequate functioning;

2.  alcohol-induced impairment of social or occupational functioning; and

3.  duration of a least one month.

**Alcohol dependence** includes the above, as well as:

1.  tolerance - defined in terms of the need for increased amounts of alcohol to achieve the same effects, or that the effect is decreased with the same amount of alcohol.

2.  withdrawal - defined as a physical reaction ("shakes" or malaise) with reduction or cessation of drinking.

The term "alcoholic" often refers to anyone who frequently, or periodically, abuses alcohol without regard for physical dependency or organ pathology. Alcoholics Anonymous (AA), (Alcoholics Anonymous World Services, 1952, 1976), a world wide self-help organization of and for alcoholics, identifies an alcoholic as one who has lost control of his life due to the use of alcohol and is powerless over alcohol. There is considerable confusion surrounding **alcoholism** and the **alcoholic**. Much of this is due to the lack of a clear distinction between the abusive use of alcohol and alcohol addiction. Light to moderate use of alcohol, in social settings, is generally acceptable. Where moderate to heavy drinking ends and **alcoholism** begins, is frequently blurred. The diagnosis of **alcoholism** usually does not occur until the disease is well advanced.

# CAUSES OF ALCOHOLISM

## *Biological Factors*

Attempts to determine the etiology of alcoholism are surrounded by controversy. The body of research evidence that some individuals may be more genetically vulnerable to alcoholism than others is growing. Familial alcoholism, that is, individuals with a close relative who is alcoholic, may account for nearly half of the cases. Researchers are attempting to identify differences in metabolic function, blood chemistry, and brain functions among alcoholics, children of alcoholics, and others. Evidence is being compiled which indicates a possible genetic link between alcoholism and antisocial personalities (sociopaths).

At the present time, physiological susceptibility, as it relates to alcoholism, is generally accepted. Alcohol consumption affects individuals differently. There are significant differences among individuals both in tolerance for alcohol and susceptibility to the development of the clinical symptoms of alcoholism. Whether such differences are due to genetics, brain defects, metabolic disorders, blood chemistry, or other factor(s) has not been determined (National Institute of Drug Abuse, 1986).

## *Personality*

Personality factors which are most predictive of the development of alcoholism in preadolescents include rebelliousness, high levels of sensation seeking, nonconformity, high tolerance for deviance, resistance to authority, a strong need for independence, low self-esteem, and feelings of lack of control (Jessor & Jessor 1977; Kandel, 1978). Hawkins, Lishner, Catalano, and Howard (1985) reported that children who use alcohol or other drugs prior to adolescence are more likely to demonstrate antisocial behaviors as compared to those who begin to use alcohol or drugs later in life. Those preadolescents who are most likely to use alcohol or other drugs are frequently those who demonstrate psychological maladjustment or emotional distress. Early use of alcohol is predictive of later alcoholism.

## Social Competence

Individuals who are at risk for the development of alcoholism are often, or believe themselves to be, socially, economically, or culturally disadvantaged. This is especially noted in adolescents who are alcoholic. It is typical for adolescent alcoholics to report feeling inadequate.

Adolescents and preadolescents who are alcoholic have frequently been abused or neglected and are often school drop-outs. They are frequently children of alcoholic parents or abusers of other drugs, lack supervision and adequate role models, or experience a combination of these factors. Many are culturally deprived in that they lack the opportunity to either develop adequate social skills or are unable to select the appropriate social strategy for a specific social situation. Consequently, they become anxious or depressed and frequently seek to control their anxiety or depression by drinking. Coping with uncomfortable situations by drinking may gradually increase tolerance for alcohol and symptoms of withdrawal may begin. In an attempt to decrease the symptoms of withdrawal, these individuals drink more; they also do so in order to try to function more adequately. The result may be dependence on alcohol (Hawkins, Lishner, & Catalano, 1985).

## Cultural Values

The community norm as it relates to the use or nonuse of alcohol may have decided effect upon an individual. In some subcultures, the regular use of alcohol is the norm and to be a nondrinker is viewed as deviant. Drinking patterns of parents and others within the community may influence the drinking behaviors of children when they become adults. Peer pressure and cultural values may contribute to the development of alcoholism in some individuals, however, many who are subjected to such pressure, and drink, never become alcoholics.

## Life Situations

Alcoholism is observed in all ethnic and cultural groups which use alcohol. Some groups drink more and at a younger age. Malone (1986) reported that regular drinking before the teen years is common among Hispanics. The death rate from cirrhosis among Mexican-Americans is three times that of the general United States population (Heien & Pompelli, 1987).

The death rate of African-Americans from cirrhosis of the liver is twice that of Whites. However, one must realize that within the Hispanic, African-American, and other subcultures, alcohol use is interwoven with the conditions under which so many live. That is, alcohol use is a part of the mix of poverty, inadequate housing, limited access to medical care, crime and delinquency, lack of employment, economic factors, limited educational opportunities, and other factors associated with discrimination. It must be noted that alcohol abuse is not limited to any ethnic, socioeconomic class, or culture. However, the more the number of risk factors present, the higher the probability of alcohol or drug abuse.

# CONSEQUENCES OF ALCOHOLISM

A detailed discussion of the consequences of alcoholism is beyond the scope of this chapter, however, the following statistics provide the basis for insight into the immensity of the problems related to alcohol abuse:

The National Institute on Alcohol Abuse and Alcoholism (NIAAA) 5th Special Report to Congress (1987) reported that up to 50% of spousal abuse cases involve alcohol use. The NIAA

**6th Special Report to Congress** (1988) reported additional alcohol related crimes: murder (49%), manslaughter (68%), suicide (20-30%), rape (52%), and child abuse which results in death (38%). The National Association for Children of Alcoholics estimates that one out of every eight adult individuals is a child of an adult alcoholic.

The National Institute of Alcohol Abuse and Alcoholism (1988), of the University of Michigan's Institute for Social Research, indicates that one in 23 high school seniors drink alcohol daily.

The **Weekly Reader National Survey on Drugs and Drinking** (Spring, 1987) reports that 51% of 6th graders experience peer pressure to drink beer, wine, or hard liquor.

The National Highway Traffic Safety Administration (1988), Fatal Accident Reporting System, revealed that in 1986, alcohol-impaired driving was the leading cause of death of young people. Alcohol-related highway accidents killed nearly 9,000 adolescents and young adults.

In a Gallup Poll, (U.S. Department of Health and Human Services, 1987), it was reported that nearly 25% of American homes have been affected by family problems related to alcohol consumption.

# THE SYMPTOMATOLOGY OF ALCOHOLISM

## Symptoms

The symptoms of alcoholism vary greatly from individual to individual. Both physical and psychological deterioration are difficult, if not impossible, to predict. Some individuals develop tolerance for alcohol at a slower rate than others. Individuals with cross-addiction (addiction to more than one substance) tend to develop alcoholism more rapidly. This is assumed to be the result of increased tolerance for alcohol resulting from increased tolerance for sedatives or narcotic drugs. Regardless of the time required to become alcoholic, alcoholism is a progressive disease.

Alcohol addiction may result in physical disabilities, even at the early stages of the disease. Motor dysfunctions, memory loss, tremors, impaired judgment, and gastritis and organ damage are often the result of alcohol abuse. Impairment in judgment, motor function, and memory (blackouts) are often obvious while the individual is engaged in a drinking bout. However, tremors, anxiety, autonomic hyperactivity, orthostatic hypotension (abnormally low blood pressure occurring when the person stands), depressed mood or irritability, gastritis, and malaise are frequently observed after cessation of, or reduction in, drinking.

Delirium may occur within one week after the reduction or cessation of heavy alcohol consumption. Individuals who are dependent on alcohol may exhibit organic hallucinosis with auditory hallucinations. Convulsions, seizures, and alcohol amnestic disorder (loss of short and/or long term memory) and, in some cases, dementia result in mild cognitive impairment in the ability to function independently.

A detailing of the physical and psychological complications associated with alcoholism may be found in the many volumes written on the subject. The diagnosis requires detailed observation as well as medical and psychological evaluation. Most of the medical complications develop in the later stages of alcoholism, and are usually reversible with abstinence and appropriate treatment. The psychological problems related to alcohol abuse may be more difficult to treat.

# DIAGNOSIS AND ASSESSMENT

## *Diagnosis*

Diagnosis of alcoholism may be either very complex or relatively simple depending upon the motivation of the individual. Alcoholism can result in symptoms which are similar to many diseases. There is no specific pattern in which the individual is affected organically. One individual may drink a relatively small amount for a short period of time and demonstrate greater organ damage than an individual who has been drinking large amounts of alcohol for a prolonged period. Many factors, such as nutrition and general health, may be related to the onset and degree of organic damage.

Alcoholism is present in every ethnic, socioeconomic, cultural, and racial group. Diagnosis must be made individually, based upon the assessment of the history of alcohol consumption, employment, and social functioning, as well as physical and psychological status. It must be accomplished with the realization that some individuals experience alcohol idiosyncratic intoxication, in which they react with marked behavior changes with only small amounts of alcohol. A history of drunkenness must be carefully evaluated. Tolerance, cross tolerance, and psychological reactions to alcohol vary greatly.

## *The Purpose of Assessment*

Alcoholism is debilitating on a personal, social, and occupational basis. Many individuals function adequately for extended periods of time while drinking. However, as tolerance increases, withdrawal symptoms also tend to increase. The alcoholic frequently finds that a desire to decrease the effects of withdrawal results in a craving for more alcohol. Unless the person ceases to drink, the effects become greater with additional physical and psychological damage.

Assessment of alcoholism is designed for evaluation of the severity of the problems associated with the alcoholism, and for development of a treatment program to assist the individual to abstain from the use of alcohol. Recovery and rehabilitation may require an extended period of time. Recidivism (a return to drinking) is very common among alcoholics and the evaluation of prior drinking behavior, including those times of abstinence, if any, must be evaluated. The assessment includes evaluation of recidivistic behaviors as to cause and patterns. Assessment should include:

1.  **Detoxification needs.** Symptoms of withdrawal are observed within a few hours after the individual ceases a period of heavy drinking. The withdrawal symptoms may be mild or so severe as to be fatal. Detoxification generally requires from 3-7 days, however, some individuals may require long term detoxification which may involve from 3-9 months.

2.  **Review or development of medical history.** Many alcoholics have histories of heavy alcohol consumption and multiple diagnoses resulting from physical problems, such as loss of appetite, accidents, excessive sweating, sexual impotence, or gastrointestinal problems. As the disease progresses, pathological changes in the brain, liver, stomach, pancreas, peripheral nerves, and heart may be noted.

3.  **Medical evaluation.** The majority of the serious medical problems, including organ change, usually develop in the later stages of alcoholism. An evaluation of current physical status will reveal the existence of possible physical alcohol-related complications and expedite medical intervention and recovery.

4.  **Psychological evaluation.** Psychosocial issues surrounding the use and abuse of alcohol are extremely varied and complex. Severe psychopathology can result from prolonged alcohol abuse. A complete psychological evaluation, including a neuropsychological examination, may be helpful in the determination of the course of treatment required. The psychological manifestations of the alcohol abuser may be highly

suggestive of underlying psychiatric disorders. It may be impossible to accurately evaluate the psychiatric condition of the addict until alcohol-induced brain dysfunction has been reduced or reversed. In addition to the evaluation of the psychological status of the individual, it is critical to assess the motivation of the alcoholic to attempt behavior change. Such change must be planned to lead to abstinence; the level of willingness to accept help through the initiation and execution of a treatment program is crucial to success.

5. **Development of a treatment plan.** The individual treatment plan is based upon the assessment of findings, taking into consideration both the deficits and the strengths of the individual. Medical, psychological, and psychosocial factors are considered.

## Assessment for Rehabilitation Services

The rehabilitation counselor can be the key to recovery and maintenance of sobriety after initial treatment. Job loss or threat of job loss and the disruption of personal relationships are, perhaps, the most frequent impetus for individuals to seek treatment for alcoholism. It is for this reason that some states have established the diagnosis of alcoholism from a functional basis. That is, when an individual's job, home, or marriage are jeopardized, or if the person is incarcerated because of alcohol ingestion, that person is diagnosed as an alcoholic. The rehabilitation counselor can serve as a conduit by which appropriate treatment can be accessed while, at the same time, providing the counseling support which is often critical to recovery.

**Focus of assessment.** The focus of the rehabilitation counselor must be on the assessment of abilities and skills related to securing or maintaining employment. During the process of assessment and evaluation for rehabilitation, the counselor may serve as an information and referral source for medical or psychological evaluation and treatment. In some instances, the client may have been referred by the physician, psychologist, or other interested party. The medical and psychological evaluations may have been accomplished and detoxification either completed or in progress. The counselor's responsibility is to assess and evaluate the client's vocational, social, educational, psychological, and medical status in relationship to employment, and the development of a plan to assist with the establishment or reestablishment of attitudes and performance skills appropriate to meaningful employment.

**Rehabilitation program assessment.** Assessment for the purpose of developing a rehabilitation program should include, but not be limited to, the following:

1. Current medical status
   a. Has detoxification been accomplished or is it in progress?
   b. Has a satisfactory nutritional status been reestablished?
   c. Are any physical or medical complications present? If so, what are they and how are they limiting?

2. Psychological status
   a. Has a psychological evaluation been completed?
   b. Do any psychological or psychiatric problems which would interfere with employment exist?
   c. Are there any indicators of cognitive dysfunction or mental illness or instability?

3. Length of sobriety
   a. How long has the client been sober?
   b. Are maintenance and support structures in place?

4. Reality orientation
   a. Are the client's perceptions of abilities realistic?
   b. Are the client's expectations realistic?
   c. Does the client view recovery in realistic terms?

5. Employment history
   a. Does the client have a negative employment history?
   b. Is the client currently employed? If so, for how long?
   c. If employed, are the job requirements consistent with the client's training?

6. Vocational planning
   a. Can the client manage the responsibility and stress of employment? If so, what types and how much can be managed?
   b. What work skills or training does the client have?
   c. Does the client demonstrate any functional employment limitations? If so, what is the nature of the limitation(s)?
   d. Are the client's employment objectives consistent with abilities?
   e. Does the client have marketable employment skills?
   f. Does the client require vocational training or retraining?
   g. Has the client committed to a program designed for maintenance of abstinence from alcohol?

   **Assessment and recovery.** There is a tendency for individuals recovering from alcoholism to be impatient and to misperceive their tolerance for stress. Stress tolerance usually increases over time, however, low tolerance for stress is not uncommon for the first several years of recovery. Support and crisis counseling is particularly important during this period. In most cases, recovery is only achieved over an extended period of time. Assessment should be ongoing. As the individual is sober for a longer time, changes will occur which may make significant differences in interest and ability to perform certain tasks. With increased abstinence, it may be in the best interest of the client to periodically review employment and vocational objectives with consideration being given to the establishment of new vocational goals. Ongoing assessment will enable the counselor to provide support and a positive influence during the entire rehabilitation process.

# TREATMENT

## Program Goals

   Treatment programs for alcoholics vary greatly based upon multidisciplinary assessment and evaluation of need. The goal of the treatment program is to enable the alcoholic to regain functional skills in all areas of life. This may be relatively simple or complex depending upon the disease stage at which the program is initiated, the degree of physical damage, psychological problems, and complications, both social and vocational. Treatment is ongoing. Most treatment programs are designed to produce changes in social interactions, work habits, and behavioral patterns and increase stress tolerance based upon experiences gained through adherence to a program plan.

## Stages of Treatment

   The treatment progresses through a series of stages:

1. Detoxification -
   > Acute - 3-7 days for mild withdrawal symptoms
   > Chronic - 3-9 months with medical supervision

2. Assessment and Evaluation -
   Determination of physical, mental, and emotional status and needs

3. Mode of Treatment -
   Inpatient
   Outpatient
   Self-help

4. Manipulation of Environmental Variables -
   Life crisis resolution
   Financial status
   Vocational planning
   Family structure

5. Type of Treatment -
   Management of organic pathology
   Medical intervention (e.g., Antabuse)
   Individual counseling
   Group therapy
   Self-help

6. Family or Significant Other Treatment -
   Family counseling
   Individual counseling
   Group therapy
   Self-help

## Family Involvement

Alcoholism is a family disease. All members of a family in which there is an alcoholic member are affected by the alcoholism. Adult children of alcoholics often experience feelings of guilt, shame, and isolation, even after they have left the home. Many who experience an alcoholic parent require support and counseling to resolve negative feelings. The organization, "Adult Children of Alcoholics" (a self-help organization), is designed to provide support through the recovery process.

## The Role of the Rehabilitation Counselor

By becoming the case manager providing the interface among the resources which are available to the client, the rehabilitation counselor often plays a crucial role in the treatment of the recovering alcoholic. The rehabilitation counselor facilitates, but seldom assumes the primary role in the rehabilitation process. A multidisciplinary treatment team consists of representatives from all areas providing services. This team assists with the initial recovery program with the physician, psychologist, or social worker who frequently may assume the lead role. After the initial stages of medical and psychological treatment, the rehabilitation counselor usually assumes lead responsibility. Help in establishing life-long preventive maintenance goals is also provided by the counselor. It is the rehabilitation counselor who provides support and assists the recovering alcoholic to become self-monitoring during vocational training and in the early stages of employment.

# FUNCTIONAL LIMITATIONS

Practicing alcoholics characteristically demonstrate progressive loss of job skills and the inability to develop new abilities. Alcoholics typically demonstrate higher rates of absenteeism, tardiness, accidents, and lower production rates than do non-alcoholics. They frequently show high levels of dependency; alcoholics often find it difficult to act effectively on their own behalf. This dependency may last well into recovery. They may seek to get others, either through manipulation or by direct request, to do things for them which they capable of doing for themselves.

Dependency may be the result of an unwillingness or inability to assume responsibility for decision-making. Additionally, the alcoholic may experience feelings of anxiety associated with decision-making or performing specific tasks due to a history of poor decision-making or failure while drinking. The rejection and isolation experienced by the practicing alcoholic often results in a lack of trust and social contacts, and an inability to establish or maintain a relationship with another person. During the process of recovery, it takes time to reestablish social contacts, trust, and enter into relationships.

The functional limitations of the recovering alcoholic depend upon both the physical and psychosocial status at the time these limitations are evaluated. The vast majority of alcoholics show marked improvement or complete recovery with abstinence, treatment, and sufficient time.

The functional limitations of the recovering alcoholic are usually more directly associated with psychosocial factors than physical factors. Impatience, inaccurate self-appraisal, unrealistic expectations, and an inability to handle work-related or personal stress are frequently more limiting than either physical or cognitive disabilities resulting from alcohol addiction.

# REHABILITATION POTENTIAL

The potential for rehabilitation is not easily assessed. The degree to which the alcoholism has advanced and effectiveness of treatment are factors for consideration in attempting to appraise rehabilitation potential. If the individual consistently relapses after attempts at detoxification, the potential is less than for one who has experienced minor physical damage and has gone through successful detoxification. While it is not common, some individuals with long histories of very heavy drinking develop brain damage to the extent that there is permanent dementia ("wet brain") and require custodial care. However, most of the complications associated with alcoholism are reversible.

Alcoholics Anonymous (AA) (Alcoholics Anonymous World Services, 1952, 1976) has established a 12-step program of recovery. This program advocates total abstinence and regular participation in a self-help support group. AA is an international organization which has provided a program plan of recovery for millions of alcoholics throughout the world. Ancillary to AA are various other self-help "anonymous" programs with specific target populations (Narcotics Anonymous, Overeaters Anonymous, among others). There are also support groups for family members and significant others (Alanon and Alateen). These support groups assist in the alcoholic's recovery program by breaking up behaviors which may contribute to the alcoholic's dependency or co-dependency. While membership in AA offers no assurance of abstinence or recovery, AA has been the recovery platform, or mainstay, for countless alcoholics and is very successful for many people.

AA is a source of support for many, but it is not effective for all. Physical, psychological, and other factor make participation in the AA program impossible for some and different approaches are needed. In some instances, medical intervention is required; in others, psychiatric treatment must be provided prior to the individual becoming capable of participation in a self-help group.

The best indicators of rehabilitation potential are the following:

1. The individual must admit to having a problem associated with alcohol consumption.

2. There must be a willingness to seek and accept help through participation in the development and execution of a treatment plan.

3. There must be a willingness to assume responsibility for one's behaviors.

4. An individual must be an active participant in an ongoing therapeutic prevention program with a willingness for lifetime participation.

5. If cross-addicted (addicted to more than one substance, i.e., cocaine, heroin, among others), there must be a willingness to abstain from use of other intoxicants, as well as alcohol.

The evaluation of rehabilitation potential must consider that most alcoholics have long histories of manipulative behavior, as well as alcohol use. Alcoholics in the advanced stages of alcoholism will do almost anything to obtain alcohol and reduce the cravings for alcohol resulting from the effects of withdrawal. It is all too frequent that the alcoholic will continue to engage in "alcoholic thinking" well into recovery. With this kind of thought process, the individual continues to set unrealistic goals and expectations and will expect these goals to be accomplished within impossible time frames. Old patterns of behavior take time to change; the counselor needs to work patiently with the client to support the long and often slow path to recovery.

Many alcoholics have "slips." That is, they revert back to drinking. Some drink as the result of thinking they are "cured," while others simply fall back into old patterns of coping behavior when confronted with change, difficult situations, or emotional stress. Constant reassessment of the treatment program will reduce the probability of such "slips." The counselor must be aware that no one can stop the alcoholic from drinking or force an individual to stay sober. Maintaining sobriety rests with the alcoholic. The counselor, a strong support system involving significant others, and willing participation in a treatment program are the best predictors of continued abstinence from alcohol.

# CASE STUDY

Sally, a 32 year-old woman, is currently undergoing detoxification at a local alcohol treatment center. Two previous attempts to become sober and maintain long-term sobriety have failed. She is married, although separated, and has two children, 3 and 6 years of age. The present attempt at sobriety was prompted by the departure of the husband due to her continued drinking. The children are living with her mother in a nearby city.

There is a history of alcoholism in Sally's family. Her father was a diagnosed alcoholic and died at the age of 47, the result of physical complications resulting from alcoholism. The mother's present husband was previously married to an alcoholic. Sally states that she feels that her parents are not sympathetic or supportive of her sobriety. Her parents indicate that they are willing to provide care for the children, but that Sally is not welcome in their home when she is drinking.

Drinking did not become a problem for Sally until she became an adult, although she began drinking at about 12 years of age. She drank secretly from her father's stock of alcohol and enjoyed the feelings she experienced. Drinking progressed in high school, but never resulted in much trouble. However, once she was expelled from a school dance due to drinking. Serious trouble from alcohol consumption began during her freshman year at college. There were frequent problems in classes due to absences. Sally had to move from her apartment on three occasions because her roommates refused to put up with her drinking. College life became impossible for her and she dropped out after the second term.

At the age of 20, Sally secured employment with a ticket agency. At this job, she met a band musician and was married within 3 weeks. Her drinking and socially unacceptable behavior resulted in a divorce about 6 months later. She enrolled in an alcohol treatment program at the time of the divorce, but left the program after 5 days. Continuing to drink, she was eventually fired from her job. Sally's parents allowed her to return home to live under the condition that she seek help for her drinking problem. She attended several meetings at a women's center and enrolled in an outpatient treatment program at a local hospital. She continued participation in the outpatient program for 3 months, but stopped when she married her current husband, who was a produce manager at a local supermarket.

Sally controlled her drinking for the next 8 years and gave birth to two children. She worked part-time at a local printing shop and did general office work. Drinking became a problem again when she was 30 years old. While at home, she would secretly drink. It soon became obvious to all around her that she was drinking. On several occasions, she would leave the children unattended and stay out all night. She lost her job and the week after her 31st birthday, her husband left after she had destroyed much of the furniture at home in a drunken rage. The mother was called and took her and the children home, and again required that Sally enter some type of treatment program.

Alcoholics Anonymous (AA) became Sally's support system; she attended meetings regularly, but continued to drink. Her mother and stepfather finally told her that she could no longer reside with them, but that they would continue to care for the children until she was capable of caring for them. Sally was angry, frustrated, and hurt. She enrolled at a county detoxification center and is currently seeking help from a counselor.

## *Questions*

1. Identify any factors which might have contributed to Sally becoming an alcoholic.

2. What are the positive factors in this case for rehabilitation?

3. As Sally's counselor, identify the first three measures you would recommend.

4. In your intervention, how would you involve Sally's significant others?

5. What types of intervention would you suggest for this individual?

# REFERENCES

Alcoholics Anonymous World Services (1952). **Twelve steps and twelve traditions.** New York: World Services.

Alcoholics Anonymous World Services (1976). **Alcoholics anonymous** (3rd ed.). New York: World Services.

American Psychiatric Association (1987). **Diagnostic and statistical manual of mental disorders** (3rd ed., revised). Washington, DC: Author.

Hawkins, J. D., Lishner, D.M., & Catalano, R.F. (1985). Childhood predictors and the prevention of adolescent substance abuse. In C.L. Jones & R. J. Battjes (Eds.), **Etiology of drug abuse: Implications for prevention** (DHHS Publication No. ADM 85-1385). Washington, DC: National Institute on Drug Abuse.

Hawkins, J.D., Lishner, D.M., Catalano, R.F. & Howard, M.O., (1985). Childhood predictors of adolescent substance abuse: Toward an empirically grounded theory. **Journal of Children in Contemporary Society, 18,** 1-2.

Heien, D., & Pompelli, G. (1987). Stress, ethnic and distribution factors in dichotomous response model of alcohol abuse. **Journal of Studies on Alcohol, 48**(5), 450-455.

Jessor R., & Jessor, S.L. (1977). **Problem behavior and psychosocial development: A longitudinal study of youth.** Orlando, FL: Academic Press.

Kandel, D.B. (1978). Convergences in prospective longitudinal surveys of drug use in normal populations. In B.D. Kandel (Ed.), **Longitudinal research on drug use.** Washington, DC: Hemisphere Publishing.

Malone, T.E. (Ed.). (1986). **Report of the secretary's task force on minority health - Volume V: Homicide, suicide, and unintentional injuries** (GPO Publication No. 491-313/44710). Washington, DC: U.S. Government Printing Office.

National Highway Traffic Safety Administration, U.S. Department of Transportation (1988). **Digest of state alcohol-highway safety related legislation** (6th ed.). Washington, DC: U.S. Government Printing Office.

National Institute of Drug Abuse (1986). Inheritance of risk to develop alcoholism. In **Genetic and biological markers in drug abuse and alcoholism** (Monograph 66, DHHS Pub. No. ADM 86-1444). Washington, DC: U.S. Government Printing Office.

National Institute on Alcohol Abuse and Alcoholism (1987). **NIAA fifth special report.** Ann Arbor, MI: University of Michigan.

National Institute on Alcohol Abuse and Alcoholism (1988). **NIAA sixth special report.** Ann Arbor, MI: University of Michigan.

U.S. Department of Health and Human Services (1987). **Sixth special report to the U.S. Congress on alcohol and health** (DHHS Pub. No. ADM 87-1519). Washington, DC: U.S. Government Printing Office.

**Weekly reader national survey on drugs and drinking** (Spring, 1987). Middletown, CT: Field Publications.

## *About the Authors*

Eugene H. Rogolsky, M.D., is Board Certified in Family Practice and is in private group practice in Sherman Oaks, California. Dr. Rogolsky is a Clinical Instructor at the University of Southern California, School of Medicine in Los Angeles, California. He is known for his work on AIDS and HIV infection, which includes numerous professional publications and presentations.

Jack Little, Ph.D., is a Professor of Education, Division of Special Education, California State University, Los Angeles, California. He coordinates the Special Education Teacher Training Program in the areas of learning handicaps and serious emotional disturbance. Dr. Little is also known for his extensive work in the area of AIDS research and case management for persons with HIV infection.

# Chapter 6

# SEXUALITY AND DISABILITY

by
*Gary A. Best, Ph.D.*

## INTRODUCTION

Sexuality and disability are both extremely complex issues. The broad category of sexuality includes not only physical/physiological functioning, but the psychosocial feelings associated with gender identity, self-worth, and social attitudes. Because maleness and femaleness is expressed as "the integration of physical, emotional, intellectual, and social aspects of an individual's personality" (Bogle, cited in Cole, 1988, pp. 277-278), the rehabilitation counselor needs to understand the interrelatedness and interaction of disability and sexuality. The complexity associated with these ideas is compounded by negative societal attitudes, which have had grave impact on the disabled person's self-esteem.

Society, particularly the media, continues to equate sex with youthful, physically active, healthy bodies. According to society's norm, in order to be happy and productive, one must be beautiful and physically active. Persons with disability are impacted by the internalization of these perpetuated false concepts of sexuality. Their self-image and worth are constantly eroded by the inability to fulfill society's gender role expectations (Person, 1989). This self-denigration infiltrates and impedes all aspects of a person's life from intimate relationships to interaction within school and the workplace.

## DISABILITY AND SEXUAL FUNCTIONING

### Identification of Disability Characteristics

The first step in adjustment toward a positive sense of sexuality is to assess the many identifying characteristics of disability pertaining to sexual function. Included in this identification of disability characteristics are the following:

1. **The identification of the specific disability and its characteristic patterns of involvement, both physical and intellectual.** This includes the degree of body involvement, range of motion, stability, chronicity, fatigue, pain, and progressiveness of the disability.

2. **Severity and level of involvement within the context of specific disability identification.** One often thinks of this concept in terms of major demarcations of mild, moderate, and severe levels of involvement. It also may include such characteristics as paresis (partial or incomplete paralysis), partial or total loss of function, amputation, paralysis, and concerns relating to physical disfigurement.

3. **Nature of disability acquisition.** Psychological adjustment and physical management may be influenced by the manner in which the person acquired the disability. Disabilities may be acquired as a result of trauma, life-threatening disease, progressive but non-life-threatening disease, congenital conditions, or conditions related to the aging process. Each present different patterns of adjustment and management.

4. **Utilization of assistive devices.** Assistive devices aid in control of fine and gross motor function, ambulation, balance, and include devices such as wheelchairs, braces, splints, prosthetic limbs, and those aids that monitor and control bodily functions such as breathing and human management of waste.

5. **Age of onset.** This characteristic is of considerable importance in adjustment to disability. Important factors in the adjustment process include length of time an individual has had a disability, age at which it was identified, and its possible progression. The impact of these characteristics on functioning and rehabilitation affect sexual adjustment. An example of the impact of age and disability can be thought of in terms of comparing two 20 year-old men, both of whom use wheelchairs for mobility, have no bowel or bladder control, and are identified as having paraplegia. One disability is the result of the birth defect, spina bifida (a congenital defect of the spinal cord); the other was a consequence of a motorcycle accident at the age of 18, in which permanent spinal cord injury occurred.

In the case of a congenital disease, such as spina bifida, "from birth or early childhood, the child will integrate the disability into all aspects of sexual development. Sexual maturation inevitably will occur within the context of the disability." It is important to note that in many situations, "chronological age of the child will not be consistent with the maturational or emotional age" (Cole, 1988, p. 279). Mobility limitations, lack of privacy, including the area of personal hygiene, and over-protection by parents, all interfere with the disabled child's learning about sexuality.

For the person with an acquired disability, Cole (1988) further notes that if "...gender role and sexual development of the individual is interrupted, additional implications are to be noted. Expectations of masculinity and femininity are already in place in an able-bodied person, and personal goals are being pursued toward acquiring the societal traits expected in order to fulfill the role of being a 'real' man or woman" (p. 279).

6. **The presence of several disabilities with multiple symptomatology.** An example may be found in cerebral palsy, where there may not only be motor involvement, but mental retardation, epilepsy, and sensory impairment. In this case, the counselor must address the interrelated issues of adjustment, sexual dysfunction, mobility, and cognitive deficits.

7. **Characteristics of chronic progressive illness.** Chronic progressive illnesses generally have multiple disability characteristics such as mobility, fatigue, vision impairment, and sensation deficits. Some examples of this type of disability are diabetes, multiple sclerosis, and lupus erythematosus acquired during adulthood. It is vital that the client have a medical evaluation, including review of medications which may often compound sexual ability and sex education or re-education.

Many of these diseases are more common to women than men and the issues of fertility, pregnancy, and child-rearing should be taken into consideration as a part of the client's counseling and education. In addition, certain diseases may be life threatening or exacerbated by pregnancy, and birth control becomes an important factor (Cole, 1988). We need to include, in this category, diseases which may be terminal or life-threatening such as certain types of cancer.

8. **The presence of depression.** The presence of depression is consistent with the process of adjusting to the changes and losses incurred with a disability. Feelings of anger, depression, and frustration are natural emotions when grieving for these losses. Roles in an interpersonal relationship may change and can be hindered by caretaking duties which impact both partners. The person with the disability may feel like "damaged goods," and no longer feel sexual which further diminishes self-worth. Untreated, these thoughts can turn into depression (Person, 1989).

## *Additional Factors*

Partners with disabilities and those who are non-disabled may encounter fears of rejection, pain, inability to perform, and accidents involving incontinence. These fears translate into anxiety and depression which can be interpreted by the non-disabled partner as rejection or lack of interest. Simple acts of affection and normal communication may be interrupted in the relationship. "Negative cycles" such as these can be lessened with increased communication and flexibility within the relationship (Sanford & Petajan, 1989).

If there is severe ongoing depression, for any reason, it may result in a lowered sexual self-esteem and in a diminished interest in sex. In this case, a physician may recommend therapeutic intervention (Sanford & Petajan, 1989).

# SEXUAL FUNCTIONING

Sexual functioning refers to those physical and physiological characteristics of sex that involve physical contact, stimulation, arousal, sexual intercourse, and orgasm. Masters and Johnson (1966) categorized these combined sexual functioning and performance activities in their identification of the sexual response cycle.

## *Phases of Sexual Response*

The excitement phase (first phase) involves physical or psychological stimuli which, when it occurs in an uninterrupted and effective manner, may result in genital arousal (penile erection or vaginal lubrication). A second phase, the plateau phase, is an advanced stage of the excitement phase which, when continued without interruption, will lead to the next step of the sexual response cycle. The next phase (third phase) is orgasm, usually associated with ejaculation and penile and perineal contractions in males, and in vaginal and perineal contractions in females. Resolution, the fourth phase, follows an intermediate stage following orgasm, the refractory period. Further arousal will not occur in this phase (may last from several moments to several hours). This final phase is the period in which the body returns to a relaxed, unstimulated state.

## *Concept of Sexuality and Disability*

The concept of sexuality, in many respects, is more difficult to understand than the above phases of sexual functioning. It is the very nature of this difficulty in understanding that complicates individual adjustment and realization of sexual self-worth. Sexuality can be considered as the total collection of characteristics that identify and communicate the sexual nature of the individual. These include gender identity, physical appearance and abilities, clothing and other body adornment and enhancement choices, and behavioral and life styles. Sexuality is not only the acceptance and self-realization of these characteristics, but the communication of these traits and the ability to receive and accept these sexual communication choices to and by others. For many individuals, the ability to integrate these characteristics with a recently acquired or long-term disability impacts on the adjustment of and adaptation to disabling conditions.

# SEXUAL DYSFUNCTION

Sexual dysfunctions are identified here as those which occur independent of the presence of specific disability characteristics and may be broadly classified as gender related. Possible dysfunctions in women are discussed first, followed by information on sexual dysfunctioning in men.

## Sexual Dysfunction in Women

In women, dysfunction may be associated with orgasmic capability (inhibited or absent), due to a variety of circumstances including the influence of personal belief systems, fear and other emotional involvement, or partner-specific relationships. In addition, women may experience dysfunction related to vaginal penetration-dyspareunia (vaginal pain during intercourse) and vaginismus (painful involuntary spasm of the muscles of the outer portions of the vagina).

## Sexual Dysfunction in Men

Male sexual dysfunctions generally are identified as those related to impotence, penile erection, and ejaculation. Impotence refers to the inability to obtain and maintain an erection for sexual penetration. Erectile ability may be situation-specific including temporary inability due to fatigue, alcohol or substance ingestion, anxiety related to performance expectations, personal belief systems regarding intercourse or masturbation, and partner specific situations. Emotional components are also important to male sexual dysfunction, and while they may be temporary and situation-specific if they occur on several occasions, they may lead to permanent dysfunction.

Ejaculation dysfunctions are most often identified with premature ejaculation - experiencing ejaculation before a desired time or occurrence. Further, retarded ejaculation also may be seen as a dysfunction - the inability to ejaculate although an erection can be obtained and maintained for sexual penetration.

Further, the effects of medications may decrease sexual drive and ability to perform in both women and men. A careful and thorough medical work-up may be helpful.

# THE CLIENT CENTERED APPROACH TO SEXUALITY

## Intervention of Client and Disability Factors

When combining the characteristics of disability and sexuality, it is important not to lose track of the reason for considering these interrelated issues: the individual client. Figure 1 presents a graphic representation of how these various components interact with the client as the center of these concentric and related issues. The client with the disability, not the disability itself, is the primary focus of the rehabilitation specialist. When considering the sexuality and sexual functioning of the client, several factors need to be taken into account. These factors should not be considered in isolation from one another or in isolation from the client, but as interactive segments of a total sphere of influence on sexual adjustment. These segments are interrelated because of their mutual ability to influence the client; hence, the client's adjustment and response to self and sexuality are impacted by each of the segments as a unit, and as they impact on one another.

**Figure 1**
**CLIENT CENTERED APPROACH TO SEXUALITY**

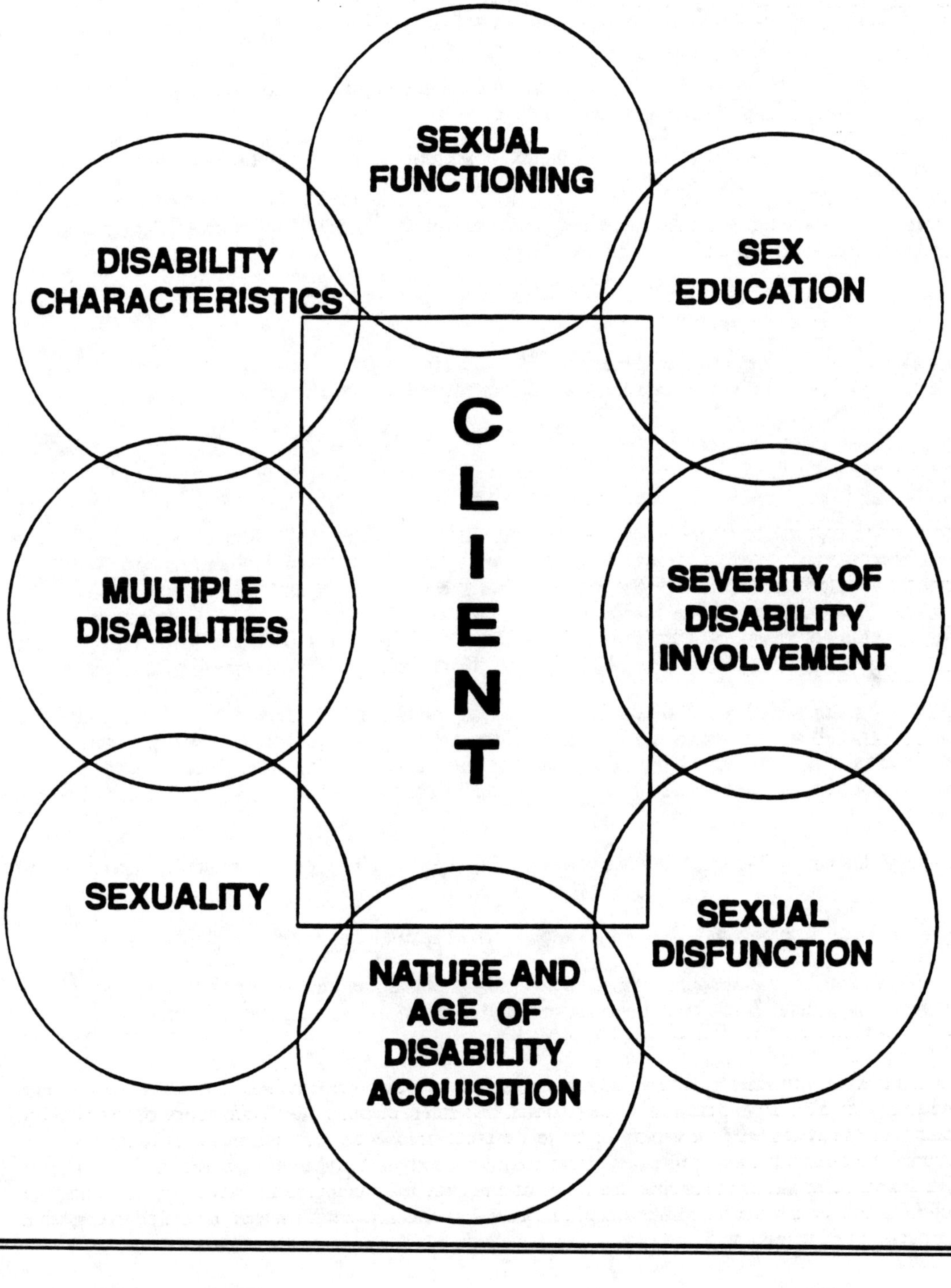

SEXUAL FUNCTIONING

DISABILITY CHARACTERISTICS

SEX EDUCATION

MULTIPLE DISABILITIES

C L I E N T

SEVERITY OF DISABILITY INVOLVEMENT

SEXUALITY

NATURE AND AGE OF DISABILITY ACQUISITION

SEXUAL DISFUNCTION

| | |
|---|---|
| **Sexuality** | the identification and communication of one's self as a sexual individual. |
| **Multiple Disabilities** | the presence of more than one disability that impacts on function and ability to manipulate the environment. |
| **Disability Characteristics** | the disability-specific limitations associated with a given diagnosis of disease, condition, or syndrome. |
| **Sexual Functioning** | the physical and psychosocial management of the individual to participate and engage in sex-related activity. |
| **Sex Education** | the education or re-education of an individual regarding sexual functioning, health, behaviors, and responsibilities. |
| **Severity of Disability Involvement** | the degree of functional limitation (physical, emotional, intellectual) associated with a given disability diagnosis. |
| **Sexual Dysfunction** | the inability to perform sexually as a result of temporary or permanent impairment or loss of function. |
| **Nature and Age of Disability Acquisition** | the impact of the nature of the disability and the age of acquisition on an individual's response to adjustment and consequent sexual well-being. |

## *Sex Education*

**Counselor knowledge and areas of concern.** Sex education is more than a collection of information about physical functioning, body parts, and sexual identity. Sex education is the recognition of the interrelatedness of these parts and the synthesis of this information. For the rehabilitation specialist, this educational synthesis should be acknowledged with the understanding of the impact on personal value systems but without the imposition of individual preference or attitude. Emotional adjustment for the client is of primary importance. Many rehabilitation counselors do not have expertise in this area and may best help the client through referral to appropriate resources.

Today, education regarding sexuality and disability must include the unbiased understanding of alternative life styles. Heterosexuality, as well as homosexuality and bisexuality, are available to and chosen by disabled and non-disabled alike. Personal and social issues related to masturbation, sexually transmitted diseases, birth control, AIDS, sexual abstinence, and alternative styles of sexual functioning are important to recognize as a part of the rehabilitation process.

Two areas of major concern for the rehabilitation counselor in responding to problems related to sexuality and disability include:

1. The education of the client who may have little or no knowledge of sexuality and sexual functioning.

2. Problems related to re-educating and counseling of those who may have had knowledge and experience as sexually active persons, but who, because of illness, injury, or disability, are sexually dysfunctional.

**Sex education programs and curricula.** Sex education as a curriculum content area should be viewed and presented in a broad context of independent life studies, often imbedded in the larger framework of "family-life education." Kempton (1988) has suggested a variety of subject matter areas to be included in the development of a sex education program. These include gender role identification; body awareness and eroticism; sexual responsibility and non-exploitative sexual behavior, with specific emphases on the need for dealing with sexuality in a responsible manner; the privacy of sexuality and the inappropriateness of sexual exploitation; differences in sexual drives; love, sex, and intimacy; marriage and parenthood; and human sexual behavior and sexual response.

There are several available curricula about sexuality and disability, most of which have common content areas. The following general topic areas are offered as a guide for consideration in the development of a sex education curriculum:

1. Parts of the body

2. General personal hygiene

3. Puberty
   a. biological changes in male/female
   b. menstruation, erections, masturbation, wet dreams

4. Social behavior and relationships
   a. differences between public/private places
   b. differences between appropriate/inappropriate behaviors

5. Human reproduction
   a. non-coital sexual behavior
   b. sexual response cycle
   c. intercourse (coitus)

6. Birth control

7. Sexual health
   a. sexually transmitted diseases
   b. AIDS (Acquired Immune Deficiency Syndrome)

8. Homosexuality and bisexuality

9. Legal/illegal sexual behavior
   a. sexual exploitation
   b. sexual abuse
   c. rape

10. Adult living life-styles
    a. the single life
    b. couples
    c. marriage
    d. group living facilities

11. Parenting/families

12. Life cycle
    a. wellness/illness
    b. aging
    c. death/dying

**Appropriate referral.** According to Szasz (1991), the physician, as part of a team managing the sexual difficulties of a person with disabilities, has three roles to perform: " . . . identifying problems that are sexual; assessing these problems; and providing psychological or surgical treatment methods in the context of the patients' rehabilitation programs" (p. 560).

The rehabilitation counselor can assist the client who is presenting a sexual problem by referral to the treating physician for a complete assessment. This assessment includes a physical examination, history taking, mental status evaluation, and investigation into sexual functioning and problems. The assessment may be conducted with the aid of a spouse or an attendant. The physician should address the individual's chief sexual concerns along with other areas of sexual functioning.

Symptoms, their duration, and the context in which they occur need to be identified. This identification will clarify whether the problem is "primary" - a life-long complaint, or "secondary" - recent and related directly to an event or a disability onset. Often, the chief complaint may be due to an undiagnosed physical ailment not involved with the obvious disability. An accurate medical history will also reveal if the person is having sexual performance difficulties due to anxiety over anticipated failure of complete performance, or related to specific disability limitations.

During an interview, the physician can address other pertinent areas concerning sexual response such as personal preferences, styles, and expectations in relation to sexual performance. The physical examination of the patient (client) will determine physical mobility, hygiene practices, including those related to assistive devices, and the structural and neurological integrity of the genitalia. Investigation of function also may be performed by the patient through bodily self-exploration at home for self-evaluation and possible referral for clinical and laboratory testing.

**Treatment.** Care and treatment of the patient/client with a disability must encompass psychological, social, and vocational rehabilitation, as well as the implementation of physical and medical management programs. This care and treatment includes listening to the patient; giving information; suggesting alternative ways of experiencing sexuality; facilitation of social skills, appearance, and self-care; prescribing birth control, assistive devices, surgery, and medications; fertility issues; and parenting counseling (Szasz, 1991).

# SOCIETAL ATTITUDES TOWARD SEXUALITY AND DISABILITY

## Societal Attitudes

This section discusses considerations of sex and sexuality of an adult with a disability and the myths about sexuality and disability. As with all topics on sexuality, it is nearly impossible and usually inappropriate to make generalizations regarding disability and sexuality.

Much of what the public has come to know or suspect about the sexuality of persons with disabilities has come through the various forms of the media - television, movies, and fictional literature. Often, these forms of mass communication have established stereotypes of expected behaviors. Society continually struggles with attitudes that imply people with disabilities are asexual and have no thoughts concerning their sexuality (Cole, 1988). "Disabled men and women are encouraged to be helpless, non-assertive, non-sexual, passive, dependent, grateful, and apologetic for a less than perfect body in a society where physical appearance is often the measure of value" (Daily cited in Cole, 1988, p. 285).

These attitudes have inhibited persons with disabilities from accepting and acknowledging their sexuality and that they can be and are sexually functional individuals. Two examples from fictional literature illustrate the statement of expectation for sexual ability and how the passage of time and social changes have begun to erode long-held stereotypes and assumptions made about persons with disabilities.

The first example is a quotation from **Lady Chatterley's Lover** by D. H. Lawrence. The first page of this novel sets the raison d'etre for Lady Chatterley's acceptance of an extramarital lover - the paraplegia of her husband due to a war injury:

> His hold on life was marvelous. He didn't die, and the bits seemed to grow together again. For two years he remained in the doctor's hands. Then he was pronounced a cure, and could return to life again, with the lower half of his body, from the hips down, paralyzed forever...Crippled for ever, knowing he could never have any children, Clifford came home to the smoky Midlands to keep the Chatterley name alive while he could (p. 1).

The assumption that can easily be made from this presentation is that those with lower body paralysis can be considered sexually nonfunctional, capable of neither genital intercourse nor reproduction. It is important to consider the wide range of understanding about how sexual functioning may be seen - from recreational to procreational experiences, to the notion that genital intercourse is but one form of physical sexual expression.

A later description of sexuality and disability in the genre of fictional literature is found in the novel by Arthur Hailey, **Overload**. This novel of the late 1970s reflects a change in the sexual role and functional ability of a person with a disability.

In the following scenario, a woman with quadriplegia involvement and near total body paralysis has a sexual encounter with a man without a disability:

> Karen was demanding, responsive, exciting, satisfying. Yes, in one sense she was passive. Her body, other than her head, was unable to move. Yet Nim could feel the effect of their lovemaking transmitting itself through her skin, vagina, breasts, and most of all her passionate cries and kisses. It was not, he thought in a flash of whimsy, at all like having sex with a mannequin...Nor was the pleasure brief. It was prolonged as if neither wanted it to end...until at last the ending came...**And for them both.** Could a quadriplegic woman have an orgasm? Emphatically, **yes**! (pp. 260-261).

While it should be emphasized that not all sexual encounters result in intercourse and orgasm, this fictional account is significant because of the specific relationship between two people, one who has a disability, and the importance of sexuality in the relationship. Further, for this woman, sexual intercourse, passion, and orgasm were appropriate, and functionally possible.

## Sexual Functioning

As noted previously, there are a myriad of factors which influence the ability of an adult with a disability to be sexually functional and to value sexuality. Age of onset and nature of the disability (progressive or static, congenital or acquired, long-term or recent onset), are important factors in this adjustment process. Previous sexual experience and disability-related characteristics, including mobility and assistive devices, medications, pain, strength, bodily function, and prostheses (such as colostomies and catheters) also need consideration. Severity of the disability and the presence of multiple disabilities, attitudes, and psychological well-being of the person with a disability and that of the partner are factors to evaluate.

## Myths About Sexuality and Disability

In addition, there is another area of concern that may interfere with the sexual expression of persons with disabilities, the myths about sexuality and disability. Cornelius, Chipouras, Makas, and Daniels (1982) identified several common myths they feel not only affect the sexuality of the person with a disability, but also impact self-concept and motivation for independent living. These **myths** include:

"Disabled people are asexual"

"Disabled people are over-sexed and have uncontrollable urges"

"Disabled people are dependent and child-like, and, thus need to be protected"

"Disability breeds disability"

"Disabled people should stay with and marry their own kind"

"If a disabled person has a sexual problem, it is almost always the result of the disability"

"If a nondisabled person has a sexual relationship with a disabled individual, it's because (s)he can't attract anyone else" (pp. 2-4).

To dispel the impact of myth and impose the rigor of fact regarding sexuality and disability, the client should consult a knowledgeable physician regarding physical characteristics of the disability as related to sexual functioning. The physical examination and consultation will provide significant information regarding a better understanding of what physiologically might be expected because of a specific disability.

Physical disability, in some respects, may be seen as a limiting factor in sexual expression and sexual functioning. Yet, it also may offer opportunities for a wider avenue of personal sexual exploration than previously known. As individuals with disabilities and their partners contemplate the role of sexuality in their lives, they learn that the most important concept and function of sexuality is that of communication.

## Sexual Activity in Persons with Disabilities

**Sexual activity.** Sexual activity is a very basic form of communication; it includes more than the stimulation and activation of the various senses. It is often much easier to engage in sexual activity than in the verbal expressions associated with this multifaceted form of communication. The ability to talk about sex - what pleases, what displeases; what hurts, what feels good; what position is more or less comfortable; what techniques may be used, all allow for the opening of a wide range of experiences. What seems to inhibit many people is the inability to discover a usable and acceptable language to express sexuality. Most commonly used words to describe body parts, body functions, and sex have been represented as "dirty." This culturally biased value system may well prevent many from experiencing satisfaction of sexual expression. As Johnson (1975) has noted " . . . most people can be led to realize that words do not really have magical powers unless we choose to invest them with such powers, and a more related, perhaps even playful, approach to terminology can be encouraged." (p. 56).

**Communication and sexual pleasure.** To experience satisfactory and enjoyable sexual functioning, it is important that the partners communicate and openly discuss those factors that will more likely enhance sexual pleasure. These areas may include such topics as:

1. **Positioning** - what position for intercourse will cause the least discomfort and assure ease of performance.

2. **Timing** - what times of the day are most likely to be associated with the highest energy levels, least amount of pain or discomfort, and the affects of disability-related medications.

3. **Intercourse alternatives** - what areas of the body other than the genitals may be found to have erogenous qualities; what method of sexual activity may be newly initiated. Oral-genital sex may be a new experience for some and is often an alternative used with, or instead of, intercourse. For some, this may be an untried method of sexual expression, and yet, one that may add to the sexual repertoire and enhancement of the pleasure of both partners.

4. **Aids** - what type of activities may enhance or ease sexual performance - the use of massage oils, pillows and other supports, vibrators, lights or mirrors to aid in visual appreciation of sexual activity by those who have limited range of motion of the head and neck.

**Sexual expression.** What should be remembered in all aspects of a sexual relationship is that it should be pleasurable to both partners, and should bring a sense of self and mutual worth to the participants. Everyone has the right to be sexually expressive in the most appropriate and responsible ways possible.

As a concluding comment, Comfort (1978) has expanded on Anderson and Cole's (1975) guidelines, which may be useful to rehabilitation practitioners and clients in learning about the sexuality of physical disability:

A stiff penis does not make a solid relationship, nor does a wet vagina.

Urinary incontinence does not mean genital incompetence.

Absence of sensation does not mean absence of feelings.

Inability to move does not mean inability to please.

The presence of deformities does not mean the absence of desire.

Inability to perform does not mean inability to enjoy.

Loss of genitals does not mean loss of sexuality. (p. 43)

# CONCLUSION

The rehabilitation counselor should keep in mind the many facets of disability that can inhibit a person's sexuality and sexual functioning. Each client is an individual with distinct views, values, and life-styles; every experience of disability is unique to that person, although symptoms across disabilities may be similar. Clients will adjust to disability at their own pace, in their own way. To facilitate the client's adjustment, an accurate, unbiased assessment should be made. The counselor's psychological support, knowledge of sex-education and information about sexuality, and expressions of validation will enhance the client's sense of health and well-being (Cole, 1988).

Defined in its narrowest sense, sexuality is the expression of our sexual urges. But it is much more than that. It is also how we feel about ourselves, how we present ourselves to others and how we fill our roles in society (Person, 1989, p. 6).

# REFERENCES

Anderson, T.P., & Cole, T.M. (1975). Sexual counseling of the physically disabled. **Postgraduate Medicine, 58(1),** 117-123.

Cole, S.S. (1988). Women, sexuality, and disabilities. **Women and Therapy, 7,** 277-294.

Comfort, A. (1978). **Sexual consequences of disability.** Philadelphia, PA: George F. Stickley.

Cornelius, D.A., Chipouras, S., Makas, E., & Daniels, S.M. (1982). **Who cares? A handbook on sex education and counseling services for disabled people** (2nd ed.). Baltimore, MD: University Park Press.

Hailey, A. (1979). **Overload.** Garden City, NY: Doubleday.

Johnson, W.R. (1975). **Sex education and counseling of special groups.** Springfield, IL: Charles C Thomas.

Kempton, W. (1988). **Sex education for persons with disabilities that hinder learning.** Santa Monica, CA: James Stanfield.

Lawrence, D.H. (1959). **Lady Chatterley's lover.** New York, NY: New American Library.

Masters, W.H., & Johnson, V.E. (1966). **Human sexual response.** Boston, MA: Little, Brown.

Person, P.S. (1989). Sexuality, self-image and you. **Arthritis Today, July-August,** 6-10.

Sanford, M.E. & Petajan, J.H. (1989). **Multiple sclerosis and your emotions.** New York: National Multiple Sclerosis Society.

Szasz, G. (1991). Sex and disability are not mutually exclusive - evaluation and management. **Western Journal of Medicine, 154,** 560-563.

## *About the Author*

Gary A. Best, Ph.D., is a Professor in the Division of Special Education at California State University, Los Angeles, located in Los Angeles, California. He is the Coordinator of the Special Education Teacher Education Program in the area of physical disabilities, and a member and certified sex educator of the American Association of Sex Educators, Counselors, and Therapists.

## *Chapter 7*

# THE ACQUIRED IMMUNODEFICIENCY SYNDROME

by
*John J. Howard, M.D., M.P.H.*

## INTRODUCTION

The first cases of the acquired immunodeficiency syndrome (AIDS) were described medically in 1981 (Gottlieb et al., 1981). Since then, tens of thousands of AIDS cases have been reported in the United States. Estimates by the Centers for Disease Control (CDC) of the United States Public Health Service suggest there may be as many as one million people in America already infected with the causative agent of AIDS, the human immunodeficiency virus (HIV). Worldwide, a similar number of Europeans and possibly millions of Africans are also infected with HIV (Quinn, Mann, Curran, & Piot, 1986). Each of these HIV-infected individuals will eventually develop AIDS (Curran et al., 1985).

Since its recognition 10 years ago, AIDS has not only had a profound impact on the medical world, but it has also affected every social institution in American life. The problems caused by the AIDS epidemic have touched families, schools, communities, businesses, courts, religious institutions, and government at all levels. AIDS has brought many controversial issues to the forefront of public discussion. These include discrimination against HIV-infected persons in housing, employment, and health care; the economic cost of providing care to persons with AIDS; the duty of government to protect its citizens from communicable diseases like AIDS; and the obligation of physicians and nurses to provide care for persons with AIDS.

The epidemic's most profound effect has been on those who have become infected with HIV. Over time, HIV causes progressive deterioration of the body's immune system, which makes the individual susceptible to many different types of life-threatening infections and tumors. Even with medical treatment, which is very often of an experimental nature, nearly all persons with AIDS eventually succumb to the disease.

As the second decade of the AIDS epidemic begins, important medical advances are occurring. The quality of life for persons with AIDS is slowly improving due to several factors. One is the positive effect newly emerging therapies are having on the course of the underlying viral infection. Another is the development of treatments for the specific infections and tumors that define the syndrome of acquired immunodeficiency. Due to medical advances, many persons with AIDS can now function at higher levels for longer periods of time than they were able to in the 1980s.

Living with AIDS requires a tremendous amount of physical and emotional energy, even for young adults, the group most commonly affected. Frequently, individuals with AIDS are not able to function at their previous high level of activity. They often must quit their jobs and join the unemployed even when they can still physically work, although at a lower functional level. Typically, persons with AIDS do not receive any type of medical or vocational rehabilitation. The reason for this may lie in the commonly held belief that persons with AIDS are not candidates for any type of medical or vocational rehabilitation because they have a "fatal disease." Fear of contagion may also play a role.

With the recognition of AIDS as a medical condition in 1981, few individuals thought that persons with AIDS would ever have any rehabilitation potential. At that time, AIDS was usually only diagnosed when the virus had already destroyed a person's immune system, and little could be done medically to prolong the patient's life. Persons with AIDS died within a short time following diagnosis.

Medical progress is quickly transforming AIDS from a severely activity-limiting condition with a very short survival time, into a chronic disabling condition with rehabilitation potential. However, limitations caused by societal discrimination continue to be a challenge.

Similar to the obstacles surrounding the development of rehabilitation programs for cancer patients in the 1960s, negative attitudes of the public and the medical community alike make rehabilitation of persons with AIDS very difficult. Such globally negative attitudes need to be replaced with an enlightened and positive approach to rehabilitative care for those with HIV disease. Many persons could benefit from early recognition of their rehabilitation potential, the establishment of therapeutic goals, and prompt referral to a rehabilitation counselor.

This chapter presents to rehabilitation professionals a comprehensive overview of the scientific and medical aspects of HIV infection and HIV disease. First, the chapter presents the modes of HIV transmission followed by a discussion of the natural history of HIV infection. Next, the clinical manifestations of HIV disease will be reviewed, including the specific infections and tumors which define the syndrome of acquired immunodeficiency or AIDS. The chapter discusses treatment strategies against HIV itself, and against different types of infections and tumors that define AIDS, and also preventive and post-infection vaccines. Lastly, this chapter focuses on the functional and vocational limitations associated with HIV disease, and on the rehabilitative potential for persons affected by the human immunodeficiency virus.

# MODES OF HIV TRANSMISSION

A newly recognized member of the lentivirus family of viruses, called the human immunodeficiency virus (HIV), causes AIDS. Lentiviruses are examples of a broad category of RNA-containing viruses, called retroviruses. Retroviruses process genetic information in a fashion that is the reverse of the way other viruses and cells do it.

By the 1970s, researchers had discovered retroviruses caused disease in several animal species. No immunosuppressive retrovirus was found to cause disease in human beings. By 1981, the first cases of an immunosuppressive disease began to appear in young homosexual males in the United States. It was similar to immunological effects seen in animal species infected with other types of retroviruses (Essex & Kanki, 1988).

Much speculation has centered on the origin of HIV; there are more questions than answers at this time. Questions abound, including when and where HIV first appeared, whether it is a new entity or a mutation of a pre-existing virus, and whether exposure to HIV through close contact with African green monkeys caused AIDS in humans. We may never know definite answers to many of these questions. Yet, the emergence of AIDS as a clinical entity supports the view that a pathogenic form of HIV was only recently introduced into the human population.

HIV infection is established in human beings through the introduction of blood cells or bodily fluids from an infected individual into the bloodstream of an uninfected individual. This occurs either through sexual contact or through blood-related contact (Friedland & Klein, 1987).

## Sexual Contact

Sexual transmission is the most common mode of HIV transmission throughout the world. Penetrative sexual intercourse involving the passage of HIV-containing white blood cells and bodily fluids, such as semen or vaginal secretions, can result in HIV transmission. The efficiency with which sexual contact transmits HIV varies with the particular type of sexual practice and with the gender of the sexual partners involved. Current epidemiologic data points to anal intercourse between two males, especially for the receptive partner, as the most efficient means of sexual transmission. Penile-vaginal intercourse also can result in HIV transmission, but at a lower level of transmissive efficiency (Peterman & Curran, 1986). Much of AIDS public health education is directed at the interruption of the sexual transmission of HIV by encouraging people to engage in "safer sex" practices (Francis & Chin, 1987).

## Blood Contact

The second means of HIV transmission is blood-related contact, which can occur in five different ways. First, blood from an HIV-infected blood donor can be transfused into an uninfected person during a medical emergency or a surgical operation. A second type of blood contact involves the transfusion of a particular blood factor from an HIV-infected blood donor to an uninfected person who has hemophilia (a blood-clotting disorder). These routes of HIV transmission will largely disappear in the future because all blood donations are now screened for the presence of HIV. Further, blood used for the preparation of clotting products for persons with hemophilia goes through a heat treatment process that inactivates HIV.

The third type of blood contact accounts for most of the blood- related HIV transmission - intravenous drug use. Intravenous drug users often share their "equipment" (e.g., needles or syringes) with other drug users. This equipment can contain minute amounts of HIV-infected blood. If an HIV-infected drug user shares "equipment" with an uninfected person, HIV transmission can occur. This route of HIV transmission is the fastest growing type of transmission in the United States today.

Fourth, HIV can be transmitted from an infected pregnant woman to her fetus. Physicians call this route of HIV transmission, maternal-fetal transmission. It is the route of HIV transmission which accounts for most of the cases of pediatric AIDS. These newborn infants become HIV-infected because their mothers became infected before giving birth through either sexual contact with an infected male partner or through their own intravenous drug use. Approximately half the infants born to HIV-infected mothers develop clinical AIDS.

Lastly, HIV can be transmitted inadvertently during an accident in health care institutions and research laboratories. The routes of transmission that occur in these occupational settings are needlestick injuries and direct skin or mucous membrane contact. For instance, HIV can be transmitted when an uninfected health care provider is stuck with a needle or cut with a scalpel, which contains blood from an HIV-infected patient (Marcus & Centers for Disease Control, 1988). Transmission of the virus also can occur when blood contaminated with HIV comes into direct contact with the abraded skin or mucous membrane of an uninfected person. In addition, HIV can be transmitted in occupational settings from an HIV-infected health care worker to an uninfected patient (Centers for Disease Control, 1990).

# THE NATURAL HISTORY OF HIV INFECTION

After HIV is transmitted to an uninfected individual through sexual or blood contact, most individuals are unaware they have become infected with HIV. A few experience a condition called acute HIV infection (Cooper et al., 1985), but the majority do not. They remain asymptomatic, and up to 14 years can go by before HIV-infected individuals experience any symptoms. During the long incubation period, infected individuals may transmit the virus to others.

## Acute HIV Infection

Acute HIV infection manifests itself as a flu-like illness, characterized by fever, body aches, swollen lymph nodes, and a faint rash. Many newly infected individuals do not experience such an acute illness following HIV transmission or attribute the illness to the "flu." Even when present, acute HIV infection lasts only a few days. A period of well-being follows during which the only sign of HIV infection is the development of antibodies to HIV. Such antibodies usually develop within 90-180 days after HIV transmission, but a minority of infected individuals can remain antibody negative for long periods of time following infection (Imagawa et al., 1989). For most individuals, the first time they realize they are infected with HIV is when they undergo a blood test for the presence of HIV antibodies and are told they are seropositive.

## HIV Antibody Formation

Development of an antibody response to the presence of HIV in the blood is the body's way of eliminating the invading virus. These antibodies are detectable throughout the course of HIV infection, and decline only late in the course of HIV disease when the person has AIDS. Unlike many of the body's other antibodies that are protective against viruses, HIV antibodies do not protect the individual against progressive destruction by HIV.

## Latent Period

HIV begins to destroy the body's immune system soon after HIV transmission occurs. An infected person can remain clinically asymptomatic for long periods after becoming infected with HIV. Yet, the virus begins to attack a pivotal infection fighting white blood cell, the CD4+ lymphocyte, soon after transmission occurs. Since this cell is responsible for coordinating the body's response to certain invading microorganisms, the slow destruction of these CD4+ cells leaves the person prone to many infections and tumors. Destruction of CD4+ cells that are critical to immune defense is the major cause of the progressive immune dysfunction, which is the hallmark of HIV infection.

The destruction of CD4+ cells, due to continuous low level viral replication, is a constant feature of the infected state (Ho, Moudgil, & Alam, 1989). At the time of initial transmission, there is a short but intense burst of HIV replication. The body forms antibodies and viral replication subsides, but not entirely. Throughout the long incubation period when infected individuals are clinically well, HIV continues to replicate, damaging CD4+ cells, and slowly reducing their numbers.

It is not clear what controls the pace of this destructive process. Research suggests that viral growth could be the result of factors internal to the virus itself or to some interaction between HIV and the body's own immune system. Also, genetic, lifestyle, and normally unrelated medical factors that vary from person to person may play a role. Included in these factors are exercise, diet, sleep patterns, and the number of colds and other infections.

Clearly, though, there is a prolonged incubation period. The incubation period of HIV infection (the period from HIV transmission to the development of symptoms for individuals who acquire HIV through sexual contact) can last from 7-14 years (Lui, Darrow, & Rutherford, 1988).

### Progressive Immunodeficiency

During this long asymptomatic incubation period, the virus is not quiescent. HIV gradually depletes the body's supply of CD4+ cells, resulting in a progressively worsening state of immunodeficiency. The particular type of immunodeficiency HIV induces is a cellular type immunodeficiency that does not impair the body's ability to manufacture antibodies to fight- off common infections like colds and flu.

Ideally, one would like to measure the rate at which the virus is replicating. Knowledge of the state of viral activity would be useful for both patient and physician. Patients would know when the virus is switching from a quiescent state to a more active one, which may herald the onset of AIDS. The physician would know if the medications given to stop viral growth were effective. There are a number of research-oriented tests available to determine the state of viral activity, such as HIV culture, p24 antigen assay, and polymerase chain reaction (PCR) testing.

More commonly, physicians use a surrogate marker of viral activity, a quantitative CD4+ cell count. During the latent period, one can deduce the rate at which immune system destruction is occurring by serially measuring the number of CD4+ cells. A declining number indicates evidence of "progression" to a more advanced state of immunodeficiency and the development of early symptomatic HIV infection. Nearly all HIV-infected individuals will eventually progress from a state of asymptomatic HIV infection to symptomatic HIV disease.

# CLINICAL MANIFESTATIONS

### Early HIV Disease

Early symptomatic HIV disease is characterized by relatively non-specific signs (what the physician notices) and symptoms (what the patient notices). These include swollen glands or lymph nodes, mild fevers, and a state of fatigue or low energy. Soon, these signs and symptoms worsen, and others make their appearance.

### AIDS-Related Complex

Moderate to severe HIV disease is often called AIDS-Related Complex or ARC. However, there is no universally accepted collection of signs and symptoms that defines ARC precisely. Individuals with ARC typically manifest several different signs and symptoms of HIV disease. These include daily fevers, night sweats, fatigue and weakness, weight loss of more than 10 pounds, intermittent diarrhea, oral thrush (yeast growing in the mouth), swollen lymph nodes, various skin conditions such as fungal rashes and herpes zoster infection or "shingles," and memory and concentration problems. Since there is no one definition of ARC, physicians often use the term to describe HIV-infected individuals with any degree of symptomatology related to HIV. Official agencies, like the Social Security Administration, often group the signs and symptoms of ARC and AIDS together to determine disability status (Social Security Administration, 1987).

### AIDS

Until very recently, the transition from early HIV disease and ARC to AIDS has been related less to the underlying level of cellular immunodeficiency and more to the clinical development of certain infections and tumors. Early in the HIV epidemic, the Centers for Disease Control epidemiologically "defined" what AIDS was to track accurately the number of persons who manifested the syndrome. According to the original CDC surveillance case definition, AIDS existed under two conditions. First, the individual must be diagnosed with one of a specific set of infections or tumors, which are moderately indicative of the presence of a cellular-type immunodeficiency. Second, the individual must not have any known medical reason to have such an infection or tumor, such as receiving chemotherapy for cancer or medications associated with the development of immunosuppression (Centers for Disease Control, 1981).

Under the 1981 epidemiologic surveillance definition of AIDS, HIV-infected individuals were said to have AIDS if they developed one out of a list of several different infections or tumors. The most common infection that HIV-infected individuals contract is a pneumonia caused by a protozoa, called **Pneumocystis carinii** pneumonia, and the most common tumor is called Kaposi's sarcoma.

Other bacterial, viral, fungal, or protozoal organisms can cause infectious diseases, the occurrence of which results in a diagnosis of AIDS. These organisms share in common an inherently low level of virulence or ability to harm human beings. Since these microorganisms rarely cause disease in persons with intact immune systems, we call them "opportunistic infections" because they take advantage of the opportunity of the body's somewhat defenseless posture caused by HIV to produce infection.

The most common tumor seen in HIV-infected persons developing AIDS is Kaposi's sarcoma. It most commonly affects the skin, resulting in a violet-colored skin tumor. Kaposi's sarcoma can also occur in lymph nodes and inside the gastrointestinal or respiratory tract. Unlike opportunistic infections, the development of Kaposi's sarcoma is not necessarily related to the level of immunodeficiency present, and HIV-infected persons with minimal immunodeficiency can develop Kaposi's sarcoma. Some researchers believe factors other than HIV infection are causal in the development of Kaposi's sarcoma. Cancers, such as non-Hodgkin's lymphoma, also qualify as an AIDS-defining tumor.

In 1987, the AIDS case definition was refined to take account of the development of the HIV antibody test (Centers for Disease Control, 1987). In 1991, the Centers for Disease Control proposed that the level of cellular immunodeficiency, as reflected in the quantitative CD4+ cell count, be used as the basis of a new definition of AIDS. Thus, according to the 1991 case definition, AIDS is present in any HIV-infected individual who has 200 or fewer CD4+ cells per cubic millimeter, even in the absence of overt symptoms.

HIV infection can affect nearly every system in the body. Of particular importance for rehabilitation professionals is the effect HIV has on the nervous system, especially on an individual's activity level and cognitive functioning.

## Neurological Manifestations

Neurological dysfunction occurs frequently in HIV infection and AIDS. As many as 20% of patients with AIDS have some neurological dysfunction as their presenting manifestation of AIDS. Often, neurological symptoms occur before other manifestations of HIV disease. Approximately 60% of persons with AIDS have neurological symptoms (Snider et al., 1983).

Common neurological problems include both opportunistic infections of the central nervous system, such as toxoplasmosis (a protozoan infection), cryptococcosis (a fungal infection), and tumors such as lymphoma. Several unexplained neurological syndromes are also frequently seen in persons with HIV infection. They include (1) meningitis, or an inflammation of the lining of the brain and spinal cord; (2) myelopathy, or spinal cord disease; (3) painful sensory neuropathies of the arms and legs; and (4) myopathies, or aching sensations in the leg muscles.

Subacute encephalitis (AIDS encephalopathy or AIDS dementia complex) is the most insidious neurological problem seen in AIDS. Clinically, one sees symptoms such as poor memory, inability to concentrate, verbal and motor slowing, affective and behavioral changes, and social apathy (Price et al., 1988). AIDS dementia complex (ADC) can adversely influence a person's ability to cope with the condition, and the potential for vocational rehabilitation. As discussed in the next section of this chapter, ADC can sometimes be controlled by treatment with an antiviral drug called zidovudine (formerly AZT).

# TREATMENT STRATEGIES

In 1984, when researchers first discovered the human immunodeficiency virus, many in medical science doubted that a drug capable of attacking the virus would be found. Previous efforts to find antiviral drugs had produced few effective agents. Further, HIV could integrate itself into the body's own genetic material, where it could remain dormant and go undetected for long periods of time. Also, it could infect a multiplicity of different tissues and cells of the body, including the brain. In 1986, zidovudine was shown to prolong the lives of persons with AIDS. New knowledge of the life cycle of HIV now makes it possible to design drugs that interrupt specific phases of the viral life cycle.

Treatment of HIV infection and AIDS is a rapidly evolving field; any discussion of the topic in written material rapidly becomes obsolete. The reason is that much of HIV treatment is medically experimental and, therefore, subject to rapid medical obsolescence. A particularly promising experimental therapy can quickly turn out to lack effectiveness or be too toxic to be useful in human beings. With these limitations in mind, treatment strategies for HIV infection and AIDS can be divided into three conceptual categories: primary, secondary, and preventive.

## Primary Treatment

Primary treatment can be directed either at interrupting the life cycle of the virus itself (antiviral therapy), or aimed at positively modulating the body's immune response to the virus (immunomodulator therapy). Both types of primary treatment are designed to control HIV growth, which in turn will prevent the development of secondary infections and tumors.

Antiviral therapy can be difficult because any therapy that interferes with HIV replication also can harm the patient in the process. The traditional way interruptive therapy works is by attacking a biochemical pathway unique to the offending organism. With bacteria, this is somewhat easy to do; in HIV, it is a formidable task. Because HIV is a virus, it uses the body's own cellular machinery to replicate itself. Thus, any drug that interferes with HIV replication also can interfere with the body's normal cell division, especially that occurring in bone marrow, which is responsible for producing new red and white blood cells.

Antiviral therapy can be categorized on where in the life cycle of the virus the chemical agent intervenes. The largest number of antiviral agents currently in use, both clinically and experimentally, interfere with an enzyme essential to HIV replication, called reverse transcriptase. The most prominent drug in this category of reverse transcriptase inhibitors is zidovudine.

In 1987, the United States Food and Drug Administration (FDA) first approved zidovudine for use in adults with AIDS, or with symptomatic HIV infection with fewer than 200 CD4+ lymphocytes. In early 1990, the FDA expanded zidovudine's use to include asymptomatic HIV-infected persons with fewer than 500 CD4+ lymphocytes (Volberding et al., 1990). Its expanded use in the large population of asymptomatic individuals with HIV infection is termed "early intervention therapy." Early intervention therapy slows progression from HIV infection to the development of AIDS (Friedland, 1990).

Primary treatment also can be directed at "boosting" the function of the body's immune system (immunomodulation). Several drugs are available that do not interrupt the life cycle of HIV within the body, but improve the immune system's ability to defend itself against HIV. For example, chemicals that are naturally produced by the cells of the body's immune system to fight infections, such as interferons and interleukins, are now synthesized in the laboratory. They can be given to HIV-infected individuals to help their immune system in overcoming HIV infection.

Another form of immunomodulation that shows promise in augmenting the body's immune defenses against HIV involves post-infection vaccination (Salk, 1987). Post-infection vaccination stimulates the body to produce higher levels of antibody against HIV, which improves the body's ability to suppress the growth of HIV (Redfield et al., 1991). This in turn may eventually deter the development of HIV disease and AIDS.

## Secondary Treatment

Secondary treatment is directed not against HIV itself, but against the specific infections and tumors that are indirectly caused by HIV. For example, secondary therapies are aimed at curing or controlling **Pneumocystis carinii** pneumonia, cryptococcal meningitis, cytomegalovirus retinitis, and the tumors associated with AIDS, such as Kaposi's sarcoma and non-Hodgkin's lymphoma. Secondary treatment is nearly always given to individuals who are also receiving primary or antiviral treatment.

Preventive therapies exist for several AIDS-defining opportunistic infections. These strategies are designed to prevent a clinical occurrence or recurrence of specific infection. A medication can be given to a person who is at risk of developing **Pneumocystis carinii** pneumonia, or to a person who already had an episode of the pneumonia, to prevent its recurrence. Steady improvement in secondary treatment modalities has greatly decreased the mortality from specific AIDS-related infections, helping to prolong the lives of individuals with AIDS.

## Preventive Strategies

The best way to combat any disease is to prevent it. Pre-infection vaccination would be the safest, simplest, and most effective way to prevent HIV infection. Vaccines have achieved enormous success against infectious diseases like polio, smallpox, yellow fever, and rubella, and development of a vaccine against HIV has become a high priority. However, development of an HIV vaccine has proven to be a great challenge for several reasons. HIV can "hide" within cells for long periods of time by integrating its own genes within the genes of the host. It also can then change the composition of its outer coat or envelope, potentially making any vaccine inadequate. Importantly, HIV infects some of the same cells any vaccine would have to activate to be effective. If these cells are activated by a vaccine, the result may be unrestrained HIV growth (Matthews & Bolognesi, 1988).

Despite these obstacles, the first anti-AIDS vaccines are now being tested in limited trials in several places in the United States. Too little information is currently available to suggest an effective vaccine will be discovered any time soon. Yet, it is still somewhat remarkable that so many candidate HIV vaccines have reached the stage of human testing trials so soon after the discovery of HIV.

# FUNCTIONAL LIMITATIONS

## Physical

HIV infection can cause disturbances in the normal functioning of many systems of the body, including mental functioning. These disturbances often progress to functional physical and mental impairments. Chief among the body's systems that can be physically impaired by HIV infection and AIDS are (1) the respiratory, gastrointestinal, and cardiac systems; (2) the musculoskeletal system; (3) the neurological system; and (4) the various sensory systems, such as the eyes. Mental impairments related to HIV infection also can cause significant functional limitations.

**Energy-restricting disorders.** Energy-restricting disorders are the most common functional impairments due to HIV disease and AIDS. The primary manifestation of HIV disease is fatigue. As HIV-related immunodeficiency progresses through time, HIV-infected individuals begin to experience a state of lowered energy that restricts daily activity. Employed individuals are frequently exhausted; often, midday rest periods or naps are necessary. Persons with advanced HIV infection must rest after only a few hours of activity. For some individuals, the activities of daily living, such as dressing, washing, cooking, bathing, and toilet needs can be restrictive since they deplete the existing energy reserve.

Besides the underlying HIV infection itself being energy restrictive, additional energy restriction can occur in individuals with cardiorespiratory diseases associated with AIDS. For example, the single most common AIDS-defining disease is **Pneumocystis carinii** pneumonia, which among other things, causes shortness of breath and fatigue during the acute episode and for many weeks after recovery. Some individuals never fully recover respiratory function following an episode of pneumonia.

HIV-infected individuals are often functionally impaired by gastrointestinal disorders. Chief among these are infectious and non-infectious diarrhea syndromes that cause prolonged bouts of profuse diarrhea and impair a person's ability to absorb vital nutrients from the diet. This malabsorption causes progressive weight loss, profound fatigue, and produces an aversion to food out of fear of triggering diarrhea.

HIV also can affect the heart, causing an inflammation of the heart muscle itself (myocarditis) or the thin lining around the heart (pericarditis). Either of these conditions can produce energy restriction by causing shortness of breath, chest pain, and fatigue.

**Musculoskeletal disorders.** Musculoskeletal disorders are the second type of physical impairment seen in HIV-infected individuals. Since HIV can produce inflammation of both muscles and nerves, many HIV-infected persons have diffuse musculoskeletal pain. Management of pain can include analgesic medications (some of which can produce drowsiness and impaired judgement). The physician may also prescribe physiotherapy, hypnosis, acupressure, and acupuncture. Sometimes, pain becomes chronic, further restricting the activities of the individual. Besides pain, musculoskeletal disorders associated with HIV can impair ambulation because of pain or muscle weakness in one or both legs. Bilateral leg myopathy can totally impair ambulation.

**Neurological disorders.** Neurological impairment related to HIV can be divided into two types: that affecting the central nervous system and that affecting the peripheral nervous system. Central nervous system impairment can cause limitations as serious as recurrent seizures to milder limitations resulting from mental slowness (see cognitive impairment below). Inflammation of peripheral nerves can result in pain and weakness, both which can restrict an individual's activities.

**Sensory disorders.** Sensory disorders may impair an HIV-infected individual. The most common example of this type of impairment is visual loss due to infection of the retina either by HIV itself or by cytomegalovirus (CMV). CMV retinitis is by far the most common type of visual impairment, usually seen in individuals with severe degrees of immunodeficiency who already have several other functional impairments. The normally sighted adult who loses any degree of vision faces physical challenges, such as loss of reading and writing skills, mobility limitations, and other daily living limitations. There are also a variety of emotional and social problems that occur with significant visual loss.

**Cognitive impairment.** Individuals who have signs of central nervous system involvement (AIDS dementia complex) manifest a myriad of cognitive impairments such as short-term memory deficits, and a decrease in concentration ability. Affective and behavioral abnormalities also can appear that can range from social withdrawal and apathy to impatience, irritability, mania, and even psychosis. Any of these mental impairments can progress, like their physical counterparts, to a stage where the individual is not capable of independent living.

## Emotional

The psychological reaction to impairments caused by HIV depends chiefly on the severity and the rate of progression of the particular impairment, and the underlying personality of the affected individual. This includes self-image and coping style. Other important factors include any neuropsychiatric changes caused by the virus itself and the reaction of those around the patient to the condition. The extent of the patient's social support network and the quality of the psychological care available to the patient also are crucial factors.

Emotional disturbances are common in HIV-infected individuals. The most common are depression and anxiety; often, patients exhibit both. Even those without any symptoms related to HIV can have feelings of guilt over becoming infected in the first place, with sadness and anxiety about their status as HIV-infected individuals. They often suffer from low self-esteem and feelings of powerlessness over the course of their lives.

Importantly, because HIV infection is a progressive condition with a poor prognosis, those affected by HIV can frequently become very anxious about what the future may hold. Each measurement of their immune system's function which reveals further deterioration, can result in increased feelings of anxiety, helplessness, and depression. Professional counseling is essential.

Psychological problems can increase at the time when a previously stable HIV-infected person develops an AIDS-defining disease like **Pneumocystis carinii** pneumonia or Kaposi's sarcoma. Any loss of function can lead to further depression. For young adults with AIDS, the losses associated with advancing disease are psychologically devastating. The loss of health, earning power, enjoyable activities, and sex life, coupled with having to experience premature old age and disability can produce profound depression and suicidal ideation.

Clearly, these primarily psychological effects of HIV infection and AIDS can either add to, or worsen, an AIDS patient's physical impairments. Disturbances of sleep, appetite, and weight are only a few of the physical effects that can be a direct result of the emotional manifestations associated with HIV disease.

## Social

All medical professionals are aware of the influence that various social factors can exert on the course of any illness. Factors such as a person's ethnic and cultural background, marital status, family support system, educational level, financial capability, and vocational background all have an effect on the provision of rehabilitation services. The greater the number of problematic social factors involved, the less likely will be the level of recovery.

One of the greatest challenges facing rehabilitation of a person with AIDS is overcoming overwhelming social limitations. A person with HIV infection, ARC, or AIDS faces more than the usual number of social obstacles to recovery.

The HIV epidemic has elicited very strong responses from many individuals in society. The reasons for this strong response to a disease are not difficult to understand. HIV transmission involves forms of behavior that are either illegal or socially taboo in most places in the United States. Groups at greatest risk for contracting AIDS, gay males and intravenous drug users, have traditionally been the subject of legal sanctions and social stigma. Further, AIDS affects a disproportionate number of Blacks and Latinos, racial and ethnic groups already the subject of various social limitations and prejudice in American society.

Because of the unique epidemiologic nature of AIDS, individuals infected with HIV are frequently ostracized by their family members, and abandoned by the society in which they live. They face discrimination in employment, housing, social services, and health care.

It is not surprising individuals with AIDS fear social interaction with their immediate family, friends, and society. Because they may withdraw socially, both their physical and social limitations combine to hinder meaningful social interaction. Their sense of isolation, in some cases, can become so severe and hopeless they commit suicide.

The situation is not entirely bleak. Many agencies have responded to the social isolation that persons with AIDS experience by setting up organizations to meet their needs for companionship, shopping assistance, meal preparation, and other activities of daily living. Volunteers staff these organizations.

# VOCATIONAL LIMITATIONS

Vocational rehabilitation services for persons with HIV-related disease are similar to those for other disorders. An individualized approach to a vocational rehabilitation work-up is crucial. Although no one type of assessment or method of evaluation can be applied in all cases, three general issues are important:

1. Is the individual able to return to the previous job or occupation?

2. Are skills or abilities of the person transferable to a new job?

3. In conjunction with the medical factors, what type of rehabilitation training needs to be conducted to facilitate reemployment? (Matheson, 1984)

The age group most commonly affected by HIV infection is young adults, ranging in age from 20-40 years. Many of these individuals are employed at the time of their AIDS diagnosis. Some have well developed vocational skills. Others are unemployed or only employed on a part-time basis. After developing HIV disease, many persons cannot continue working at the same level of activity. Many have to quit their jobs because of development of functional impairments; many resign or are fired after the employer learns the nature of their condition. These individuals are candidates for vocational assessment and possible rehabilitation.

During vocational evaluation, several physical, emotional, and social factors associated with HIV disease need to be kept in mind. Some of these can be particularly disabling in the vocational environment. First, individuals with HIV disease have different levels of medical stability. Unlike impairments that reach a level of permanence before the process of vocational rehabilitation begins, impairments associated with HIV disease are progressively and inherently unstable. The only major difference between persons is their relative rate of instability. Some individuals have conditions that are sufficiently stable as not to interfere with work. Others have a disease state that interferes with work to a greater or lesser extent. The rehabilitation counselor needs to assess the relative medical stability of each individual.

Second, an important factor that can be particularly handicapping in the vocational environment is the lack of physical endurance to work a full day. As discussed in the previous section on functional limitations, there are many causes for a person with HIV disease to have fatigue. A rehabilitation counselor can assess physical tolerance for work by ascertaining the person's daily energy patterns. The counselor needs to investigate the energy requirements expended in the home environment. Assistance in home management activities may save energy that can be used for work.

Third, individuals with HIV disease can develop various cognitive impairments secondary to the effect HIV can have on the central nervous system. Clearly, moderate to severe degrees of AIDS dementia complex manifested by memory deficits, lack of coordination, and poor concentration ability can be handicapping in all work environments. The counselor needs to be aware that cognitive impairments can exist in all HIV-infected persons and neuropsychological testing should be a part of the evaluation.

Fourth, emotional factors such as depression and anxiety, can interfere with a successful outcome of vocational rehabilitation. Motivation to work should be explicitly determined. Also, the rehabilitation counselor needs to assess the individual's level of emotional adjustment. It is not advisable to place a person with AIDS in a vocational situation before emotional adjustment to the disease has occurred.

Fifth, the presence of skin lesions on the face or other exposed surfaces of the body from Kaposi's sarcoma may be a source of great embarrassment for patients and impede vocational rehabilitation. The application of cosmetics to cover such lesions may allow a person to overcome reluctance to enter the work environment.

Lastly, there are two social factors that are particularly disabling for anyone trying to re-enter the vocational environment after being diagnosed with any form of HIV disease. The most important relates to the incorrect perception by many people that HIV-infected individuals pose a communicable disease risk when they are in the workplace. The only possible risk of HIV transmission in the workplace is if an accident occurs resulting in blood from the HIV-infected individual coming into direct contact with an open wound of an uninfected co-worker. This is an unlikely occurrence, which can be anticipated, and appropriate safety steps can be planned.

Another important social factor is the prejudice directed toward individuals with HIV infection, based on personal judgements about their sexual behavior or drug use. This factor can severely limit the vocational rehabilitation of individuals with HIV disease; the rehabilitation counselor needs to be aware of the reality of its existence.

# REHABILITATION POTENTIAL

The rehabilitation potential of individuals affected by HIV depends in large part on the level of their underlying immunodeficiency, and the presence of any physical limitations arising from specific disorders. Individuals with greater degrees of immunodeficiency, as measured by reductions in their level of CD4+ cells in the blood, have less residual capacity for rehabilitation. The severity of various physical impairments frequently increases with increasing degrees of immunodeficiency. Still, many persons with HIV disease and severe immunodeficiency manifest significant capacities for rehabilitation.

A positive attribute of most persons with HIV disease in terms of rehabilitation potential is age. Since HIV primarily affects previously healthy young adults, very significant reductions in strength and capacity for work have to occur before these persons have little rehabilitation potential. Only a minority of persons with AIDS are in this category and usually only after having the condition for several years. The vast majority of individuals affected by HIV disease have enough residual physical, mental, emotional, and educational capabilities to respond favorably to vocational rehabilitation.

An additional positive factor contributing to rehabilitation potential is the absence of any spinal cord damage, complete loss of appendages, reduction in arm or leg mobility, or other severely disabling neuromuscular impairment. All ambulatory individuals with HIV disease have enough residual neuromuscular capacity to engage in at least sedentary categories of work. Those with energy-restricting disorders usually have enough residual capacity to engage in light to medium categories of work.

It is important to emphasize the rehabilitation potential of persons with HIV disease needs to be thoroughly assessed on an individual basis. Many persons with AIDS have rehabilitation potential. A counselor needs to conduct an adequate and thorough assessment of remaining strengths, capacities, and skills. As medical science improves the quality and length of life for those with HIV disease, rehabilitation professionals will be called upon more frequently to help in restoring ability to live and work as fully as possible.

# CASE STUDY

Mr. James Dexter is a 29 year-old male oil refinery worker. Although he did not finish high school, he completed most of the 12th grade. His job title is oil-field equipment mechanic (petroleum production), D.O.T. # 629.381-014. The job involves installation, maintenance, and repair of oil well drilling machinery and equipment. He uses handtools and power tools, and reads diagrams and schematics. The job involves disassembly and reassembly of equipment such as pumps, transmissions, and diesel engines, to make repairs. Occasionally, the mechanic does welding and soldering, as needed. All oil refinery mechanics run tests to insure the equipment is fully functional. This type of work takes 1-2 years to learn proficiently and involves occasional lifting of 50 pounds with repetitive lifting and carrying of 25 pounds. Mr. Dexter has worked as an oil-field equipment mechanic for 6 years. Before this job, he worked in the construction field. The construction job is classified as a construction worker II (construction), D.O.T. # 869.687-026. This work did not involve any skills and required lifting of up to 120 pounds occasionally and 75 pounds repetitively. The job responsibilities included loading and unloading of building materials, tools, and supplies. It also involved digging, spreading, and leveling dirt and gravel, using a pick and shovel. Mr. Dexter held this job for 4 years.

In 1986, Mr. Dexter developed a painful tingling sensation on the left side of his chest, followed the next day by water blisters in the same area. He was diagnosed with "shingles" or herpes zoster. His physician advised him the herpes zoster was a sign of an impaired immune system. He thought no more about it; after 4 weeks, the shingles resolved.

In late 1988, he began to develop feelings of fatigue at work, especially when climbing the "cracking" towers at the oil refinery. Gradually, his fatigue worsened and his work performance began to decline. He never felt rested, even after a good night's sleep. His boss told him to "shape-up" or he would be fired. In January of 1989, he noticed fatigue when climbing the towers at the refinery. Shortly after that, he started having night sweats. Finally, when he developed a dry cough and a fever of 102° F., he went to see a physician. The physician diagnosed pneumonia and admitted Mr. Dexter to the hospital the same day.

A thorough medical history revealed he had been in good health all his life, except for a broken leg in 1985. He has been married for several years and has three young children. He and his wife were having marital difficulties. He denied sexual contact with other men, the use of intravenous drugs, or a history of hemophilia. When hospitalized in 1985 for the broken leg, he noted the doctors "tore" a major blood vessel in his leg when they reduced the fracture. Because of this, he was given one pint of blood.

Mr. Dexter's pneumonia turned out to be caused by **Pneumocystis carinii**. His doctors became suspicious and ordered an HIV antibody test. He had a positive HIV antibody test and, on laboratory analysis, was severely immunodeficient. His wife tested negative for the HIV antibody and so did their youngest child, who was conceived after James received the blood transfusion.

During his hospitalization, he had intermittent diarrhea; no cause was found. There was a loss of weight of about 30 pounds. Also, he developed CMV retinitis in the left eye, which left him with a 50% visual loss in that eye. He was hospitalized for a total of 6 weeks. After an emotional 3 weeks, his wife moved out and took the children with her. She made it clear she wanted a divorce.

When his wife and children left, he considered suicide. His physician recommended emotional counseling, but Mr. Dexter turned it down. After 3 months of convalescence, Mr. Dexter felt much better and wanted to return to work. He takes a short nap during the middle of the day, but feels he can work an 8-hour shift. The physician restricts him to a maximum of light work activity.

He wants to return to his previous work because he thinks he is physically fit to do the work. He is very concerned and would like to return to work to support himself and his family. He recently received a letter from the oil company terminating his employment.

## Questions

1.  What is the nature of Mr. Dexter's HIV-related disease, and what are the possible physical limitations associated with his medical condition that can influence his rehabilitation potential?

2.  What emotional limitations does Mr. Dexter have that need to be addressed during the process of rehabilitation?

3.  Discuss the social limitations of Mr. Dexter's medical condition.

4.  What is Mr. Dexter's rehabilitation potential? Discuss the possibility of return to previous work.

5.  Give a vocational profile including age category, educational level, skill and exertional level of previous work, occupationally significant characteristics, and skills. Note if any of the skills are transferable and if so, to what jobs.

# REFERENCES

Centers for Disease Control (1990). Possible transmission of human immunodeficiency virus to a patient during an invasive dental procedure. **Morbidity and Mortality Weekly Report, 39,** 489-493.

Centers for Disease Control (1987). Revision of the CDC surveillance case definition for acquired immunodeficiency syndrome. **Morbidity and Mortality Weekly Report, 36,** 1S-15S.

Centers for Disease Control (1981). Surveillance case definition for the acquired immunodeficiency syndrome. **Morbidity and Mortality Weekly Report, 30,** 305.

Cooper, D.A., Maclean, P., Finlayson, R., Michelmore, H.M., Gold., J., Donovan, B., Barnes, T.G., Brooke, P., & Penny, R. (1985). Acute AIDS retrovirus infection. Definition of a clinical illness associated with seroconversion. **Lancet, 1,** 537-540.

Curran, J.W., Morgan, W.M., Hardy, A.M., Jaffe, H.W., Darrow, W.W., & Dowdle, W.R. (1985). The epidemiology of AIDS: Current status and future prospects. **Science, 229,** 1352-1357.

Essex, M., & Kanki, P.J. (1988). The origins of the AIDS virus. **Scientific American, 259,** 64-71.

Francis, D.P., & Chin, J. (1987). The prevention of acquired immunodeficiency syndrome in the United States: An objective strategy for medicine, public health, business and the community. **Journal of the American Medical Association, 257,** 1357-1366.

Friedland, G.H. (1990). Early treatment for HIV: The time has come. New England Journal of Medicine, 322, 1000-1002.

Friedland, G.H., & Klein, R.S. (1987). Transmission of the human immunodeficiency virus. **New England Journal of Medicine, 317,** 1125-1135.

Gottlieb, M.S., Schroff, R., Schanker, H.M., Weisman, J.O., Fan, P.T., Wolf, R.A., & Saxon, A. (1981). **Pneumocystis carinii** pneumonia and mucosal candidiasis in previously healthy homosexual men: Evidence of a new acquired cellular immunodeficiency. New England Journal of Medicine, 305, 1425-1431.

Ho, D.D., Moudgil, T., & Alam, M. (1989). Quantitation of human immunodeficiency virus type 1 in the blood of infected persons. **New England Journal of Medicine, 321,** 1621-1625.

Imagawa, D.T., Lee, M.H., Wolinsky, S.M., Sano, K., Morales, F., Kwok, S.,Snisnky, J.J., Nishanian, P.G., Giergy, J., & Fahey, J.L. (1989). Human immunodeficiency virus type 1 infection in homosexual men who remain seronegative for prolonged periods. **New England Journal of Medicine, 320,** 1458-1462.

Lui, K.J., Darrow, W.W., & Rutherford, G.W. (1988). A model-based estimate of the mean incubation period for AIDS in homosexual men. **Science, 240,** 1333-1335.

Marcus, R., & Centers for Disease Control (CDC) Cooperative Needlestick Surveillance Group (1988). Surveillance of health care workers exposed to blood from patients infected with the human immunodeficiency virus. **New England Journal of Medicine, 319,** 1118-1122.

Matheson, L. (1984). **Work capacity evaluation: Interdisciplinary approach to industrial rehabilitation.** Anaheim, CA: Employment and Rehabilitation Institute of California.

Matthews, T.J., & Bolognesi, D.P. (1988). AIDS vaccines. **Scientific American, 258,** 120-127.

Peterman, T.A., & Curran, J.W. (1986). Sexual transmission of human immunodeficiency virus. **Journal of the American Medical Association, 256,** 2222-2226.

Price, R.Q., Brew, B., Sidtis, J., Rosenblum, M., Scheck, A.C., & Clearly, P. (1988). The brain in AIDS: Central nervous system HIV-1 infection and AIDS dementia complex. **Science, 239,** 586-592.

Quinn, T.C., Mann, J.M., Curran, J.W., & Piot, P. (1986). Aids in Africa: An epidemiologic paradigm. **Science, 234,** 955- 963.

Redfield, R.R., Birx, D.L., Ketter, N., Tramont, E., Polanis, V., Davis, C., Brundage, J.F., Smith, G., Johnson, S., Fowler, A., Wierzba, T., Shafferman, A., Voilvovitz, F., Oster, C., Burke, D., & The Military Medical Consortium for Applied Retroviral Research (1991). Phase I evaluation of the safety and immunogenicity of vaccination with recombinant human immunodeficiency virus infection. **New England Journal of Medicine, 324,** 1677-1687.

Salk, J. (1987). Prospects for the control of AIDS by immunizing seropositive individuals. **Nature, 327,** 473-476.

Social Security Administration (1987). **Evaluation of acquired immunodeficiency disease syndrome (AIDS) and AIDS-related complex (ARC).** Section 24525.000 et seq. Washington, DC: Author.

Snider, W.D., Simpson, D.M., Nelson, S., Gold, J.W.M., Metrolla, C.E., & Posner, J.B. (1983). Neurological complication of acquired immune deficiency syndrome: Analysis of 50 patients. **Annals of Neurology, 14,** 403-418.

Volberding, P.A., Lagakos, S.W., Koch, M.A., Pettinelli, C., Myers, M.W., Booth, D.K., Belfour, H.H., Jr., Reichman, R.C., Varlett, J.A., & Hirsch, M.S. (1990). Zidovudine in asymptomatic human immunodeficiency virus infection. A controlled trial in persons with fewer than 500 CD4 - positive cells per cubic millimeter. **New England Journal of Medicine, 322,** 941-949.

### *About the Author*

John J. Howard, M.D., M.P.H., is an Assistant Professor in the College of Medicine at the University of California, Irvine, California.

## Chapter 8

# COPING WITH PHYSICAL DISABILITY - A BIOPSYCHOSOCIAL APPROACH

by
*Carol Beardmore, Ph.D.*

## INTRODUCTION

When a catastrophic accident or a chronic, progressive disease resulting in physical disability confronts a person, the individual most typically is faced with profound life stress and crisis. While the event itself is a stressor, a crisis occurs when characteristic coping mechanisms, which already exist in the person's behavioral repertoire, are ineffective in resolving the crisis. For some individuals, having a health problem may be stressful but not necessarily create a crisis. For example, having an appendectomy may be stressful, but once the surgery is over and the person is recovering, the stress ends. A different reaction occurs when there is a catastrophic accident which results in significant and permanent disability. An example is an injury to the spinal cord that results in paraplegia or quadriplegia.

Each person is unique and responds in a different way to the stresses of life. Anxiety, depression, anger, denial, and grief are typical reactions to catastrophic injury and loss. Psychologically healthy people typically react in positive ways, while emotionally disturbed people react in unhealthy and dysfunctional ways. Appraisal of the event will influence a person's reaction to it. The meaning of the illness or injury and the person's stage of life also will determine how the individual responds (Carter & McGoldrick, 1988). An event that is devastating to one individual may not be for another.

Historically, much of the psychological literature has focused on stages of adjustment that an individual passes through in adapting to physical disability. More recently, Moos and Shaeffer (1984) have described strategies and adaptive tasks employed by people faced with acute health crises. Many people faced with acute health crises adjust in a satisfactory manner. Others become despondent and experience severe psychological sequelae. Still others experience tremendous psychological growth and are able to create an opportunity out of a catastrophic event.

This chapter addresses the biological, psychological, and social aspects of coping with a disability. The stages of emotional response to disability are described from early realization of disability through acknowledgement and adaptation. This is followed by a discussion of coping, including appraisal-focused coping, problem-focused coping, and emotion-focused coping. The chapter reviews adaptive tasks of the person who has experienced a catastrophic, disabling accident or a chronic, progressive illness including illness-related behavior and general methods of adaptation. The final section describes the role of the rehabilitation counselor and offers suggestions when working with an individual who is not adapting well to disability.

# STAGES OF EMOTIONAL RESPONSE

It may be more helpful to think of the stages of emotional response as psychological states or reactions that are part of the process of adaptation. Not every individual with a disability will experience every stage and not necessarily in this sequence. The more typical sequence is as follows (see Table 1) (Shontz, 1975):

---

## Table 1
## STAGES OF EMOTIONAL RESPONSES

**The Pre-Impact Phase**
    Substages:
        Prelude Stage - Approach
        Warning Stage - Avoidance

**The Impact Phase**
    Substages:
        Shock Stage - Detachment
        Encounter (Realization) Stage - Approach

**The Post-Impact Phase**
    Substages:
        Defensive Retreat Stage - Avoidance
        Acknowledgment Stage - Approach and Avoidance
        Adaptation Stage

---

## The Pre-Impact Phase

When the first signs and symptoms of a chronic, progressive illness occur, the individual and family try to make sense out of what is happening. The response during this period is important in that it sets the tone for later responses to the crisis. The pre-impact phase is especially applicable in the case of chronic disease where the onset may be slow and symptoms are intermittent. Two sub-stages, prelude and warning, comprise the pre-impact phase (Shontz, 1975).

**Prelude stage.** The prelude stage begins with the first indication that something is seriously wrong. The prelude phase is an attempt to approach the event by appraising it in familiar terms. For example, a person with undiagnosed rheumatoid arthritis may begin to experience increased aches, pains, fevers, and chills. The person is likely to continue life as usual, perhaps believing that it is only a temporary illness, such as the flu. As the symptoms increase, the individual becomes more aware that something serious may be occurring. The person may rationalize that the pain is due to a temporary event, such as overexertion. These reactions are realistic since early symptoms of rheumatoid arthritis may resemble the flu or physical strain. Initially, the person pays little attention to the symptoms and deals with them by using strategies that have been effective in the past.

**Warning stage.** When it becomes apparent the individual's typical mode of adaptation is inadequate, the warning stage begins. This is a transitional period where the person is reluctant to relinquish the former appraisal and coping strategies, but is also resistant to confront the reality of the situation. While the prelude stage represents an attempt to approach the situation in terms of the familiar, the warning stage is an attempt to avoid the threatening situation by employing the same coping mechanisms. The warning stage, which may overlap with the prelude stage, is ambiguous and conflicting for the individual, and produces a higher level of tension. Between denial and realization, there may occur a period of rationalization, where the individual is becoming aware of the condition, but is not ready to deal with it.

During this period, the person vacillates between the previous appraisal, rationalization, and accepting a new diagnosis. A more knowledgeable person is capable of reappraising the situation and moving more rapidly from the prelude stage, through the warning stage to the impact phase. The warning stage leaves little doubt about the serious nature of the symptoms. Once this realization is made, the impact phase begins.

## The Impact Phase

The warning stage (part of the pre-impact phase) and the impact phase are likely to overlap somewhat as long as there is some ambiguity about the diagnosis. When the crisis is acute and comes without warning, the individual will skip the pre-impact phase and enter the shock stage of the impact phase.

Often in the chronic progressive diseases, such as the rheumatic diseases and various neurological disorders, long periods elapse between the onset of symptoms and the confirmation of a definitive diagnosis. Uncertainty can be a very disconcerting period for individuals. While they know that something is definitely wrong, the answers remain unknown, and they continue to live in an ambiguous state. The impact phase, consisting of the substages of shock and encounter, begins when there is a definitive diagnosis, or when a sudden catastrophic injury occurs. While the person intellectually accepts the diagnosis, seldom are all the implications understood. Feelings of helplessness, despair, and loss may occur once there is a diagnosis and an understanding of a disabling condition or an explanation of the permanent physical limitations. Situational depression and anxiety are common.

**Shock stage.** Shock is more likely to occur in cases of sudden, traumatic onset when the crisis comes without warning, such as in spinal cord injury or sudden amputation of a limb. Shock is less likely to occur when the onset has been gradual. As an example, rheumatoid arthritis (a chronic, progressive disease) usually has a gradual onset. Patients may experience shock when first diagnosed. When symptoms have persisted for a prolonged period and the patient has been to many physicians before receiving a definitive diagnosis, the emotional reaction when told of the condition may be one of relief rather than shock. More typically, the person feels relief in having found a reason for the symptoms. Confirmation that the problem is physical and not psychological frequently brings relief. While it is helpful for health professionals to conceptualize adjustment to disability in terms of certain stages, there are exceptions.

Shontz (1975) describes shock as a depersonalized emergency reaction. During this period, the individual experiences muted emotional reactions. Rather than believing this is happening, the person may feel more like a detached observer. While this period is brief, it is striking and not easily forgotten. This is an appropriate time for the rehabilitation counselor to have initial contact with the client. It is a time for listening, establishing rapport, and forming a professional relationship. At this point, it is usually too early to begin vocational counseling.

**Encounter (realization) stage.** This is the second substage within the impact phase. At this point, the person begins to approach and recognize the reality of the situation. Realization is an emotionally painful period in which the person experiences feelings of anxiety, depression, panic, disorganization, helplessness, and loss of control. These symptoms are similar to post-traumatic stress disorder described in the American Psychiatric Association's DSM-III-R (1987). Such a diagnosis applies to some patients who have experienced events that are not typically part of the realm of usual human experiences. For example, burn survivors sometimes report flashbacks and nightmares about the accident. Reliving the impact experience provides an outlet for discharge of emotional energy. At this time, the patient fears possible death, critical loss, and unpredictable changes. Anger about the injustice of the situation and depression related to loss are also common emotional reactions.

Appropriate interventions by the rehabilitation counselor include showing empathy and understanding. The counselor can offer realistic reassurance and provide emotional support by actively listening and expressing sincere interest. It is important to remember that grieving about loss and an appropriate display of emotions are part of the healing process.

## The Post-Impact Phase

**Defensive retreat stage.** When the emotional response of realization becomes too intense and intolerable, the person may withdraw into defensive retreat. This enables avoidance of overwhelming feelings and anxiety. The defense mechanism of denial temporarily protects against this.

Defensive retreat is characterized by avoidance of reality. The person with a complete spinal cord injury may believe it will be possible to walk again. An individual with rheumatoid arthritis stops taking medications and believes there will be a sudden cure. Out of desperation, some people go to unqualified individuals and take unproven remedies that supposedly will cure their disease. Anxiety reduction, which serves as a very powerful reinforcer, perpetuates this stage.

Some patients retreat into illness. Initially, this does not pose a problem for health care providers since these patients tend to be passive and comply with treatment plans. A problem arises, however, when the time comes for active participation in a rehabilitation program.

When an injury or illness produces a crisis state, one can expect some degree of defensive retreat. Flight into health or illness serves a dual purpose (Shontz, 1975). First, it defends the individual from the continuous threat of psychological disorganization. Secondly, it allows emotional growth to take place by providing a haven for exploration of the broader implications of the crisis. During this stage, the individual will benefit from empathy, understanding, and acceptance by the health care professional who can assist the person with facing reality. The longer the denial persists, the more difficult it will be to confront the situation realistically.

The period of retreat is an inappropriate time for the rehabilitation counselor to initiate vocational rehabilitation services. Contact at this time is inappropriate in that it may create overwhelming psychological distress.

Breaking down denial prematurely may create problems with the rehabilitation counselor/client relationship. The sudden loss of denial resulting in overwhelming anxiety may be associated directly with the counselor. Consequently, the client will remember this emotional pain and may reject counseling in the future. The counselor needs to work around the anxiety and depression, be realistic and sensitive, and be careful not to destroy hope, which helps maintain motivation for rehabilitation.

**Acknowledgment stage.** Acknowledgment is the final stage, before adaptation, and involves a series of both approaches and avoidances that diminish in intensity and become increasingly longer over time. These prolonged phases allow psychological reorganization and stability to occur (Shontz, 1975). During acknowledgment, the individual gains an accurate understanding of the disability and its limitations. Both emotional and intellectual components comprise this understanding. Depression may ensue as the person grieves losses.

It is common for health care professionals to confuse depression with lack of motivation. To say a client is unmotivated is judgmental and implies that the depressed person is deliberately refusing to work. Loss of energy is one symptom of depression. Other symptoms include insomnia, poor appetite, loss of interest in usual activities, poor attention and concentration, loss of sexual desire, and inability to derive pleasure from activities. It is critical the rehabilitation counselor and other health care professionals accurately identify the signs of depression.

Some persons have suicidal ideation and intent. This can be assessed by asking directly if there have been thoughts of suicide. If there is an affirmative answer to this question, it is important to learn if there is a plan and, if so, does the person have the means to carry out the plan. Suicidal ideation is fairly common among people with disabilities. Loss of hope is highly correlated with suicidal ideation. There is a vast difference between suicidal thoughts and actions. Severely depressed persons who actively have suicidal thoughts need immediate referral to appropriate mental health professionals. Psychiatric hospitalization may be required for the individual who is contemplating suicide.

Most depression is not this severe. Sadness is a normal part of the grieving process. It is helpful to validate the client's feelings and to acknowledge the emotional reactions to loss and disability. Health care professionals are advised to show empathy, not sympathy. Empathy lets the person know the helping professional understands, while sympathy is condescending and reinforces depressive behavior. On the other hand, one should not force depression if it does not occur. A person can grieve without becoming depressed, when there is no loss of self-esteem. By setting short-term, accomplishable goals, the client can experience success. This helps alleviate depression and builds self-esteem.

With each new gain, the person may have to face another challenge. For example, the woman with rheumatoid arthritis learns to live with pain and deformity. As the disease progresses, she fatigues easily and must use a wheelchair for mobility. She notices people staring at her and assumes they are pitying her. This individual may feel despair, decide to avoid the public, and retreat to the safety of her home. If acknowledgment (a series of both approaches and avoidances) continues, she will again give up, retreat, and forge ahead with new behaviors, which may again precipitate despair and retreat. This process is ongoing. With each repetition of the cycle, the person attains a higher level of psychological organization.

If the individual fails to abandon retreat, there will be a delay of the acknowledgment stage. This occurs if the person maintains denial or adopts the sick role. If fearful of failure, the person may want to be certain of success before making an open commitment to change.

**Adaptation stage.** Adaptation occurs when the person has worked through the emotional reaction to the disability. The focus, in this stage, is on abilities rather than disabilities. This means learning to live with functional limitations while maximizing one's potential. The rehabilitation professional guides the individual to be realistic about these limitations. It is the function of the counselor to empower the client to use abilities in maximizing potential as it relates to activities of daily life and employment.


# COPING STRATEGIES


Moos and Shaeffer (1986) have organized coping strategies into three major categories (see Table 2). Appraisal-focused coping (1) is existential in nature in that there is an effort to understand and find meaning in the crisis. Problem-focused coping (2) reflects an effort to deal with the tangible reality of the situation and take active steps to make the situation more tolerable and satisfying. Emotion-focused coping (3) allows one to maintain affective homeostasis (state of equilibrium) with the ultimate goal of achieving a resigned acceptance of the disease or disability.


## Appraisal-Focused Coping


**Logical analysis and mental preparation.** This involves breaking the overwhelming aspect of the crisis into its component parts. One then focuses on one part of the crisis at a time, relies on past experience, mentally rehearses various measures that might be taken, and anticipates probable consequences. By focusing on a small manageable component, the crisis can be faced one step at a time. This is similar to the Alcoholics Anonymous belief in taking one day at a time. Recalling an instance when one was able to cope with a similar situation, helps the person build confidence. This strategy is particularly helpful when facing a difficult medical procedure.

**Table 2**
**COPING STRATEGIES**

**Appraisal-Focused Coping**
    Logical analysis and mental preparation
    Cognitive restructuring
    Cognitive avoidance or denial

**Problem-Focused Coping**
    Seeking information and support
    Taking problem-solving action
    Identifying alternative rewards

**Emotion-Focused Coping**
    Affective regulation
    Emotional discharge
    Resigned acceptance

An anticipatory mourning process takes place when preparing for an anticipated loss. It involves grieving for what is going to happen in the future and for how it will affect self-image. Anticipatory grieving will follow a pattern which may include depression, anxiety, numbness, yearning, despair, and psychological reorganization (Parks, 1986).

When a health crisis occurs, especially when there is a disease without a known cause or cure, it is helpful to find meaning in life's unpredictable and uncontrollable events. Victor Frankl (1959), an existential psychiatrist, survived the Nazi Holocaust only to discover he had lost most of his family. In his writing, he noted that those who did not give up while in the concentration camp were able to do so by finding meaning and purpose in life. Often religious faith or the belief that one will be a better person because of the crisis, helps a person cope. Some individuals believe their disease or disability teaches patience and tolerance which were lacking before the crisis.

**Cognitive restructuring** is a cognitive behavioral technique that people frequently employ. It is a method by which they alter their thinking about the catastrophic events that have occurred. Such phrases as, "It could be worse" and "I look around and see so many who are worse off than I", are examples of restructuring one's attitude about disability. Clients apply these procedures in an attempt to cope with loss. It is a method which allows the client to replace negative, self-defeating perceptions with positive self-supporting perceptions (Cormier & Cormier, 1991).

**Cognitive avoidance or denial** is similar to the previously discussed stage of defensive retreat (part of the post-impact phase). It enables the individual to minimize or deny the serious nature of the disability, serves to reduce overwhelming anxiety, and provides time to mobilize psychological strength to face difficult situations.

## Problem-Focused Coping

**Seeking information and support.** This involves becoming knowledgeable about the disease or disability. The individual gathers information about various treatments, medications, and possible surgery. One evaluates the positive and negative consequences of each. The person reads magazine and newspaper articles about the condition and questions physicians to obtain as much information as possible.

There are support groups throughout the country for most of the common disabilities. For example, the Arthritis Self-Help Course (Lorig, 1986) is a time-limited course that provides information and support to people with arthritis. It consists of six sessions and covers such topics as pain management, diet, medication, surgery, depression, stress, and relaxation techniques. The course conveys the idea that the individual exerts control over the course of the disease by the choices that are made concerning treatment options. Even though a person may have an incurable disease, control remains with the individual through the decisions and choices one makes. People can benefit from hearing how others with the same or similar diseases cope and handle problems.

**Taking problem-solving action.** This requires taking definitive steps in caring for oneself. Dressing a wound, wearing a pressure garment to reduce burn scars, daily exercises for cardiac fitness, and modifying one's home to make it wheelchair accessible are examples of tangible problem-solving action. Ability to do these tasks independently can raise one's confidence and self-esteem and help the individual compensate for losses.

**Identifying alternative rewards** involves finding short- term goals and activities that replace permanent losses and provide a source of satisfaction and accomplishment. For some persons, this involves providing information and help for others with similar disabilities. One young woman, diagnosed with rheumatoid arthritis while still in her 20s, formed a support group for those under 40 who have arthritis. Although no longer able to work because of her disease, she is active in the local Arthritis Foundation and serves on the Board of Directors.

A school teacher who is a burn survivor, designed her own reentry plan to return to the classroom after her injury. She now helps children with burns return to classroom settings using the same techniques. Working as an image consultant, she also teaches the use of corrective cosmetics to camouflage burn scars. It is her philosophy that this skill will increase self-esteem so a person is better able to face people in the community and eventually return to work. By becoming a role model for other burn survivors, this woman is pursuing activities that give additional meaning to her life.

## Emotion-Focused Coping

**Affective regulation.** This involves the ability to be in control of one's emotions and to maintain hope in the face of stressful situations. Real life systematic desensitization occurs as the person with deformity or disfigurement gradually goes out into the public, first with family, then with friends, and eventually alone. Thus, they desensitize their own and others' reactions to disability or disfigurement.

**Emotional discharge.** At the opposite continuum of affective regulation is emotional discharge. People need to vent anger, frustration, and despair. Emotional discharge may take different forms, such as emotional outbursts or non-compliance with treatment programs. Each person needs to find ways to release frustration. Following periods of acting out, people frequently experience remorse.

**Resigned acceptance.** The process is complete when the person reaches resigned acceptance (adaptation) of the situation. The individual comes to terms with the disease, disability, or deformity and learns to cope. The condition is emotionally and intellectually accepted with the realization it cannot be changed. At this point, the phases of mourning the loss of the previous self-image are complete.

Judith Viorst, in her book, **Necessary Losses** (1987) notes that, in the course of life, we leave and are left and let go of much that we love. Losing is the price we pay for living. It is also the source of much of our growth and gain. Growth occurs through the realization and acceptance of the disability. The gains achieved by the client depend on the ability to discover freedoms, choices, and opportunities, and the willingness to transform these into realities.

# ADAPTIVE TASKS

According to the principles of cognitive behavioral therapy, how an individual interprets or appraises a situation is as important as the situation itself. Consequently, how the person appraises injury, disease, and disability is likely to have as great an impact as the actual disability (Lazarus, 1981). Self-efficacy (Bandura, 1982, 1989) is the belief that individuals have the ability to succeed and to control the future by the choices they make. Such an orientation is consistent with active participation in a rehabilitation program and the determination to master tasks and goals throughout the process.

Moos and Shaeffer (1984) have delineated seven major adaptive tasks employed by people faced with acute health crises. Three of these tasks relate to illness and four are general and apply to any type of life crisis. Table 3 illustrates these major adaptive tasks (Moos & Shaeffer, 1984):

---

## Table 3
## MAJOR ADAPTIVE TASKS

### Illness-Related Adaptive Tasks

Dealing with pain, functional limitations, and other symptoms

Dealing with the hospital environment and special treatment procedures

Developing and maintaining adequate relationships with health care staff

### General Adaptive Tasks

Preserving a reasonable emotional balance by managing disturbing
feelings aroused by illness and disability

Preserving a satisfactory self-image and maintaining a sense of
mastery and competence

Sustaining relationships with family and friends

Preparing for an uncertain future

---

## Illness-Related Adaptive Tasks

**Dealing with pain, functional limitations, and other symptoms.** Pain, weakness, restrictions in mobility including paralysis, vertigo, nausea, deformity or facial disfigurement, and shortness of breath are just a few of the symptoms that may require adaptation. Anticipating a medical crisis and being able to control some of the symptoms facilitates adaptation.

**Dealing with the hospital environment and special treatment procedures.** While sophisticated medical technology is able to prolong life, in some instances the treatment or "cure" may be perceived as more traumatic than the disease or injury itself. Some surgical procedures (such as mastectomy or colostomy), the use of braces and assistive devices, and amputation involve a significant alteration of body image. Treatment for cancer, such as radiation and chemotherapy, produces side-effects such as nausea, vomiting, and loss of hair, that are extremely difficult for patients to accept. CAT (computerized axial tomography) scans and MRI (magnetic resonance imaging), state of the art imaging procedures requiring immobility and confinement in a tunnel-like space, produce claustrophobia in some individuals. Hospital and recovery rooms, intensive, surgical and critical care units, and oncology waiting rooms can be very stressful and unsettling for both patients and their families.

Separation from the family leaves the individual feeling alone, alienated, and isolated. To reduce the anxiety produced by unfamiliar medical procedures, it is helpful for hospital staff to carefully explain what will be occurring. Many people want significant others to be involved in this process. When the treatment procedure involves pain and disfigurement, it is best to be truthful and honest, while demonstrating sensitivity and concern. Knowing what to expect can have a tranquilizing effect on a patient, considering the patient's fantasy is often far worse than reality. People sense when information is being withheld and this often causes them to expect the worst.

**Developing and maintaining adequate relationships with health care staff.** During periods of hospitalization, especially following surgery or due to a disability, the patient is very dependent upon hospital staff. Having to depend on hospital staff for very basic needs may leave the patient feeling helpless and powerless (Beisser, 1989). For example, needing to use a bedpan can be degrading and demeaning. At times, when patients feel angry with nursing staff, they are reluctant to express these feelings for fear of retaliation. Asking for pain medication often becomes a major issue, especially if medical staff members become judgmental and decide the medication is not necessary. Patients may feel uncomfortable about asking questions when they do not understand medical terminology. A person who lacked confidence before hospitalization can feel intimidated by medical staff upon whom they have to depend for basic physical needs.

## General Adaptive Tasks

**Preserving a reasonable emotional balance by managing disturbing feelings aroused by illness and disability.** The person with a chronic disease or disability may experience a wide range of emotions. Anger is common and patients may ask, "Why me?" If they feel in some way responsible for their misfortune, guilt may be experienced. In trying to rationalize why this happened, especially when there is a disease with no known cause, individuals sometimes consider the disease punishment for perceived past sins. Anxiety and apprehension about an unknown future also are typical. Embarrassment may occur with altered body image. Depression and mourning frequently occur over loss of function, loss of a body part, or the inability to integrate the former sense of self with a new self-image.

Feelings of alienation and isolation also contribute to depression. Maintaining a positive attitude in the face of overwhelming misfortune is an important task for the client. The rehabilitation counselor can help the individual maintain this attitude by presenting viable career alternatives when the client is no longer able to perform the duties of previous employment.

**Preserving a satisfactory self-image and maintaining a sense of mastery and competence.** Loss of function and change in physical appearance will require the person to alter self-image. When there is visible scarring, disfigurement, or the need for assistive devices, it is also necessary to change one's body image. This may produce an "identity crisis" and necessitate an alteration in values and lifestyle. A person with noticeable facial scarring from a burn will learn to place less value on physical attractiveness. Changes in body image raise issues of sexual concern. These individuals fear they will no longer be sexually attractive or loved. Ability to grieve enables some persons to come to terms with altered body image and accept the new image.

Individuals who rely on mechanical or assistive devices also experience a change in body image. This includes people who must depend on such devices as wheelchairs, braces, splints, respirators, hemodialysis, and pacemakers. Persons with severe arthritis often have artificial joint replacements to relieve pain and improve function. Some use humor effectively to adapt to change.

A person who was independent prior to a disabling accident or illness may have difficulty adapting to a more dependent role, especially during periods of lengthy hospitalization. The patient who has been dependent while hospitalized, requires a period of transition to be more independent outside the hospital environment. Once home, there may be additional adaptation to role and lifestyle changes. People with severe disabilities need to find an acceptable balance between doing all they can within their limitations and asking for and accepting help when necessary. The person can maintain a sense of control by taking an active role in making decisions that affect the direction one's life is taking.

**Sustaining relationships with family and friends.** Physical separation from family and friends during periods of hospitalization often results in the person experiencing feelings of loneliness and alienation. The nature of one's role in the family may change as the result of functional limitations. For example, a male laborer who sustains a severe spinal cord injury will be unable to return to the same job and may have to accept that his wife will now have to help provide financial support for the family. The very traditional, older homemaker with arthritis may no longer be able to perform household tasks and may have to depend on her husband to do what she regards as her responsibility. These shifts in responsibility may result in a loss of self-esteem and lead to tension in many relationships.

Communication may be difficult. Family and friends often do not know what to say or how to behave. A person may be ashamed or embarrassed to ask for help. Yet, resentment builds up when help is not forthcoming. During hospitalization, it is beneficial for patients to form close, although temporary, relationships with hospital staff. These relationships can enhance self-esteem as the patient comes to the realization that acceptance occurs regardless of disease or disability. These relationships also enable patients to obtain information which is valuable for making decisions regarding medical care and for obtaining emotional support and reassurance.

**Preparing for an uncertain future.** Uncertainty about the future generally results in anticipatory anxiety. Loss of body parts or physical function generally results in mourning or grieving over the loss. While new medical procedures may prolong life, they alter the quality of life. The individual who focuses on remaining abilities, while putting the losses in the appropriate perspective, will be better able to proceed to the stage of adaptation. Realistic hope that future procedures or medical discoveries will restore some of the loss will enable the individual with a disability to face the future with increased hope.

# THE ROLE OF THE REHABILITATION COUNSELOR

Rehabilitation requires a holistic approach that incorporates a biopsychosocial orientation. By considering biological, psychological, and social information about the client, treatment plans can incorporate all aspects of the person's life and establish meaningful goals. Within a rehabilitation facility, the holistic approach allows the health care team, including the rehabilitation counselor, to provide maximum assistance to the client. Ideally, the client is a member of the team and integrally involved in establishing meaningful goals which also consider family and lifestyles. Included in the program is an understanding of the determinants of behavior and various coping styles. The disease state, emotional status, social, vocational, and financial factors are considered (Green, 1985).

It is extremely important for the rehabilitation counselor to become involved with the patient soon after injury or disease onset. The initial task is to form a supportive relationship and establish rapport. The counselor needs to communicate with the client at an understanding and empathic level; timing in early intervention is crucial. During periods of denial and avoidance, it is best to provide support and let the individual know vocational rehabilitation services are available. To make plans or to set short or long-term goals during these phases is usually inappropriate since it may create overwhelming anxiety by forcing the patient to acknowledge the seriousness of the condition (Wright, 1983).

Once the rehabilitation counselor establishes rapport, the next step in the counseling process is to perform a careful assessment which should consider past, present, and potential levels of functioning. Knowledge of "premorbid personality" (the personality that was present before the injury or disease) and level of psychological functioning is critical. A general psychological principle that applies in most cases is that past behavior is the best predictor of future behavior. Consequently, the best predictor of future employment potential is past psychological functioning and previous work history.

By actively listening to the patient and truly hearing what is said, the counselor can demonstrate empathy and support. This is a prerequisite for establishing rapport and developing a therapeutic relationship. It also enables the counselor to understand what the person wants and needs in the future. In this way, the counselor can collaborate with the client to establish goals. When the client is part of the goal-setting process, it provides a sense of empowerment and control. The accomplishment of these goals is more likely to occur with the involvement of the individual. Client participation and involvement with the decision-making process is vital to future success. By becoming actively involved in one's own rehabilitation process, the client recognizes there are choices to be made and that these choices will impact the future.

The counselor may be asking, "What if I let the client make the decision and the choices are unrealistic and reflect denial?" Clients may fail, especially when confronted with new and challenging situations. It may be the only way for the person to gain proper perspective and become more realistic. It does not help to accuse the client of being unrealistic and in denial. Neither does it help to predict failure. Denial will dissipate if the counselor allows the patient to learn from experience. At that time, the rehabilitation counselor and client will be ready to work collaboratively to establish more appropriate goals.

Of course, the counselor does not want to deliberately set the client up for failure. Yet, some failure may be inevitable in the initial stages of counseling. This is the time to let the individual experiment with work samples and try out new behaviors. If a crisis occurs, the counselor needs to demonstrate sensitivity. It is important to validate the client's feelings and provide emotional support.

When failure does occur, the rehabilitation counselor should not take the failure personally. Failure is part of the process by which the client truly begins to understand the functional limitations, learns to accept the disability, and begins to face reality. Counselor and client can work together to establish modest, realistic, and accomplishable goals, allowing for the experience of success.

Working collaboratively with the client requires that the counselor ask appropriate questions to determine real needs and desires. It is important to avoid making assumptions, since these are more likely to reflect the counselor's agenda than that of the client. Providing emotional support and helping the client problem-solve are key ingredients to successful intervention. The counselor can become a client advocate. If the client is working, it may be necessary to visit the workplace and meet the employer to explain special problems and issues. Working with the employer can facilitate modifying the work environment to accommodate the disability.

Behavior modification techniques are effective in easing the transition from home to workplace. Behavioral rehearsal, role playing, and modeling are useful for preparing the client to face fearful expectations and to develop appropriate behaviors currently not part of the behavioral repertoire. Fading techniques can be used in "supported employment" by sending a job coach to the place of employment with the client. The employee can gradually increase the number of working hours performed independently, while decreasing the time spent with the job coach.

Finally, the rehabilitation counselor may need to find creative and ingenious ways to help a client succeed (Yost & Corbishley, 1987). By becoming the client's advocate during the difficult and trying times, the counselor can empower the client to regain self-esteem. With the assistance of the counselor, the client can begin to achieve a sense of control over life and develop a positive self-image. The role of the rehabilitation counselor is crucial in assisting the individual with a disability to face a life crisis and return to being a productive member of society.

# CASE STUDY

The client, Mr. Sidney Donaldson, is a neat appearing 35 year-old male who suffers from rheumatoid arthritis involving multiple joints, a dermatological disorder involving the fingernails and toenails, hypertension, and a dysthymic disorder. During the initial rehabilitation counseling interview, Mr. Donaldson was articulate and knowledgeable. Although he appears to be a very sensible person, there are signs of anxiety, depression, and preoccupation with the recently diagnosed arthritis.

Mr. Donaldson describes a need for counseling and guidance, but does not express his feelings, nor give any indication as to his inner conflicts and emotions; denial and rationalization are very much in evidence. His arthritis symptoms caused him to stop working one year ago. While improved since that time, he has been advised against returning to his previous and long-held occupation of journeyman terrazo worker (D.O.T.#: 861.381-046). The treating physician restricts him to light work. Mr. Donaldson is interested in remaining in this field, but has no idea as to the type of job for which he could qualify that does not involve strenuous physical exertion, prolonged walking and standing, and emotional strain. He feels his condition will improve.

The **Dictionary of Occupational Titles** (U.S. Department of Labor, 1991) describes this job as follow:

**861.381-045 Terrazzo Worker (construction) alternate titles: artificial-marble worker; floor grinder.**

Applies cement, sand, pigment, and marble chips to floors, stairways, and cabinet fixtures to attain durable and decorative surfacing, according to specifications and drawings: spreads roofing paper on surface of foundation. Spreads mixture of sand, cement, and water over surface with trowel to form terrazzo base. Cuts metal division strips and presses them into terrazzo base so that top edges form desired design or pattern and defines level of finished floor surface. Spreads mixture of marble chips, cement, pigment, and water over terrazzo base to form finished surface, using float and trowel. Scatters marble chips over finished surface. Pushes roller over surface to imbed chips. Allows surface to dry, and pushes electric-powered surfacing machine over floor to grind and polish terrazzo surface. Grinds curved surfaces and areas inaccessible to surfacing machine, such as stairways and cabinet tops, with portable hand grinder. May precast terrazzo blocks in wooden forms. May perform finishing operations only and be designated Terrazzo Polisher (construction) (p. 897).

This job involves lifting a maximum of 50 pounds with repetitive lifting and carrying of 25 pounds. The job takes 2-4 years to learn proficiently.

Before this occupation, Mr. Donaldson worked for a large aerospace corporation, first as a lathe operator (3 years) and then as an assistant drafter (1 year). As a lathe operator he lifted and carried a maximum of 30 pounds; it took 6 months to learn this machine operator job, a job that physically required continuous standing and occasional walking. The drafter position was sedentary work activity and involved limited skills.

There is not a pressing financial problem because Mr. Donaldson receives Social Security Disability Insurance benefits, private insurance benefits, and a Veterans Administration service-connected disability pension. He is the sole source of income for his wife and their one dependent child.

Mr. Donaldson attended school through the 11th grade and went on to prepare for his GED examination while serving in the military. He was about one month from completing the requirements for the GED when he lost interest.

In addition to the medical information noted above, Mr. Donaldson has service-connected bilateral ankle injuries. Medical management of all diagnosed physical problems is excellent, according to the client. The emotional problems need intervention and treatment if Mr. Donaldson is to succeed in vocational rehabilitation.

## Questions

1. Provide a vocational profile for this client, including age category, educational level, and work history (skill levels and exertional categories).

2. As the rehabilitation counselor, what additional medical information, if any, would you like to receive?

3. Evaluate this case from the standpoint of the "Stages of Emotional Response" discussed in this chapter.

4. Discuss a holistic approach to this case incorporating a biopsychosocial orientation.

5. Describe possible rehabilitation services you will provide, including an analysis of occupationally significant characteristics as they relate to the medical conditions, and transferability of work skills.

# REFERENCES

American Psychiatric Association (1987). **Diagnostic and statistical manual of mental disorders (DSM-III-R)** (3rd ed.). Washington, DC: Author.

Bandura, A. (1982). Self-efficacy mechanism in human agency. **American Psychologist, 37,** 122-147.

Bandura, A. (1989). Human agency in social cognitive theory. **American Psychologist, 44,** 1175-1183.

Beisser, A.R. (1989) **Flying without wings: Personal reflections on being disabled.** New York: Doubleday.

Carter, B., & McGoldrick, M. (Eds.). (1988). **The changing family life cycle** (2nd ed.). New York, NY: Gardner Press.

Cormier, W.H., & Cormier, L.S. (1991). **Interviewing strategies for helpers.** Pacific Grove, CA: Brooks/Cole.

Frankl, V.E. (1959). **Man's search for meaning.** New York, NY: Pocket Books.

Green, S.A. (1985). **Mind and body: The psychology of physical illness.** Washington, DC: American Psychiatric Press.

Lazarus, A.A. (1981). The stress and coping paradigm. In C. Eisdorfer, D. Cohen, A. Kleinman, & P. Maxim (Eds.), **Theoretical bases for psychopathology.** New York: Spectrum.

Lorig, K. (1986). **Arthritis self-help course: Leader's manual and reference materials.** Atlanta, GA: Arthritis Foundation.

Moos, R.H., & Shaeffer, J.A. (1984). The crisis of physical illness: An overview and conceptual approach. In R.H. Moos (Ed.), **Coping with physical illness 2: New perspectives.** New York: Plenum Press.

Moos, R.H., & Shaeffer, J.A. (1986). Life transitions and crises: A conceptual overview. In R.H. Moos & J.A. Shaeffer (Eds.), **Coping with life crises: An integrated approach.** New York: Plenum Press.

Parks, C.M. (1986). **Bereavement: Studies of grief in adult life** (2nd ed.). London, England: Tavistock.

Shontz, F.C. (1975). **The psychological aspects of physical illness and disability.** New York, NY: Macmillan.

U.S. Department of Labor (1991). **Dictionary of occupational titles** (4th ed., revised). Washington, DC: Author.

Viorst, Judith (1987). **Necessary losses.** New York, NY:Ballantine Books.

Wright, B.A. (1983). **Physical disability - A psychosocial approach.** New York, NY: Harper & Row.

Yost, E.B., & Corbishley, M.A. (1987). **Career counseling, a psychological approach**. San Francisco, CA: Jossey-Bass.

## *About the Author*

Carol Beardmore, Ph.D., is a clinical psychologist on the Arthritis Service and the Plastic and Reconstructive Surgery Service at Rancho Los Amigos Medical Center in Downey, California.

# Chapter 9

# PLASTIC AND RECONSTRUCTIVE SURGERY

by
*Neil E. Klein, M.D.*

## INTRODUCTION

To evaluate disability properly, it is essential to understand plastic and reconstructive surgery, as this surgical subspecialty concerns itself with wound healing. To know how a wound will heal is to know, in part, how the patient will recover and the potential for return to employment. In the specialty of plastic and reconstructive surgery, the word **plastic** refers not to the use of artificial materials for surgery, but to the Greek word "plastikos" meaning to mold or shape. The plastic surgeon uses knowledge of the wound healing process to correct deformities and aid function to overcome disabilities.

Plastic surgery is a broad field that encompasses many areas of anatomy and body systems. The common denominator of wound healing expertise relates the various subunits of plastic surgery. These areas include burns, hand surgery, congenital anomalies, head and neck cancer, reconstruction of deformities and defects in all areas of the body and, perhaps best known, cosmetic surgery.

Of major concern, along with the surgical aspect, is the rehabilitation of the patient. It is not enough merely to do surgery to enhance healing, but to reestablish function and minimize limitations as well. For this reason, plastic surgeons often work closely with psychologists, physical and occupational therapists, speech therapists, rehabilitation counselors, social workers, and other professionals. On many occasions, treatment of persons needing plastic and reconstructive surgery involves the team approach. The goal of the team is to provide maximum function for the patient following injury, tumor treatment, or correction of congenital deformity.

## WOUND HEALING

Wound healing is the way the body repairs itself following a physical insult. There is no proven method to accelerate healing of a wound. Only the body can heal the wound; all the surgeon can do is remove impediments to healing. These impediments include infection, dead tissue, poor vascular (blood) supply to the injured tissues, or a general health problem of the patient that is preventing wound healing, such as a metabolic or immune disease or severe malnutrition. To help heal the wound, one must recognize the problem, correct it, and allow the body to heal itself (Peacock & Van Winkle, 1976).

The surgeon cleans and closes a simple traumatic wound. In more complex or long standing wounds, dead or severely damaged tissue must be cut away or removed by other debridement (cleaning) processes. Infection can be treated with antibiotics either systemically (by mouth or by injection) or topically (applying the antibiotic directly to the tissues).

Tumors must be surgically removed or occasionally treated with chemotherapy or radiation. The plastic and reconstructive surgeon can then treat the resulting defect or wound.

## Types of Wounds

Wounds may be classified by how they are likely to heal. A simple laceration or cut is sutured directly in a straight line and heals by primary intention. A wound that is missing tissue so that the skin edges of the wound cannot be brought together (such as the wound created by removal of a tumor, a significant burn, or a gouging type injury) heals by secondary intention. In other cases where the wound defect created by the injury is too large to heal on its own, the plastic and reconstructive surgeon may need to transfer tissue from another part of the body to cover the wound.

As previously mentioned, science is incapable of speeding the healing of wounds, but the surgeon can aid the healing process by removing impediments to healing. Significant impediments to healing, such as the physical size of the wound or the covering of tissues that wounds cannot grow easily across such as bone or bare tendon, can be aided by surgery. In these cases, wound closure can be augmented by using reconstructive techniques such as skin grafts or flaps. Again, these procedures do not speed wound healing, but simply provide the raw material needed for the body to heal itself.

## Scar and Epithelialization

**Scar.** The actual material of wound healing is scar, a specialized protein that pours into a wound shortly following injury to hold the wound together. For example, in the process of primary intention healing of a simple cut in the skin (Figure 1), the physician first cleanses the wound. The cleansing process is crucial to healing as it minimizes the chances of infection by mechanical removal of contaminants and infectious agents. Next, the physician brings together the edges of the wound, either by sutures, or by simple bandage if the wound is small. The surrounding tissue starts to attract fibroblasts, which are the cells that make collagen (Peacock & Van Winkle, 1976).

Collagen, a glue-like protein, is the chemical of scar. Figure 1 illustrates a sharply cut wound through the skin into the fat layer. In the second part of the illustration, the wound has been sutured and scar is beginning to strengthen the bonding of the wound edges. The uppermost layer of skin heals by epithelialization (production of epithelial cells), a regenerative process.

During the early days following a wound (injury), the collagen (the protein glue-like substance) is soft and weak. That is why young wounds may fall apart or pull apart if the physician removes the sutures too early. Gradually, the collagen toughens by creating more chemical bonding within itself and the scar becomes stronger. One calls this process scar maturation. For a scar to fully mature, it takes from 6 months to 2 years, depending on a person's own physiology. During this period, the scar may be red, tender, pruritic (itchy), swollen, and unsightly. As the scar matures and toughens, the metabolism within it decreases. Thus, there is less itching and swelling, and the blood supply lessens, so the redness diminishes. When the scar is fully mature, it ideally will be a fine line that is difficult to detect.

Scars do not always heal in a fine line. Some people have a physiological make-up that tends to produce unattractive or thickened scars known as hypertrophic scars or, in more severe forms, keloids. These may be aesthetically undesirable, painful, and pruritic. Also, a scar in a bad location such as across a joint may tighten and create a contracture (tightening or shrinkage) impairing motion in that joint. **Contraction** is a normal occurrence of

## Figure 1
## HEALING BY PRIMARY INTENTION

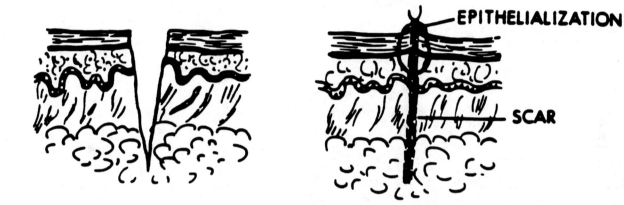

**Figures 1-7 drawn by Ms. Crista Osterberg.

scar maturation. All scars contract as they strengthen. **Contracture,** however, may be a pathological problem one sees when normal scar contraction takes place in an unfavorable location. For example, it may involve shortening of the tissues around a joint and prevent full range of motion of that joint. Scar contractures often need to be treated by therapy or surgical release. Scar contracture is a common aftereffect of burns involving joints.

**Epithelialization.** This is an important phenomenon of wound healing. Epithelialization occurs whenever a wound breaks the skin in both primary and secondary intention healing. It takes place concurrently with the early phases of scar formation in healing by primary intention. It is the process by which the top layer of skin heals itself. The uppermost layer of skin can heal itself by this regenerative process, as opposed to the deeper layers that must be repaired by the body's scarring. While the deeper layers are laying down scar, the germinal or formative cells of the skin are making new skin cells. These new cells migrate across the top of the healing wound until the approaching layers from either side touch and close the wound. This process is called epithelialization.

The germinal epithelial cells are located in the basal layer of skin and within all of the dermal elements of skin such as hair follicles, sebaceous tissue, and oil glands (Figure 2). That is why in a partial thickness or 2nd degree burn or scrape, where some deeper skin dermal elements are left behind, the skin regenerates or reepithelializes without the need for surgical closure (Figure 3). In Figure 2, normal skin is depicted. The black line designated "a" is the location of the basal cell layer or regenerative layer. This layer, as previously noted, lines the skin and all hair follicles and dermal elements.

## Figure 2
## NORMAL SKIN

Note basal layer (a) lining skin and dermal elements.

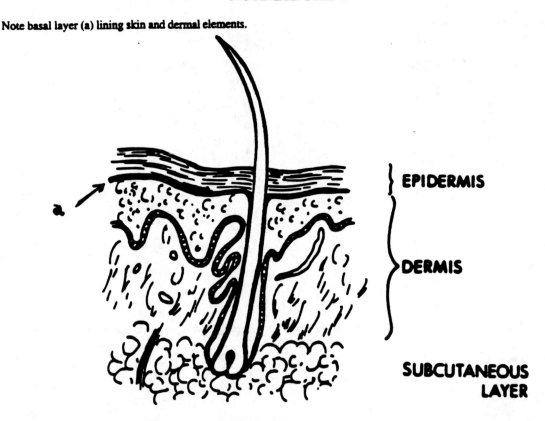

EPIDERMIS

DERMIS

SUBCUTANEOUS LAYER

Whether a wound or burn is full thickness (3rd degree) or partial thickness (2nd degree) is determined by how much of this layer is left behind (see Table 1). Visualize a scraping wound of the skin that takes away the top layers of skin down to the deep dermis or fat. Such a wound can be seen in the demonstration Figure 3A. The epithelial cells will grow from the basal layer and remaining hair follicles as seen in Figure 3B to cover the open areas healing the wound by the process of epithelialization. All skin in mammals has hair follicles or dermal elements which can provide epithelial for partial thickness injuries to heal by epithelialization. The more superficial the wound, the more dermal elements are left. That is why a superficial wound (partial thickness) will epithelialize more quickly. A very superficial wound, such as a minor scrape or "skinned knee" for example, will epithelialize so quickly there is no

# Figure 3
## EPITHELIALIZATION

Epithelial cells grow from basal layer of adjacent healthy skin and dermal elements.

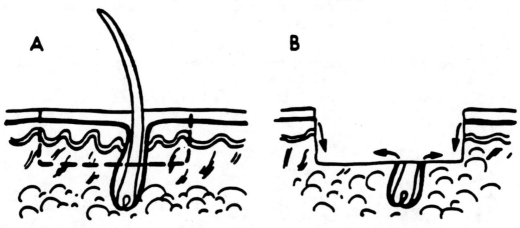

**A**

**B**

# Table 1
## CLASSIFICATION OF BURNS

| | |
|---|---|
| **Superficial**<br>(1st degree burn) | Epidermis (upper most layer) only. |
| **Partial -Thickness**<br>(2nd degree burn) | Epidermis and dermis (inner portion of the skin). |
| **Full-Thickness**<br>(3rd degree burn) | Destruction of the entire skin epidermis and dermis. |
| (4th degree burn) | Extends deeply into subcutaneous fat, muscle, bone, or deeper tissue. |

time for scar formation. Scrapes or superficial partial thickness (2nd degree) burns will heal with minimal scar or possibly no visible scar.

Healing by secondary intention may occur when there is a wound with full thickness skin loss into the subcutaneous fat or deeper layers leaving behind no dermal elements or hair follicles (Figure 4). In this situation, the scar develops similarly to what occurs in primary intention but as the sides of the wound are not together, the open wound edges cannot stick to themselves. The scar in this open wound bed will now contract as normal scar always does, but the contraction will continue until the wound edges touch.

## Figure 4
## HEALING BY SECONDARY INTENTION

Contraction of the wound

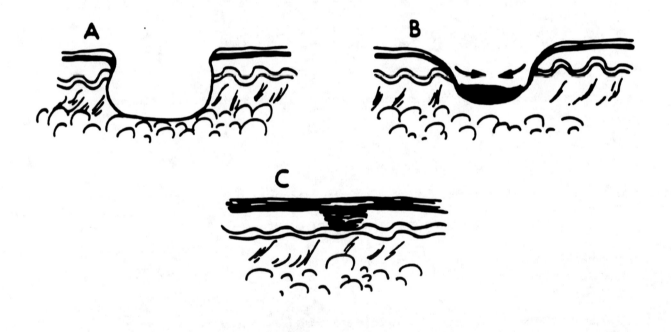

Epithelialization will occur simultaneously covering this bed of scar with a new top layer of skin; yet, the epithelium must grow from the edges only, as there are no dermal elements left in the full thickness wound, since all structures of the skin have been destroyed or removed. Examples of this type of wound are the full thickness skin loss or 3rd degree burn, or very deep gouging wound. Due to the extensive destruction of tissue and the slow nature of scar contraction, healing by secondary intention takes longer. When epithelialization takes place from the wound edges only, the healing process takes longer than if dermal elements are present within the wound, such as in a partial thickness injury.

If the wound is too large to heal by itself or if there is a physical impediment to healing such as bone in the wound, healing by secondary intention cannot occur and reconstructive surgery is required. This type of wound is said to have a defect, since it has a deficiency of tissue. It is the job of the plastic and reconstructive surgeon to identify the actual tissue deficit and decide how to close the defect by replacing the appropriate tissues.

## Surgical Closure of Wounds

The first step in closing a wound is to determine if the wound is clean and if the patient is in general good health. Infection, if present in the wound, must be treated. Dead tissue is debrided (cleaned out). Also, the patient must be metabolically capable of wound healing (Krizek, 1976). When these basic factors are under control, the surgeon assesses the wound for repair. If the wound is simple and small, the surgeon will close it directly. If it is more complex, the surgeon must determine the simplest, most effective means of wound closure. The surgeon will have to evaluate what tissue is missing and to what extent. Once these factors have been determined, one must decide on the method of wound closure. The plastic surgeon has two basic techniques available to close wounds. These are skin grafts and flaps.

## Figure 5
## SKIN GRAFTING

(A) Defect to be grafted         (B)Blood vessels from defect supply the skin graft

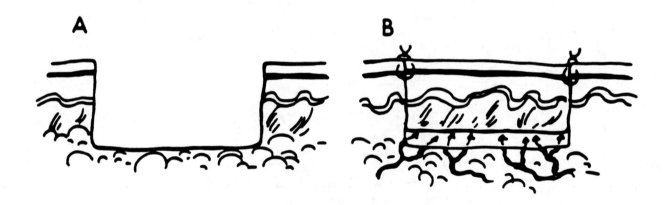

**Grafts.** If a small amount of tissue is missing, grafting can be done. A graft is tissue that is transplanted or implanted in a part of the body to repair a defect. The surgeon takes a graft from an area of the body that can spare it, known as the donor site, and transfers it to the deficient area known as the recipient site. Only tissue from one's own body may be used, except in special cases such as heart or kidney transplants. Many kinds of tissue may be grafted (McCarthy, 1990). The most common is skin. An example is skin grafting performed to cover a burn site. Other tissues commonly grafted are bone, tendon, and nerve.

A graft must be limited in its size or thickness because it takes its blood supply from the recipient site (Figure 5). Figure 5A shows a wound defect requiring a graft. Note the full thickness wound with no residual dermal elements. Here a skin graft was chosen because the wound was too large to await healing by secondary intention. Figure 5B shows the skin graft in place and the blood supply going into the donor skin from the recipient bed. Note that the skin graft itself (in the illustration) is a thin shave of skin consisting of only dermis and above layers. Full thickness skin grafting or composite tissue grafting may be done in special circumstances but require special techniques to be successful. A skin graft is very thin, on the order of 10-15 thousandths of an inch; a bone graft is merely chips of bone wherein cells grow and form a solid structural support.

---

### Figure 6
### FLAPS

A flap carries its own blood supply

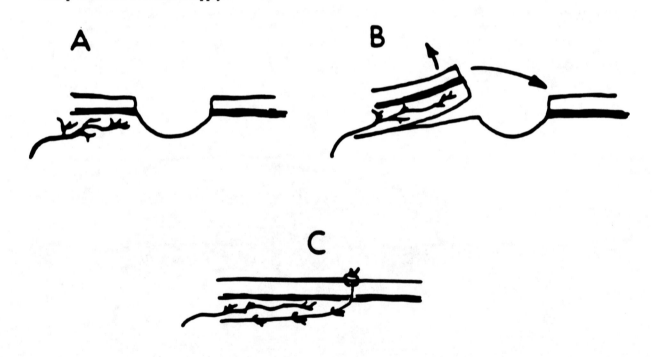

---

**Flaps.** If the surgeon needs larger quantities of donor tissue, tissue with its own blood supply (a flap) must be used. Since a flap has its own blood supply, thickness is not a problem, however, the surgery is more complex. A flap must be cut from tissue near the wound and rotated or transposed into the defect (Figure 6). In Figure 6A, a defect is seen with its nearby blood supply shown as the arborized line coming in from the left. The flap can be pictured as the tissue adjacent to the defect, as it is being freed from its bed with respect to the integrity of its blood supply (Figure 6B). Once this tissue is elevated and the surgeon is sure it is alive and healthy and unrestrained enough to move easily into the defect, the flap can be transferred and sutured over the defect (Figure 6C) and allowed to heal in its new location.

If for any reason this procedure cannot be performed (e.g., the local tissue is too scarred to use), the surgeon must resort to a very complex microsurgical technique called a free flap procedure (Figure 7). In free flap surgery, the surgeon proceeds only when the following criteria are met:

## Figure 7
## FREE FLAPS

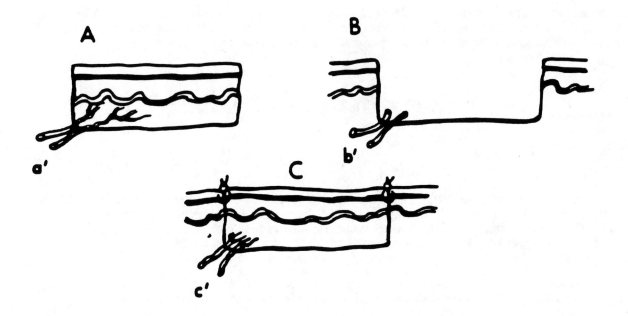

(A) Free flap taken from distant donor site with its blood supply (a' supplying artery and draining vein)
(B) Recipient site and recipient artery and vein (b')
(C) Anastamosis (connecting of hollow tubes or vessels) (c') of artery and vein with flap sutured in place

1. the donor site can spare the tissue

2. the artery bringing blood into the tissue and the vein draining the tissue can be identified

3. an artery and vein of appropriate size can be identified near the recipient site.

After the criteria are met, the surgeon attaches the free flap's blood vessels to the recipient vessels using microsurgery (Figure 7C). The surgeon will use this donor tissue for the reconstruction, assured that the donor tissue will now survive at the new site.

A simple wound will probably have sutures in place from 2 days to 2 weeks, depending on the site and the tension placed on the wound edges. The acute discomfort from an injury usually lasts only a few days, but immature wounds often may be swollen or scars may be tender for much longer periods of time. Wounds near joints may need prolonged immobilization to prevent separation.

Skin grafts frequently require about one week to ensure growth of the blood supply from the recipient bed into the new skin. The donor site, from which the thin layers of skin was shared, may take as long as 2-3 weeks to reepithelialize. Complex grafts or flaps may require several days to weeks of hospitalization and healing time is dependent on location, size of defects, and type of tissue replaced.

After the wound is strong enough to allow the person to use the injured part, the rehabilitation counselor may begin intervention. As each patient is different, it is important to communicate regularly with the surgeon to check on the progress of healing. Medical complications can occur at any time, but are less likely as time elapses.


# SPECIFIC AREAS OF WOUND HEALING


## Burns

A burn can be devastating in its effect. Emotional, physical, and socio-economic ramifications can alter a patient's life in catastrophic proportions. We classify burns as full thickness or 3rd degree when all layers of the skin are destroyed. Figure 8 illustrates pathological scar contractures secondary to full thickness burns. Partial thickness or 2nd degree burns, depending on the depth, leave dermal elements to allow reepithelialization. Burns are 1st degree if superficial and cause only reddening of the skin with rarely any serious sequelae.

Burns may be caused by fire, electricity, or contact with hot substances that transmit heat. Chemical burns may result in similar wounds, but also are associated with special problems particular to the damaging chemical.

After assessment of depth, the physician evaluates the amount of the body damaged. This is often expressed as a percentage of total body surface area. While the total body surface area percentage burn is important in evaluating a disability, it must be remembered that a small area of burn may result in a severe disability if an important structure is injured. If the burn affects a hand, foot, eye, or face, the consequences may be severe. Even a small burn on the face that causes no functional damage may distort the features or leave a scar that causes serious emotional problems which cannot be ignored.

# Figure 8

Pathological scar contractures secondary to full-thickness (3rd degree) burns.

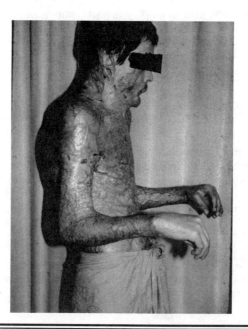

Large body surface area burns may involve many body systems and cause the patient's death. Survivors of such burns will have lived through weeks to months in the hospital, enduring many surgical procedures just to remove the dead tissue and cover the defects with skin. The problem of coverage is compounded when a patient has a large burn and much less healthy skin available for grafting. Long periods of time are required to allow for healing until donor sites can be reharvested (used again). Remember, the surgeon can use only the person's own tissues for grafts or flaps. Skin taken from other human donors or animals may be helpful for temporary coverage but cannot be left in place as it will be rejected by the body.

Hospitalization consists of painful debridements, prolonged periods of immobility, concern about survival, and anxiety about the future. Depression and other emotional problems may complicate recovery by diminishing motivation. Even after these problems are resolved, many patients will need further surgery to reconstruct areas that were postponed while life-saving measures were taken. Scar contractures that limit function need surgical release and skin grafting. Compressive garments may then be prescribed for months to years (Carle Medical Communications, 1989). Pressure garments apply compression to healing surfaces and may flatten these, providing some comfort to symptoms of immature scars. Physical deformities, facial scarring, loss of self-esteem, and other factors complicate the life of the survivor of a major burn. The recovering burn survivor requires a compassionate long-term approach to therapy. Some permanent disability is invariably present.

Smaller burns are, of course, less of a problem but often the stigma of scarring may complicate an apparently simple burn. The surgeon always considers psychosocial effects of scars on the face or hands when evaluating patients following seemingly minor burns. If the burn occurs on a child, the surgeon may make different decisions than if the burn occurs on an adult (Carvajal & Parks, 1988; McLaughlin, 1990).

## Hand

Another chapter in this book discusses hand surgery, which is a sub-specialty of plastic and reconstructive surgery. The surgeon's skill must combine a knowledge of healing with the need to preserve function. A hand that does not move and lacks strength restricts gainful employment. Principles of wound healing must be matched with medical and surgical techniques to allow as much range of motion as possible in moving anatomical structures. Tissues need to heal and yet move and glide, as in tendons, or flex as in joints. The surgeon uses knowledge of scar chemistry and properties of healing to achieve maximum return of function. Many professionals consider this field of endeavor the essence of wound healing.

## Congenital Anomalies

When helping children with congenital anomalies, the plastic and reconstructive surgeon may work in many areas of the body. These areas include cleft lip and palate, hand anomalies, congenital problems of the trunk, anomalies of the genitalia, among other problems. The surgeon first identifies the deficiency and then assesses how to repair it and what tissues will be used. The cleft lip may have a small or large deficiency of tissue. The surgeon accurately measures the defect and uses local tissues to match skin color and texture. Plastic surgeons treat major anomalies of the head and neck as well. These involve combined cranio-facial surgeries that may revise the facial skeleton, and procedures that enter the brain cavity of the skull.

In hand anomalies, function is all important. Children often learn to compensate for disability at an early age and usually develop skills that allow them to function even prior to a surgeon's intervention. These adapted skills have to be taken into consideration when planning surgical corrections.

## General Reconstructive Surgery

Head and neck tumors, skin cancer, and breast diseases are also treated in the field of plastic and reconstructive surgery. The principles remain the same: remove the tumor, identify the defect, and use proven techniques to replace or reconstruct deficiencies.

The plastic and reconstructive surgeon evaluates and treats deficiencies and defects of the abdominal wall and of the extremities. Osteomyelitis (infection of the bone) of the leg may occur following open fractures, as often seen in the tibia. This chronic disease is resistant to treatment and challenges the skills of the surgeon, as it is very difficult to eradicate. In addition, the lower part of the leg presents a difficult area of the body to cover with a flap. The lack of local tissue for use in flaps frequently requires free flap surgery. Scar from injury and infection invariably complicates surgery. Yet, modern reconstructive surgery has turned a once near hopeless medical problem into a highly manageable and treatable condition.

## Cosmetic Surgery

No writing on plastic and reconstructive surgery is complete without the mention of cosmetic surgery. Once thought of as the province of the wealthy and vain, cosmetic surgery is now widely accepted in our culture. As people realize that disability is often a function of how we perceive ourselves, surgery to aid self-esteem has become more acceptable and popular. The plastic and reconstructive surgeon uses the same skills and knowledge acquired in the healing of those with major deformities to treat aesthetic problems.

These may be problems of the aging face or deformities of the nose, cheeks, or chin. Breasts can be made larger, smaller, or more shapely; body contouring with liposuction, and abdominoplasty or thigh and buttock lifts are common. As with reconstructive surgery, cosmetic surgery is designed to attain the physical as well as the emotional well-being of the patient.

# FUNCTIONAL LIMITATIONS

Functional limitations can be classified as both physical and emotional. The physical limitations are often easier to assess, yet, the emotional or psychological are of equal importance.

## *Physical Limitations*

As stated at the beginning of this chapter, plastic surgeons work closely with other professionals, using a team approach to treatment. An individual needing plastic and reconstructive surgery will frequently have major physical disabilities. The goal of the team is to provide maximum restoration of function.

Individuals with lower extremity problems may have limitations in ambulation. Often, surgical intervention can restore some function, but other individuals will have limitations in standing, walking, climbing, and carrying weights. The rehabilitation counselor must be aware, understand, and plan within these limitations. When functional limitations are not clearly addressed in medical reports, it is appropriate for the counselor to contact the treating physician for clarification.

There are a number of conditions that can result in functional limitations of the upper extremities. These can affect manual dexterity, fine eye-hand coordination, lifting and carrying, and similar activities. A contracture involves tightening of tissue around a joint and may limit full range of motion of the affected joint. The development of a contracture limits range of motion, and results in functional limitation in physical activity. The reconstructive surgeon attempts to minimize contracture and thereby maximize function. At the point when the rehabilitation counselor and client begin to establish vocational goals, the counselor may benefit from consultation with the treating physician. For example, if limitations of movement of the hands caused by contracture are interfering with a specific vocational goal, the physician may be able to increase functions to a certain needed movement through minor surgical intervention. As part of the overall treatment, the physician also prescribes additional physical or occupational therapy.

There is a common tendency in severe burns to form contractures. The burn survivor may be required to wear compression garments up to 2 years following injury to minimize both contracture and scarring. These garments are hot and uncomfortable. Additionally, they are strange and unusual in appearance. The counselor can comfort these clients in their physical and emotional adjustment to these unnatural appearing garments that are crucial to medical rehabilitation (Carle Medical Communications, 1989; Colmano & Tempereau, 1989).

## *Emotional Complications*

Treatment of the psychological impact of severe disability and disfigurement is an important aspect of the rehabilitation process. The surgeon must be sensitive to the psychological and social factors involved in the individual case. Some individuals will need referral for psychological counseling to help alleviate depression and anxiety. These emotional symptoms can persist long after achievement of the surgical goals (Felton, Perkins, & Lewin, 1966).

Many months of medical isolation to prevent infection may lead to social isolation from family, friends, and the community. This situation may further aggravate the emotional impact of the injury on the individual. The impact of this separation is often overlooked or minimized (McLaughlin, 1990).

Additionally, the reactions of a person may not be proportional to the severity of the injury. Relatively small injuries or disfigurements may result in serious psychosocial disability (McLaughlin, 1990; Wright, 1983). In providing services to a variety of clients, counselors need to remember there is no correlation between the amount of disability and the person's reaction to that disability.

Persons with clearly visible, severe disfigurement may have become socially isolated as a result; education or work may be disrupted. In these cases, restoration of self-image is as important as the physical aspects of reconstruction (Colmano & Tempereau, 1989; Irons & Irons, 1989; Wright, 1983).

Colmano and Tempereau (1989) described factors that tend to help patients recover emotionally from severe burns and disfigurement. These individuals typically fear the loss of independence, re-entering society, and being viewed in public. The authors recommend patients be treated by a multidisciplinary treatment team since these professionals must address patients' emotional, spiritual, and physical needs in a holistic manner.

Because of the immediate and often life-threatening medical needs of the patient, professionals providing treatment often overlook the patient's personal feelings and emotional concerns (Irons & Irons, 1989). A part of the rehabilitation function of the counselor is to be aware of and deal with the emotional concerns of the individual. Early intervention on the part of the counselor can provide timely and necessary support in the vocational and psychosocial readjustment process. Much of the counselor's time in the early intervention phase of rehabilitation may be well spent in helping the person rebuild self-esteem and confidence and in eliminating destructive and negative ideas of self-perception.

# REHABILITATION POTENTIAL

One of the primary purposes of plastic and reconstructive surgery is to restore function. Clearly, medical and surgical restoration to the best functional capacity can lead to a decrease in functional limitations and thus improve the individual's rehabilitation potential. Plastic and reconstructive surgery may help to minimize disfigurement and assist the person in adjustment to disability and interacting with the public.

Rehabilitation potential for individuals who have had plastic or reconstructive surgery varies, depending on the area of the body affected and the extent of functional limitations that remain. Both the counselor and client can work together to develop a rehabilitation plan emphasizing the person's abilities while considering the limitations.

An individual who has had reconstructive surgery and is proceeding in vocational rehabilitation may well have gone through a long period of intense physical and emotional upheaval. The procedures are often painful, complicated, and difficult, and the net results less than a return of normal function or appearance. The counselor needs patience and empathy in working with an individual who has recently experienced loss of function or disfigurement.

The person who has survived severe burns frequently may have unrealized rehabilitation potential. As previously noted, persons who have had severe burns may need to wear compressive garments for up to 2 years, in order to minimize scarring. These garments, especially when worn on the face and arms, create a challenge not only to the client, but to the rehabilitation counselor as well. Most of these individuals do not return to work during this time because of the reactions of other people to the appearance of these garments. The counselor may need to be actively involved with potential employers in explaining the nature and purpose of the garments. For people wearing gloves, manual dexterity is affected and the individual must be careful not to use substances that will damage the gloves as they are expensive and not easy to replace. The face mask may seem threatening and make jobs dealing with the public difficult or inappropriate.

Many persons with severe facial disfigurement due to burns stay at home because of fear of the reaction of others. Potential referrals can be found through interaction with local burn centers and hospitals providing care for individuals with severe burns. The counselor may need to take a proactive position and meet these individuals in the hospital or the home to discuss the benefits of rehabilitation services. These people often have surprising rehabilitation potential and could benefit from provision of vocational services.

The multidisciplinary approach to catastrophic injury is most effective in maximizing rehabilitation potential. It has become more common practice to have a rehabilitation counselor on the "team," which includes physicians, nurses, physical therapists, occupational therapists, recreation therapists, social workers, and psychologists. Through this type of early intervention, the person can more easily visualize the goal of returning to work as quickly as possible. This approach will also assist the person with catastrophic injury to achieve independence that is so crucial in the total rehabilitation process.

The counselor can serve as a bridge between the person and the current or potential employer. Potential employers must be sensitive to and understand such aspects as recovery time, possibilities of multiple surgeries, functional limitations, the wearing of pressure garments, and reasonable accommodation.

Some individuals, despite severe disfigurement, still want to work with the public; others would rather avoid public contact. The counselor through understanding of the feelings of the individual, can carefully provide appropriate guidance and support toward a realistic occupational goal. The client's desires and goals must always be given primary and serious consideration when developing rehabilitation possibilities.

## Summary

In evaluation of people with deformities and resulting disabilities, understanding the role of plastic and reconstructive surgery is essential. The knowledge of how wounds heal will allow the rehabilitation counselor to be better informed when dealing with the treating physicians and surgeons, more accurate in predicting work status and disability, and more understanding in dealing with clients. Each client is unique with different physiological and psychological characteristics. When evaluating the person who has had or is currently undergoing plastic or reconstructive surgery, the counselor must take all of these factors into consideration.

# CASE STUDY

Mr. Ricardo Hernandez is a 22 year-old male who, while attempting to prime a carburetor with gasoline, had his shirt and coat catch fire. He suffered deep partial-thickness (2nd degree) and full-thickness (3rd degree) burns over 33% of his body. These burns involved his trunk from the waist up, both arms and hands, face, and neck. Treatment at a burn center required 3 months of hospitalization. Mr. Hernandez has contractures of his hands, elbows, and axillae. The facial features are deformed and there are contractures around the mouth, preventing full opening of the mouth. The physicians have kept his eyes closed to prevent the lids from scarring open. There is distortion of facial features, including the nose which has been partially burned away. Fifty percent of his scalp has been burned causing baldness.

Mr. Hernandez was an apprentice baker prior to the injury, and is married with one son, 3 years of age. He completed the eleventh grade and a training program in baking. For the last month, he has been home from the hospital. There has just been a medical and vocational rehabilitation staff consultation with Mr. Hernandez, his wife, and child. Following careful interviews and assessment by all team members, the following problems are observed.

## I. Physical problems

Both eyes bandaged due to scar contractures of the upper and lower eyelids.

Perioral scar contracture of the mouth.

Deformity of the nose.

Flexion contracture of the neck.

Alopecia (baldness) 50% of the scalp.

Scar contractures flexion of the interphalangeal joints of both hands, all digits.

First webspace contracture of both thumbs.

Flexion contracture of both elbows.

Contracture of both axillae, anterior and posterior.

## II. Emotional problems

Anxiety and depression.

Inability to sleep regularly.

Impotence.

Fears he will be unable to see when his eye bandages are removed.

Concerns regarding inability to use his hands or return to work and earn a living.

Inability to keep up with rent payments.

Family seems more distant.

His son is frightened of him.

Has had thoughts of suicide.

The plastic and reconstructive surgeon has come up with a plan for surgical intervention. It is felt that after three surgical procedures, the top priority physical problems will be markedly improved.

## Questions

1. When should rehabilitation counseling begin?

2. Outline a vocational profile for this individual including age category, educational level, work history (exertional and skill levels), occupationally significant characteristics, and transferable skills, if any.

3. What types of employment positions will be available assuming Mr. Hernandez will have marked residual decreases in strength and range of motion of the hands and arms?

4. What can be done to accommodate his facial disfigurement which will be severe, even following the most favorable surgical outcome?

5. How can the rehabilitation counselor help Ricardo deal with his compressive garments and compressive facial mask?

6. How can the rehabilitation counselor help Mr. Hernandez with his emotional problems?

# REFERENCES

Carle Medical Communications (1989). **Remodeling the scars: A burn patients' guide to compression garments** [Videotape]. Urbana, IL: Author.

Carvajal, H.F., & Parks, D.H. (1988). **Burns in children: Pediatric burn management.** Chicago, IL: Year Book Medical Publishers.

Colmano, M. (Director), & Tempereau, M. (Producer) (1989). **Reservoirs of strength: A burn recovery film** [Videotape]. North Hollywood, CA: The B.P. Company.

Felton, J.S., Perkins, D.C., & Lewin, M. (1966). **A survey of medicine and medical practice for the rehabilitation counselor.** Washington, DC: U.S. Department of Health, Education, and Welfare.

Irons, E., & Irons, T.R. (1989). Counseling for the catastrophically disabled: A critical need in the medical model. **Journal of Applied Rehabilitation Counseling, 20,** 39-41.

Krizek, T.J. (1976). **Symposium on basic science in plastic surgery** (Vol. 15). St. Louis, MO: C.V. Mosby.

McCarthy, J.G. (Ed.). (1990). **Plastic surgery** (Vol. 1). Philadelphia, PA: W.B. Saunders.

McLaughlin, E.G. (1990). **Critical care of the burn patient: A case study approach.** Rockville, MD: Aspen.

Peacock, E.E., & Van Winkle, W. (1976). **Wound repair** (2nd ed.). Philadelphia, PA: W.B. Saunders.

Wright, B.A. (1983). **Physical disability - A psychosocial approach** (2nd ed.). New York: Harper and Row.

## About the Author

Neil E. Klein, M.D., F.A.C.S., is a plastic and reconstructive surgeon in private practice and the Chief of the Medical Staff at Downey Community Hospital in Downey, California. He is an Assistant Professor of Surgery at the University of Southern California in Los Angeles, California, and the former Chairperson of the Division of Plastic Surgery at Rancho Los Amigos Medical Center, a Los Angeles County rehabilitation facility.

# Chapter 10

# IMAGE OF PEOPLE WITH VISIBLE DISFIGUREMENT AND DISABILITIES

by
*Barbara Kammerer-Quayle, M.A.*

## THE MASTER PASSION, THE HUNGER FOR SELF-APPROVAL

*Time somebody told me*
*That I am lovely, good and real*
*That my beauty could make hearts stand still*
*It's time somebody told me*
*That my love is so complete*
*That my mind is quick and full of wit*
*That my loving is just too good to quit*
*Time somebody told me*
*How much they want and need me*
*How much my spirit helps set them free*
*How much my eyes shine full of the white light*
*How good it feels to hold me tight*
*Time somebody told me*
*So I had a talk with myself*
*just me--nobody else*
*Cause it was time somebody told me.*

-by C. Tillery Banks (date and source unknown).

# THE TOTAL IMAGE CENTER

As a result of personal rehabilitation experience (the author had severe burns from an automobile accident that occurred in 1977) and years of learning and personal growth regarding image enhancement and communication, I began the first hospital-based "Center for Image Enhancement" in the United States. A healthy body image is essential to a positive self-concept and self-esteem. Corrective cosmetics, color analysis, clothing coordination, and STEPS to self-esteem are offered to adults, teens, and children with disfigurements and disabilities.

State agencies recognize the importance of the Center for Image Enhancement to the future of patients; the center has received many honors and awards. Results of research projects and oral presentations are well received at national and international meetings. More importantly, training on this subject is presented to assist other medical centers to begin similar programs to aid their rehabilitation of patients. The goals of the program include supporting rehabilitation centers throughout the United States to adopt this therapeutic intervention as a standard.

A facial disfigurement, whether congenital or acquired, causes a disadvantage in terms of one's ease of movement in social situations, in school, and in the workplace. In general, those with disfigurement have a diminished quality of life. Disfigurement is often given less significance and importance in rehabilitation because it is regarded as cosmetic and not functional. Disfigurement causes as much of an impairment in one's life as does a functional impairment (Dion, Berscheild, & Walster, 1972; Elks, 1990).

# APPEARANCE ENHANCEMENT: A VITAL NEED

It is crucial that rehabilitation professionals address the vital impact of appearance and the improvement of self-image of people with facial and other disfigurements and disabilities. Appearance and image are frequently avoided or ignored by counselors and other helping professionals. They may be uncomfortable due to a societal value system that gives appearance great importance. They also may not possess the skills or expertise to appropriately advise individuals with disfigurement. A person's appearance is an important factor which determines how one interacts with society. Society often judges facial and bodily disfigurement by an implied standard of how people "should" look and what is considered "normal." Therapists and the public need greater understanding of how to help people cope and develop skills in this area.

Because we live in a society in which personal appearance makes a difference in the reactions we receive from others, there is a need for programs focusing on the enhancement of appearance and self-esteem. According to various writers (Dion, Berscheild, & Walster, 1972; Elks, 1990; Macgregor, 1979), we live in a world in which a person's face serves as a criterion of the person. Society has stereotypes that suggest that "desired" facial configuration, features, and expressions also indicate such qualities as acceptable personality, intelligence, character traits, and temperament. People who are seen as physically attractive are also viewed as more socially desirable, likely to find better employment, marry earlier, have more successful marriages, and be better parents. These factors influence us in our response and our interactions with persons who have disfigurement.

The person whose facial and bodily features deviate from the norm not only receives differential treatment, but often becomes the object of negative judgments and prejudice. Social acceptability of one's appearance is a major goal for a person with any disfigurement. The importance of social acceptance is basic to the establishment of normal peer relationships, healthy psychological adjustment, and success in school and career.

Reconstructive and plastic surgery greatly improves the appearance of individuals with traumatic disfigurement or congenital birth abnormality. Yet, restoring an individual's face to perfect symmetry and uniform skin tones is often impossible. For many, it will mean only a change from conspicuously unattractive to less conspicuously unattractive. Any person with disfigurement often experiences conscious and unconscious expectations of rejection.

Initial encounters with other people is a critical time for a person with disfigurement. These interactions offer the greatest social vulnerability and possibilities of rejection. The support of family and friends is beneficial and, at times, crucial during the adjustment process.

# GOALS OF REHABILITATION

No easy answers or perfect solutions prevail for the complications surrounding a disfigurement. Macgregor (1979) states the primary goal of rehabilitation is to prevent potentially devastating social and psychological consequences. The first step is to seek early treatment from a plastic and reconstructive surgeon to minimize the damage. Second, both patient and family need to access the support and guidance of professionals familiar with emotional stress problems caused by disfigurement or disability. Third, society needs educational programs to dispel the myths and misconceptions about the causes of facial anomalies, and the notions that link them with negative character traits. A fourth goal, which involves the core of human interaction, is the need for modification of societal attitudes and responses toward those who happen to look different.

A successful attitude change is difficult because society equates disfigurement with imperfection, which often results in responses of fear, rejection, or discomfort. We live in a society dedicated to "first impressions"; these frequently create false judgments.

Research shows that most people react negatively to facial disfigurement (Dion, Berscheild, & Walster, 1972; Kleck & Stenta, 1985). Graham and Kligman (1987), noted pioneers in the psychology of cosmetic treatment, suggested that rejection by society of individuals with facial disfigurement is more drastic than for individuals with functional impairment. The needs of the latter group are usually more easily accepted and understood. Canfield (1989) believes that through our actions, we are constantly teaching others how to respond to us. This author suggests if we do not like how people respond to us, we need to change our message by behaving in more positive ways.

Given societal prejudices regarding visible disfigurement and disability, a goal of rehabilitation for a person with disfigurement or disability is to establish a positive and attractive outer image and a positive self-esteem or inner image. The field of rehabilitation seldom focuses on the subject of appearance. Counselors may have feelings of inadequacy about the right approach to take with clients, due to a lack of training regarding image and communication skills.

Those involved with the rehabilitation of clients with either facial disfigurement or physical disability must examine these issues. People spend a significant amount of money yearly to enhance their outer image for a variety of reasons. Some people want to look their best to promote themselves in the work place. Others strive to interact more effectively in social situations; still others attempt to achieve higher self-worth. Books, classes, and audio and video tapes are available on "dressing for success," "power dressing," "creating your professional image" and "building greater self-esteem." The able-bodied and "the beautiful people" enroll by the thousands to learn concepts and techniques that bring rewards from an attractive personal appearance and effective communication skills.

Appearance enhancement techniques include general grooming, diet, exercise, hair styles, nail care, eye wear, corrective cosmetics, color analysis, dental care, plastic surgery, clothing and accessories, posture, voice training, and eye contact. To include these skills within the rehabilitation programs of persons with facial disfigurement and physical disability is essential for optimal results.

# A PERSONAL EXPERIENCE

As a burn survivor since 1977, I have had first hand experience that many people with facial disfigurement encounter. While in the acute care phase of burn treatment, the primary aim is survival. The recovery or rehabilitation phase begins with the reality of what a facial disfigurement means in terms of interacting with the public. People react with a combination of fear, curiosity, rejection, and avoidance.

The residuals of my burn left me facially disfigured and disabled in the use of my hands. I quickly realized I had lost the image I once had of myself, both internally and externally. Soon, I learned the difficulties and the diminished value I possessed because of my disfigurement and physical disability. How does one create a new image? I desired an image I liked and one that enabled me to mainstream comfortably through life. This was not an issue addressed within any forms of therapy, except psychotherapy. Being included was my goal and the techniques and tools to reach it were left to me to discover.

## Coping with the Public

I remember episodes in restaurants when individuals would stare so intently that even direct eye contact would not deter them. Occasionally, I would spontaneously wave at a person to break the constant gaze. People sometimes would get up and move if I occupied a seat next to them in a waiting area. Others chose to stand if the only available seating was next to me. And then there were comments such as "You can take off the mask, Halloween is over," "Is she going to be okay?" and "Mommy, Mommy, look at that lady's face!"

While some people seemed somewhat unaffected by my facial disfigurement, others had visible reactions such as double-takes, shocked expressions, or rapid turns in another direction to avoid any contact. Many reacted in a negative way to touching my hands.

Because of the burn injury, the fingers on my right hand were amputated and the fingers on my left hand are misshapen. Some people avoid shaking my right hand which I am capable of and prefer. I have learned to be assertive in this gesture, although it is a bit awkward. When beginning to dance, a few men have grasped my wrist and not my hand, to lead me. I feel both shocked and hurt when this occurs and assume they are either very sensitive and afraid they may hurt my hand or very uncomfortable and fearful about touching my hand. It is necessary to explain that it is all right to touch my hand, and I place it in my partner's hand so it is not extended like an unwanted part of my body.

There were times when I felt as if men looked past me or through me as if I were not present. It was a terrible feeling, and I remembered that before my injury, this would never have happened.

## Communicating a Positive Image

I wanted desperately to "fit in" and look as attractive as possible. Even during the reconstructive surgery process and the wearing of pressure garments on my face and body to minimize scarring, I still wanted to look my best. Though I felt extremely insecure, I did not want others to know. I wanted people to realize that beyond the disfigurement, there was a real person who is worth knowing.

Only a small percentage of communication is verbal. According to most experts in this field, 95% of communication is nonverbal and has more influence on people than what is communicated verbally. Our facial expressions, eyes and mouth movements, how we sit, stand, or walk, arm and hand gestures, and the volume and intonation of our voice convey messages beyond the words that we speak. There are "techniques and tools" of communication that make a difference in interactions and responses and give power and confidence that can change the quality of relationships and life.

# DEVELOPING STEPS TO SELF-ESTEEM

## Posture

The "techniques and tools" of communicating a positive self-image have made my life easier. I intentionally walk with my rib cage lifted and my head up to allow my **posture** to convey confidence. By slumping my shoulders and leaning my head downward, people assume I do not like myself and am uncomfortable about my appearance. To some degree, both are true, but clearly not the message I want to convey.

## Eye Contact

Another "technique" I incorporate into daily life is the positive influence of **eye contact**. Whether dealing with a waitress in a restaurant, a clerk in a department store, or an attendant at a gas station, I look straight into the person's eyes as I speak to them. When I connect with another's eyes, the two of us interact more easily and comfortably. When an individual looks away or down to avoid another person's eyes, the message communicated is that the person is ill at ease and not comfortable. I have observed many situations and various reactions of the public to my disfigurement and disability, and realize I have a large role to play in the responses I receive from others. A person can influence acceptance or rejection by others.

## Tone of Voice

Another "technique" I find helpful is **tone of voice**. When I speak in a warm, enthusiastic, and confident tone, people seem to relax and feel at ease. No one enjoys listening to a person who speaks in a weak, self-effacing monotone voice. The intonation used when speaking influences a listener's response to the message. If people feel I am comfortable with myself, they can relax and react authentically.

## Smile

Proverbs, song lyrics, and advertising slogans all advocate a smile. Some of these include "let a smile be your umbrella" or "a smile is the lighting system of the face and the heating of the heart."

The power of a **smile** is overwhelming. An individual with facial disfigurement or physical disability who smiles has a great advantage. A smile can dispel the fears of strangers, eliminate apprehensions, and communicate the message of being approachable, loveable, and all right. For those with facial scarring, a smile softens the appearance of the face and diminishes the effect of the scars. In many situations, a smile can break barriers or end stigmas that may exist.

In a practical sense, a smile used as a behavioral technique can produce positive results, lift the spirits, and increase one's energy and self-esteem. Stand in front of a bathroom mirror without a smile on your face and look at your image steadily for 30 seconds. Now, change your facial expression to your friendliest and warmest smile and again look at your image steadily for 30 seconds. You will notice a difference in how vibrant and radiant you look and how much more energetic and alive you feel. A smile seems to improve not only our appearance, but our feelings.

Some people still look at me a little too long for comfort. An effective method to break their gaze and diminish my discomfort has been to look directly into the person's eyes and smile sincerely and warmly. The result always amazes me and seems like magic. This is a powerful behavioral skill to teach people during their re-entry into society.

"Men are disturbed, not by things, but by the view they take of them." (Epictetus).

The behavioral "techniques and tools" of communication that I learned - posture, eye contact, tone of voice, and a smile - are incorporated into a patient program entitled "STEPS to Self-Esteem" (see Figure 1).

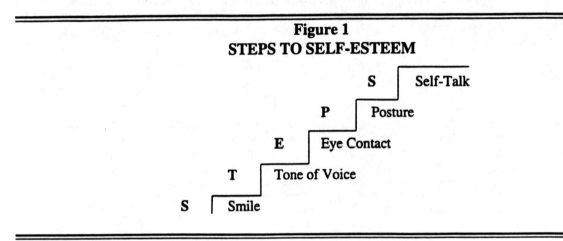

**Figure 1**
**STEPS TO SELF-ESTEEM**

S — Self-Talk
P — Posture
E — Eye Contact
T — Tone of Voice
S — Smile

## Self-Talk

The final S in **STEPS** represents **self-talk**. Self-talk is the constant conversation we have about ourselves and our circumstances throughout the day and has a direct affect on how we act and feel. The result is always the same - the things we say to ourselves determine how we live our lives.

For those who have a disfigurement or disability, this model (STEPS) program is basic to a successful rehabilitation program. It is not just the task of psychologists to begin and to continue to use this model, but all health care professionals can incorporate it into their work with patients.

According to Ellis (1973), a rational-emotive therapist, there are other factors at work that determine emotional and behavioral responses to life situations that influence our thoughts and belief systems. The words we use are extremely powerful in meaning and in the concepts and emotions they evoke. Slaikeu and Lawhood (1985) called these words and the emotions they conjure, "self-talk." Self-talk is a powerful force at work in our lives. It seems wise to understand it and use it to our advantage - especially in times of crisis.

**Positive self-talk: A rehabilitation essential.** Self-talk has permeated such fields as psychology, neuropsychology, education, and psychiatry. It is recognized as a powerful force for self-transformation. An essential strategy of rehabilitation is to enable people to build in a new manner and on a foundation that perhaps they previously lacked. When persons are in the crisis period, realizing their physical mobility may be limited or their body will be disfigured, life looks negative. Self-talk at this time reflects negative thinking and feeling. Changing their thoughts to positive ones will produce a positive change in feelings and behaviors. How people think about themselves, their therapies, and their future, directly affects how they act and feel.

**Self-talk awareness.** Every phase of rehabilitation can benefit from repeated positive thoughts and images; it gives individuals a chance to begin thinking and acting in ways that are more conducive to an optimal outcome. Positive self-talk starts with a statement that clarifies the goal of the individual to overcome a situation and learn from it. Early in recovery from a disabling event, individuals often use self-defeating phrases such as, "I can't do it!"

"I'm too afraid," "It's impossible," or "I'll never be able to go on." Phrases like these keep one in a hopeless and helpless situation. To change this verbalization of negative thinking, rehabilitation counselors must be conscious of its impact and incorporate self-talk awareness into therapy sessions. Within every recovery process, there is an opportunity to develop, learn new skills, and rebuild and live fully in ways not previously perceived.

When a crisis occurs, everything associated with it is usually negative. My crises have more often than not marked a new course for my life, which is more fulfilling and more exciting than anything in the past. The special features of the crisis include being suddenly cut off from past patterns, habits, and interdependencies. Along with the distress and pain is freedom... "freedom to build again with a new foundation and modern structure using wisdom you didn't have the last time you built" (Furnas, 1981). The above quote is by a noted plastic and reconstructive surgeon, Dr. David W. Furnas, and is his response regarding a crisis in his own life. These words provide strength and a new perspective to an individual facing a life crisis. We see clearly that it is not what happens to us in life, but our attitude and our self-talk regarding what happens.

Using empowering statements regularly such as "I'm getting stronger every day!" "I can do it!" or "I will be home again" (if hospitalized), will produce effective and lasting results. This process of recovery requires a committed interdisciplinary approach by rehabilitation therapists.

**Positive imagery.** An effective interdisciplinary approach is the use of positive self-talk coupled with the use of positive imagery. Self-talk uses the left side of the brain (the language center), while mental images make use of the right side (the image center). Sports psychology uses these techniques extensively with athletes to improve individual and team ability. Similar techniques can be incorporated into rehabilitation programs to maximize results for patients (Gawain, 1978).

Cousins (1979), Simonton (1978), Siegel (1989), and other researchers have done work on the mind/body connection and its affect on health and well-being. Some evidence exists that these approaches produce positive results for cancer, arthritis, asthma, and other chronic illnesses. Although not empirically proven, rehabilitation clients may benefit from use of these approaches.

# CORRECTIVE COSMETICS: AN ADJUNCT TO PLASTIC SURGERY

## *Corrective Cosmetics as a Therapeutic Tool*

This can be a therapeutic aid for both the person with disfigurement and the individual with a physical disability. When a change in appearance occurs, an individual often suffers both psychological and social damage. Although plastic and reconstructive surgery can often rebuild the facial features, such as ears, nose, and eyelids, there are limitations. Perfect symmetry is usually not possible. Often, skin discoloration from scars and suture lines cannot be corrected surgically. At this point, corrective cosmetic techniques can improve the overall appearance.

As previously stated, Graham and Kligman (1987) suggested that people with facial disfigurement suffer more rejection than people with functional impairment. The needs of the latter group are usually more easily accepted and understood. Many individuals give greater significance to cosmetic results than to increased functioning. In other words, how I look may have a greater impact than what I can do.

Through our actions, we are constantly teaching others how to respond to us. Canfield (1989) suggested that by thinking and behaving in a positive manner, we will influence how other people respond to us. Graham and Kligman (1987), and Canfield (1989) make a strong case for learning corrective cosmetic techniques to aid the facially disfigured.

Most burn centers and rehabilitation programs give minimal concern to, or overlook, corrective cosmetics. Much of the neglect in this area has been through not having information or the resources to obtain this information. Recently, cosmetic companies have been producing a variety of corrective cosmetic products. Training courses are available to teach techniques to "normalize" the appearance of persons with visible disfigurement and physical disability.

Research indicates the important psychological benefits for the cosmetic user. Use of cosmetics provides a beneficial effect on how others perceive a person and on self-perception (Graham & Juochar, 1981). If the general population receives benefits from cosmetic makeup, persons with facial disfigurement may receive even greater benefits.

**Corrective cosmetics and the consumer.** The consumer will find cosmetic products to conceal imperfections in the skin caused by either trauma, disease, or birth anomaly. Some examples of imperfections are birthmarks, cleft lip, scarring due to burn injuries or other accidents, vitiligo, lupus, scleroderma, hemangioma, and cancer. Terms such as paramedical, camouflage, concealer, and cover color all refer to corrective cosmetics.

A corrective cosmetic differs from standard liquid makeup in its increased opaque consistency. This serves to completely cover even the most extreme discoloration. It adheres to the skin better than normal liquid foundation products. It has a major limitation in its inability to correct the third dimensional element of a scar. It cannot change the raised areas of scars, nor the depressed or pitted areas.

## Creating a Normalized Appearance

Because of my facial disfigurement, I had a stronger need and desire to "fit in" with the rest of society. Besides the scar lines from numerous skin grafts, uneven skin tones presented a challenge. Careful application of a corrective cosmetic product enabled me to create one color for my skin. By using makeup that had the appropriate undertone for my skin color, I also looked healthier.

**Eyebrows.** The burn injury also left me without eyebrows and an asymmetrical lip line. I learned to draw feather-like strokes with a special slim-line mechanical eyebrow pencil to give the illusion of the fine hair of eyebrows. This technique takes some practice but, once mastered, provides a natural appearance that adds to facial symmetry. When an individual has consistent color of skin and the facial features others do, moving about in public places becomes easier and more comfortable. People seem to more frequently notice when a facial feature is missing. Another positive result is increased confidence and self-esteem.

Figure 2 are pictures of two individuals before the application of corrective cosmetics and subsequent to the application of makeup. Both these people suffered burn injuries.

Learning to enhance and bring attention to more attractive features also reduces the focus on scarred areas. Since eyes are a center of communication, application of eye makeup enhances and draws the viewer's attention to the eyes. Eye makeup applied moderately in the correct subtle tones creates harmony and balance to the face. The compliment should be "you look well today" not "your eye makeup is pretty."

**Lip line.** Creating a symmetrical lip line requires a three-step process. The first is to apply a corrective cosmetic product to cover any scarred areas. Second, use of a mechanical lip pencil to draw an even lip line creates a symmetrical mouth. The final step is application of a lip color that harmonizes with facial tones.

Providing rehabilitation clients with this type of intervention can increase self-esteem and motivate them toward a successful transition into the community and work place. Greater long-term progress for individuals may result from making a cosmetic program an integral part of the rehabilitation strategy. These techniques are used for both women and men.

# Figure 2
## APPLICATION OF CORRECTIVE COSMETICS

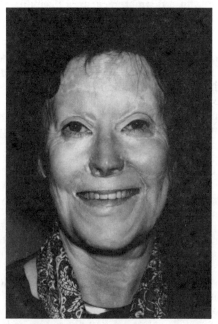

Picture without makeup

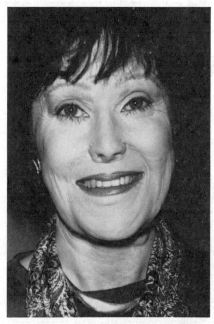

Picture with corrective cosmetics

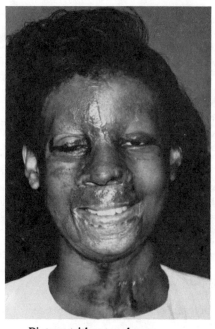

Picture without makeup

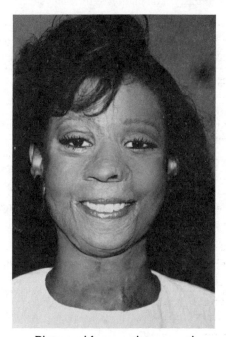

Picture with corrective cosmetics

## Color Analysis to Create Harmony

An additional dimension to enhance the appearance of a person with a disfigurement or a disability is **color analysis**. A trained consultant determines what colors of clothing will make a person look the healthiest and create a sense of well-being and confidence.

**Psychological impact of color**. The fields of advertising, the automotive industry, home furnishings, food and restaurants, and fashions recognize the influence of color and its importance as a vital tool. Color wields such strength that, according to the Wagner Institute for Color Research, color alone comprises 60% of a customer's decision to purchase an item. Quality, craftsmanship, cost, guarantee, reliability, and other factors account for the remaining 40% (Wagner, 1988). In addition, research substantiates the psychological impact of color. Colors cause us to experience calm or anxiety, move slowly or quickly, purchase or reject products, and show a healthy, radiant or an unhealthy, lifeless appearance.

The use of colors is a rehabilitation tool for people with disabilities and disfigurements. Colors that do not harmonize with the undertones of the skin and the colors of hair and eyes cause the scars on the face to be highly accentuated. When colors are draped around the face and shoulders that harmonize with skin tone, hair and eyes, the scarring appears less pronounced and less visible. The scars are then not the primary focus.

**Enhancing appearance**. Pinckney (1984), an international expert in the field of color analysis, states that the colors worn (particularly near the face) can create an optimal appearance and an inner feeling of well-being. The colors that best enhance one's appearance are based on a seasonal concept of wardrobe planning. Pinckney, who is also a pioneer in the field of wardrobe analysis, divides colors into two types: warm and cool. The warm or cool concept is the universal basis for all color systems and theories. An individual can wear any color; it is the coolness or warmness as well as the darkness and lightness of the color that makes the difference. Color analysis uses a system of seasonal names (winter, summer, spring, and autumn) to divide colors. The colors are first divided by undertones. Winter and summer possess a blue undertone, while spring and autumn possess a yellow undertone. The colors are divided again based on clarity. Winter and spring are vivid and clear; summer and autumn are dusty and muted.

The message from color analysis is that people can wear any color and look satisfactory. Color analysis technology, however, enables a person to go from satisfactory to outstanding. The seasonal color concept in wardrobe selection offers other benefits besides looking and feeling better. This approach saves time and money by allowing an individual to purchase clothing that not only looks well on them, but also coordinates with other wardrobe pieces.

Throughout the country, a variety of people utilize the seasonal color concept approach to wardrobe planning. Professionals in many fields of work from sales and the corporate world to medicine and education use this technique to feel and look their best. With this knowledge available, people who have disfigurement or disability can add to self-esteem and influence how others respond to them. Wagner (1988) believes color is an important element in personal presentation and is often the first characteristic people see.

A person with a scarred, paralyzed body, or with an amputation will need time to accept this new state and learn to feel comfortable and self-confident. The feelings that individuals had about their bodies before the alteration will dramatically influence how they experience their bodies afterward.

In the world of rehabilitation, professionals give primary significance to a person's transition from hospital to community. They help individuals develop new images of themselves and resolve the losses of former self-image. This has both psychological and social implications.

## Clothing Coordination Techniques

Before my burn injury, I was proud of my proportions, weight, and general muscle tone. After the burn injury changed the color and texture of my skin, I felt my body was unacceptable. Because of scarring on my back and arms due to the burns and scarring on my legs from skin used as donor sites, I felt limited in the clothing I could or would wear. I wanted to wear long sleeves in winter and summer to hide my scars. Pants covered the scars on my legs and occasionally, if I wore opaque hose, I would venture into a skirt or dress. My statement clearly indicated I did not love my body and wanted to hide it. There were no programs available at that time to help me enhance my image through corrective cosmetics and clothing coordination.

A healthy body image is essential to healthy self-esteem. Acceptance of a new self requires time, work, and healing. Eventually, I saw the scars as only a small part of who I am. Then, I ventured into short sleeves, skirts, sheer hose, shorts, and finally, a bathing suit. I learned the clothes I chose to wear gave me and others a distinct message about how I felt toward myself. I consciously learned to project a clear image that said who I was and that I liked myself.

Individuals can learn to use **clothes** to their advantage to create their best image, and to send a positive message about themselves. The public often concludes they have an accurate picture of an individual based on the message clothing transmits.

## Controlling the Non-Verbal Message

Since only 5% of our communication is verbal, according to Jack Canfield (1989), a national self-esteem expert, the greatest message we send to others is nonverbal. Besides the message we project with corrective cosmetics, color, clothing, and the STEPS to Self-Esteem, we also send other messages with hair, eyeglasses, nails, shoes, teeth, and general grooming.

To create an image of health, vitality, and harmony demands learning new skills and using them to meet specific goals. These skills enhance an individual's attractiveness.

Some people feel it is shallow to be concerned about image and how one looks. They believe a person should not care what others think of their outer image. This concept is unrealistic. Experts on this subject (Canfield, 1989; Dion, Berscheild, & Walster, 1972; Elks, 1990) concluded that people do pass judgment on others based upon initial impressions. In rehabilitation facilities and in the public, I have frequently seen individuals with disfigurements and disabilities wearing clothes, colors, and hair styles that say, "I do not feel good about myself, why bother." If people do not feel good and secure about themselves, it is revealed in many other ways. They do not project confidence, are not spontaneous, and are withdrawn.

Whether able-bodied or disabled, we are constantly teaching others how to respond to us through nonverbal communication. From my personal and professional experience, I have seen lives improve because the message being communicated has changed. The impact of image enhancement can create a more positive inner and external image for persons with disability or disfigurement. Rehabilitation counselors can help provide these important skills and behaviors through appropriate referrals and by learning these skills themselves.

Health care professionals who model healthy living habits, positive communication skills, and image enhancement techniques will have a greater impact on their clients. They will model, teach, and support clients in creating healthy, positive images and in developing positive self-esteem, coping skills, and attractive images.

# REFERENCES

Canfield, J. (1989). **How to build self-esteem** (audio cassette seminar). Pacific Palisades, CA: Self-Esteem Seminars.

Cousins, N. (1979). **Anatomy of an illness**. New York, NY: W.W. Norton.

Dion, K., Berscheild, E., & Walster, E. (1972). What is beautiful is good. **Journal of Personality and Social Psychology, 24**, 285-290.

Elks, M. (1990). Another look at facial disfigurement. **Journal of Rehabilitation, 56**, 36-40.

Ellis, A. (1973). **Humanistic psychotherapy**. New York, NY: McGraw-Hill.

Furnas, D.W. (1989). **Who's who, in America** (45th ed, Vol. I, p. 1070). Chicago, IL: Marquis Who's Who.

Gawain, S. (1978). **Creative visualization**. Mill Valley, CA: Whatever Publishing Company.

Graham, J.A., & Kligman, A. (1987). Cosmetic therapy for the patient with facial disfigurement. **Ear, Nose, and Throat Journal, 66**, 43-48.

Graham, J.A., & Juochar, A.J. (1981). **International Journal of Cosmetic Sciences, 3**, 197-208.

Kleck, R.E., & Stenta, A.C. (1985). Physical deviance and the perception of social outcomes. In J.A. Graham & A. Kligman (Eds.), **The psychology of cosmetic treatment** (pp. 161-179). New York, NY: Praeger.

Macgregor, F.C. (1979). **After plastic surgery: Adaptation and adjustment**. New York, NY: F. Bergin.

Pinckney, G. (1984). **New image for women**. Washington, DC: Acroplis Books.

Siegel, B. (1989). **Peace, love, and healing**. New York: Harper and Row.

Simonton, C., (1978). **Getting well again**. New York, NY:Bantam Books.

Slaikeu, K., & Lawhood, S. (1985). **The phoenix factor: Surviving and growing through personal crisis**. Boston, MA: Houghton Mifflin.

Stoop, D. (1982). **Self-talk: Key to personal growth**. Old Tappan, NJ: Fleming H. Revell.

Wagner, C. (1988). **The Wagner color response report**. Santa Barbara, CA: Wagner Institute for Color Research.

## *About the Author*

Barbara Kammerer-Quayle, M.A., directs the Center for Image Enhancement and School Reentry Program at Rancho Los Amigos Medical Center in Downey, California. She has a Masters degree in counseling psychology and a teaching credential, and is also a qualified corrective cosmetic, color, and image consultant. The California Governor's Committee for Employment of Disabled Persons awarded her the Governor's Trophy in 1988, and in 1989, she was inducted into the Governor's Hall of Fame for People with Disabilities.

# Chapter 11

# PSYCHIATRIC DISABILITIES

by
*Kathryn D. Bishop, Ph.D.*
*and*
*Mary A. Falvey, Ph.D.*

## INTRODUCTION

This chapter includes a basic overview of common psychiatric disabilities and a description of a service delivery model intended to meet the vocational needs of individuals with long-term mental illness. Specifically, a description of four main diagnostic categories and accompanying behaviors will be discussed with a historical perspective of treatment or intervention strategies commonly practiced with people who have mental illness. This chapter describes characteristics of effective rehabilitation services for this population and how supported employment, as a service delivery option, is used as an effective rehabilitation strategy for individuals with long-term mental illness.

Four main diagnostic categories of psychiatric disabilities discussed include psychoses, neuroses, personality disorders, and common "other" examples of disorders. Each of these categories are defined and discussed briefly to familiarize the rehabilitation counselor with common terminology and symptoms experienced by clients with specific diagnoses. It is important to realize that, although an individual might be given a specific diagnosis, the person will have a unique history of life experiences, symptoms, treatments, and support systems. This unique history means no two individuals will have the same rehabilitation needs despite similar diagnoses or symptom manifestations. Anthony and Jansen (1984) stressed that diagnosis and vocational outcome are not necessarily correlated. Diagnosis should be used to determine the **medical** eligibility for service and not to predict the likelihood of success. Each client needs to be treated as an individual and provided with support specific to individual needs, not a diagnostic label.

## Psychoses

**Schizophrenia.** One describes a diagnosis of a psychotic disorder as a loss of identification with reality. Schizophrenia, one psychotic disorder, is characterized by extreme distortions of reality. Some prominent features of schizophrenia include retreat from reality, emotional blunting, and disturbed thinking, varying in severity from individual to individual (Atwood & Chester, 1987). Manifestations of schizophrenia may include hallucinations, delusions, withdrawal, loss of self-control, and bizarre behavior. Schizophrenia is estimated to affect 1% of the population in the United States and constitutes the largest group of diagnosed individuals. About 50% of those reside in psychiatric hospitals (President's Commission on Mental Health, 1987). Schizophrenia is a serious condition and affects social, emotional, vocational functioning, and causes great individual discomfort.

Professionals often treat individuals diagnosed as having schizophrenia with psychoactive drugs. The complexity of this disorder, and the range of severity and manifestations paired with the infancy of the psychopharmacological field, result in inconsistent outcomes of drug-related treatments. Side effects from specific drugs or drug combinations may complicate the individual's daily functioning. In some cases, drug therapy successfully facilitates a person's ability to gain stability and function more independently in the community. The rehabilitation counselor must be familiar with a client's prescribed medications and encourage correct and consistent use of those medications.

**Affective disorders.** This is another common category of psychoses. Disturbances of mood characterize the affective disorders. An individual may experience a unipolar disorder, either manic or depressive, or a bipolar disorder of both manic and depressive experiences at different times. Manic episodes include an extreme **increase** in thought processes and activity, whereas depressive episodes result in an extreme **decrease** in thought processes and activity. An episode of a specific affective disorder can last from a few weeks to a year and is usually recurring. The episodes can be recognized through behavior reflecting sheer joy, unending energy, and inflated self-esteem with mania, to utter sadness, complete loss of energy, and feelings of worthlessness with depression. People with affective disorders are frequently treated with medications.

## Neuroses

Neuroses are similar to psychoses except that they are milder in nature and the person remains in contact with reality. Anxiety, obsessive-compulsive behaviors, and phobias are common types of neuroses. The pattern of any of these neuroses will vary greatly among individuals and from episode to episode. Some people may experience neuroses at a level not considered a severe disability and may not be eligible for vocational rehabilitation services. What one person experiences through a specific type of neurosis may be entirely different than what another person experiences with the same type of neurosis.

**Anxiety.** Anxiety is often classified as either a generalized anxiety disorder or a panic disorder. One usually experiences anxiety on a daily basis. Symptoms may consist of loss of sleep and appetite, rapid heart rate, dizziness and fainting, tremors, diarrhea, vomiting, tension, and general uneasiness (Atwood & Chester, 1987). People with this disorder seem unable to relax and focus incessantly on real or imagined mistakes, regrets, and worries and anticipation of potential future problems. Individuals having a generalized anxiety disorder may feel socially, emotionally, and vocationally inadequate.

**Panic disorders.** These disorders are less chronic in nature and more acute. A person with a panic attack may experience extreme terror or apprehensiveness for a few minutes to a few hours. These panic attacks manifest themselves without any obvious cause or warning.

Besides the possible physical symptoms of increased heart rate, difficulty in breathing, profuse sweating, chest pains, and an imminent feeling of death, the individual experiences a loss of control. A combination of the powerful physical reactions and the intense psychological disturbances lead to a tremendously terrifying experience for the individual. The frequency of the attacks vary among individuals but can range from several times a day to less than once a month. The fact that attacks can come at any time and that the individual anticipates disaster, may result in a reluctance to leave the security of home or a safe, familiar place.

**Obsessive-compulsive disorders.** People with obsessive-compulsive disorders think thoughts they do not want to or behave in ways they do not want. Although these people recognize the behavior as bizarre, unhealthy, illegal, or irrational, they cannot control it. Obsessive thoughts seem to come from nowhere and may focus on a variety of topics. The individual may not always act out obsessive thoughts, but the thoughts disturb the person and impede the ability to function in everyday life activities. Compulsive behavior is repetitive and ritualistic in nature, and although perceived as bizarre, seems purposeful. Often, compulsive behavior is designed to prevent the occurrence in actuality of the obsessive thought. For example, an individual may obsess on the thought of burning the house down. The person may then spend hours a day ritualistically unplugging appliances, rechecking stove switches, testing smoke detectors, and watering down the roof of the house. Although the individual does not experience pleasure from the behavior, there occurs a temporary reduction in tension.

**Phobias.** A phobia is an extreme, irrational fear, which greatly affects and interferes with a person's life. Although all people have certain fears that affect behavior, an individual diagnosed as phobic experiences a fear or fears to such an irrational extent that life becomes seriously disrupted. Phobias are classified as either simple, social, or agoraphobia.

Simple phobias include a fear of objects, situations, or conditions (e.g., certain animals, heights, or diseases). Social phobias are fears of social situations such as public engagements, dates, and meeting new people. Agoraphobia is a fear of leaving a familiar setting and an intense fear of open spaces. These phobias may result in physical and emotional symptoms similar to those experienced in panic attacks. The difference one experiences is that phobias are in relation to specific stimuli and panic attacks are random and unpredictable. Without support, the fears or avoidance behaviors may dominate the individual's life.

## Personality Disorders

Personality disorders are categorized as disturbances of behavior rather than as symptoms. Personality disorders, as all psychiatric disabilities, are complex, diverse, and not well understood. A personality disorder diagnosis can be based on inflexible or maladaptive personality traits that can lead to serious impairment in social and vocational functioning. Although some individuals may have one specific type of personality disorder, multiple diagnoses, or personality disorders may be evident based upon predominant personality traits. Personality disorders may be paired with mood disorders. The specific expression of the personality disorder should be of greater concern to the rehabilitation professional than the specific diagnosis. Knowledge of the disability manifestations will help the counselor provide the appropriate support toward the goal of successful employment.

**Antisocial personality disorders.** A diagnosis of antisocial personality disorder most likely means an individual displays overt, negative behavior, which disrupts those around the person. A person diagnosed as having an antisocial personality disorder for example, appears to need immediate self-gratification even at the expense of others. Although they possess much personal charm, they seem to have an undeveloped conscience and, therefore, consistently exhibit antisocial behaviors that persist.

**Passive-aggressive and passive-dependent personalities.** These disorders also belong in this category. As the label implies, individuals who have these personality disorders exhibit aggressive or dependent behaviors through passive means. For example, a person who is passive-aggressive may express extreme dislike for a particular job through blatant inefficiency. People who experience personality disorders may or may not be aware of their behaviors and the purposes they serve.

**Borderline personality disorders.** These involve basic identity disturbances that can be related to self-image, gender identity, or goals (Webb, DiClemente, Johnstone, Sanders & Perley, 1981). A person with a borderline personality disorder most likely has a long history of chronicity. Symptoms might include lack of anger control, impulsive and self-damaging acts, and intensely unstable interpersonal relationships. After reviewing several studies on predicting global outcome for people with a diagnosis of borderline personality disorder, Paris (1988) found there is a consistent lack of predictability of outcome. The documented lack of deterioration and lack of improvement should serve as encouragement for the rehabilitation counselor to focus on individual needs and means of support as opposed to methods of treatment.

## Other Common Disabilities

Post-traumatic stress syndrome, substance abuse, eating disorders, and sexual dysfunction also may be considered psychiatric disabilities. An individual who experiences one of these disabilities may demonstrate how someone, who at one point was exhibiting behaviors that were considered appropriate and adaptive, can change their pattern and have serious maladaptive problems. Although each of these disabilities is unique in nature, this unofficial group of diagnoses may have the potential for the most complete recovery in the sense of becoming symptom free.

For example, an individual who is a substance abuser may receive successful detoxification treatment and be free from abuse-related behaviors, whereas a person with schizophrenia may have a lifelong condition. It is important to realize, however, that while some disorders may seem milder in nature, they can still serve to interfere seriously with the everyday life of the individual.

## Value of Diagnoses

Although it is of value for rehabilitation counselors and other service providers to have a basic understanding of clinical diagnoses, the role of the counselor is to provide the most appropriate support for the client and individual needs. The important aspect is not to know everything about a specific diagnosis but to know as much as one can about a specific individual. The clinical perspective on psychiatric disabilities is limited in its ability to describe, predict, and treat individuals in a common fashion. As rehabilitation counselors, it is important to maintain contact with all professionals involved with the client and maintain a focus of providing support within the community and in an employment setting. Individuals may not be completely symptom free.

Clients do not have to be cured (i.e., symptom free) to benefit from effective rehabilitation services. Practitioners may need special attitudes, knowledge, and skills to enhance the full employment potential of each individual (Danley, Rogers & Nevas (in press)).

# HISTORICAL PERSPECTIVE OF SERVICES

## Normalization

During the mid-1800s, citizens concerned with societal well-being began advocating for segregation of people with psychiatric disabilities. The intent of this segregation was two-fold. First, was the perceived need to protect society from people considered deviant. Second, there was the perception that individuals considered deviant should be protected from the potential harassment and abuse of the insensitive majority in society. In response to these well-intended concerns, public policy developed institutions to house and care for individuals with severe disabilities of all types, including mental and physical.

It was not until the 1960s that a philosophical shift began to occur that called for the recognition of the value and dignity of all human beings. Basic to this philosophy was the principle of normalization. Wolfensberger (1972) introduced the principle of normalization to the United States and defined the goal of normalization as supporting individuals with disabilities to achieve those "traits, behaviors, appearances, roles, and statuses that a society considers to be appropriate and desirable in different social contexts and situations" (Flynn & Nitsch, 1980, p. 5). To achieve the goals of normalization, individuals with disabilities need the same opportunities, experiences, and routines afforded nondisabled persons. Two main components of normalization essential to the achievement of this goal are **integration** and **status**.

**Integration.** One achieves integration through physical proximity (physical integration) and voluntary interaction (social integration) with nondisabled people in fully accessible environments. Ideally, integration results in the development of ongoing personal interactions, which will vary in nature from casual acquaintances to intimate relationships.

**Status.** The second component of the principle of normalization is status. Status is defined by a person's roles and responsibilities and the success of meeting the specific demands involved in these areas. Wolfensberger (1980) emphasized one determines and measures status by members of a specific society based upon the values of that society. One achieves status by successfully assuming and maintaining roles and responsibilities the society values.

In order for people with disabilities to meet the goals for normalization, a major shift of focus in service delivery was necessary.

## Employment

An outcome of the shifting focus in service delivery was to provide vocational rehabilitation services to people with disabilities in hopes of achieving employment outcomes. For people with psychiatric disabilities, this focus on employment outcomes was slower than for people with developmental disabilities, such as mental retardation. Campbell (1989) stated that treatment programs for people with psychiatric disabilities, although non-institutionalized, stressed an overall level of wellness and social independence and not employment.

**Social independence and well-being.** The goal of creating social independence and well-being without a focus on employment is nearly impossible in contemporary American society. Work is a normalized, valued part of our society, and according to Kiernan and Stark (1986), is an essential component of the well-being of adults in this society. Anthony and Blanch (1987) supported this notion by pointing out that the "symptoms of chronic unemployment, i.e., social withdrawal, passivity, lethargy, and isolation, seem to mirror some of the symptoms of a chronic mental impairment" (p. 5).

**Work history.** The vocational history of people with psychiatric disabilities is dismal at best. Anthony and Blanch (1987) generously estimated 15% of people with serious psychiatric disabilities are competitively employed part or full-time. Another factor in unemployment may be a potential pattern of professional interventions and treatments, which can possibly inhibit successful outcomes. In a review of research attempting to predict the vocational capacity of people with chronic psychiatric disabilities, Anthony and Jansen (1984) drew the following conclusions:

1. "Psychiatric symptomatology is a poor predictor of future work performance" (p. 538). Specific symptoms or symptom patterns, therefore, have no direct bearing on potential work performance.

2. "Diagnostic category is a poor predictor of future work performance" (p. 539). One's capacity to work is not correlated with a specific diagnosis.

3. "Intelligence, aptitude, and personality tests are a poor predictor of future work performance" (p. 539). Traditional methods of assessment fail to correlate with work performance.

4. "A person's ability to function in one environment (e.g., a community setting) is not predictive of a person's ability to function in a different type of environment (e.g., a work setting)" (p. 539). Evaluation and reports of an individual's success or failure in non-work settings do not correlate with potential success or failure in work settings.

5. "There is little or no correlation between a person's symptomatology and functional skills" (p. 540). Knowledge of an individual's clinically defined and expressed symptoms does not provide knowledge of an individual's skills or abilities.

6. "The best clinical predictors of future work performance are ratings of a person's work adjustment skills exhibited in a work-related setting" (p. 540). Measures of work adjustment skills as demonstrated in work settings are good predictors of future success in employment.

7. "The best clinical predictors of future work performance is the person's prior employment history" (p. 541). This finding stresses the importance of supporting individuals with psychiatric disabilities to develop work histories.

8. "A significant predictor of future work performance is a person's ability to get along or function socially with others" (p. 541). This strengthens the argument for providing integrated services for people with

psychiatric disabilities, allowing them to develop the social skills necessary to function socially in work environments.

9. "The best paper-and-pencil test predictors of future vocational performance are tests that measure a person's ego-strength or self-concept in the role of worker" (p. 542). This finding argues against treatment programs or interventions aimed at protecting the individual from employment in the guise of the individual's fragility as a worker.

The findings delineated by Anthony and Jansen (1984) have profound implications for the delivery of services to people with psychiatric disabilities and the measures by which some agencies determine eligibility for job placement services. The initial shift away from state institutions for people with psychiatric disabilities leads to treatment and intervention in smaller psychiatric hospitals. Hospital-based vocational programs were an attempt to provide long-term patients with a sense of productivity and, by that, increase self-esteem.

**Hospital-based programs.** In a review of studies examining the relationship between hospital-based vocational programs and employment outcomes, Bond and Boyer (1987) found no positive relationship between participation in the work programs and post-hospital employment. There were concerns such programs may have created "institutional dependency" when some studies demonstrated rehospitalization rates were higher for those who participated in the work programs than for those who did not (Barbee, Berry & Micek, 1969). Other problems with hospital placements which may or may not have work-based programs, include diminishing work habits and employment skills, outdated skills, and interfering behaviors resulting from medication side effects (Evans, Souma, & Maier, 1989).

**Sheltered workshops.** Another vocational option for people with psychiatric disabilities has been sheltered workshops. These workshops have proven to be permanent placements as opposed to the intended temporary skill-building placement. Rudrud, Ziarnik, Bernstein, and Ferrara (1984) found only 3% of individuals placed in sheltered workshops for 2 years or more become competitively employed. Because the individuals in sheltered workshops do not typically become competitively employed, they also have no opportunity for interaction with nondisabled peers. This further inhibits their ability to learn socially valued interaction skills and develop important interpersonal relationships. In a study on workshop outcomes for individuals with all types of disabilities, Whitehead (1977) found people with psychiatric disabilities were the least successful and earned an average of $0.45 per hour.

**Psychosocial rehabilitation.** A more recent philosophy of rehabilitation, psychosocial rehabilitation, has provided the impetus for a significant change in service provision for people with psychiatric disabilities. The psychosocial rehabilitation model was based upon aspects of physical rehabilitation, psychiatric rehabilitation, vocational rehabilitation, and societal rehabilitation. Psychosocial rehabilitation emphasizes factors such as normalized settings, experiential learning, and individual strengths. The goals of psychosocial rehabilitation are pragmatic, such as avoiding rehospitalization and functioning in the community through obtaining competitive employment and independent living options (Bond, 1987).

Psychosocial rehabilitation programs generally offer a continuum of vocational services. These services are levels of work experiences including prevocational work crews and transitional employment programs (group, then individual placement), leading to competitive employment or supported employment. Prevocational work crews tend to be organized in such a way as to provide small groups of individuals work responsibilities necessary to maintain operation of the service provision agency and may be considered volunteer assignments. Concerns about prevocational work crew arrangements are that they again may be creating institutional dependency and lack the opportunity for true integration and full employment status.

**Transitional employment programs.** These programs often have two phases, group placement and individual placement. The first step or group placement phase of transitional employment involves a small group of individuals with psychiatric disabilities working for pay in a regular community business for a limited period. After this period in a group placement, a client should move into the second phase, which is an individualized temporary placement or series of individual placements, with placements contracted by the service provision agency. These placements may be designed as permanent contracts between the employer and the agency. Yet, the specific individuals to fill the positions would change as clients flow through the transitional continuum. After a period of time (typically 3-9 months), a client would move into a competitive employment position. All phases of transitional employment include paid employment for participants.

Although transitional employment programs were extremely positive new options for providing more normalized services to individuals with psychiatric disabilities, the employment outcomes were not as significant as expected. Bond, Dincin, Setze, and Witheridge (1984) have shown that although transitional employment programs demonstrated a decrease in rehospitalization rates of participants, there was not a significant increase in competitive employment outcomes.

As transitional employment programs were being developed and evaluated for people with psychiatric disabilities, vocational services were also changing for people with developmental disabilities, such as mental retardation. The service providers in the developmental disabilities field were developing, implementing, researching, and legislating for a new service delivery option called supported employment.

# SUPPORTED EMPLOYMENT

## *Definition and Legislation*

The United States Rehabilitation Services Administration defines supported employment as "competitive work in an integrated work setting with ongoing support for individuals with severe disabilities for whom competitive employment (a) has not traditionally occurred, or (b) has been interrupted or intermittent as a result of severe disabilities" (34 C.F.R. Part 363.7). The Federal Register, August 14, 1987, stated that supported employment contains three elements (1) competitive work; (2) an integrated work setting; and (3) the provision of ongoing support services. The proposed regulations state competitive work means work performed at least an average of 20 hours a week and compensated in compliance with the Fair Labor Standards Act. The Fair Labor Standards Act allows employers to pay employees with disabilities wages commensurate with nondisabled employees performing the same tasks based on the employee's productivity. Employers may pay workers less than the prevailing wage if they can establish and maintain sufficient documentation of differing productivity levels.

Supported employment as an initiative emerged in the regulations of the Office of Special Education and Rehabilitative Services (OSERS) in 1984. A series of 1986 amendments to the Rehabilitation Act of 1973 (P.L. 99-506) provides for supported employment to be an option in all rehabilitation services. The intent of this law is to provide more employment opportunities for people with severe disabilities and specifically includes people with severe psychiatric disabilities. P.L. 99-506 authorizes the use of rehabilitation funds for providing supported employment services meeting the federal criteria.

An important distinction between supported employment and traditional vocational services is the difference between the "readiness approach" exemplified in transitional employment programs and the "support approach" in supported employment. Bellamy, Rhodes, and Albin (1986) provide a clear distinction between these two approaches:

> Both approaches strive for the ultimate objective of a decent life in the community that includes productive work, independence, and social integration. The readiness approach of many current services addresses this goal by attempting to 'fix' the individual by providing therapy, training, and related services in anticipation of a productive future. Supported employment (the support approach) provides immediate opportunities for work and community participation while offering a level of support reflective of an individual's needs. (p. 132)

Another difference between transitional employment programs and supported employment is the issue of time limitations. Transitional employment is a temporary program, with gradual but marked progress toward independent, competitive employment as the outcome. Supported employment, however, provides ongoing support with no time restrictions and with the assumption an individual may require certain types or levels of support for the duration of employment.

## Components of Supported Employment

The main components of supported employment include: marketing and job development, job match (client assessment and job analysis), job coaching, and follow along services (McDaniel & Flippo, 1986; Moon, Goodall, Barcus, & Brookes, 1986; Robinson, Andrew, Bishop, Dutton, & LaMar, 1988). The idea was first introduced for people with developmental disabilities and characterized as a place and train approach. The basic implementation called for a functional assessment (assessing real work skills, and interest in real work settings) of a client and an analysis of potential job sites to create a job match. A job coach (a representative of the service agency) learns the particular job that has been identified as appropriate for the client, then trains the individual to do the job. As the supported employee gains skills and independence, the job coach then fades support; some workers may need permanent support for some parts of the job. Follow- along services are provided to ensure the supported employee is maintaining adequate work performance and is receiving any other services which may be necessary (e.g., independent living skills, mobility training).

**Implementation.** The implementation of supported employment services for people with psychiatric disabilities, although similar to those for people with developmental disabilities, differs in subtle but important ways. The place and train approach is adapted and characterized as the "choose, get, keep" model of service provision (Danley & Anthony, 1987). A very critical aspect of "choose, get, keep" is the full and active involvement of the client in all the phases of supported employment, emphasizing client choice at all times.

**Client assessment.** The initial component of supported employment for people with disabilities is one of assessment, choice, and match between the interests, aptitudes, and needs of a client and the job itself. For people with psychiatric disabilities, assessment consists of the individual, an interdisciplinary team, and significant members of the person's life working together to ascertain the type of employment and support most suitable for the individual to be successfully employed.

As opposed to traditional methods used for vocational evaluation, the value of this type of assessment is setting appropriate vocational objectives and empowering individuals to make their own choices. Traditional vocational evaluation methods have not demonstrated a positive correlation to vocational outcomes and may serve only to frustrate the client and slow down the rehabilitation process.

**Work environment analysis.** The second aspect of the job matching process is an assessment of the potential work environment. For people with developmental disabilities, the focus of the workplace analysis in on the tasks required. For people with psychiatric disabilities, the focus is on work environment personalities and social realities of the workplace. Isbister and Donaldson (1987) identified the components of social realities as:

1) purpose of the organization
2) criteria by which performance is measured
3) location of authority
4) base of power
5) decision-making style
6) leadership style
7) focus of the evaluation of membership
8) valued motives of members (p. 49)

People with psychiatric disabilities may have the skills to be employed in managerial positions, or may be looking at entry-level positions. Whatever the case, a thorough understanding of the potential place of employment is necessary.

**Job development.** Job development and placement for people with psychiatric disabilities may also differ from that of services for people with developmental disabilities. The stigma associated with a psychiatric disability, in a sense, is more negative than that of a developmental disability. Whereas society might react inappropriately to a person with a developmental disability with pity or infantile responses, society reacts to a person with a psychiatric disability with fear or intimidation. Unfortunately, the media does little to promote change in such misconceptions by promoting horror films and other public images of sensational terror related to mental illness. Yet, through ensuring the support of the agency and providing a realistic profile of a potential worker, employers are willing to provide supported employment opportunities. Good job developers are providing a service to employers that will benefit both the supported employee and the business itself.

In supported employment for people with psychiatric disabilities, the involvement of the client at the job development stage may be an option. The individual may only need support in writing a resume, practicing interview techniques, completing job applications, and identifying job openings. With this type of support, the individual may then seek a job without the service agency ever becoming directly involved with the employer.

**Job coaching.** The job coaching process will vary greatly based on individual need. Support from a job coach may range from full-time on-the-job support to weekly lunchtime meetings to monthly telephone conversations. Although some individuals may need actual job-task training, others may need support for work-related behaviors such as attendance and punctuality, appropriate dress and hygiene, or social interactions. Others may need support, which is indirectly related to the work environment such as coping strategies, maintaining consistent intake of medications, coordinating other related services, or individual or group counseling. Occasionally, job coaches actually do the work of a supported employee for a period of weeks or months while the employee receives intensive treatment in a psychiatric hospital.

**Follow-along support.** This service will vary and may resemble job coaching services to a certain extent. Follow-along support ensures that a particular individual is experiencing success over time; contact with the service agency is still maintained. This contact may lead to supporting the individual in requesting raises or promotions or in job changes. It also serves to assure the supported employee has stable connections and easy access to support for any area of need.

Rehabilitation counselors are rarely in the role of providing supported employment services to individuals with disabilities. They do serve a critical role in referring clients to appropriate supported employment agencies. A study by Harold Russell Associated (1985) (cited in Danley & Mellen, 1987), lists critical functions associated with an agency's ability to provide effective supported employment services. The functions of management listed as critical were knowledge and skills in:

1) program marketing
2) program planning and development
3) business management
4) private sector operations
5) funding mechanisms
6) staff training and supervision
7) public relations

Danley and Mellen (1987) outlined the competencies of job coaches or direct service providers in three major categories: attitudes, skills, and knowledge. Attitudes include belief systems and values that reflect the philosophy of psychosocial rehabilitation. Such attitudes include treating every individual with respect and dignity and incorporating the individual's active participation and decision-making into all processes. Valuing the support of friends and family of the individual is also important, as is maintaining appropriate expectations of the supported employee regarding work performance and behavior. Some skills of a job coach include effective communication, teaching, advocacy, evaluation, nonaversive behavior management, and functional assessment. The knowledge expected of a job coach includes employer requirements, Social Security disability policies, rights of an individual with disabilities, and basic information specific to psychiatric disabilities, including symptomatology and psychopharmacology.

# REHABILITATION POTENTIAL

The rehabilitation potential for persons with psychiatric disabilities seems limited only by the systems, agencies, and individuals who provide support. As service providers become more skilled at the components of supported employment implementation, the success of supported employees will become greater. The rehabilitation of persons with psychiatric disabilities requires the full support of a range of community service agencies. The cooperation and collaboration of those agencies allow a more effective support system for individuals than does maintaining separate systems of service provision. Success of supported employment for persons with psychiatric disabilities also relies on the awareness that supported employment is a service, not a program. Such a service provides for individuals based on needs, interests, and talents. Supported employment service offers each person an individualized program and does not attempt to offer a standardized program. The more adept service providers become at realizing the needs of a very heterogeneous population, the greater the opportunity for individualized services.

Although there have been significant changes in the delivery of services to people with psychiatric disabilities, we are far from reaching the goal of maximizing the potential of each individual. Systems barriers impose limitations that need to be overcome (Anthony & Blanch, 1987; Nobel & Collignon, 1987). Those systems barriers that impede the expanded delivery of supported employment include the historically poor collaboration between various funding and service provision agencies. The problems associated with the established poor collaboration are apparent in problems associated with joint funding, data collection and documentation, priority areas of interest, and enormous caseloads.

The cost effectiveness of supported employment for people with psychiatric disabilities has yet to be established. Although there is some evidence in developmental disabilities that supported employment is cost-effective in the long-term, the initial costs may be high. Many professionals view the initial costs as a barrier to developing services. The cost effectiveness of supported employment for people with psychiatric disabilities becomes further complicated because there is no systematic evidence, which allows a comparison of supported employment costs and benefits to those of other treatment or intervention models.

# SUMMARY

This chapter provides a basic overview of common psychiatric disabilities. It describes psychoses, neuroses, personality disorders, and other common disabilities. Included, is an overview of vocational services for people with psychiatric disabilities including hospital-based programs, sheltered workshops, prevocational work programs, transitional employment programs, and supported employment services.

Another purpose of this chapter is to provide rehabilitation counselors with a basic awareness of supported employment services for people with psychiatric disabilities. Supported employment services consist of providing whatever support an individual may need to obtain and maintain competitive employment in the community. Components of supported employment as provided by a service agency include marketing and job development, client assessment, workplace analysis, job coaching, and follow-along services. Supported employment services are provided through a "place and train" approach which empowers an individual with a severe psychiatric disability to choose, get, and keep a job. The chapter discusses the rehabilitation potential of persons with psychiatric disabilities related to systems issues and service provider skills, as opposed to individual client characteristics.

# CASE STUDY

Kristen is a 30 year-old woman who has a sporadic work history of menial jobs such as kitchen attendant, housekeeping cleaner, and factory assembler, with frequent periods of unemployment since she was 18 years of age. She successfully conpleted high school but has no additional education or training. Living alone in an apartment in the city, Kristen had been unemployed for the past 3½ years. One year ago, a neighbor took her to see a physician who referred her for mental health services. Kristen complained of being unable to function on her own because she was spending up to 6 hours of her waking day washing her hands. By washing and scrubbing her hands with such vigor and frequency, they were constantly raw and bleeding.

She claimed she had lost her last job because she was either late for work or did not make it to work at all. Unable to stop washing her hands before she went to bed, she spent many sleepless nights awake in the bathroom and often was too tired to go to work. Also, she would wash her hands for an hour or more in the morning, causing her to be late. At work, she often failed to return from breaks and lunch and would be found in the washroom scrubbing her hands.

This client was diagnosed as having an obsessive-compulsive disorder. She was referred to a day treatment program for people with psychiatric disabilities. Jubala House has an open door policy which means that clients come and go as they please. The House operates from 8:00 a.m. to 3:00 p.m. and consists of providing the clients with arts and crafts activities and indoor recreation options such as card games and billiards. Twice a week, clients are encouraged to participate in small group therapy sessions with a counselor. Garret, a rehabilitation counselor intern, is associated with Jubala House and waits for the clients to be ready to go back to work, then helps them apply for jobs.

For the first few weeks Kristen participated at Jubala House, getting there at different times of the day depending on how much she could control her hand washing behavior. Morgan, the social worker in the program, would help Kristen stop washing her hands whenever she had problems at the House. The social worker noted in her weekly reports that Kristen was a quiet, pleasant young woman who seemed intimidated by the behaviors of some of the other clients. Kristen was very interested, from a distance, in the problems of the other clients at the facility and looked forward to attending the therapy sessions. She expressed frustration at not being able to stop washing her hands - that she could just never get them clean enough, particularly clean enough to kill the germs that she could not see.

Kristen became friends with another woman, Lauren, in the program who was also labeled as having an obsessive-compulsive disorder. One of the things that Kristen learned about Lauren was that she had trouble leaving her house because she was never certain she had properly locked the doors and windows. These two women made some nice art projects at Jubala House and talked in the corner about the other clients.

Although Kristen enjoyed Lauren's friendship, she began to get discouraged about her own lack of productivity in life and her poor financial status. In addition, Kristen found herself checking and rechecking the doors and windows in her own apartment to make sure she had locked them. Kristen began to attend Jubala House less and less frequently, her hand washing and door checking was increasing, and she just could not get herself out of the house. On the days she did attend, she was bored with the projects and tired of the mess. She began to sneak across the street to use the restroom at the library to wash her hands for extended periods of time.

Garret, who was completing his master's degree in rehabilitation counseling, made an appointment to meet with Kristen at her apartment to discuss a project on which he was working. He was taking a class on supported employment, and with his professors' help, had received state funding to get some services started through Jubala House. Garret wanted Kristen to be one of the first clients to become involved. They discussed what type of jobs Kristen would be interested in, and what hours might be best for her to work. Kristen was afraid to miss the group counseling sessions at Jubala House, but was very excited about the possibility of securing a real job once again. Garret went through the newspaper want ads with Kristen; he then went to look into several of the job openings they had identified.

Two weeks later, Kristen became employed at the Adam Street Lab as a laboratory assistant. Garret had agreed to work as the job coach until enough people had been placed through Jubala House and a new person could be hired as a job coach. Kristen was trained for the job by one of the lab technicians and no one at the lab but the supervisor knew of her disability. Garret and Kristen had agreed that he would call her in the morning to remind her to stop washing her hands. The fact that the telephone was ringing would cause her to interrupt her behavior and leave the bathroom. She was then able to finish getting ready for work. They also devised a checklist so that as Kristen locked each window and door, she could check it off on the list and then glance at the list every time she felt uneasy about whether she secured each opening. At the lab, there was only one restroom, so Kristen rarely had the opportunity to spend long periods of time without being disturbed. Her supervisor also checked occasionally to make sure she was not having difficulties. Because the lab was a sterile environment and Kristen was kept very busy, she had little time or need for excessive washing.

Evenings were still a problem because Garret had classes and a life outside of work, so he was not always available. Kristen's friend Lauren, and Morgan, the social worker, each agreed to call her with some regularity at night to interrupt her handwashing. At the same time, Garret and Kristen were working one morning a week on developing a new, more normal hand washing ritual that Kristen could use to feel that she was washing as effectively but with much greater efficiency. Kristen is thrilled with her job and the friends she has made at work. Although she occasionally has difficulty at night, she rarely misses a day of work. She does want to begin group therapy sessions again and is looking into trying to find financial support for evening therapy sessions.

## Questions

1. Assign Kristen a vocational profile including age category, educational level, and work history.

2. Identify occupationally significant characteristics of the lab assistant position. List the potential strengths and weaknesses of this position with regard to her specific disability.

3. What were the major factors interfering with Kristen's ability to maintain employment? Did these factors relate to competence?

4. List the concerns you have with the day treatment program (Jubala House).

5. What other support strategies might be used to enhance Kristen's overall quality of life?

6. How might rehabilitation and mental health service providers better coordinate their services to respond to the issues you listed in #5.

# REFERENCES

Anthony, W.A., & Blanch, A. (1987). Supported employment for persons who are psychiatrically disabled: A historical and conceptual perspective. **Psychosocial Rehabilitation Journal, 11**(2), 5-44.

Anthony, W.A., & Jansen, M.A. (1984). Predicting the vocational capacity of the chronically mentally ill. **American Psychologist, 39**(5), 537-544.

Atwood, J.D., & Chester, R. (1987). **Treatment techniques for common mental disorders.** London, England: Jason Aronson.

Barbee, M.S., Berry K.L., & Micek, L.A. (1969). Relationship of work therapy to psychiatric length of stay and readmission. **Journal of Consulting and Clinical Psychology, 33**, 735-738.

Bellamy, G.T., Rhodes, L.E., & Albin, J.M. (1986). Supported employment. In W. Kiernan & J. Stark (Eds.), **Pathways to employment for adults with developmental disabilities** (pp. 129-138). Baltimore, MD: Paul H. Brookes.

Bond, G.R. (1987). Supported work as a modification of the transitional employment model for clients with psychiatric disabilities. **Psychosocial Rehabilitation Journal, 11**(2), 55-74.

Bond, G.R., & Boyer, S.L. (1987). Rehabilitation programs and outcomes. In J.A. Bell & M.D. Bell (Eds.), **Vocational rehabilitation for persons with prolonged psychiatric disorders.** Baltimore, MD: The Johns Hopkins University.

Bond, G.R., Dincin, J., Setze, P.J., & Witheridge, T.F. (1984). The effectiveness of psychiatric rehabilitation: A summary of research at Thresholds. **Psychosocial Rehabilitation Journal, 7**, 6-22.

Campbell, J.F. (1989). Employment programs for people with a psychiatric disability: An overview. **Community Support Network News, 6**(2), 1 & 11.

Danley, K.S., & Anthony, W.A. (1987). The choose-get-keep model: Serving severely psychiatrically disabled people. **American Rehabilitation, 13**(4), 6-9.

Danley, K.S., & Mellen, V. (1987). Training and personnel issues of supported employment programs which serve persons who are severely mentally ill. **Psychosocial Rehabilitation Journal, 11**(2), 87-102.

Danley, K.S., Rogers, E.S., & Nevas, D.B. (in press). An overview of a psychiatric rehabilitation approach to vocational rehabilitation. In M. Farkas & W. Anthony (Eds), **Psychiatric rehabilitation program: Putting theory into practice.** Baltimore, MD: The Johns Hopkins University.

Evans, B., Souma, A., & Maier, G.J. (1989). A vocational assessment and training program for individuals in an inpatient forensic mental health center. **Psychosocial Rehabilitation Journal, 13**(2), 61-69.

**Federal Register.** (1987, August, 14). Washington, DC: U.S. Government Printing Office.

Flynn, R., & Nitsch, K.E. (1980). **Normalization, social integration, and community services.** Austin, TX: Pro-ed.

Isbister, F., & Donaldson, G. (1987). Supported employment for individuals who are mentally ill: Program development. **Psychosocial Rehabilitation Journal, 11**(2), 45-54.

Kiernan, W.E., & Stark, J.A. (1986). The adult with developmental disabilities. In W.E. Kiernan & J.A. Stark (Eds.), **Pathways to employment for adults with developmental disabilities** (pp. 3-8). Baltimore, MD: Paul H. Brookes.

McDaniel, R., & Flippo, K. (1986). **Telesis: Supported employment resource manuals.** San Francisco, CA: University of San Francisco, Rehabilitation Administration.

Moon, M.S., Goodall, D., Barcus, M., & Brookes, V. (1986). **The supported work model of competitive employment for citizens with severe handicaps: A guide for the job trainer** (2nd ed.). Richmond, VA: Virginia Commonwealth University, Rehabilitation Research and Training Center.

Nobel, J.H., & Collignon, F.C. (1988). Systems barriers to supported employment for person with chronic mental illness. In P. Wehman & S. Moon (Eds.), **Vocational rehabilitation and supported employment** (pp. 325-340). Baltimore, MD: Paul H. Brookes.

Paris, J. (1988). Follow-up studies of borderline personality disorder: A critical review. **Journal of Personality Disorders, 2**(3), 189-197.

President's Commission on Mental Health (1978). **Report to the President**. Washington, DC: U.S. Government Printing Office.

Robinson, R.C., Andrew, P., Bishop, K.D., Dutton, D.L., & LaMar, K. (1988). **Supported employment: An overview**. San Francisco, CA: University of San Francisco, Rehabilitation Administration.

Rudrud, E.H., Ziarnik, J.P., Bernstein, G.S., & Ferrara, J.M. (1984). **Proactive vocational habilitation**. Baltimore, MD: Paul H. Brookes.

Webb, L.J., DiClemente, C.C., Johnstone, E.E., Sanders, J.L., & Perley, R.A. (1981). **DSM-III training guide**. New York: Brunner/Mazel.

Whitehead, C.W. (1977). **Sheltered workshop study: A nationwide report on sheltered workshops and their employment of handicapped individuals**. Workshop Survey, Vol. 1, U.S. Department of Labor Service Publication. Washington, DC: U.S. Government Printing Office.

Wolfensberger, W. (1972). **The principle of normalization in human services**. Toronto, Canada: National Institute on Mental Retardation.

Wolfensberger, W. (1980). The definition of normalization: Update, problems, disagreements, and misunderstandings. In R. Flynn & K. Nitsch (Eds.), **Normalization, social integration, and community services** (pp. 71-115). Austin, TX: Pro-Ed.

## *About the Authors*

Kathryn D. Bishop, Ph.D., is an Assistant Professor in Special Education at the University of San Diego in San Diego, California. She has worked in the area of supported employment as a direct service provider and national trainer for the past 7 years.

Mary A. Falvey, Ph.D., is a Professor of Special Education at California State University, Los Angeles, California. She has authored several books on community-based intervention and is a consultant with many school districts throughout the country.

## Chapter 12

# MENTAL RETARDATION

by
*Mary A. Falvey, Ph.D.,*
*Kathryn D. Bishop, Ph.D.*
*and*
*Susann Terry Gage, M.A.*

## INTRODUCTION

Changes in services, expectations, and personal values over the past several decades have significantly affected the quality of life for persons with mental retardation. This chapter discusses programs, services, and support for these individuals. The framework of the chapter includes definition, prevalence, and etiology of mental retardation; the specific learning characteristics generally observed in these persons; and rehabilitation potential. We encourage rehabilitation personnel to consider the information presented in the hope that they may develop better quality programs, services, and support for their clients with mental retardation.

## DEFINITION OF MENTAL RETARDATION

Definitions of mental retardation usually are based on the individual's mental and functional limitations. The American Association of Mental Deficiency (AAMD - now called AAMR, American Association of Mental Retardation) developed a frequently used definition. The AAMR's definition of mental retardation is as follows: "Mental retardation refers to significantly subaverage general functioning existing concurrently with deficits in adaptive behavior, and manifested during the development period" (Grossman, 1977, p. 5).

Instead of defining mental retardation by a person's limitations, some have discussed the importance of identifying the person's needs and placing the burden of responsibility on society to meet those needs (Falvey, 1989). Specifically, Marc Gold (1980), who developed the Try Another Way System, discussed mental retardation by noting one should consider:

> . . . The level of power needed in the training process required for (the individual) to learn, and not by limitations in what he or she can learn. The height of a retarded person's level of functioning is determined by the availability of training technology and the amount of resources society is willing to allocate and not by significant limitations in biological potential. (p. 5)

People with mental retardation are not a homogeneous group. The degree of **development delay** (mental retardation) ranges from mild to moderate, from severe to profound. A person with mild mental retardation has an

I.Q. of between 50-75, while a person with moderate mental retardation has any I.Q. of 30-50. An individual with severe mental retardation has an I.Q. of 20-30, and a person with profound mental retardation (who often has other accompanying disabilities such as physical or sensory disabilities) has an I.Q. of 20 or below.

The manifestation of the degree of developmental delay has a relationship to the **assistance**, **support**, and **instructional** opportunities a person with mental retardation has available. Secondly, the interests and strengths of persons with mental retardation are as extensive and varied as nondisabled persons. Thirdly, the personalities of individuals with mental retardation are as diverse as nondisabled persons throughout society (e.g., quiet, shy, boisterous, gregarious, friendly, and withdrawn).

# PREVALENCE OF MENTAL RETARDATION

The prevalence of mental retardation is " . . . approximately 3% of school-age population and approximately 1-2% of pre-school and post-school age populations" (Brimer, 1990, p. 25). The variations of these figures are directly related to the labeling and classifying procedures used in school programs. Pre-schoolers and adults with mild to moderate mental retardation, may not be labeled or in any way considered different. Traditionally, schools have grouped and classified school-age students into discrete and distinct ability levels, often labeling students as mentally retarded who would otherwise go unlabeled in preschool and adult years. This explains the slightly higher percentage of mentally retarded in the school-age population.

## *Gender Differences*

The gender difference, in terms of prevalence, is significant. Although there is some disagreement about the specific percentages, research generally supports the notion there are more males than females diagnosed as mentally retarded. There appear to be two possible explanations. (1) Sex-linked recessive conditions are more frequently associated with males, and (2) society places on males more often than females stereotypic sex roles, which tend to influence diagnoses and labels. For example, society often reinforces males for masculinity and aggressiveness, while reinforcing females more often for being polite, quiet, and shy. Aggressive behavior in students often leads to "testing" and subsequent labeling. Boys who are aggressive and mildly retarded have a greater chance of being identified as retarded rather than girls who are mildly retarded, quiet, and well-behaved (MacMillian, 1982).

## *Race and Economic Status*

Race and economic status variations have been more prevalent in the past. Major litigation and legislation (Larry P. v. Riles and Diana v. State Board of Education, Public Law 94-142, 1975) have made it more difficult to incorrectly identify mental retardation in members of minority groups. During the 1960s, there was a disproportionate number of school-age students identified as mentally retarded from certain minority groups (i.e., Blacks and Hispanics). A primary method of identifying mental retardation was the use of intelligence quotient (I.Q.) tests. In the past, professionals have criticized I.Q. tests as culturally and linguistically biased in favor of White, middle-class children. Researchers consider invalid and of little use the results of these tests given to children that are not members of the White middle class community. For vocational rehabilitation planning, I.Q. scores are of little value (Brown et al., 1983).

# ETIOLOGY OF MENTAL RETARDATION

There are many known causes of mental retardation, although some cases have no known or recognizable etiology. Researchers have identified genetic and physical factors as the causes of mental retardation. Down's Syndrome is the most frequently observed genetic factor influencing mental retardation. In 1866, Dr. Langdon Down, a physician, identified Down's Syndrome, known as Trisomy XXI, and characterized by extra genetic material in the 21st chromosome. Maternal age is a factor in the prevalence of Down's Syndrome. The older the mother, particularly over the age of 35, the higher the possibility the baby may have Down's Syndrome. One sees other developmental problems, such as respiratory and heart abnormalities, with Down's Syndrome. The degree of mental retardation observed in persons with Down's Syndrome ranges from mild to profound.

## PKU

In 1934, Dr. Asbjourn Folling, a Norwegian physician, discovered phenylketonuria (PKU) as a cause of mental retardation. PKU is a sign of deficiency in the production of phenylalanine hydroxylase, an enzyme necessary in the metabolism of phenylalanine, an essential amino acid. Brain damage occurs with the buildup of phenylalanine in the blood. In 1959, Dr. Robert Guthrie developed a screening test for newborns that physicians routinely use today to detect PKU. When a physician identifies PKU in a newborn, a phenylalanine-restricted diet is started. The degree of mental retardation varies significantly for persons with treated versus untreated PKU; dietary restrictions during the primary years are essential and generally decrease the degree of mental retardation.

## Tay-Sachs Disease

Tay-Sachs disease also causes mental retardation. This disease is a lipid metabolic disorder that is most often found in persons of Jewish descent. Besides mental retardation, it causes a progressive deterioration of nervous tissue and generally results in death at an early age.

## Physical Factors

There are several physical factors, besides the specific genetic factors, that influence the presence of mental retardation. Beginning with the prenatal stages of development, the mother's general eating habits and physical health are critical. Chronic maternal illness, such as diabetes, may impair fetal development. Maternal use of alcohol, drugs, tobacco, and exposure to environmental pollution during pregnancy increase the probability of mental retardation and additional disorders. Maternal infections and viruses such as rubella, perinatal cytomegalovirus infection (CMV), meningoencephalitis, syphilis, and toxoplasmosis can influence fetal development and result in mental retardation. Fetal exposure to radiation during development can cause genetic mutations resulting in mental retardation.

During childbirth, several factors can increase the possibility of mental retardation. Cephalopelvic disproportion is when the size of the birth canal is too narrow for the presenting infant's head. This condition can result in brain damage. Other factors include prematurity, accidental physical trauma, asphyxia, hypoglycemia, infection, blood cell or blood type diseases, and Rh factor blood incompatibilities between mother and baby.

Following birth of the baby, there are factors that can increase the probability of mental retardation. These include malnutrition, acquired traumatic brain injury, infection, and chemicals (e.g., pesticides, drug abuse, and metal poisoning). When physicians rule out specific syndromes and causes, they often cite other pre-, peri- (during), and post-pregnancy conditions which may result in mental retardation.

# NORMALIZATION

## *Institutionalization*

During the nineteenth and early part of the twentieth centuries, society created institutions for mentally retarded persons. In the last three decades, organized coalitions of parents and the "normalization" principle played a significant role in developing community-based services as an alternative to institutionalization.

During the 1950s, parents formed an organization called the National Association for Retarded Children (later renamed the National Association for Retarded Citizens). These parents rejected institutionalization for their children. Local chapters of the Association of Retarded Citizens developed throughout the United States. Many of these chapters and other informal networks organized programs and services. Until the 1970s, public schools excluded most children with mental retardation. Parents had to raise money and volunteer their time in order for their children to receive other services available in the community.

## *Services and Support - The Principle of Normalization*

Besides this parent movement, the director of the Danish Mental Retardation Service, Bank-Mikkelsen, in 1959, helped develop Danish law that reflected the "normalization" principle. The normalization principle simply states that persons with mental retardation must be able to " . . . obtain an existence as close to normal as possible" (Wolfensberger, 1980, p. 7). Nirje (1969) published the first systematic statement of normalization in the world literature. In 1972, Wolfensberger applied the normalization principle to North Americans with mental retardation and the society in which they lived.

**Deinstitutionalization.** The normalization principle has been a strong driving force in establishing the deinstitutionalization movement. This movement involves placing persons from institutions into the community. Biklen and Knoll (1987) identified the major problems with institutions and other larger congregate facilities, and the primary reasons for deinstitutionalizing people with mental retardation.

*   institutions are the most expensive way of providing residential or any other services to people with mental retardation.

*   institutions do not offer warm, homelike individualized environments necessary for full human development.

*   institutions do not provide opportunities for interaction with members of the community.

*   institutions do not allow for positive community living experiences and for development of skills needed for community life.

*   Institutions perpetuate and enforce the image that people with mental retardation are oddities.

*   people residing in institutions do not have the opportunities to learn adaptive behavior from functioning non-institutionalized people.

*   institutionalized people model their behavior after other people living in the institution; these behaviors are often maladaptive.

*   institutions provide a minimum of social and recreational activities and interaction; when they do, it is often demeaning and age inappropriate.

Besides the above, institutional living does not offer opportunities for vocational development. One does not see typical jobs performed nor are there opportunities to learn about employment through observation. Most, if not all, of the people living in institutions are unemployed. Few have ever had the opportunity to become gainfully employed. Discussion of work is nonexistent; normal vocational development does not occur for institutionalized individuals.

**Homelike settings.** As an alternative, state and local communities and parent organizations developed group homes, board and care homes, and foster homes to create homelike settings for persons with mental retardation. These settings were less restrictive and more normalizing than institutional residences. In terms of the normalization principle, more needs to be done to create living opportunities and arrangements that are homes, not institutions. Facilities should hire staff to help community interaction for persons with mental retardation (Knoll & Ford, 1987).

**Self-advocacy.** The normalization principle also had an impact on the development of the self-advocacy movement. The self-advocacy movement involves " . . . people with disabilities asserting their sworn rights and interests, usually without others' help" (Turnbull, Turnbull, Bronicki, Summers, & Roeder-Gordon, 1989, p. 314). Two self-advocacy international networks (i.e., People First and United Together) have been formed and are becoming more influential and powerful, particularly concerning employment advocacy, fair working conditions, and financial compensation.

## *Legislation and Normalization*

**The Rehabilitation Act of 1973.** Professionals often refer to Section 504 of the 1973 Rehabilitation Act as the "civil rights" bill for individuals with disabilities. This legislation requires public and private employers, educators, and service providers to use nondiscriminatory and affirmative action practices.

**The Education of All Handicapped Children Act of 1975.** This act ensured a free and appropriate education in the least restrictive environment for people between the ages of 3-21. The least restrictive environment mandates education of students in the presence of their nondisabled peers and within the general education program to the "maximum extent appropriate." Research has consistently supported maximum integration of all students in "regular" education programs (Falvey, 1989; Lipsky & Gardner, 1989; Sailor et al., 1989; Stainback, Stainback & Forest, 1989).

**The Developmental Disabilities Assistance Act and the Bill of Rights Act of 1978.** This legislation provided assistance to states to support individuals with developmental disabilities by designing and implementing Individualized Habilitation Plans (IHP). Many amendments to this act have clearly specified the rights of and services for persons with developmental disabilities. In relationship to rehabilitation and habilitation services for adults, legislation passed in 1984 reauthorized supported employment as " . . . renumerative, competitive employment in an integrated community environment that meets three requirements:

(1) the person is unlikely to earn a salary at or above minimum wage because of the severity of his or her disability;

(2) the work site employs primarily persons without disabilities; and

(3) the person is likely to need ongoing support such as supervision, training, and transportation to sustain paid employment" (Brimer, 1990, p. 222).

**The 1987 Developmental Disabilities Act.** The stated goals for the 1987 Developmental Disabilities Act were..."[to] assure that persons with developmental disabilities receive the care, treatment, and other services necessary to enable them to achieve their maximum potential through increased independence, productivity, and integration into the community, ...

and

[to] establish and operate a system which coordinates monitors, plans, and evaluates services which ensure the protection of the legal and human rights of persons with developmental disabilities."

**Social Security Act amendments.** In 1987, Congress amended the Social Security Act to provide a work incentive program within the Supplemental Security Income (SSI) program. Before these amendments, the SSI regulations were fostering dependency and discouraging people from acquiring an income because they would lose their Medicare coverage (medical insurance) and all financial support. The new program allowed the SSI recipient to receive Medicare benefits if the employer does not provide equivalent comprehensive medical coverage. Also, the income level of the worker who qualifies for SSI is higher than in past years. Most persons with mental retardation qualify for SSI benefits and have been more likely to obtain employment since these changes in the Social Security Act.

**The Americans with Disabilities Act.** Congress passed the Americans with Disabilities Act (ADA) in 1990. This act has broad implications concerning employment, transportation, public accommodations, state and local government, and telecommunications. The most important area for persons with mental retardation is employment. The ADA specifies that employers may not discriminate against an individual with a disability in hiring or promotion. Employers will need to provide reasonable accommodation, including job modification and restructuring to individuals with disabilities. All large employers (those who employ 25 or more) must comply by July of 1992; smaller employers (15-24 employees) need to comply by July of 1994. Enactment of the ADA will help rehabilitation counselors facilitate obtaining competitive employment for clients with mental retardation.

# FUNCTIONAL LIMITATIONS

The most salient learning characteristics of persons with mental retardation are slower rates of learning skills than their typical peers, and difficulty in generalizing or transferring information learned in one situation to another. One should not misinterpret this slower learning rate and difficulty in generalizing as an inability to learn or acquire new skills. It does mean people with mental retardation need to be taught specific skills in the environment in which an individual would naturally perform these skills. For example, teaching public transportation skills should include using the public transportation system in the person's community; one needs to teach job-related skills in a "real" work environment.

Persons with mental retardation have been characterized, at times, as not capable of learning or having reached a "plateau" (Falvey, 1989). When a person's learning has reached a plateau, it may be an indication that different services and support are necessary. The learning possibilities and potential of persons with mental retardation are directly dependent upon the commitment of services and support society is willing to commit, as opposed to limitations inherent in the disability itself.

## *Learned Helplessness*

A phenomenon repeatedly observed in institutions and segregated schools, workshops, and activity centers is "learned helplessness" (Payne & Patton, 1981). This phenomenon is "...a pattern of submissiveness which develops when the victims repeatedly discover that their actions are of no consequence, that outcomes are beyond their control" (Payne & Patton, 1981, pp. 299-300). The person then learns not to demonstrate skill proficiency, independence, or sometimes even awareness of the surroundings. This phenomenon has a similar effect to that of the self-fulfilling prophecy (Rosenthal & Jacobson, 1968).

The self-fulfilling prophecy states that most people's opinions and expectations about themselves are influenced in a significant way by those around them. If teachers, social workers, rehabilitation counselors, and job coaches believe an individual student or client is unable to learn, that person probably will not learn. Yet, if the same group of supportive professionals hold expectations the individual can learn and be successful, the chances for a successful outcome will be greatly enhanced (Wehman, 1981).

## *Environmental Factors*

The environment plays a significant role in influencing the success and employability of an individual with mental retardation. The traditional model that adult service agencies provided was vocational training in a "train and place" model, such as occurs in a sheltered workshop. Practitioners designed this model to train the client in a simulated job setting first and then place the client on a job. Because clients with mental retardation do not generalize well across settings, this model did not generally result in employment of persons with mental retardation in integrated community jobs. The recently developed "place and train" model has resulted in a significantly greater number of employed clients with mental retardation in integrated community job settings. These two models will be discussed further later in the chapter.

## *Societal Discrimination*

Society has, over the years, discriminated against those with mental retardation, primarily due to ignorance and stereotypical incorrect information. Until recently, most employers did not have life experiences with persons with mental retardation. As a result, much work is being done to change the attitudes and expectations of employers. A most effective way to change employers' attitudes and expectations is observation of other employers who have hired individuals with metal retardation. This experience often results in more positive attitudes and raises expectations of what a person with that label is capable of performing.

Society is slowly changing its negative attitudes toward individuals with metal retardation to one that is more accepting and positive. There are several reasons for this change. As schools include children with mental retardation in the same classrooms as typical children, teachers, administrators, children, and parents are influenced in accepting children with differences and valuing their differences. Supported employment, which involves placing clients in "real" jobs in the community and providing them with the needed instruction in that setting, has positively influenced employers, co-workers, and members of the community. Although there still exists ignorance about and discrimination against persons with mental retardation in the work force, those attitudes are changing.

# REHABILITATION POTENTIAL

## *The Supported Employment Model*

Research over the past several decades has influenced changes in the delivery of services. In 1972, Gold demonstrated that persons with severe mental retardation, who were deaf and blind, could assemble complex electronic circuit boards. Hunter and Bellamy (1977) taught persons with profound mental retardation to assemble harnesses. This, and other research findings, lead to teaching persons with mental retardation work skills that could be used for competitive, gainful employment. Supported employment is the term used to describe the provision of employment in community job settings while simultaneously receiving support or assistance to do the job. Research and legislation have helped expand the concept and implementation of supported employment. Rehabilitation counselors throughout the country are currently using the principles of supported employment.

**Traditional services.** The traditional service options available to most adults with mental retardation before 1980 was a developmental center, work activity center, or sheltered workshop. Professionals have criticized these settings because they generally do not provide "real" work in actual work environments. The assumption of sheltered work environments was to get people ready for real work. Bellamy (1983) conducted a national survey and concluded that sheltered workshops took too much time training people for competitive employment. According to his research, people with mental retardation spent an average of 37 years in adult developmental centers, 10 years in work activity centers, and 9 years in sheltered workshops. Since most persons with mental retardation "graduate" from school at approximately age 21, they would be, on the average, 77 years old before entering competitive employment. According to Bellamy, the supported employment model has been extremely successful in placing persons with severe disabilities in competitive, gainful employment.

**Anti-habilitative characteristics of workshops.** According to Bishop and Falvey (1989), there are several anti-habilitative characteristics of sheltered workshops that do not exist in supported employment:

1. Work performed often requires minimal learning on the part of the workers.

2. Sheltered workshops often retain the best workers for the more demanding work, instead of training them for nonsheltered vocational environments.

3. Adequate time is not available for training workers in nonsheltered environments.

4. Personnel often lack training in critical areas, such as effective teaching methods, production, and providing "real" job training.

5. "Down time" or "dead time" is frequent.

6. Practitioners often base formal vocational evaluations on inferences, not on actual observation of the client in real community jobs.

7. All the students/clients receiving training have disabilities and, therefore, they have no contact with nondisabled workers.

8. Inappropriate assumptions are made that persons in sheltered workshops and activity centers "enjoy" or are more competent at tasks that involve sitting or standing at tables and using predominantly fine motor and coordination skills.

9. Tasks vary according to the contracts secured, not according to the client's training needs.

10. Equipment is often out of date and in poor condition, resulting in worthless training.

11. Frequently, the workshop does not follow normal workdays or workweeks. Consequently, persons in workshops or at centers do not have sufficient opportunities to build endurance. Historically, workshops and work activity centers have interrupted work periods, particularly at holiday times, with events such as dances, that feature age-inappropriate music.

12. Workshop personnel do not develop systematic strategies to assists clients in making the transition to less restrictive work settings.

13. Irrelevant exit requirements or prerequisite skill requirements are often higher than requirements in "real" community jobs.

**Characteristics of supported employment.** Supported employment is an alternative to sheltered workshop training. The characteristics of supported employment services follow below:

**\*Place and Train:** This characteristic refers to developing services that reverse the traditional method of "train and place." "Place and train" involves placing a person on the job regardless of job readiness, and training that person to perform that job and services. A job coach must be made available to support a person in the job in order for the "place and train" model to be successful (Falvey, Bishop, Grenot-Scheyer, & Coots, 1988).

**\*Integrated Job Settings**: Job settings used for training must be job settings used for nondisabled employees. In addition, these integrated job settings should not create a disproportionate number of employees with disabilities. The integrated job setting should reflect the natural proportion of persons who do not have disabilities in the community. The rehabilitation counselor needs to make every effort to encourage interactions, relationships, and ultimately friendships to develop between the trainee with mental retardation and co-workers (Brown et al., 1984).

**\*Individual Placements**: Job placements should be based on the trainees' preferences and strengths and should be accessible to them. One must make a good job match at the time of job placement (McDaniel & Flippo, 1986).

**\*Meaningful Work**: This characteristic implies that rehabilitation counselors need to avoid providing makeshift work or otherwise made up jobs that persons who do not have disabilities would not perform (Brown et al., 1983).

**\*Job Development and Marketing**: This service involves systematically accessing existing jobs, modifying existing jobs, and creating new jobs. This service is essential in the delivery of supported employment and should be provided by individuals who have knowledge of the local job market and credibility with employers. Interactions with potential employers must be conducted in a business-like manner (Bishop & Falvey, 1989).

**\*Job Coaching**: This service involves providing systematic instruction on the job and teaching job-related skills, including social skills. In addition, job coaches provide instruction in the client's home or community setting in areas related to work. These include getting ready for work, using public transportation for work, depositing and budgeting paychecks, and developing social networks and friendships within the community. The job coach provides instruction in a salient enough way for the client to develop the required skills, but also in a subtle enough way so as not to embarrass or discourage the client. If the client is not doing the job correctly, the job coach provides additional instruction. When a client fails to show up for work, the job coach will come in and perform the actual work activity.

One enhances the rehabilitation potential of persons with mental retardation by providing the support to access and maintain employment, housing, and other community services and activities. Supported employment services across the United States and within other countries (e.g., Canada and Italy) have successfully placed millions of persons with mental retardation. Many have been provided with the support to live where they wish and with whom they want, accessing their neighborhoods and communities, while receiving sufficient support to be successful.

Attitudes of people in the community have changed over the years leading to greater acceptance of their neighbors with mental retardation. Technology has also influenced successful integration of persons with mental retardation into the community. Simple adaptations such as calculators, computers, and other technological adaptations, such as voice synthesizers and other electronic communication aides, have greatly enhanced the participation of persons with mental retardation.

# SUMMARY

This chapter provides the rehabilitation counselor with an overview of issues related to mental retardation. The most critical concept is that the degree of participation and potential of persons with mental retardation is dependent upon society's commitment and willingness to support these people in work, housing, and within the community. This chapter includes historical perspectives of services and provides a description of current service trends. The most effective service delivery system that supports persons with mental retardation in employment is the supported employment model.

# CASE STUDY

Anthony is a 25-year old man who had spent the last 12 years of his life in an institution. His day, while in the institution, consisted of being lifted from bed, having his clothes changed, being fed pureed foods, and sitting in front of a television set for hours. He also attended a classroom called "school" where he listened to preschool music and put pegs in a peg board. Seldom did anyone speak to him except to give him instructions. He had no friends and never left the institution until, one day, a social worker came to his room and asked if he wanted to share an apartment with two other men in a city 20 miles away. Although Anthony had very little reaction to anything that went on around him, he smiled and looked straight at the social worker when she was talking to him. A week later, he moved into the apartment and began learning about living, working, and recreating in the community.

Anthony was multihandicapped. This diagnosis included profound mental retardation, cerebral palsy, and a significant visual loss. He used a wheelchair and an attendant to push his chair to get around. The attendant provided him with support in basic self-care skills. Once he was living in the community, the social worker referred him to the supported employment agency in that area to assist him in obtaining and maintaining employment. A job developer and a job coach visited him at his apartment to begin the task of helping him secure employment. Anthony was learning to use his new picture communication aid, provided through rehabilitation services. The job developer and the job coach relied on his responses when he used his communication aid, his facial expressions, and overall body language.

They spent 30 minutes in the apartment watching him participate with the support of his attendant in various tasks around the apartment. For the next hour, they went out in the neighborhood to observe Anthony's reactions to various stimuli and to determine potential job possibilities within a reasonable distance from his apartment. Two blocks away was a recycling center with a sign in the window advertising "Help Wanted." Since they were in the neighborhood, they all went in to inquire about the job. The center supervisor indicated they needed someone to sort the cans and other items being delivered to the recycling center. The job developer suggested to the company supervisor that she consider employing two people with developmental disabilities to do the job. Together, with the support of their job coach, they could be very successful on the job. The supervisor was reluctant since she lacked experience hiring or working with people with developmental disabilities. The job developer gave her the names and telephone numbers of other employers who had hired employees with developmental disabilities and encouraged her to contact them.

A week later the recycling center supervisor contacted the job developer and stated she would like to hire Anthony and the other client identified in the original conversation. The recycling center hired both Anthony and the other client, Nathan; the supported employment agency provided a job coach for support.

A year later, both Anthony and Nathan were still working at the center; the employer was very enthusiastic about their employment. With the support of a job coach, Nathan and Anthony share the job tasks of sorting and classifying the items brought into the center. In addition, both have become friends and have developed good relationships with their co-workers, both at work and off the job. The quality of life for Anthony has been greatly enhanced. He shows greater interest in his life and surroundings; Anthony smiles and laughs much more.

## *Questions*

1. What are the possible causes of Anthony's mental retardation?

2. Identify the major problems with institutional living and the primary reasons for deinstitutionalizing people such as Anthony.

3. Describe advantages of supported employment over sheltered workshop employment.

4. Discuss the roles and functions of the job coach in supported employment. If Anthony or Nathan were not performing the work correctly or did not show up for work, how would the job coach proceed?

# REFERENCES

Bellamy, G.T. (1983). **Competitive employment training.** Paper presented at a conference of the California Chapter of the Association for the Severely Handicapped, San Diego, CA.

Biklen, D., & Knoll, J. (1987). The disabled minority. In S. Taylor, D. Biklen, & J. Knoll (Eds.), **Community integration for people with severe disabilities** (pp. 3-24). New York: Teachers College Press.

Bishop, K.D. & Falvey, M.A. (1989). Employment skills. In M.A. Falvey, **Community-based curriculum: Instructional strategies for students with severe handicaps** (pp. 165-188). Baltimore, MD: Paul H. Brooks.

Brimer, R.W. (1990). **Students with severe disabilities: Current perspectives and practices.** Mountain View, CA: Mayfield.

Brown, L., Shiraga, B., Ford, A., VanDeventer, P., Nesbit, J., Loomis, R., & Sweet, M. (1983). Teaching severely handicapped students to perform meaningful work in nonsheltered vocational environments. In L. Brown, J. Nesbit, A. Ford, M. Sweet, R. Loomis, & P. VanDeventer (Eds.), **Educational programs for severely handicapped students** (Vol 13, pp. 1-100). Madison, WI: Madison Metropolitan School District.

Brown, L., Shiraga, B., York, J., Kessler, K., Strohm, B., Rogan, P., Sweet, M., Zanella, K., VanDeventer, P., & Loomis, R., (1984). Integrated work opportunities for adults with severe handicaps: The extended training option. **Journal of the Association for Persons with Severe Handicaps,** 9(4), 262-269.

Falvey, M.A. (1989). **Community-based curriculum: Instructional strategies for students with severe handicaps** (2nd ed.). Baltimore, MD: Paul H. Brookes.

Falvey, M.A., Bishop, K. D., Grenot-Scheyer, M., & Coots, J. (1988). Issues and trends in mental retardation. In S. Calculator & J. Bedrosian (Eds.), **Communication assessment and interventions for adults with mental retardation** (pp. 45-65). Boston, MA: College Hill.

Gold, M.W. (1972). Task analysis at a complex assembly task by the blind. **Exceptional Children, 43,** 78-84.

Gold, M.W. (1980). **Try another way training manual.** Champaign, IL: Research Press.

Grossman, H.J. (Ed.). (1977). **Manual on terminology and classification in mental retardation**. Washington, DC: American Association on Mental Deficiency.

Hunter, J., & Bellamy, G.T. (1977). Cable harness construction for severely retarded adults: A demonstration of training techniques. **American Association for the Education of Severely and Profoundly Handicapped Review, 1**(7), 2-13.

Knoll, J., & Ford, A. (1987). Beyond caregiving: A reconceptualization of the role of the residential service provider. In S. Taylor, D. Biklen & J. Knoll (Eds.), **Community integration for people with severe disabilities** (pp. 129-146). New York: Teachers College.

Lipsky, D., & Gardner, W. (1989). **Beyond separate education: Quality education for all**. Baltimore, MD: Paul H. Brookes.

MacMillian, D.L. (1982). **Mental retardation in school and society** (2nd ed.). Boston, MA: Little, Brown.

McDaniel, R.H., & Flippo, K. (1986). **Telesis: Supported employment resource manuals**. San Francisco, CA: University of San Francisco, Rehabilitation Administration.

Nirje, B. (1969). The normalization principle and its management implications. In R. Kugel & W. Wolfensberger (Eds), **Changing patterns in residential services for the mentally retarded** (pp. 51-57). Washington, DC: U.S. Government Printing Office.

Payne, J.S., & Patton, J.R. (1981). **Mental retardation**. Columbus, OH: Charles E. Merrill.

Rosenthal, R., & Jacobson, L.F. (1968). **Pygmalian in the classroom**. New York, NY: Holt, Rinehardt & Winston.

Sailor, W., Anderson, J.L., Halvorsen, A.T., Doering, K., Filler, J., & Goetz, L. (1989). **The comprehensive local school: Regular education for all students**. Baltimore, MD: Paul H. Brookes.

Stainback, S., Stainback, W., & Forest, M. (Eds.). (1989). **Educating all students in the mainstream of regular education**. Baltimore, MD: Paul H. Brookes.

Turnbull, H.R., Turnbull, A.P., Bronicki, G.J., Summers, J.A., & Roeder-Gordon, C. (1989). **Disability and the family: A guide to decisions for adulthood**. Baltimore, MD: Paul H. Brookes.

Wehman, P. (1981). **Competitive employment: New horizons for severely disabled individuals**. Baltimore, MD: Paul H. Brookes.

Wolfensberger, W. (1980). A brief overview of the principle of normalization. In R.J. Flynn & K.E. Kitsch (Eds.), **Normalization, social integration and community services** (pp. 7-30). Baltimore, MD: University Park Press.

## *About the Authors*

Mary A. Falvey, Ph.D., is a Professor of Special Education at California State University, Los Angeles, California. She has authored several books on community-based intervention and is a consultant with many school districts throughout the country.

Kathryn D. Bishop, Ph.D., is an Assistant Professor in Special Education at the University of San Diego in San Diego, California. She has worked in the area of supported employment as a direct service provider and national trainer for the past 7 years.

Susann Terry Gage, M.A., is currently working on her Ph.D. in Special Education in the Joint Doctoral Program at California State University, Los Angeles, California, and the University of California, Los Angeles. She has worked with several school districts within Los Angeles County.

# Chapter 13

# CHRONIC PAIN SYNDROMES AND THEIR TREATMENT

by
*Jack Pinsky, M.D.*

## INTRODUCTION

Rehabilitation counselors will see individuals with core problems of chronic pain. This chapter can assist the counselor in working with these problematic cases.

Pain is a subjective, personal, and perceptual experience which eludes a comprehensive definition that would fit all of its occurrences and expressions seen in humans. Usually, the central nervous system (CNS) allows an individual to become aware of noxious (injurious) body (soma) events or significant dysfunctions of the soma by relaying signals that the brain receives and interprets as pain. Noxious stimuli generate specific coded signals that enter the nervous system; these are signals, not pain signals and certainly not pain. Pain itself is a perception, an event that occurs in the brain.

The brain is capable of perceiving pain in response to any type of event, whether or not it is a noxious event. The extreme range of inciting inputs, of varying types and intensities, can result in pain. This contributes to making pain a highly subjective experience that is difficult to conceptualize, define, and classify in a fixed way.

### Definitions

A general broad definition of "pain" adopted by the International Association for the Study of Pain (IASP) (1986) is the following: "Pain is an unpleasant sensory and emotional experience associated with actual or potential tissue damage, or, described in terms of such damage" (p. S217).

The broad range of this definition includes readily explained experiences of pain associated with known tissue trauma or active disease. Typical experiences of pain occur with these readily identifiable disorders in which there are actual changes in tissue behavior or structure (objective findings) that produce noxious input. Examples of this include radiculitis (inflammation of spinal nerve roots) that can result from impingement of intervertebral disc material on nerve roots, and pain that accompanies inflammatory joint and connective tissue responses to many injuries and diseases.

The IASP definition also serves to include more incompletely understood pain disorders. Some of these are phantom limb pain, central pain (e.g., post-stroke pain), atypical facial neuralgias (facial pain that does not correspond to the clinical pattern of a specific nerve disorder), and post-herpetic neuralgia (pain that persists after a herpes zoster infection). Others include fibrositis (presumed inflammation of the whitish sheaths that cover muscle and allied tissues), fibromyalgia (non-specific aching, pain, tenderness, and stiffness around joints and soft tissues), and enthesopathies (pain at the site of tendon or muscle attachment).

The IASP pain definition also encompasses pain experienced in mental disorders that do not have any known noxious, somatic source. A conversion disorder (hysterical neurosis) or the conversion symptoms of pain that may accompany other mental states, are examples of this. Pain is a common symptom in mood disorders, such as depressions and unresolved grief reactions. It can be incorporated into delusional states. Pain as a part of mental dysfunction or disorders rarely has any somatic, noxious source.

## Description

The common and necessary component of all the painful conditions noted above, and others, is **perception**; this is always a brain event. Yet, pain is experienced as an event of the body. Pain and its location is determined in the brain because of the complete, intricate, and many-leveled connections between the non-nervous systems, the peripheral nervous system, and the central nervous system. When these systems are intact, pain will always be a body-labeled experience in which we name a body part(s) that hurts, whether or not there are noxious signals coming from the hurtful area.

Pain is the most common symptom that brings people for medical evaluation and relief. **Acute** pain is part of an important biological warning system that tells us of a change. It tells us that something has gone amiss, helps us to identify what that is, and begins the process of seeking a resolution to the problem. In medicine, there are many rapid and effective ways to alleviate acute pain and to resolve the problem that generated the process. An individual's history of pain onset, its location, and its qualities provide valuable information for the diagnostic search for the presence, absence, and seriousness of specific inciting events. This is heavily involved in the therapeutic decisions that are made in medical care. We use many terms to describe pain. It is important to distinguish between **acute** (short-term) and **chronic** (long-standing) pain. These terms refer only to the length of time the pain has been present; they are not intended to denote the intensity of the pain or the severity of the problem.

When pain has been present for longer than 6 months, it is arbitrarily regarded as chronic. It is this type of pain and its clinical expressions that takes the largest toll in human suffering, health care delivery problems, and costs. This chapter will focus on this aspect of pain.

# CHRONIC PAIN

## Classification

A difficult and unresolved problem in the fields of pain medicine and rehabilitation is the classification of chronic pain. Major obstacles to the resolution of the problem include not only distinctions between **acute** and **chronic**, but also those between chronic pain and chronic diseases (Crue, 1983).

There are medical disorders that have acute and intermittent pain while the disorder itself is regarded as being chronically present. Migraine headache is one such disorder. The same general model of pain is frequently seen in rheumatoid arthritis. When there is inflammation, there is acute pain. There may be no pain experienced while the underlying chronic disease remains stable or worsens over time without the presence of inflammation.

When there is active cancer, pain associated with this pathology can be ongoing, unrelenting, and in this sense chronic, as a direct result of the activity and location of the disease. This is an instance of a chronic disease resulting in a form of chronic pain, in contrast to those chronic disorders discussed above.

Pain in the absence of any known noxious source in the periphery is the most difficult for both sufferers and clinicians to accept conceptually (i.e., **real** pain felt elsewhere in the body can have the central nervous system as its sole source). Yet, this kind of chronic pain in the absence of the perennial peripheral or systemic markers for **acute** pain remains consistent with the accepted general definition of pain put forth by the IASP.

A part of the body lost through injury or surgery can be experienced as continuing to be present after all healing of the injury has taken place. This phantom sensation can be present for different tissues, but most commonly is in relation to a missing limb. Phantom limb pain occurs in a significant number of people losing limbs. This condition is the classic example of chronic pain that can be continuously present without any remaining disease activity, unhealed tissue injury, or remaining inflammation.

In addition, chronic pain is often not a static state and changes occur with time. This includes the extensiveness of the suffering and its impact on the sufferer and those in the person's social sphere (Black, 1975). The rehabilitation counselor needs to be aware of these dynamic characteristics that are part of the chronic problem. One can understand more about the nature of a person's struggle with chronic pain by observing its impact on life than from repeatedly trying to quantify the intensity of the pain.

There are large numbers of people who experience pain over long periods of time without it changing, in major ways, how they function in life. Their pain may be daily and, in this sense, constant. Conversely, there are large numbers of people who suffer regularly with pain and cannot maintain their usual levels of functioning. Both these groups are people that have chronic pain. The rehabilitation counselor will see both types of individuals.

Because of these differences, the concept of the **chronic intractable benign pain syndrome** (CIBPS) was introduced (Crue & Pinsky, 1981; Pinsky, 1978). Distinguishing between the two states, chronic pain and the chronic pain syndromes, helps us better understand the different ways that chronic pain appears as a major symptom that disrupts the life process. It also helps us promote the most appropriate treatment interventions to relieve the suffering and impairment resulting from chronic pain.

## Chronic Intractable Benign Pain Syndrome (CIBPS)

This syndrome refers to the human problem in which the intensity, duration, and unremitting nature of non-cancer (**benign**) pain cannot be reasonably explained on the basis of unresolved tissue injury or known disease activity. The pain and its attendant suffering process has usually persisted for more than 6 months (can be less) in people in whom malingering (a conscious mental process of feigning illness or medical impairment) is not present.

Under these conditions, the major characteristic that distinguishes this as a particular syndrome is the extreme place of pain in the person's life. The counselor should be alerted to the possible presence of this syndrome when the client has persistent and constant complaints of pain expressed during counseling sessions. In addition to the pain and associated symptoms, another main feature of this syndrome is that of reported loss of or decreased physical and psychosocial functioning because of body pain and the additional problems related to it (see Figure 1).

The CIBPS will be the focus of this chapter. Within this category are the bulk of pain patients who are the most difficult to treat and rehabilitate; it is the most costly of all pain and suffering problems in both human and economic terms.

There is much controversy about the medical classification of these chronic pain syndromes. Conceptual differences about chronic pain are the source of this controversy when it occurs among physicians and between patients and physicians. This involves different explanations that are given about the reasons for the pain and its constancy over time. Each explanation serves as the main basis for the direction of treatment. All agree that the pain is real. In many patients, the physician, on physical examination, can find some evidence consistent with the pain complaint. However, it is often very clear that these may not be sufficient to be considered the source of the full pain syndrome.

---

## Figure 1
## CHRONIC INTRACTABLE BENIGN PAIN SYNDROME (CIBPS)

**The CIBPS is defined as a chronic and major problem with pain that has become a major life focus and:**

> cannot be shown to be significantly causally related to the here-and-now with an active pathoanatomic or pathophysiologic process, or a mental disorder with a major thought disorder.
>
> has an antecedent history of generally ineffective medical and surgical interventions for the pain problem.
>
> has come to be accompanied by significantly disturbed work and psychosocial functioning that includes the pain complaint with associated epiphenomena.

**Common epiphenomena of CIBPS include:**

> drug dependency or abuse, of varying severities, with their attendant central nervous system, psychosocial, and medical care adverse side effects.
>
> history of multiple surgeries or pharmacological treatments (often polypharmacy) with their own morbid side effects, separate from drug dependency issues;
>
> escalating physical inactivity secondary to increased pain and the belief that chronic pain of increased intensity is a signal of increasing bodily damage;
>
> dysphoric and lasting mood and affect changes;
>
> conflicts with medical care personnel (physicians, nurses, therapists, technicians) with resulting treatment outcome dissatisfaction, disguised and misplaced blame and more general hostilities;
>
> increasing hopelessness and helplessness as constant pain and increasing dysphoria does not give way in the face of mounting numbers of newer or different therapies;
>
> interpersonal conflict with significant others that often leads to serious dysfunction in or breaches of relationships;
>
> escalating psychosocial withdrawal with increased loss of anticipated and actual gratification from these interactions;
>
> decreasing ability to obtain pleasure from different areas of the life process (relative anhedonia) contributing to profound demoralization and, at times, siginificant depression;
>
> decrease in feelings of self-esteem, self-worth, and self-confidence.

---

If at least 7 of these 10 epiphenomenal conditions prevail when there is chronic pain, as described above, it is reasonable to regard the condition as a CIBPS.

---

When there is a CIBPS, it is not necessary to prove the absence of any findings in the soma that may be related to the pain. However, history of the problem, extent of the central complaint of pain, and its self-ascribed or observed impairments, provide a clinical picture of far greater complexity than can be explained only by the usual standard medical evaluations. These conceptual differences continue to delay the development of a realistic and accurate classification for the syndrome (CIBPS), whose existence is repeatedly validated by direct clinical observations. This will surface regularly as a dilemma for the rehabilitation counselor and the client.

## Classification Problems of CIBPS

Conceptual conflict about the places held by somatic and psychologic factors in chronic pain syndromes is omnipresent. Medical diagnoses and treatment, medical insurance, responsibilities for payment, legal proceedings, and workers' compensation and rehabilitation efforts are all affected by these conceptual differences. This conflict state is enhanced by the absence of an officially accepted definition and diagnostic classification for CIBPS. There is no specific classification of chronic pain syndromes in the current **International Classification of Diseases** (Commission on Professional and Hospital Activities, 1980).

The medical diagnoses used must be based on the idea of some form of tissue pathology or mental disorder. This perpetuates the idea that specific pathology or presumed pathophysiology of some kind is persistently and actively present in the soma or in the central nervous system, accounting for the syndrome's presence. In contrast to this, CIBPS is regarded by some as psychogenic in nature or not believed as existing at all.

A comprehensive understanding of the person who has the presenting symptoms will lead to a more complete understanding of the pain problem, its classification, and the most reasonable approach to treatment. Many medical diagnoses, like CIBPS, cannot be established solely with objective (physical) findings. The evolution of the pain problem and the patient's life history are of critical importance, even though they lack the same type of objectivity as an x-ray or laboratory test.

All major aspects of the patient's life are significant to understand the origin of the pain problem and how it developed into a full chronic pain syndrome. The rehabilitation counselor will find it difficult, if not impossible, to have the client focus on vocational issues until there is at least some change in the client's and treater's understanding of these different contributing issues.

The same clinical rigor in assessing objective medical information should be applied to discovering historical life events that may be pertinent. When an intractable chronic pain problem is present, such terms as "psychogenic origin" or phrases such as "clearly a product of disordered thought" should not be used in a patient's medical record. Expressions of mental events that are part of the clinical picture must be pursued in order to understand their roles in the chronic process. When a patient has CIBPS, the pain and its consequences become the central focus of the sufferer's existence. The pain is real and not consciously fabricated. All aspects of the patient's life history including intrapsychic, psychosocial, and physical event patterns are of paramount importance in understanding the extent of the suffering with pain and should be directly considered in the diagnosis and treatment plan (Pinsky, 1978, 1984).

The **Diagnostic and Statistical Manual for Mental Disorders** (American Psychiatric Association, 1987) classification of somatoform pain disorder attempts to bring all poorly documented chronic pain under a mental disorder paradigm. It is too conceptually limited to be useful because of the range of exclusions of physical and other mental dysfunctioning that are very frequently integral parts of CIBPS. Also, it tends to require or imply more cause and effect relationship between specific psychological events and the chronic pain than usually can be discovered.

The ramifications of including psychiatric diagnoses along with organic diagnoses are manifold. This can affect patients and their treaters as well as others involved in assessment and treatment in less direct, but vital ways. This includes insurers, rehabilitationists, attorneys, and agencies involved in assessing disability.

There is universal agreement that chronic pain syndromes often include potent and disturbing psychologic symptomatology. However, there is considerable variation among patients, physicians, and paramedical treaters in their abilities or inclinations to identify the symptoms and decreased physical functioning as being significantly generated or maintained by psychological determinants. This is also the case for insurance payers whose administrative and fiduciary systems more easily accept labels of a physical nature, than psychological labels for claims made for problems of chronic pain. In fact, payment for treatment may be contested or withheld when there is a psychiatric tinge to a person's problem with pain. Perhaps this discrimination exists because an organically-based diagnosis gives the illusion of being more easily understood and having a clearer resolution.

Nonetheless, chronic pain syndromes are medical problems regardless of the difficulty of diagnosis. Again, Figure 1 is a descriptive summary of CIBPS, its most frequent components, and a proposed model for its establishment as a diagnosis that is realistic. The adoption of a specific ICD-CM (**International Classification of Diseases, Clinical Modification**) diagnostic category for CIBPS will be a step toward an improved and useful diagnostic classification and help to avoid inappropriate treatments. This is being pursued by the American Academy of Pain Medicine (Pinsky, 1991).

# IMPAIRMENT AND DISABILITY ISSUES

## *Areas of Evaluation*

There are three general areas of evaluation of a person with a complaint of chronic pain. These areas have been outlined because they represent the most recent federal government positions about chronic pain, impairment, and disability (Osterweis, Kleinman, & Mechanic, 1987).

1. Extent of impairment of function that accompanies physical tissue damage in parts of the body that are specifically related to the pain complaint.

2. Complaints of chronic pain that seem disproportionate in their intensity and constancy to that of the documentable physical damage or outside the limit of normal recovery time.

3. The behavioral manifestations of pain (including verbal) that include the preoccupation and persistency of the complaints, a history of repeated evaluations, and multiple types of failed treatment attempts. Also included are persistent and excessive use of analgesics or some other psychoactive medication; impaired physical movements; facial grimaces; and sleep, eating, and sexual dysfunctions.

These three areas of evaluation require results that determine that there is impairment of a significant degree with lasting restriction of activities of daily living, social functioning, and other functional limitations in performing work activities before disability with chronic pain is declared.

## *Impairment and Disability-Chronic Pain vs CIBPS*

The criteria used for chronic pain to be considered a disability are similar to the components of CIBPS presented in Figure 1. There is one striking difference in that the list of criteria for CIBPS begins with "no known significant lesion in the here-and-now" (an unidentifiable cause) that can account for the extent of the impairment caused by the chronic pain.

According to the criteria used by the federal governmental agency for disability with chronic pain, there **must** be some evidence of physical damage. There is a built-in irony to this situation in that at least two-thirds of those having CIBPS will have **some** physical findings that can be related to their chronic pain. It is approximately this percentage of people who have musculoskeletal problems with some physical findings. In addition, individuals have often gone through multiple invasive diagnostic and treatment procedures that have left residuals of abnormal physical signs and symptoms, including pain.

Even with this high level of similarity between chronic pain (as outlined for disability evaluation) and CIBPS (as clinically described), there is reluctance to recognize CIBPS as a syndrome. This seems to be largely the result of opposition to any concept of chronic pain that is perceived as diminishing the direct "cause and effect" connection of chronic pain with active tissue damage or disease. There is also the concern that if we recognize chronic pain as a legitimate syndrome, it may be used inappropriately as a diagnostic dumping ground for another poorly understood set of medical problems. Anticipatory worry about the inappropriate use of a legitimate diagnostic category should not be the basis for its exclusion.

# PSYCHOSOCIAL ASPECTS OF CIBPS

It is usual and understandable to focus on psychological factors in many chronic medical problems because these factors often contribute to the maintenance of the severity of symptoms and the chronicity of the suffering (Mechanic, 1986). When chronicity of pain is part of a person's experience, it is easier to attribute the psychological malfunctioning to this chronicity. The roles of pain itself and the determinants that produce chronicity and the full syndrome, CIBPS, become difficult for all involved to separate. Biological, psychological, and social elements have regularly been found to profoundly affect chronic pain and its clinical course (Blackwell & Gutman, 1986; Osterweis et al., 1987; Pinsky, 1978, 1984).

## Dysphoria, Affect, Emotion, and Cognition

Individuals with CIBPS vary considerably in their abilities to recognize and express emotions and related feeling states. For this reason, a more general **dysphoria** is expressed that includes dejection, disaffection, unhappiness, and dissatisfaction with life or self. This is often manifested as an underestimation of self on any or every level (Campbell, 1981). When asked to list commonly experienced affects, emotions, and thoughts, these individuals at first are surprised at how limited their list seems (see Figure 2). The size of the list varies among different groups of pain peers, but the emotions and feeling states named remain fairly stable. It is then that they begin to take note of the subtle variations in the items on their list and often realize for the first time the extremely large number of combinations of feeling states that can occur from limited emotions and affect-laden thoughts.

A mix of thoughts, feelings, and ideas about their pain is present in people who have CIBPS. This mix has a rather distinctive pattern as part of a person's dynamic state. Changing interactions among the components of the mix can play a large role in determining the type and degree of symptoms and other behaviors. Because of the focus on chronic pain, it is not unusual for dysphoria (e.g., anxiety and depression) to take on atypical expressions; as such, the person may not be as responsive to the more usual treatment approaches. This may be accompanied by a firmly held belief that dysphoria would disappear if the pain were to go away.

---

### Figure 2
### COMMON THOUGHTS & EMOTIONS IN PEOPLE WITH CIBPS

| Affects/Emotions | Cognitive Constructs |
|---|---|
| Anger/rage | Abandonment |
| Anxiety | Alienation |
| Depression | Dependency |
| Fear | Disease and death |
| Grief and mourning | Future |
| Guilt | Loss |
| Hostility | Mental illness |
| Shame | Past |
| Remembered pain | |

---

One may view **acute** pain as a biologically useful signal of the danger of present or impending tissue damage. If this presence no longer exists in a significant way (CIBPS), there is no such danger. What then can be the usefulness of this expression of chronic pain? One view of CIBPS that attempts to understand and explain this **usefulness** involves some variations of Rado's concepts of **psychodynamic adaptation** (Pinsky, 1979; Senescu, 1975).

Long-standing patterns of adapting to strong emotional forces are present and are often referred to as "pre-morbid personality" (personality structure before the onset of pain). These characteristics determine to some degree the "fit" of CIBPS for any one individual.

Figure 3 is a schematic of possible determinants of the CIBPS as **attempts** at a form of psychological adaptation. It involves an interaction of affect, emotion, cognition, and need. The first three of these have been discussed; the concept of need now will be introduced. Needs represent a prominent motivational base for behavior (i.e., they are the basis for individual tendencies to move in the direction of goals). These needs may be linked to instinctual or developmental (learned) sources and are regarded to be present from early phases of human development. They may vary in their intensity and forms of expression and remain closely linked to emotions. These expressions may clearly exhibit the nature of the need or conceal and distort it. Loss of the sense of being able to gain specific need fulfillment will lead to attempts to adapt to this sense of loss, often at great human cost.

The items in the columns labeled **adaptive** and **adaptive failure** in Figure 3, represent the types of negative psychological forces that can be present and be affected by the presence of CIBPS. CIBPS may be developed in part

## Figure 3
## THE CHRONIC INTRACTABLE BENIGN PAIN SYNDROME (CIBPS) ATTEMPTED ADAPTATION TO DYSPHORIA, AFFECT, EMOTION, AND NEED

| ADAPTIVE | ADAPTIVE FAILURE |
|---|---|
| Dysphoria Binding or discharge related to: | Dysphoria Breakthrough: |
| Anxiety, fear | Anxiety, fear, tension |
| Depression | Demoralization |
| Anger, hostility | Depression |
| Shame | Sustained anger, hostility |
| Guilt | Unresolved grief response |
| Loss, unresolved grief | Drug dependence and abuse disorders |
| Hypochondriacal preoccupation | Other somatic disorders |
| Rejection and alienation | |
| Fulfillment of needs not otherwise met: | Increase of superimposed pathophysiological deficiencies: |
| Acceptance by others | Pharmacologic toxicity pattern |
| Special belonging | Deficits or dysesthesias from polysurgery |
| Nurture by others | Severe physical deconditioning |
| | Problems consequent to musculoskeletal disuse |
| Maintenance of self-esteem: | |
| Martyr role | |
| Psychosocial manipulation, control of personal environment | |
| Exercise of interpersonal power | |
| Avoidance of stigma and fear of mental illness | |

by the premorbid existence of these psychological forces. This is not an exhaustive list of these conditions, but this schema of CIBPS gives an overview of the complicated states that are encountered with this syndrome.

The outcome of any one attempt to adapt to the presence or anticipation of any lasting pain is largely determined (in a negative or positive way) by mental defense mechanisms and the coping abilities they allow to develop (Vaillant, 1988). The kinds of human support systems available to the individual are also critical factors for adaptive success. Some or all of these determinants of adaptation are often impaired in chronic medical syndromes. The need to protect oneself from unpleasant or threatening feeling states can be sufficiently strong so that CIBPS can serve as a defense against even **more** painful states. The combination of the avoidance of painful affects with the need gratification met through the existence of impairments can become a resultant motivational force sufficiently powerful to maintain the syndrome.

It is very difficult for people with these syndromes to be able to consciously address the existence, let alone the contents, of these troubled dynamic states. It should be recognized that the forces depicted as feelings and needs are part of an individual's internal milieu, of which the person largely is not consciously aware. The types and directions of goals and behavior they generate are often rationalized as having concrete meanings related only to their physically experienced and described pain and suffering.

When chronicity of pain is entrenched, it is understandable that psychologic malfunction is attributed to the pain itself. However, there is abundant clinical experience suggesting that psychologic factors **can** be causative in the **maintenance** or even the genesis of chronic pain (Szasz, 1975). Again, it must be through careful medical and medical psychology evaluations that these different patterns are determined.

It is crucial for the rehabilitation counselor to understand the complexity of this syndrome and not ignore any of the major contributing factors. Through this, the counselor can gain further insight into the client's behavior.

# UNIMODAL TREATMENT CONSIDERATIONS

Most frequently, one or two modalities of treatment are in place or have been tried in a serial fashion, one replacing another that has failed. These are usually somatically-based approaches because of patients' and treaters' exclusively somatic understanding of the chronic problems as described above. The most often used types of treatment can be categorized as **non-invasive** and **invasive**.

## Non-Invasive Treatments

Procedures such as transcutaneous electrical nerve stimulation (TENS), applied heat or cold, and other physical therapy modalities may provide some transient relief that may be helpful in acute, subacute, or chronic pain, but rarely contribute to significant change in CIBPS. While acupuncture is technically invasive, its therapeutic results along with those of non-invasive acupressure, also seem to have minimum effect when there is CIBPS. Psychotherapy for CIBPS will be more fully covered in the section on multimodal and interdisciplinary treatment, below.

## Invasive Treatments

**Nerve blocks.** Periodic neural blocking procedures (nerve blocks) can provide some decrease of pain for short intervals or help verify an already suspected diagnosis. They vary in their anatomical approach, based on the physical findings or on where the patient describes the location of the pain. The chemical agents used in these procedures are local anesthetics and cortisone-like drugs. The rationale is to break the noxious signal pattern and treat the **presumed** to be present inflammation. Again, the model for **acute** pain is frequently misapplied in the presence of CIBPS.

**CNS stimulation procedures and neurosurgery.** Direct central nervous system stimulation procedures and neurolytic or ablative neurosurgical procedures are more clinically extensive attempts to alleviate chronic pain. These all carry their own problems and some have significantly serious risks for the patient. They also often require the complexities of regular and long-term medical monitoring and follow-up. Any one may be helpful in specific cases as a "last resort" clinical situation in which less drastic treatment efforts were not medically tolerated or repeatedly failed to provide any relief. While there is a working rationale for attacking specific central nervous system targets, the exact mechanisms by which they produce positive results remain uncertain.

**Pharmacologic treatment.** This is considered an invasive treatment on a chemical basis in contrast to the physically invasive techniques described. The potential seriousness of this type of invasive approach is determined both by the extent of any medication use and the class of drugs to which it belongs, and by the physiological health of the person being treated. The presence of other illnesses, aging, and idiosyncratic (individual) drug reactions can and does limit the use of many medications.

**Analgesic medications.** The use of analgesic medications for pain, both non-narcotic and narcotic, are widespread when there is chronic pain; and, often they do not provide the relief that one might anticipate from their use when the pain is acute. Also, there are the particular physiological and psychological problems of **tolerance** and **dependence** that can occur regularly with long-term use of narcotic medications. There is a renewed and growing medical interest in the selection and study of patients with chronic pain who may be well managed with long-term oral opioids, under close medical supervision (Portenoy, 1990).

There are complicated relationships between pain, depression, anxiety, and fear when CIBPS is present, so that standard pharmacological regimens cannot be expected to have predictable effectiveness. Drugs that mainly act to lessen symptoms of one affect or mood over another, can often decrease or increase the subjective pain experience. Also, drugs that relieve symptoms of anxiety are generally of the class that also produce tolerance and dependency that contribute to serious drug dependency problems. There is interest in the use of tricyclic antidepressant agents for chronic pain states. When the pain states are accompanied by a major depressive disorder, these medications are effective in relieving the depression and may or may not alleviate the pain or other problems of the chronic pain syndrome. They may help lessen some symptoms, such as interrupted sleep (Pilowsky, 1975).

The tricyclic antidepressants have been helpful specifically in alleviating some pain in people suffering with post-herpes zoster neuralgia ("shingles") or diabetic retinopatnhy. There are ideas about how this occurs that involve our as yet imperfect and limited knowledge of central nervous system neurochemistry.

For these reasons, if it is medically tolerated, a trial with these drugs is often indicated. They may be effective in the treatment and management of some patients with chronic pain. Yet, these drugs have not provided a definitive answer to the problem of pain for the majority of people who suffer with the full chronic pain syndrome.

# MULTIMODAL AND INTERDISCIPLINARY TREATMENT

Treatment history is marked by many different somatic and pharmacologic treatment trials and failures when CIBPS is present. CIBPS patients respond best to a multimodal and interdisciplinary treatment approach that is medically-based (Jensen et al., 1991; Pinsky, 1991).

This approach involves a structured treatment program staffed by a team of professionals who have had training and experience in working with people who have CIBPS. The programs may be outpatient or inpatient, but all need to be of sufficient intensity and internal consistency. In the past 7 years, there has been a steady move toward the outpatient intensive treatment programs that have a full 5-day-a-week treatment schedule continuing for at least 3 or 4 weeks. There are variations on this schema that are dependent on specifics of the patient population and expertise of the medical director and the treatment team personnel. The components of this type of approach are similar in most facilities in which it is offered. The areas most variable among facilities include the extensiveness of the medical direction, the inclusion of invasive methods other than medication, and the form and intensity of psychotherapy.

## Physical Modalities of Treatment

Attention to and knowledge of the physical aspects of the patient's complaints are essential for a therapeutic relationship to develop in pain medicine treatment. This translates into non-specific but active physical and occupational therapies. Occasionally, some special exercises need to be continued along with this approach. Improving the general level of physical conditioning and increasing stamina are the major goals. If this physical therapy is neglected, patients who have great difficulties seeing themselves in a psychological light will have even less inclination and motivation to attend to the psychological and psychosocial components of treatment.

## Psychological Treatment

Of all the modalities used, a psychotherapeutic approach to treatment is generally the most difficult to develop and apply. An early psychodynamic and psychosocial understanding of the patient's problem with pain translates most usefully into an appropriate psychotherapeutic approach. With this as an overall guide to understanding of the problem, a **group psychotherapy** format has been the most useful in the treatment of CIBPS, when it is in the context of a generally therapeutic milieu. It should be sufficiently intense and operationally pragmatic so as to achieve an optimal match with the specific group of patients. The dynamics that occur between pain peers are most helpful in the psychological and psychosocial facets of this treatment, and the group psychotherapy fosters development of these dynamics. A more specific description of this type of group psychotherapy has been reported (Pinsky & Crue, 1984).

The composition of the group and its dynamics varies from group to group. The therapist needs to be knowledgeable in pain medicine or medical psychology to work effectively with this population.

## Psychophysiological Treatment

These are modalities of treatment that focus on the general goal of trying to achieve an increased ability of the patient to modulate the perception of pain. The patient is trained in techniques that aim at improving the abilities to modulate sensations and normal physiological events. Modalities such as skeletal muscle relaxation procedures, autogenic training, and electronic physiological feedback (biofeedback) are all useful avenues in which patients actively attempt, to learn in another way, about the soma/central nervous system interactions occurring in themselves. Learning to modulate these interactions serves as one model for attenuating the pain experience. Each modality by itself most likely does not have a specific effect, but can help a person gain a sense of mastery in the central nervous system/soma sphere and can increase well-being, self-esteem and hence, contribute to the alleviation of the CIBPS.

## Medication Management

A time-contingent medication regimen rather than one that is "as needed" helps significantly when there are or have been problems with medication use. There is a general benefit to this regimen when the patient is unaware of the exact medication being taken. Subsequent disclosure prior to completion of the intensive treatment program allows sufficient time for interaction with the team about the medication changes that have occurred. The extent and sophistication of the medications available has been reported, as have long-term outcome studies of drug use (Pinsky, 1983). Inpatient treatment may be required specifically for serious drug use problems prior to the actual start of a pain medicine structured program, particularly if parenteral (injectable) medications are being used.

## Rehabilitation Counseling

The rehabilitation counselor is included as part of the treatment team when return to work has been identified by the patient as a treatment goal. When this is the case, it will facilitate a more smooth transition from the pain medicine treatment program to the provision of vocational rehabilitation and return to work. Early intervention by the counselor can help enhance the motivation of the person interested in returning to gainful employment.

## Treatment Outcome

Multimodal treatment, with a major emphasis on group therapy, helps patients discover they have other feeling states, and that the sources of dysphoria they experience can adversely affect their pain. The advance of this process seems to be central to a lasting therapeutic outcome. With therapeutic movement, patients become more multifaceted in their view of themselves; this contributes to a diminished focus on the pain experience.

In this pain peer group setting, consistent and firm encouragement of patients to examine stressful and conflictive areas in their lives, often results in a decrease in resistance to approach some of these psychological issues. This tends to improve the patient's use of coping abilities.

Patients become increasingly open to recognizing in themselves other human problems and conflicts, and focus less importance on their identity as chronic pain patients. This is not the substitution of one concern for another. It begins the resolution of conflicting feelings related to the pain problem and the adaptation to the life forces represented by CIBPS. This treatment experience encourages patients to be less fearful of any residual pain and to increase understanding as well as become more responsible for changing their pain experience. With this comes a sense of mastery that is accompanied by an increase in self-esteem and all of its positive benefits, including success in educational and vocational pursuits.

# SUMMARY

If we have been medically accurate and determined that there no longer is a significantly active pathophysiological process present in a particular individual, there is no known reason why the person with CIBPS must continue to have constant pain. The diagnostic and therapeutic processes described in this chapter provide a basis for individuals with chronic pain to begin to use newly gained affective and cognitive experiences that are unique for them and are powerful sources to help gain lasting pain relief.

The treatment approach described is the core of a persuasive therapeutic model for the patient with chronic pain. A successful result is reflected in the patient emerging from a chronic intractable pain syndrome, even if there remains some residual pain. The rehabilitation counselor can aid immeasurably in evaluating, encouraging, and developing return to work goals for many of these individuals.

# CASE STUDY

Mr. Gregory Kraft is a 50 year-old married man with three children, ages 13, 15, and 17, who all live at home with him and his wife. Because of discipline problems in school, he only completed the 7th grade. While working for a utility company, he fell and injured his lower back. Mr. Kraft was a meter reader for the Metropolitan Water and Power Company. The **Dictionary of Occupational Titles** (1991) describes the position of meter reader as follow:

**D.O.T.#209.567-101 METER READER (utilities; waterworks)**

Reads electric, gas, water, or steam consumption meters and records volume used by residential and commercial consumers: Walks or drives truck over established route and takes readings of meter dials. Inspects meters and connections for defects, damage, and unauthorized connections. Indicates irregularities on forms for necessary action by servicing department. Verifies reading to locate abnormal consumption and records reason for fluctuations. Turns service off for nonpayment of charges in vacant premises, or on for new occupants. Collects bills in area. Returns route book to business office for billing purposes. May be designated according to type of meter read as electric-meter reader (utilities); gas-meter reader (utilities); steam-meter reader (utilities); water-meter reader (waterworks).

This job involves lifting a maximum of 15 pounds occasionally, with frequent lifting and carrying of 2-5 pounds. It typically takes 1-3 months to learn this job.

This worker had been employed by this company in the same capacity for 15 years when he was injured. There was some generalized lower back soreness that grew worse; pain began to radiate into his left buttocks and down the back of the left leg.

After 5 days of bed rest prescribed by his family physician, the pain did not diminish. Orthopedic consultation and examination led to a diagnosis of radiculitis (inflammation of a spinal nerve root, accompanied by pain and increased sensitivity) of the left first sacral nerve root (S1). A lumbar spine CT (computerized tomography) scan indicated a ruptured L5-S1 (Lumbar 5-Sacral 1) disk that was irritating the S1 nerve root. A lumbar laminectomy and diskectomy were performed 2 weeks following his injury; the recovery was without complications. Physical therapy began gradually after the third postoperative week.  ·

The original pain complaints were alleviated by the surgery and Mr. Kraft did well until approximately 6 weeks after surgery, when pain of the same intensity reappeared. This seemed to be made worse by active physical therapy maneuvers and any physical activity, continuous sitting, or prolonged standing. He again needed potent pain medication for this pain.

There was an orthopedic re-evaluation, showing no new or additional findings other than the S1 nerve root irritability and some paraspinal muscle spasm. Three months after surgery, a magnetic resonance imaging (MRI) procedure was done on his lumbar spine. It showed what appeared to be scar tissue in the area of the S1 nerve root on the left (also the area of his recent surgery). It was not definitively determined whether or not there was some disk material present in addition to the scar tissue. His pain intensified without any changes in its location or qualities and his use of prescribed pain medications escalated, while his level of ambulation and physical activity steadily decreased.

The possibility of residual disk material being an irritative focus led to a second laminectomy. At this surgery, scar tissue was verified, but there was only slight evidence for the presence of disk material. There was surgical removal of scar without risking injury to the nerve root or the lining of the spinal canal to which scar was adhered. Again, Mr. Kraft had a quick and uneventful surgical recovery, with some leg pain relief that lasted for about 6 weeks at which time the leg pain began to return. It quickly became constant. The low back pain did not diminish on this occasion. His lumbar spine was mechanically stable and showed only the evidence of his recent surgeries, when evaluated radiologically.

Mr. Kraft has not worked since the industrial accident. After 6 months, he began to worry about the financial well-being of his family and became increasingly demoralized while his opioid pain medicine use gradually escalated. He reported insomnia, irritability, and had angry outbursts directed at his family. The treating physician recommended an intensive pain medicine treatment program after an early trial at vocational rehabilitation evaluation failed.

After a comprehensive evaluation, Mr. Kraft agreed to enter a pain treatment program. The multimodal and treatment team nature of this program is described earlier in this chapter. During the 4 weeks that he participated in the program, he made steady progress in his physical activities and his demoralization gave way to new and constructive assessments regarding abilities, self-concept, and residual pain. He came to realize that his residual chronic pain was not associated with any new or increased damage to his back or nervous system. This was accompanied by a gradual weaning from opioids. A month after completing the program, he joined his employer in a rehabilitation effort that enabled him to gain managerial skills and a return to employment. At one year follow-up, he had missed only 2 days of work because of acute muscle spasm in his lower back; his low back and leg pain was gradually diminishing in intensity and had stopped interfering with usual life activities and his ability to enjoy life.

## Questions

1. Provide a vocational profile for Mr. Gregory Kraft, including age category, education level, and work history (exertional and skill levels).

2. Identify the occupationally significant characteristics and skills (if any) of the work of a meter reader.

3. Discuss the chronic intractable benign pain syndrome (CIBPS) and Mr. Kraft's adaptation to the psychosocial aspects, including affects, emotions, and needs.

4. If the employer was unable to return Mr. Kraft to work, outline other vocational rehabilitation possibilities. Include a transferable skills analysis (if there are transferable skills) in your answer.

## REFERENCES

American Psychiatric Association (1987). **Diagnostic and statistical manual of mental disorders** (3rd ed., revised). Washington, DC: Author.

Black, R.J. (1975). The chronic pain syndrome. **Surgical Clinics of North America, 55,** 999.

Blackwell, B., & Gutmann, M. (1986). The management of chronic illness behavior. In S. McHugh & T.M. Vallis (Eds.), **Illness behavior** (pp. 401-408). New York: Plenum Press.

Campbell, R.J. (1981). **Psychiatric dictionary** (5th ed.). New York: Oxford University Press.

Commission on Professional and Hospital Activities (1980). **The international classification of diseases, clinical modification** (9th rev.). Ann Arbor, MI: Author.

Crue, B.L., Jr. (1983). The peripheralist and centralist views of chronic pain. **Seminars in Neurology, 3**(4), 331-339.

Crue, B.L., & Pinsky, J.J. (1981). Chronic pain syndrome: Four aspects of the problem. In L.K.Y. Ng (Ed.), **Research Monograph Series, New approaches to treatment of chronic pain: A review of multidisciplinary pain clinics and pain centers** (Research Monograph Series, No. 36, DHHS Publication No. ADM 81-1089). Rockville, MD: National Institute on Drug Abuse.

International Association for the Study of Pain (1986). Definition of pain. **Pain, 3,** S217.

Jensen, M.P., Turner, J.A., Romano, J.M., & Karoly, P. (1991). Coping with chronic pain: A critical review of the literature. **Pain, 47,** 249-283.

Mechanic, D. (1986). Illness behavior: An overview. In S. McHugh & T.M. Vallis (Eds.), **Illness Behavior-Part II** (pp. 101-109). New York: Plenum Press.

Osterweis, M., Kleinman, A., Mechanic, D., & the Clinical, Behavioral, and Public Policy Perspectives, Institute of Medicine, Committee on Pain, Disability, and Chronic Illness Behavior (Eds.) (1987). **Pain and disability: Clinical, behavioral and public policy perspectives.** Washington, DC: National Academy Press.

Pilowsky, I. (1975). Psychiatry and the pain clinic. **American Journal of Psychiatry, 133,** 752-756.

Pinsky, J.J. (1978). Chronic, intractable benign pain: A syndrome and its treatment with intensive short-term group psychotherapy. **Journal of Human Stress, 4,** 17.

Pinsky, J.J. (1979). Aspects of the psychology of pain. In B.L. Crue, Jr. (Ed.), **Chronic Pain** (pp. 301-314). New York: SP Medical and Scientific Books.

Pinsky, J.J. (1983). Psychodynamic understanding and treatment of the chronic intractable benign pain syndrome: Treatment outcomes. **Seminars in Neurology, 3**(4), 346-354.

Pinsky, J.J. (1991). Treatment of chronic pain syndromes. **The Clinical Journal of Pain, 7,** 175-176.

Pinsky, J.J., & Crue, B.L. (1984). Intensive group psychotherapy. In P.D. Wall & R. Melzack (Eds.), **Textbook of pain** (pp. 823-831). New York: Churchill Livingstone.

Portenoy, R.K. (1990). Chronic opioid therapy in non-malignant pain. **Journal of Pain Symptom Management,** 5(S15), S46-62.

Senescu, R.A. (1975). Sandor Rado. In A.M. Freedman, H.I. Kaplan, & B.J. Sadock (Eds.), **Comprehensive textbook of psychiatry/II** (2nd ed., pp. 613-619). Baltimore, MD: Williams and Wilkins.

Szasz, T.S. (1975). **Pain and pleasure.** New York: Basic Books.

U.S. Department of Labor (1991). **Dictionary of occupational titles** (4th ed., revised). Washington, DC: Author.

Vaillant, G.E. (1988). Defense Mechanisms. In A.M. Nicholi, Jr. (Ed.), **The new Harvard guide to psychiatry** (pp. 200-207). Cambridge, MA: Belknap Press of Harvard University Press.

## *About the Author*

Jack Pinsky, M.D., is a psychiatrist and an Associate Clinical Professor in the Department of Neurosurgery, California College of Medicine, University of California, Irvine (UCI), and Director of Pain Medicine, UCI Medical Center, Orange, California. He is a Clinical Associate Professor of Neurosurgery (Algology), University of Southern California School of Medicine, Los Angeles, California. A founding officer and past-president of the American Academy of Pain Medicine, he is currently an Associate Editor for the **Clinical Journal of Pain.**

# Chapter 14

# HEARING DISABILITIES

by
*Marita M. Danek, Ph.D.*
*and*
*Michael D. Seidman, M.D.*

## INTRODUCTION

Hearing impairments are the most common form of chronic physical disability in the United States today. Persons with hearing loss are an exceedingly diverse group. The loss may be mild or severe. It may be present at birth, occur throughout life and during old age. Hearing loss may present formidable educational, social, and vocational barriers or be a minor nuisance.

This chapter addresses chronic hearing loss and its implications for individuals through the lifespan. It addresses characteristics of persons with varying degrees and types of hearing loss, and identifies medical and rehabilitation interventions that enhance the capacity of individuals to function at work and in the community.

### Definitions

There are no universally accepted definitions of the terms "hearing impaired," "deaf," and "hard-of-hearing." Professionals, consumers, and the public have somewhat different interpretations of this terminology. The term "hearing impairment" is typically used to refer to any degree of decreased sensitivity to sounds. This definition includes a decreased ability to interpret auditory input correctly. Many individuals use the terms "hearing impaired" and "deaf" interchangeably, although deafness is more specific and describes more profound or severe hearing loss. In recent years, the term "hearing impaired" has become increasingly unacceptable to consumers and professionals alike.

Deafness is a rare condition among the working-age population, although its incidence increases dramatically with age. From a medical perspective, deafness means to have no perception of sound; it is the complete inability to discriminate or perceive sounds. A hard-of-hearing person has a lesser degree of hearing loss.

The state-federal rehabilitation system makes a distinction between deafness and other hearing impairments based on functional limitations that diminish the individual's capacity to engage in gainful employment or to live independently. These include degree of loss, age at onset, and etiology. Deafness is a "hearing impairment of such severity that the individual must depend primarily on visual communication such as writing, lip reading, manual communication, and gestures." A hard-of-hearing individual has a "functional loss, but not to the extent that the individual must depend primarily upon visual communication" (Rehabilitation Services Administration, 1986, pp. 15, 26, & 27).

Deaf persons, particularly individuals who have been deaf from an early age, define deafness in socio-cultural terms; deafness is not a disability, but a culturally defining condition (National Institute on Deafness and Other Communication Disorders, 1989). From the perspective of deaf persons, "deafness" results from cultural aspects of the disability in which group similarities, values, needs, and communication modality are more important than the degree of hearing loss. A person who is culturally deaf can use American Sign Language (ASL) and is a member of the Deaf Community.

Recently, two consumer groups, the World Federation of the Deaf (WFD) and the International Federation of Hard-of-Hearing people (IFHOH), clarified the distinction between "deaf" and "hard-of-hearing" individuals:

> Deaf and Hard-of-Hearing Individuals have, over a period of time, developed separate and distinct group identities and, as a result, separate specialized vocabularies. Deaf people seek to utilize their visual skills for communication while hard-of-hearing persons seek ways to retain their listening and speaking skills. ("Joint Declaration," 1991, p. 6)

Although these distinctions point to the richness of perspectives in the field, they may contribute to confusion in the minds of policy makers and the public. The lack of universally accepted definitions frequently pose problems in data gathering and reporting, valid comparisons across research studies, justification of public funding for programs and services, and individual eligibility for educational and rehabilitation programs. For example, the state-federal rehabilitation system bases priority of services on the severity of an individual's disability. Deaf persons (as defined by that system) are automatically considered severely disabled; hard-of-hearing persons are not unless they meet additional criteria.

## Prevalence

A hearing loss may be due to disorders involving any of the auditory pathways. Therefore, cerumen (wax) impaction in the external ear, fluid in the middle ear, inner ear pathology, auditory nerve abnormality or abnormalities within various parts of the brain responsible for the perception, understanding, and interpretation of sound all can cause varying degrees and severity of impairments.

Specific information regarding the prevalence of hearing impaired persons is difficult to interpret. The closest estimates suggest that more than 30 million Americans have some form of hearing loss. As the population ages, this number rapidly increases. In the United States, 23% of the population between 65-75 years has a hearing loss, and 40% of the population, 75 years and above, is affected. This number can be appreciated more when one considers that in 1980, 11% of the population was 76 years or older. This number will increase to nearly 21% by the year 2030 (Johns et al., 1989). Table 1 summarizes the trend of aging and hearing loss.

If we accept the definition of deafness as a hearing impairment that interferes with the ability to understand normal conversation, approximately 0.2 % of the working-age population (ages 15-64) are deaf. Among those persons 65 years of age and older, 0.7 % are deaf (Department of the Census, 1986).

Hearing impairments occur in approximately 1 out of every 1000 live births. In contrast, roughly 25% of elderly people have hearing impairments. Although the older population is more often affected by hearing loss, it is prelingually deaf persons (persons who have lost hearing before the age of speech) who tend to experience the most severe difficulties and represent the greatest challenge to the rehabilitation counselor. This population has difficulty acquiring skills in written and spoken English and consequently may encounter considerable barriers in educational and vocational endeavors.

**Table 1**

## ESTIMATES OF THE REPORTED PREVALENCE OF HEARING IMPAIRMENTS IN THE POPULATION BY AGE GROUP, UNITED STATES, 1987

| Age Group | Number | Rate per Thousand |
|---|---|---|
| **Total** | **20,994,000** | **88.0** |
| Under 18 years | 1,012,000 | 16.0 |
| 18-44 years | 5,529,000 | 54.1 |
| 45-64 years | 6,098,000 | 135.6 |
| 65-74 years | 4,582,000 | 264.7 |
| 75 years and over | 3,773,000 | 348.0 |

From National Center for Health Statistics, Data from the National Health Survey, Series 10, Number 166, Table 57, 1988.

## *Causes*

To understand the etiology of hearing loss, one must first have a basic understanding of the hearing mechanism. The auditory system is usually described in three sections: the external, the middle, and the inner ear. Aural communication begins with a sound. Sound is a wave form of pressure that travels through the surrounding medium (be it air, water, or another substance). These sound waves then travel through the external ear canal and strike the tympanic membrane (eardrum) causing it to vibrate. This portion of the ear constitutes the external (outer) ear. Congenital defects (obstructions) of the auricle or ear canal, for example, can and do contribute to hearing loss. The middle ear exists between the tympanic membrane and the inside surface of the stapes bone. The middle ear consists of a space that contains three of the smallest bones in the body. These bones (ossicles) are the malleus (hammer), the incus (anvil), and the stapes (stirrup).

Once a sound wave strikes the tympanic membrane, the eardrum transfers the vibration to the malleus, thus conducting the sound energy or pressure to the incus and stapes. The stapes forms the end of the middle ear. From here, the sound energy moves across the oval window (a very thin membrane that separates the stapes from the inner ear) into the inner ear. Within the inner ear is the cochlea. The cochlea contains the organ of Corti that transforms fluid pulsations generated from the sound, into nerve impulses. These impulses are then transferred via the cochleo-vestibular nerve to the brain stem and up to the auditory cortex, which is within the temporal lobe of the brain. The inner ear also contains the organ of equilibrium (the vestibular system) that consists of three semicircular canals and five neuroepithelial structures (nerve-like tissues), which interpret motion and gravitational forces. Information from the vestibular system is conducted through the vestibular portion of the cochleo-vestibular nerve (auditory nerve-cranial nerve VIII).

This highly abbreviated description (Paparella & Shumrick, 1980) of the hearing process reveals the many different areas within the hearing system that can function in a decreased or abnormal capacity, and produce a hearing impairment. The next section will review types of hearing loss.

# TYPES OF HEARING LOSS

Hearing losses are usually described as (1) conductive, (2) sensorineural, and (3) mixed (a combination of both). A conductive loss is due to disorders of the external or middle ear and means that the mechanism for bringing a sound wave into the inner ear is not functioning. This problem may have a simple cause such as cerumen (wax) impaction or fluid in the middle ear, frequently occurring after an ear infection. Yet, it might be a more severe cause such as being born without an external ear (agenesis of the auricle) and possibly without the ear canal. Sensorineural hearing loss (SNHL) is the most common type of hearing loss and is usually a more serious loss. It occurs because of abnormalities of the neural pathway. A common form of SNHL is due to excessive noise. SNHL is the type of hearing loss that is least amenable to medical treatment. It is the type of hearing loss that demands the most from the allied health professionals. As the name implies, a mixed hearing loss is a combination of the two hearing losses described; consequently, it may be the most severe.

The complexities and intricacies of the auditory system contribute to the varied and multiple causes of hearing loss. The major causes of hearing loss are sensorineural. Yet, conductive losses are significant in number and also contribute to hearing impairment. Conductive losses are typically less severe and often can be corrected by medical or surgical intervention. Sensorineural losses are often more severe and not usually correctable through surgery. The following section discusses the major causes of hearing impairments.

## Presbycusis

Presbycusis is a term that describes the hearing loss associated with the normal aging process and is the most common cause of hearing loss. Typically, presbycusis begins in the mid to late 40s age range. However, it can and probably does begin even earlier. The loss is characterized by involvement of the high frequencies, usually 3000 Hz. and above. Although the actual cause for the hearing loss is not technically known, pathological studies show loss of hair cells and damage to the supporting cells within the organ of Corti (nerve tissue within the inner ear).

Presbycusis is an irreversible loss; it does not improve and usually progresses with advancing age. As one loses the high frequency sounds, one also tends not to understand or discriminate words as well. The most common explanation for this loss in discrimination is that the sounds that impart meaning to words tend to be high frequency sounds such as ta, ss, and ff. Thus, the rehabilitation counselor should avoid speaking loudly to a person with presbycusis. This would only serve to obscure intelligible sounds for the older listener.

## Heredity

Heredity contributes significantly to causes of hearing impairment. The following is a brief discussion of the more commonly encountered hereditary syndromes that may affect hearing.

Ushers' syndrome is inherited in an autosomal recessive pattern. In this syndrome, the person experiences a hearing impairment at birth, followed by progressive blindness secondary to retinitis pigmentosa. It accounts for approximately 10% of hereditary deafness.

One inherits Waardenburg syndrome in an autosomal dominant pattern with variable expressivity. It accounts for approximately 1-7% of hereditary deafness. The syndrome is characterized by widely spaced medial canthi (eyes spaced far apart), flat nasal root, confluent eyebrows (very thick eyebrows that almost meet), heterochromia (different colored irises), a white forelock of hair, and sensorineural hearing loss. Alports' syndrome is inherited in an autosomally dominant pattern. There is a high frequency hearing loss that may be progressive. Renal (kidney) manifestations include hematuria (blood or red blood cells in the urine) and nephritis (inflammation of the kidneys). It is of interest that renal transplant may reverse the hearing loss.

Pendreds' disease is an autosomal recessive disorder that accounts for 10% of all hereditary deafness. In this syndrome, bilateral sensorineural hearing loss occurs secondary to atrophy of the organ of Corti in the inner ear. These individuals have thyroid gland involvement.

Jervell-Lange-Nielsen syndrome is characterized by hearing loss and cardiac abnormalities. Males more often have this condition. Cardiac problems associated with this syndrome may pose considerable vocational and independent living challenges and, not infrequently, individuals with this syndrome may die secondary to cardiac problems.

There are many other inherited hearing disorders. Interested persons are referred to any standard otolaryngological text for further information.

Congenital malformations of the middle and inner ear also can be a cause of mild to severe hearing impairments. A more common congenital abnormality of the cochlea is Mondinis' deformity. This is characterized by underdevelopment of the cochlea. Typically, these individuals have a moderate hearing loss. This can be diagnosed via computerized tomographic scanning (CT scan). Other less frequently encountered cochlear abnormalities, such as Michel's, Scheibe's, and Alexander's deformities, also may cause SNHL.

## Trauma

Trauma is a major factor responsible for hearing impairment today; noise-induced hearing loss accounts for most traumatic hearing loss. Noise-induced hearing loss has plagued society for thousands of years. The first concerns of noise related hearing loss dates back to 600 B.C. when the Sybarites forbade metal work and the keeping of roosters within the city limits (English, 1986). During the first century, Pliny the elder noted that "persons living near the cataracts of the Nile were stricken deaf" (Paparella & Shumrick, 1980). Acoustic trauma is directly related to the energy level and frequency of the sound stimulus. Early noise experiments showed that the longer the exposure to a damaging noise level, the greater the cochlear damage (Davis, 1953). Exposure to noise is a widespread problem that has a substantial impact on the prevalence of hearing loss among the working population.

Noise-induced hearing loss (NIHL) is 1 of 10 leading work-related diseases and injuries (Centers for Disease Control, 1983). This problem is escalating with an estimated 835 million dollars in workers' compensation paid for occupationally induced hearing loss from 1978-1987 ("Leads from the MMWR", 1988). Recent estimates suggest that between 7.4-10.2 million people work in areas where the level of noise presents an increased risk of hearing loss (85 dB or higher) (Simpson & Bruce, 1981).

Noise can cause varying degrees of hearing impairment. Blast or impulse noise of 120 dB and greater typically damages the cochlea by causing disruption of the organ of Corti from the basilar membrane. Lower levels of sound (i.e., 85-120 dB SPL) may lead to alteration and decreases in hair cell number within the organ of Corti. The actual etiology of this is not well understood, but many experiments have shown metabolic and biochemical alterations. Prevention and education about NIHL is the best resolution to lessen the future loss of hearing in susceptible persons (National Institute for Occupational Safety and Health, 1988).

## Infections

Infectious causes are very important in the etiology of hearing loss. One of the most widely known is maternal rubella, which attacks the auditory system of the fetus, leading to potentially severe hearing impairment. Other more common infections, including otitis media, can cause hearing loss. Usually otitis media leads to the accumulation of fluid within the middle ear, and this in itself causes hearing loss. Though the loss may only be about 20 dB, in a child who is beginning to learn speech, it can impede the development of speech and language. Other infections such as mumps, measles, varicella zoster (chicken pox), cytomegalovirus, influenza B, tuberculosis, and Lassa fever may cause permanent hearing loss. Meningitis, or inflammation of the meninges (lining) in the brain, has been a common cause of hearing loss, especially before the advent of antibiotic therapy.

## Tumors

Other causes of hearing loss include tumors of the brain (e.g., cerebello-pontine angle). The most common of these tumors is the acoustic neuroma. Although this is a benign tumor, it causes hearing loss. Patients with neurofibromatosis (a disease that leads to the formation of multiple tumors in nerve tissue) also can develop acoustic neuromas, which potentially will lead to irreversible hearing loss.

The growth of acoustic neuromas are typically slow (Wazen, Silverstein, Norrell, & Bessa, 1985). It is important to diagnose these tumors early since they usually can be surgically removed in the earlier stages, and thus spare some amount of useful hearing. In addition, early intervention poses less risk to the facial nerve. When tumors are diagnosed after hearing or speech discrimination becomes poor, hearing does not improve after the removal of the tumors since the initial nerve damage has already been done.

## Meniere's Disease

Meniere's disease, a disorder characterized by fluctuating sensorineural hearing loss, tinnitus, vertigo, and aural fullness is caused by endolymphatic hydrops (increased fluid pressure in the organ of equilibrium). Although this is a sensorineural type hearing loss, if diagnosed early, medical treatment may slow the progression. Severe cases that fail medical management may need surgical intervention. Surgery is aimed at alleviating vertigo, which may be more incapacitating than the hearing loss.

## Additional Distinctions

Severity and type of hearing loss obviously have considerable impact on an individual's general functioning. Another crucial factor is the age at onset of the loss. Prelingual deafness refers to deafness that was present at birth or occurred before acquisition of language or speech, typically at age 3 or earlier. A prevocational loss is one that occurs before an individual's entry into the workforce (at around age 19 or before). The implications of when the loss occurred are functionally very important. Prelingual deafness implies that a major sensory organ for acquiring and processing information does not exist for the developing person. Information must be obtained primarily through visual methods. Naturally, a person with a prevocational loss has normal speech and communicates well up to this point in life. Rehabilitation needs of the individual will vary considerably, based not only on the age at onset, but also on the degree of loss, and other characteristics of the individual, such as abilities, personality, and interests.

# EVALUATION

## Medical Evaluation

The key to diagnosis of a hearing impairment is to recognize that a problem exists. This is not always easy, especially when one considers the newborn child that may appear normal in every respect but has a profound hearing loss. Physicians do not routinely test all infants for hearing capacity; to do so is not medically feasible. Yet, there are certain situations that should raise the suspicion that a hearing loss may exist. Some indicators are a family history of this condition, serious infections or other problems during pregnancy, detection of birth trauma, and any other physical abnormalities in the newborn (Paparella & Shumrick, 1980).

When one becomes aware a child has a hearing loss, a referral to a qualified otolaryngologist (ear, nose and throat, head and neck surgeon) is necessary. The otolaryngologist will take a detailed history to find out the potential causes of the hearing loss and possible medical treatment. It is important to identify the cause of the hearing loss, age at onset, severity, and potential for progression as early as possible, and to attempt to find the site of the lesion responsible for the hearing loss, if one is present.

Once the physician obtains the medical and family history, not only is a complete head and neck examination performed, but the physician evaluates the total person beyond the region of the head and neck. It is important to observe the person as a whole. The otolaryngologist notes facial symmetry, the space between the eyes, the shape of the head, and the level of the ears. These seemingly subtle findings may lead to the recognition of a particular syndrome responsible for the hearing impairment.

After the specialist conducts a general observation, an examination of the auricles is done to be sure they have developed normally. Next, one does an examination of the external auditory canals, and tympanic membranes.

A thorough head and neck examination will note any other malformations. The physician then refers the patient to a qualified audiologist. An audiological examination usually delineates the degree of the hearing impairment and the potential for medical or surgical intervention. The audiologist carefully conducts several tests under specified conditions, to evaluate the function of the auditory system. An evaluation is conducted in conjunction with the otolaryngologist to prescribe the most beneficial aid to help the patient conduct activities of daily living. The audiologist uses an audiometer to test hearing, and audiograms to report the findings of audiological testing.

Audiograms of individuals with normal hearing and various types of hearing loss are shown in Figures 1, 2, and 3. A standard audiogram plots decibels on the Y axis and frequencies on the X axis. A decibel is a logarithmic unit that expresses sound intensity. Zero on the decibel scale is the baseline for normal hearing. Each time one increases the scale by 10 decibels, one increases the intensity of sound by a factor of 10, hence the logarithmic scale. The higher the decibels, the more power is required to hear a specific sound; this signifies a greater hearing loss. Frequency is measured in hertz (Hz.) or cycles per second. Low frequencies, i.e., 250 Hz, are sounds like a fog horn or a base singer. High frequencies; i.e., 8000 Hz., are sounds like a bird chirping or a soprano singing. For speech, the important frequencies are between 500 Hz and 2000 Hz. Hearing loss in this frequency range is particularly detrimental to everyday communication.

If necessary, auditory brain stem response (ABR) can be conducted without the active participation of the patient. The ABR or Brainstem Auditory Evoked Potentials (BAEP) assesses the retrocochlear auditory system; that is, it tests the integrity of the hearing mechanism from the area past the cochlea (i.e., the auditory nerve through the auditory cortex). It is particularly useful in the assessment of unilateral sensorineural hearing losses, or in individuals who cannot easily cooperate. It is an excellent test to evaluate and help diagnose an acoustic neuroma.

It is imperative to perform a number of laboratory tests. Most otolaryngologists will begin by recommendation of a routine complete blood count, a creatinine, a thyroid screening test, a urinalysis, and other evaluations as indicated. Occasionally, it is important to rule out an autoimmune disorder, such as systemic lupus erythematosus.

There are many factors that can complicate the diagnosis in hearing-related disorders. One of these is age. An infant or young child before the attainment of language skills, can be perceived as normal, yet have a hearing impairment. Most major medical institutions have an audiologist on staff with a specific interest in pediatrics. The most useful testing for an infant with suspected hearing loss is the ABR because the infant does not need to contribute anything to the examination process and the testing can be conducted while the infant is asleep or quiet. For the slightly older child who is not yet speaking, audiologists use warble tones in an attempt to have the child look in the direction of the released tone. This gives an indication that the child may be hearing sounds. Yet, the child could be deaf in one ear and still be able to respond to a warble tone.

# Figure 1

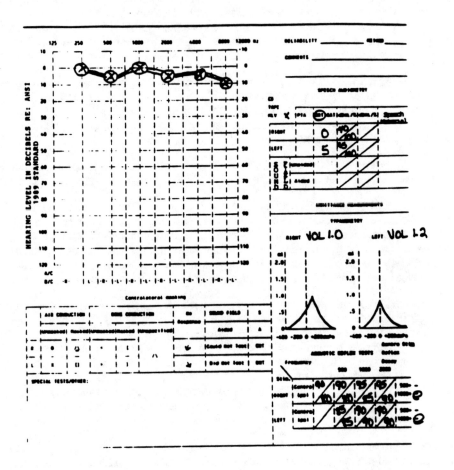

Normal Hearing

Some of these problems also occur in persons with mental impairments. These people may not be able to communicate what sounds they are hearing. An ophthalmological evaluation is frequently recommended for individuals with hearing loss. These persons must rely more heavily or entirely on sight for their communication needs. Any decrease in visual acuity must be medically corrected, if possible, and become part of counseling and service planning. This examination also may detect Usher's syndrome and other visual problems secondary to genetic deafness or deafness associated with congenital rubella syndrome.

The otolaryngologist and audiologist work with the rehabilitation counselor to address modifications in the person's environment, which will promote competency at work and in the community. The gathering of additional diagnostic information by the rehabilitation counselor takes into consideration two factors: (1) how this information will be used and (2) whether the anticipated benefits will justify the time and expense necessary to obtain such information.

# Figure 2

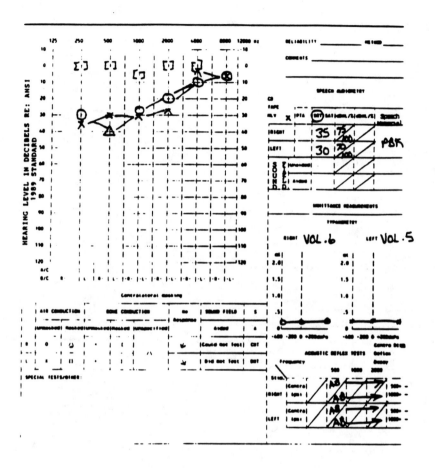

Conductive Hearing Loss

Assessment for rehabilitation purposes considers not only the individual, but also the individual's environment, perceptions, and interactions (Szymanski, Dunn, & Parker, 1989). Rehabilitation counselors work in a variety of settings; the agency or facility may require certain diagnostic information for purposes of program eligibility. Other information will be optional or recommended. The state-federal rehabilitation system typically requires a general medical examination, an otolaryngological evaluation, and in some states, audiological or ophthalmological examinations to determine eligibility for vocational rehabilitation services.

Other evaluative information that might be appropriate to obtain includes psychological testing, vocational evaluation, and an assessment of the client's expressive and receptive communication skills including speech, reading, writing, and type of sign communication, if any. All cases should have a comprehensive case study to determine psychosocial functioning, educational and vocational history, and current level of functioning. A professional who is knowledgeable about the implications of hearing loss and can communicate using the client's preferred mode of communication, is the best person to conduct the evaluations.

## Figure 3

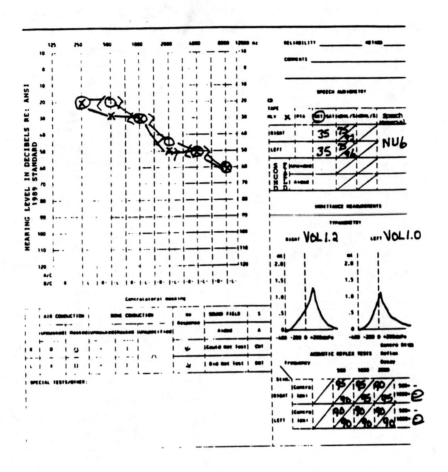

Sensorineural Hearing Loss

### Psychological Evaluation

A psychological evaluation is not used routinely with any deaf or hard-of-hearing person. These evaluations are informative when the counselor suspects a significant deviation from the norm in terms of intellectual, social, or personal functioning that may have an impact on rehabilitation planning and outcome. If the counselor only needs information on vocational interests and aptitudes, a vocational evaluation may provide a more comprehensive measure of these dimensions.

The expertise of the clinical psychologist who conducts the psychological evaluation is critical because misdiagnoses of persons with hearing impairments are prevalent. Some standardized tests frequently used in a psychological evaluation include measures of intelligence, personality, vocational interests and aptitudes, and educational achievement.

**Intelligence tests.** Deaf and hard-of-hearing persons have a normal range of intelligence. Nonverbal intelligence tests are used with persons who are prevocationally deafened or hard-of-hearing. For this population, verbal intelligence tests only measure limitations in English language usage, not intelligence. Two tests that have norms for persons with hearing loss are the Hiskey-Nebraska Test of Learning Aptitude and the Leiter International Performance Scale.

**Personality tests.** The use of personality tests with prevocationally deaf and hard-of-hearing persons requires extreme care. Not only do the hearing impaired person's English language limitations distort responses, but there is some question that the tests themselves measure factors not appropriate for this population. For example, the statement "I sometimes hear voices" on the Minnesota Multiphasic Personality Inventory (MMPI) would be answered positively by some deaf and hard-of-hearing persons.

Persons who become deaf or hard-of-hearing in adulthood may experience more withdrawal and depression due to the loss of social networks. The psychologist is sensitive to this possibility when interpreting the results of standardized tests and to "masked" depression, which may present as hypochondriasis (multiple physical complaints without an organic basis).

**Vocational interest and aptitude.** Many vocational aptitude tests depend on verbal skills. Of those that use performance measures, few have well-established norms for persons with hearing loss. The General Aptitude Test Battery (GATB) has norms for persons who are deaf, but they are based on small sample sizes. The Geist Picture Interest Inventory (Revised) (GEIST-R) and the Wide Range Interest and Opinion Test-Revised (WRIOT-R) are frequently used with hearing impaired populations. The GEIST-R has norms for males who are deaf, but has a restricted range of occupational choices. The WRIOT-R does not have norms for individuals who are deaf or hard-of-hearing and has major standardization weaknesses. Holland's Self-Directed Search-Form Easy can be used as a career assessment instrument with deaf high school students if certain administrative conditions are met (Darnell, 1991).

Vocational aptitude and interest tests should be used with caution and only for exploratory purposes in counseling persons with hearing loss. One should never use these test results as sole indicators for planning purposes.

**Educational achievement.** Because acquiring English language skills poses such difficulty for hearing impaired children, the academic achievement of hearing impaired youth lags behind their hearing counterparts, particularly in reading comprehension (Allen, 1986). The most appropriate educational achievement test is the Stanford Achievement Test, 8th edition, because of its specific subtests with deaf norms in reading, spelling, language, concepts of number, mathematics computation, and mathematics applications. The mean reading scores of deaf high school students taking the Stanford Achievement Test are approximately at the third grade level; mathematics computation scores are about at the sixth to seventh grade level.

Persons who develop hearing loss in adulthood will have scores that more closely parallel the norms for hearing people. The counselor will usually be able to obtain relevant achievement test scores from high school records rather than asking for this as part of the psychological evaluation. As a measure of potential functioning for an older person, educational achievement is less important.

## Vocational Evaluation

Over the past two decades, vocational evaluation has gradually replaced traditional aptitude testing. It offers more realistic, hands-on appraisal under simulated working conditions. Vocational evaluation systems that show particular promise for hearing impaired persons include the JEVS (Jewish Employment and Vocational Service) work samples, the Singer, the TOWER (Testing, Orientation, and Work Evaluation in Rehabilitation) and the VALPAR Component Work Sample Series. The VALPAR has norms for persons with congenital deafness with severe to profound losses. Few vocational evaluation systems have been validated on actual employment criteria and, therefore, should be used judiciously with recognition of their limitations.

## Communication Assessment

Communication skills are an integral component of vocational competence and the capacity to participate fully in community life. People with varying degrees of hearing loss occurring at different stages in their lives will experience communication barriers when interacting with hearing persons. This is the common denominator of persons with hearing loss although prelingually deafened individuals with profound or severe loss will experience more problems with spoken and written language.

There is a natural tendency to use speech less as hearing acuity decreases since speech intelligibility decreases in proportion to hearing loss. For a child with a severe or profound hearing loss, the acquisition of English language skills must be developed artificially in a formalized instructional setting. Persons with early and severe hearing loss will frequently demonstrate considerable weakness in English language usage. Yet, they are likely to have a fluent grasp of American Sign Language (ASL), which is syntactically different from English.

Most individuals with early severe to profound hearing loss use ASL to communicate as adults, despite the communication modality used at home and school during their developmental years (Stokoe, 1978). Conversely, less than one percent of later onset deafened or hard-of-hearing persons ever learn to use any form of sign language with ease (Stone & Fennell, 1990).

There is no communication profile that taps all components of communication competency in hearing impaired persons. The National Technical Institute for the Deaf (NTID) Communication Skills Profile uses separate scales to measure reading comprehension, speech intelligibility, writing skills, speechreading with and without sound, hearing discrimination, manual reception, and simultaneous reception. However, it does not measure ASL skills and it measures each dimension out of context.

The counselor cannot assume that the prelingually deaf person will know ASL. Lack of ASL competency or peculiar use of signs in a prelingually deaf person with exposure to the deaf community during the developmental years may suggest a thought disorder or learning disability, including aphasia. If this is a possibility, a neuropsychological assessment is helpful.

## Case History and Demographic Data

The rehabilitation counselor has the primary responsibility for integrating reports with differing results into a comprehensive case study. Frequently, very useful information can be obtained from the hearing impaired person or the family, without recourse to expensive and time consuming testing. The time spent gathering historical and demographic information will be well spent if the counselor systematically explores relevant psychosocial, educational, and vocational data. This data may be used as the basis for planning formal diagnostics, if necessary. Again, individuals with hearing loss cannot be studied in isolation but should be assessed in terms of their environment, perceptions, and interactions. The following is a summary of the parameters that should be considered.

**Psychosocial history and current level of functioning.** The hearing impaired child frequently faces an overwhelming communication barrier during the developmental years. Over 90% of children who are deaf are born into families in which both parents have normal hearing. This means that these children are frequently socially isolated, even within their families; the social development of children who are deaf may lag in comparison with their hearing peers. There are considerable variations in social skill attainment among prevocationally deafened persons, as there are among hearing people; these competencies depend considerably on opportunities and interventions afforded during the developmental years.

A person who was born deaf or became deaf at an early age never had to experience the feeling of loss and concomitant adjustment that a person with a later-onset hearing loss experiences. A later-onset deafened person often must painfully reevaluate many of life's major decisions because of the communication limitations caused by the hearing loss. Individuals with moderate hearing loss may deny this loss or the implications of the loss by trying to "pass" for hearing while complaining that others do not speak sufficiently loud. Many of these individuals present greater rehabilitation challenges and are more severely disabled than the individual who has always been deaf. Hard-of-hearing persons, despite the age at onset of the hearing loss, often find themselves straddling the deaf world and the hearing world and fitting into neither.

For vocational rehabilitation purposes, the counselor needs to be familiar with the following personal and social issues of the client.

1. Personal adaptation: How is the hearing loss perceived? Is the person's identification as a deaf or hard-of-hearing person consistent with level of functioning? Is the loss denied or over-compensated?

2. Family background: What are the attitudes of family members toward the hearing loss? What is the person's relationship with other family members? Is the mode of communication within the family appropriate? What goals does the family have for the person with a hearing loss and how consistent are these with the person's goals?

3. Social support systems: What is the person's capacity to form and maintain relationships? Have any relationships changed with the onset of the hearing loss and why?

4. Recreational interests: What is the nature and extent of the person's leisure activities?

5. Activities of daily living: What is the person's capacity for independent functioning in life's major activities? Is there an awareness of assistive devices such as TDDs and relay services, flashing lights, television decoders, and alarm systems? Have there been any recent changes in daily living routine (eating, sleeping, work, study, or recreation)?

6. Overall impression: What is the individual's adjustment to life's demands? What is the capacity to handle frustration? What is the person's stress tolerance?

**Educational history.** Early and appropriate educational intervention can improve many developmental and experiential deficits associated with prelingual deafness. In the past two decades, regular public schools have been increasingly responsible for the education of youth who have hearing impairments. This is a marked change from the traditional residential school or special day program. This change has placed demands on schools to provide appropriate services and hire qualified staff to deliver such services. These include teachers, counselors, interpreters, speech pathologists, and related personnel as mandated by the 1975 Individuals with Disabilities Education Act and its 1990 amendments. Some school systems have met this challenge better than others.

Hard-of-hearing youth may be under-identified and under-served in school systems and thus may not be placed in and benefit from special education services. Hard-of-hearing adolescents may refuse to wear the visible signs of a hearing loss (hearing aids). This compromises their ability to take full advantage of oral instruction in a regular school system.

Many deaf youths in residential or public school programs fail to complete high school. Only 52% graduate high school, while 19% receive a certificate and another 29% drop out or "age out" (Allen, Rawlings, & Schildroth, 1989). Few prelingually deaf youths ever attend college.

Educational issues are more relevant when working with the younger person. Issues to explore include:

1. What type of institutions did the individual attend? What was the individual's attitude toward these institutions? Prelingually deaf persons who attend residential schools usually have positive attitudes toward this experience. What is the individual's attitude toward specific subjects, teachers, and classmates? What subjects were liked most and least? What were the reasons for leaving or changing schools? Were any vocationally relevant skills developed?

2. Is the individual's academic record an accurate reflection of ability?

3. What types of additional training does the person's educational history suggest or contraindicate?

**Vocational history.** Educational achievement or lack of it ultimately shapes and limits the type and level of occupation in which an individual may engage. Persons with severe or profound hearing loss have historically been under-represented in professional and administrative positions and over-represented in skilled, semi-skilled, and unskilled occupations. This discrepancy is a challenge to our society and we must find ways to remedy this problem. Recent legislative enactments such as Title V of the Rehabilitation Act of 1973 and the Americans with Disabilities Act of 1990, and increased public awareness have enhanced employment opportunities for persons born deaf or deafened at an early age.

Many persons deafened in adulthood may be threatened with job loss or removed from supervisory positions. This possibility is an additional assault on the person's self-esteem and well-being. The potential for job restructuring, job modification services, and reasonable accommodation should be determined for these individuals.

Some vocational issues to explore include the following:

1. What is the individual's work history? What were the reasons for career or job changes? What is the person's attitude toward each job? What skills were used on each job? How did the person handle any periods of unemployment?

2. What is the individual's current vocational choice? Is it consistent with abilities and potential? What other factors are relevant to this choice (e.g., financial obligations, labor market trends in area)?

3. How well can the person use a decision-making process for vocational choice? Are there financial disincentives to work (e.g., SSI, SSDI, and Medicaid)? Are the person's major sources of job satisfaction intrinsic or extrinsic? Is vocational indecision a symptom of more pervasive problems? How do significant others (e.g., family, friends, and teachers) perceive the individual's vocational choice?

4. What type of job restructuring or modification will increase the individual's employability?

5. What kinds of reasonable accommodation increase employability or promotion possibilities?

6. Will the person need vocational or work adjustment training or help with job seeking skills?

# INTERVENTION

## *Medical Intervention*

There are many hearing impairments that can be medically or surgically improved. Conductive hearing impairments occur because of abnormalities or defects within all or part of the conductive mechanism of the external or middle ear. The most basic problem is cerumen (wax) impaction; with the simple removal of the wax by a physician, the ear canal is cleared and hearing is improved. Patients may have a congenital narrowing (stenosis) of the external auditory canal or they may have complete absence of the canal (atresia). These situations can be improved through surgical intervention (Paparella & Shumrick, 1980).

Acute suppurative otitis media is a common infection seen most commonly in young children. By the age of 5, 80% of all children have had at least one ear infection. As part of the pathological process in an acute ear infection, there is a stage where the middle ear becomes filled with fluid. The fluid may persist for up to 2 weeks following the normal course of a middle ear infection. During this period, the affected individual will have a conductive hearing loss. Typically, a physician can treat this condition with appropriately prescribed antibiotics. If a child has serous otitis media (middle ear fluid) for more than 3 months despite appropriate antibiotic therapy, there is some indication to proceed with myringotomy and pressure equalizing tubes.

The American Academy of Otolaryngology-Head and Neck Surgery has guidelines that suggest that after six ear infections per year or four ear infections each year for 2 consecutive years, or middle ear fluid for more that 3 months duration, it may be recommended to proceed with myringotomy and placement of pressure equalizing tubes.

Operative intervention exists for many other ear conditions that may lead to hearing loss. For example, people who have perforated ear drums can undergo a tympanoplasty to patch the hole in the tympanic membrane. Patients with otosclerosis (fixation of the stapes bone) can undergo a stapedectomy in an attempt to improve hearing.

There are many assistive devices that improve the ability of the hearing impaired person to live a more normal life. An example is the use of hearing aids. Hearing aids will not help everyone, but in those people who have mild to moderate hearing loss, amplification may be all they need to function normally.

Several styles of hearing aids are available today. There are many factors that must be considered when selecting the appropriate aid for the individual. These include the degree and type of hearing loss, the size and shape of the ear, and the lifestyle of the patient. The most popular hearing aid is the "all in the ear" hearing aid. This type of device fills the ear and is flush with the outer ear. It is appropriate for mild hearing losses but may not have the required power for severe losses. Another version of this hearing device is the canal aid, which is appropriate for mild to moderate hearing loss. A third style is the behind the ear hearing aid, consisting of the hearing aid and the earmold that channels the sound into the ear. This type of aid is designed for any degree of hearing loss.

Other devices, such as assistive listening devices or telecommunication equipment, are used to amplify sounds from everyday activities. These include telephone amplifiers, alerting devices (i.e., a flashing light activated by a crying infant or a doorbell), and infrared or FM systems for persons who are more severely hearing impaired. Infrared systems can be installed in theaters; they amplify sound only for the hearing impaired listener.

The Food and Drug Administration (FDA) has approved cochlear implants, under certain situations, to improve hearing in patients who have profound bilateral sensorineural deafness that cannot benefit from hearing aids. As of this writing, they have been approved for people 2 years of age or older who have postlingual hearing loss. The FDA is allowing the implant for certain individuals with prelingual deafness as well. This is because patients need to have developed linguistic skills to benefit from cochlear implant. The cochlear implant does not provide normal hearing and one must be familiar with sounds and speech to benefit from the implant.

Before implantation, potential candidates have thorough and rigorous medical, psychological, and motivational testing. Individuals who have successful implants can expect partial hearing. There are other implantable aids. These include bone conduction aids used in patients who have conductive losses. There are also electromagnetic semi-implantable hearing devices called Electromagnetic Ossicular Replacement Devices (EORD).

The internist or pediatrician typically treats acute conditions, such as acute ear infection; these problems are usually self-limiting. Chronic problems such as serous otitis media or chronic suppurative otitis media require more intensive follow-up evaluation and treatment by a qualified otolaryngologist. Also, persons who have hearing loss should be seen at least annually to have repeat audiologic testing to be sure the loss is not progressing.

It is imperative for persons with hearing impairments and even people with normal hearing to preserve their present hearing capacity. Situations that expose the individual to noisy environments need to be avoided. If exposure to these situations cannot be prevented, then protective devices must be worn, such as ear plugs or preferably ear muffs designed to impede the penetration of noise.

## Vocational Intervention

Many persons who have been deaf or hard-of-hearing from an early age will have difficulties making satisfactory vocational adjustment due to experiential deficits, environmental barriers, or a combination of both. Counselors need to guard against paternalism and stereotyping, and individually plan rehabilitation interventions.

Any intervention should ultimately empower the individual and promote independence, responsibility, and autonomy, not dependency.

Rehabilitation counselors can work with the individual with hearing loss to help identify appropriate work settings, develop job seeking skills, practice mock interviews, and explain worksite modifications when necessary (e.g., special lighting requirements, the use of interpreters, assistive devices and alerting systems, and minimization of exposure to noise). They should also provide information that clarifies employment rights under the Rehabilitation Act of 1973 and the 1990 Americans with Disabilities Act.

Individuals who experience a hearing loss in adulthood may benefit from career counseling to decide if career change is necessary or desirable. Often, these individuals will require supportive counseling and practical advice on explaining the consequences of the hearing loss to co-workers and supervisors. Counselors may provide consultation at the worksite with the person with a hearing loss and the employer to discuss job modifications, assistive devices (e.g., telecommunication devices, telephone amplifiers, audioloops, and signaling systems), or other reasonable accommodation. Sometimes a simple reassignment of work responsibilities or the addition of assistive technology at work may minimize the impact of hearing loss on work performance and relationships with co-workers.

## Social Intervention

Rehabilitation counselors have specialized training to help with adjustment to loss issues for persons with disabilities. Counseling for adaptation to hearing loss is typically not necessary or appropriate for the individual who has had the loss from an early age. These individuals have never experienced the abrupt disruption of all that is predictable and familiar in life due to hearing loss. Instead, they have mastered various developmental tasks with a core identity as a person who is deaf. The counseling needs of these individuals revolve around adjustment to an environment that is created by and for hearing persons. These individuals may have limited experience, lack social skills, or possess limited coping or independent living skills. They may need or request personal adjustment counseling from the rehabilitation counselor around issues such as the use of interpreters, appropriate assertion of rights, and participation in community and work life.

The person who sustains a hearing loss in adulthood experiences a very real loss of all that is familiar: a sense of self, social relationships, vocational and personal competency, and sometimes economic security. They may withdraw from personal interaction and social situations and experience anxiety and depression. This group can benefit from, and should be encouraged to participate in, speech reading and auditory training to use residual hearing because they have already heard sound and know the structure of language. Persons who become deaf later in life and hard-of-hearing persons do not utilize these services to the most beneficial extent. This is possibly due to lack of information or, perhaps, fear of inability to master new skills.

Family counseling is particularly important for the later-onset deafened adult. It should be approached from an information sharing, supportive perspective which focuses on personal and environmental strengths and thereby maintains the individual's self-esteem. Self-help or "coping" groups of peers are often helpful. Several organizations such as Self-Help for Hard of Hearing Persons, Inc. (SHHH) and the Association of Late-Deafened Adults (ALDA) offer such groups.

## Specialized Rehabilitation Personnel

**The RCD (rehabilitation counselor for the deaf).** The past few decades have witnessed the emergence of the rehabilitation counselor who specializes in working with persons with hearing loss. Although this specialty originally developed because of the unique communication needs of deaf persons who use sign language, communication skills, in and of themselves, are not sufficient to adequately meet the needs of clients with hearing loss. Rehabilitation counselors who specialize in working with deaf and hard-of-hearing individuals possess generic competencies in rehabilitation counseling and specialized skills and knowledge in assessment and intervention with this diverse population.

All state rehabilitation agencies now hire specialists in deafness in response to the Rehabilitation Act Amendments of 1978 that mandated hiring personnel who can use the client's preferred mode of communication. The amendments also require that the annual review of the Individualized Written Rehabilitation Plan (IWRP) be performed in the client's preferred mode of communication. Still, state hiring standards are inconsistent, due to a serious shortage of qualified personnel.

**Interpreters.** The use of interpreters in educational and rehabilitation settings has become standard practice over the past two decades. Section 504 of the Rehabilitation Act of 1973 encompasses interpreter services as a "reasonable accommodation." The Rehabilitation Act amendments of 1978 mandate hiring of personnel (either interpreters or counselors) in programs funded under the Act who can use the client's method of communication. This includes sign language, oral, or cued speech. Cued speech is a "phonemically-based system used in conjunction with speechreading, comprised of eight handshapes representing consonant sounds, and four positions about the face representing vowel sounds" (Kipila & Williams-Scott, 1990, p. 71).

The passage of the Americans with Disabilities Act further insures access to interpreters as a reasonable accommodation for persons with hearing loss. An emerging issue is whether sufficient numbers of qualified interpreters will be available to meet this expanded need. The qualifications of rehabilitation counselors and interpreters for persons with hearing loss are crucial. It is the responsibility of service programs and facilities to be aware of professional standards and carefully follow these standards in recruiting and hiring staff.

# PROGNOSIS

Hearing loss related to conductive problems is typically treatable, either medically or surgically, and the outcome is usually favorable. In contrast, sensorineural hearing loss is progressive and less amenable to medical or surgical treatment. Individuals with hearing loss can benefit from major advances today in medical, educational, and rehabilitation strategies that provide access to full participation in community life and work. Legislation has recently increased opportunities for all persons with disabilities, including individuals with hearing loss.

## The Americans with Disabilities Act and Persons with Hearing Loss

The Americans with Disabilities Act (ADA) became a reality in 1990. The ADA provides civil rights protection for people with disabilities in private sector employment, state and local government services, privately owned and public accommodations, and telecommunication relay services.

Under the ADA, telephone companies offering service to the public must provide 24-hour telephone relay services to persons with hearing loss. This allows persons with hearing loss who use TDDs or similar devices to communicate with anyone who has a telephone.

Employers with 15-25 employees need to provide reasonable accommodation to all persons with disabilities, including persons with hearing loss, starting in 1994. In July of 1992, employers with more than 25 employees needed to provide reasonable accommodation. Examples of accommodation for persons with hearing loss include qualified interpreters, amplified telephones, telecommunication devices, and worksite adaptations, such as audioloops. Major renovations and new construction must be accessible for people with hearing loss by using, for example, audioloops in meeting rooms and emergency flashing lights and alarms.

# RESOURCES

There are many organizations and associations for persons with hearing loss and professionals who work with these individuals. The following list includes most of the major organizations.

Alexander Graham Bell Association for the Deaf, 3417 Volta Place, N.W., Washington, D.C. 20007. The 100-year old Alexander Graham Bell Association for the Deaf is an international, nonprofit organization serving professional, parent, and hearing impaired members through the diffusion of knowledge on aspects of deafness. The Association promotes opportunities for children with hearing loss to learn to communicate through speech.

American Academy of Otolaryngology - Head and Neck Surgery, One Prince Street, Alexandria, Virginia 22314. The purpose of the Academy is to advance the art and science of medicine as related to otolaryngology-head and neck surgery. The Academy represents the specialty to the public, the government, and other medical specialties. They coordinate and strengthen research efforts in the specialty and represent the socioeconomic concerns of the membership, whenever appropriate. Services provided by the Academy include continuing medical education for physicians, public education through public service campaigns, patient information leaflets, and patient education videotapes. The Academy also issues monthly publications including a newsletter, "The Bulletin," and a scientific journal, Otolaryngology - Head and Neck Surgery. A Directory lists all Academy members.

American Society for Deaf Children (ASDC), 814 Thayer Avenue, Silver Spring, Maryland 20910. The purpose of ASDC is to provide information and support for parents and families with children who are deaf or hard-of-hearing. Services include workshops, information and referral services, biennial conventions, and a newsletter, "Endeavor," published six times a year.

American Tinnitus Association, Post Office Box 5, Portland, Oregon 97207. The purpose of this association is to distribute information, and support research and educational activities relating to the treatment of tinnitus and other problems affecting the ear. The Association provides a worldwide network of referral clinics and self-help groups, bibliography service, and public education. It publishes a quarterly news magazine, "Tinnitus Today."

Association of Late-Deafened Adults (ALDA), Post Office Box 468, Marshall Hills, Massachusetts 02051. This Association provides support for late-deafened people, their families, and friends. It also provides help in the identification of late-deafened adults, serves as a resource and information network, and works to increase public awareness of the special needs of late-deafened adults. Their services include self-help and support groups, social activities, outreach, advocacy, consultation, and a newsletter," ALDA News."

Conference of Educational Administrators Serving the Deaf (CEASD), 2253 Main Street, Buffalo, New York 14214. The purpose of CEASD is to maintain effective programs for meeting the educational needs of hearing impaired children and adults. CEASD provides a forum for administrators, conducts legislative advocacy, and works toward establishment and maintenance of educational standards.

Convention of American Instructors of the Deaf (CAID), Post Office Box 2025, Austin, Texas 78768-2025. CAID maintains a professional organization for teachers, administrators, educational interpreters, residential personnel, and other professionals involved in education of children with hearing loss. Their members work in residential, public, and private schools across the United States and Canada and provide united efforts to supply quality and effectiveness in education of these children. Services include biennial conventions, regional meetings, networking of professionals with shared interests through Special Interest Groups (SIGs), and advocacy for national and state legislation concerning persons who are deaf. CAID publishes the "American Annals of the Deaf."

Deafness Research Foundation (DRF), 9 East 38th Street, New York, New York 10016. The purpose of DRF is to direct public support and attention to basic and clinical research on the causes, treatment, and prevention of deafness and other hearing disabilities. It is a national, voluntary, non-profit health organization providing grants for medical and scientific research and public education and information.

National Association of the Deaf (NAD), 814 Thayer Avenue, Silver Spring, Maryland 20902. NAD is the oldest and largest consumer organization of people with disabilities in the United States serving more than 22 million deaf and hard-of-hearing people in America. The mission of the NAD is to assure that a comprehensive coordinated system of services is accessible to all persons with hearing losses, enabling them to achieve their maximum potential through increased independence, productivity, and integration into the community. Services include public information, publications, youth programs, a legal defense fund, conventions, and periodicals.

National Cued Speech Association, Post Office Box 31345, Raleigh, North Carolina 27622. This is an organization of hearing impaired persons, families, and professionals who support the use of cued speech, a sound-based visual communication system. The Association is committed to improving literacy and provides information, guidance, family support, and assurance of quality through certification standards for cued speech instructors, interpreters, and transliterators.

National Technical Institute for the Deaf (NTID) at Rochester Institute of Technology (RIT), One Lomb Memorial Drive, Post Office Box 9887, Rochester, New York 14623-0887. NTID represents the first effort to educate large numbers of students who are deaf within a college campus planned primarily for hearing students. NTID academic programs lead to certificates, diplomas, and associate degrees from RIT. RIT offers an associate degree in Educational Interpreting for hearing students.

New York League for the Hard of Hearing, 71 West 23rd Street, New York, New York 10010. The League is the oldest, not-for-profit hearing rehabilitation agency in this country. It offers a comprehensive program of rehabilitation services including audiology, communication therapies, educational management, public education and community outreach, recreation, technical services, otology, mental health services, psychological and social work services, career counseling, and job placement.

Self Help for Hard of Hearing People (SHHH), Inc., 7800 Wisconsin Avenue, Bethesda, Maryland 20814. SHHH, Inc. is a volunteer, international organization of hard-of-hearing people, their relatives, and friends. It has 250 chapters throughout the United States and in 17 other countries with over 40,000 members. It is a non-profit, educational organization devoted to the welfare and interests of those who cannot hear well, using their residual hearing, speech, and speechreading to communicate. Services include information and referral, local support groups, an assistive devices center (in Bethesda, Maryland), a bimonthly journal about hearing loss, "SHHH Journal", and special publications, including books, information series, and video and audio tapes.


# CASE STUDY


Ms. Maria Espinoza is a self-referral to the Department of Rehabilitation. She is a 49 year-old married Latino woman who works as a personal care aide for an elderly woman in the woman's home. She holds a Bachelor of Arts degree in Architecture from a university in South America and wishes to obtain more appropriate employment. Both of the Espinoza's children are grown and living independently.

At the age of 27, Maria developed a moderate to profound sensorineural hearing loss of unknown origin. The loss is permanent and not reversible or correctable by surgery. When using her hearing aids, her hearing is improved from 45 dB HTL to 15 dB HTL.

Ms. Espinoza relies on speech reading to communicate. The family communicates in the Spanish language. Her husband loses his temper with her because of her difficulty dealing with the public. She speaks broken English with a very thick Spanish accent that is difficult to understand due to the nasality caused by her deafness. Maria stressed that her receptive English is much better than people realize. Ms. Espinoza's relatives seem to question her hearing loss because of inconsistencies as to what she can and cannot hear; she cannot explain why her hearing loss seems to fluctuate.

For 5 years, Maria was employed as a drafter in South America. She had a one year job in drafting when she arrived in the United States. Both jobs were performed primarily in a seated position with lifting and carrying of minimal weights up to a maximum of 10 pounds. More recent work experience has consisted of housecleaning, babysitting, and office cleaning. She stated she has difficulties working in a noisy environment - it gives her headaches. Maria is motivated to work in a position more commensurate with her training and background.

## Questions

1. Assign Ms. Maria Espinoza a vocational profile, including age category, education level, and work history (including skill and exertional level for all jobs). Discuss occupationally significant characteristics as related to this disability and transferability of skills.

2. Would additional medical evaluation(s) be appropriate for Maria? What specific medical information would be most helpful in rehabilitation planning?

3. Should Maria learn sign language to improve her ability to communicate? Discuss.

4. What family services might the rehabilitation counselor provide? What is your assessment of her support system?

5. What additional information about Ms. Espinoza's work history would be helpful in her rehabilitation planning?

6. Would a vocational evaluation be appropriate for Maria? What information from a vocational evaluation would be most helpful in her rehabilitation planning?

7. What job modifications or accommodations would assist Ms. Espinoza in adjusting to a work environment?

# REFERENCES

Allen, T. (1986). Patterns of academic achievement among hearing impaired students: 1974 and 1983. In A. Schildroth & M. Karchmer (Eds.), **Deaf children in America** (pp. 161-206). San Diego, CA: College-Hill.

Allen, T., Rawlings, B., & Schildroth, A. (Eds.). (1989). **Deaf students and the school-to-work transition.** Baltimore, MD: Paul H. Brooks.

Centers for Disease Control (1983). Leading work-related diseases and injuries - United States. **Morbidity and Mortality Weekly Report, 34,** 24-26.

Darnell, W. (1991). **A study of the vocational characteristics of deaf high school students using Holland's Self-Directed Search-Form Easy.** Unpublished doctoral dissertation. University of Maryland, College Park, MD.

Davis, H. (1953). **Acoustic Trauma in the Guinea Pig.** WADC Technical Report (pp. 48-53). Dayton, OH: Wright Patterson Air Force Base.

Department of Commerce, Bureau of the Census (1984). Projections of the population of the United States, by age, sex, and race: 1983 to 2080. **Current Population Reports,** Population Estimates and Projections, (Series P-25, Number 952). Washington, D.C.: Author.

Department of the Census (1986). Disability, functional limitation, and health insurance coverage: 1984/85, Data from the Survey of Income and Program Participation, **Current Population Reports**, (Series P-70, Number 8). Washington, D.C.: Author.

English, G. (1986). Hearing loss from acoustic energy. **Otolaryngology** (2nd ed.). Philadelphia, PA: Harper & Row.

Johns, M., Brackman, D.E., Kimmelman, C., Papsidero, M.J., Koopman, C.F., Jr., & Loury, M. (1989). Goals and mechanisms for training otolaryngologists in the area of geriatric medicine. **Otolaryngology-Head and Neck Surgery, 100**(4), 262-265.

Joint declaration issued to clarify the terms "deaf and hard of hearing" (1991), **SHHH Journal, 12**(1), 6.

Kipila, E., & Williams-Scott, B. (1990). Cued speech: A response to "controversy within sign language." In M.D. Garretson (Ed.), **Communication issues among deaf people** (pp. 71-74). Silver Spring, MD: National Association of the Deaf.

Leads from the MMWR: Self-reported hearing loss among workers potentially exposed to industrial noise - United States. (1988, April 15). Reported by: Surveillance Branch, Division of Surveillance, Hazard Evaluations, and Field Studies.

National Institute for Occupational Safety and Health; Division of Health Interview Statistics, National Center for Health Statistics, CDC (1988). **Journal of the American Medical Association, 259**(15), 2213-2217.

National Institute on Deafness and Other Communication Disorders (1989). **National strategic research plan: A draft report of the task force.** Bethesda, MD: National Institute of Health.

Paparella, M.M., & Shumrick, D.A. (1980). **Otolaryngology** (2nd ed.). Philadelphia, PA: W.B. Saunders.

Rehabilitation Services Administration (1986). **Instructions for the RSA-911 Reporting System.** Washington, DC: Department of Education, OSERS/RSA.

Simpson, M., & Bruce, R. (1981). **The extent of the noise problem,** (BBN Report No. 3318R). Washington, DC: Bolt, Beranek, and Newman.

Stokoe, W.C. (1978). **Sign language structure: An outline of the visual communication systems of the American deaf.** Studies in linguistics: Occasional papers 8. Buffalo, NY: University of Buffalo.

Stone, H., & Fennell, D. (1990). Rehabilitation services for hard of hearing persons. In D. Watson (Ed.), **Model state plan for the vocational rehabilitation of individuals who are deaf and hard of hearing** (pp. 75-80). Little Rock, AK: Research and Training Center on Deafness and Hearing Impairment.

Szymanski, E.M., Dunn, C., & Parker, R.M. (1989). Rehabilitation of persons with learning disabilities: An ecological framework. **Rehabilitation Counseling Bulletin, 33**, 38-53.

Wazen, J., Silverstein, H., Norrell, H., & Bessa, B. (1985). Pre-operative and post-operative growth rates in acoustic neuromas with CT scans. **Otolaryngology - Head and Neck Surgery, 92**(2), 151-155.

## About the Authors

Marita M. Danek, Ph.D., is Professor and Co-director of the Rehabilitation Counselor Education Program (deafness emphasis) at Gallaudet University in Washington, D.C.. She is a former Switzer Scholar, a co-recipient of the 1986 Rehabilitation Educator of the Year award, a co-recipient of the 1990 Association for Counselor Education and Supervision Research Award, and a recipient of the 1991 Human Resources Award from the Maryland Rehabilitation Association.

Michael D. Seidman, M.D., received his medical degree from the University of Michigan and completed his residency in Otolaryngology, Head and Neck Surgery, at Henry Ford Hospital in Detroit, Michigan where he was honored as the Most Outstanding Resident. In 1990, he was awarded the American Academy of Otolaryngology - Head and Neck Surgery Resident Training Award grant to study the protective effects of investigational drugs on noise-induced hearing loss. He completed his fellowship training in neurotology/skull base surgery at the Ear Research Foundation in Sarasota, Florida. Dr. Seidman is currently an Assistant Professor in the Department of Otolaryngology, Case Western Reserve Medical School/Henry Ford Hospital in Detroit, Michigan.

# Chapter 15

# VISUAL DISABILITIES

by
*William C. Panek, M.D.*

## INTRODUCTION

The disability associated with blindness or visual loss is complex. It relates both to the actual sense of sight itself and the interaction of this sense with the other senses, with the total physical and psychological make up of the individual (Duane, 1988). A well functioning person uses all the senses and body functions as an integrated whole to interact with the environment. A loss or decrease of one part of this whole, such as loss of the sense of sight, will lead to a degree of impairment directly related to the ability of the individual to adapt to the loss.

An ophthalmologist is a physician who specializes in disease and surgery of the eye. In this chapter, ophthalmologist and physician are used interchangeably. The role of the rehabilitation counselor working with persons with visual loss is to facilitate maximum productivity and independence.

When dealing with visual disability, a tendency of government agencies, physicians, and therapists has been to define blindness and visual loss by set criteria. These criteria are based usually on visual acuity and field of remaining vision. While this approach does not address the duration of visual disability or functional abilities of the individual, it does set a standard that allows communication between the various agencies and professionals working with people who are visually impaired.

### Definition

In 1966, the World Health Organization compiled a list of 65 national definitions of blindness. Of these, only three nations used the dictionary definition of blindness, "total absence of sight." The remaining countries had criteria based on a best corrected visual acuity level and the loss of a defined amount of the field of vision. In the United States, legal blindness is defined as central visual acuity of 20/200 or less in the better eye, or a residual field of 20 degrees or less in the better eye. A more practical approach to defining blindness and visual impairment is to assume there is a large range of levels of visual impairment from mild impairment to complete loss of sight. The professional using the definition would have the option of defining the particular threshold as "blind" for a particular purpose. This would give the definition flexibility, making it more functional and helpful.

Father Carroll, a renowned figure in the field of visual rehabilitation, once commented that "more people are blinded by definition than any other cause." While legal imperatives require exact definitions, the rehabilitation counselor can define each visually impaired person's status in terms of overall functional abilities. A given individual with 20/400 vision may be better adapted to certain tasks than another with 20/20 vision.

## Prevalence

Visual loss has become an increasingly significant health problem. With the changing demographics of the American population, chronic disease and subsequent impairment have increased. The National Center for Health Statistics studied the prevalence of 10 types of physical impairment. It found visual loss had the second highest rate and the largest increase in rate per thousand population between 1971 and 1977. In 1977, 11.4 million people had some form of visual loss; 1.4 million were unable to read ordinary newsprint with corrective lenses (Greenblatt, 1988). The expectation is an even greater number of people will become visually impaired in the future due to the gradual increase in the life-span. Physicians, therapists, institutions, and government agencies, which interact with individuals who have impairments, need to be aware of this phenomenon. The psychological, sociological, and economic implications of the need for preparedness are obvious.

# THE EYE AND VISUAL FUNCTION

## The Eye

Knowledge of the visual system is important in helping the rehabilitation counselor understand the physical disability experienced by the patient. Malfunctions of different components of the system can cause totally different degrees of impairment, with a marked variability in residual functional ability. By becoming aware of the anatomic correlations between disease and physical impairment, the counselor can better understand the specific physical restrictions and rehabilitation potential of each individual (Vaughan, Asbury, & Tabbara, 1989).

The eye (see Figure 1) is a sophisticated organ, which can be compared to a video camera. Optical surfaces precisely focus visual input or light rays from the environment that are passed through a transparent media onto a receptor surface and transmitted through a cable for central processing.

In the human, this delicate camera resides in a protective bony socket of the skull known as the orbit. Soft, flexible tissues surround the orbit. This encasement provides protection from the jarring and direct trauma that other external body structures constantly endure.

Besides the protection afforded by the orbit and its contents, the eyelids also protect the front ocular surface. These movable, intermittently closing folds of skin act as a protective barrier and play a vital role in surface rewetting. With each blink, the front of the "camera" receives a fresh wash and a new tear film.

Covering the outer eye and the inner aspect of both eyelids is a thin filmy tissue layer called the conjunctiva. Beneath the conjunctiva is a strong, white collagenous layer known as the sclera. At the front of the eye, the sclera blends into the crystal clear, watch glass-like cornea. The cornea is the primary light focusing surface of the eye.

Behind the cornea is the anterior chamber, filled with a clear fluid called aqueous humor. Aqueous humor provides nutrients to the avascular (void of blood vessels), transparent tissues of the inner eye. The iris serves as the back wall of the anterior chamber and limits the amount of light entering the eye through a closeable aperture in its center known as the pupil. It is the colored portion of the eye around the pupil. In the anterior chamber angle formed by the iris and cornea is the drain site, the trabecular meshwork, through which aqueous humor exits the eye.

Directly behind the pupil is the crystalline lens, a transparent biconvex body, which with the cornea, contributes to the focusing power of the eye. This lens has the ability in younger people to change shape, and as such, changes a person's focus from distant to near, and vice versa. An individual loses this flexibility with advancing age. Behind the lens is the vitreous jell. Lining this cavity is the film-like retina, a neural tissue, which receives light energy

## Figure 1
## THE EYE

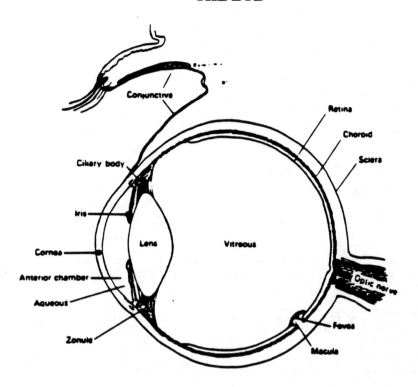

Conjunctiva

Retina

Choroid

Sclera

Ciliary body

Iris

Lens

Vitreous

Cornea

Anterior chamber

Aqueous

Optic nerve

Zonule

Fovea

Macula

From **Manual for eye examination and diagnosis** (3rd ed.) by M.W. Leitman, 1988, Oradel, NJ: Medical Economics Books. Reprinted by permission of Blackwell Scientific Publication, Inc.

focused through the eye's optical system. The retina transmits the visual message through nerve fibers into the optic nerve and ultimately to the brain.

## Visual Function

The eye is the window of the human organism to the outside world. It allows a person to interact with and be aware of stimuli that are physically far removed. Specific visual properties that aid in this function are central visual acuity, contrast sensitivity, visual field or side vision, binocular vision, color vision, and night vision.

Central visual acuity is a result of precise "picture taking" by the macula or central retina. The eye focuses on the object of regard at this very sensitive retinal area. The special anatomy of the macula allows the fine vision necessary to do intricate distant and near tasks.

A standard of measurement of central vision is Snellen acuity. In the Snellen test of acuity, which is almost universally accepted, the ophthalmologist tests the person at a defined distance from a chart containing figures that are of gradually increasing size. Distance visual acuity is the ratio of the distance of the subject from the standard eye chart (usually 20 feet) to the distance at which the letters seen could be seen by persons with normal vision. As an example, 20/80 vision indicates the subject reads at 20 feet what a person with normal vision could read at 80 feet. Most visual acuity charts have images ranging from 20/10 to 20/400. The physician tests patients with visual loss who do not have adequate retinal sensitivity or exposure to allow visualization of 20/400 by finger counting ability from 3-10 feet. One tests progressively worse visual acuity by hand motion (HM), light perception (LP), and finally, no light perception (NLP).

Contrast sensitivity is the ability of the retina to discern variations in the intensity of stimuli. Contrast measurement is the person's ability to see the difference between brightness "peaks" and darkness "valleys." It may be useful in predicting glare response, mobility performance, reading capability with magnification, the preferred eye in certain bilateral disease, and face perception. While central visual acuity tests the ability to discern fine detail, contrast sensitivity may give a more accurate assessment of overall functional capability, an important consideration in vision rehabilitation. The person with central vision, which is inadequate for reading, may have good contrast sensitivity, allowing safe functioning in the individual's environment for most other tasks. Conversely, the person with good central acuity in a high contrast reading situation, but who otherwise has poor contrast sensitivity, may be at risk driving or even walking across the street.

The retina, outside the macula, provides the visual field or side vision. While this peripheral portion of the retina is not capable of the fine acuity manifested by the macula, it is still very sensitive, especially to movement. It is this peripheral retina that provides information about the total surroundings, allowing safe travel while a person's attention is held on a forward target.

The physician conducts testing of the visual field through perimetry. Perimetry is measurement of the scope of the field of vision. The most simple type of perimetry is confrontation (how many fingers do you see?). While not sophisticated, this form of visual field testing often yields useful information.

Recent innovations in computer hardware and software have led to the development of automated threshold perimetry. In this test, now standard in ophthalmic practice, the physician tests multiple points in the field of vision with varying light intensities. One then determines a threshold value for each point. This type of perimetry allows precise reproductivity testing of the field of vision. It is helpful in defining an individual's functional capability status, and thus provides information about the ability to move freely about in the environment.

Binocular vision is the functional state in which both eyes fixate on a single object, resulting in a single perceived image. Because of complex relationships between adjacent retinal images, binocular vision is usually also associated with depth perception. Additionally, with both eyes working together, the total field of vision is larger, allowing additional awareness of the environment. Malfunction of the binocular system (loss of alignment) can lead to suppression of vision in children under the age of 8 and double vision in adolescents and adults.

Color vision, processed by the cones (cells) in the central retina, is an important function; yet, lack of it is usually not a true disability. Color vision deficit is more common in males than females, and is usually only partial, involving certain hues of color. Total color blindness is rare and may be associated with retinal pathology and an associated decrease in visual acuity.

A second type of retinal cells, the rods, which perceive only black and white images, also make up the peripheral retina. The rods are responsible for visual functioning in the dark. Impairments of the peripheral retina can markedly impair night vision and mobility. Night vision can be tested clinically through dark adaptation studies and visual field examination.

# MALFUNCTION OF THE VISUAL SYSTEM

With understanding how the normal eye functions, we can now discuss important pathological processes that affect the visual system and lead to visual loss and disability (Andreoli, Carpenter, Plum, & Smith, 1990; Schroeder,

Krupp, Tierney, & McPhee, 1990). The rehabilitation counselor will encounter these conditions either as the primary condition or as a secondary illness.

## Periocular Tissue

Because the normal ocular surface requires constant rewetting, malposition of the lids may lead to corneal drying, exposure, and erosion. While changes that occur with aging can cause such lid dysfunction, another common cause is trauma. Periocular (around the eye) scarring secondary to injury can lead to fixed, non-mobile lids that are incapable of the quick, smooth blinking necessary to protect the front surfaces of the eyes.

Abnormal turning-in of the eyelid is entropion; abnormal turning-out is ectropion. Both conditions, as with scarring, threaten the ocular surface integrity and visual loss may follow. Treatment of diseases of the periocular tissue involves plastic surgical repair and restoration of the anatomy to as normal a position as possible.

## Ocular Media

Opacification (clouding) of the transparent ocular media can interfere with the transmission of light into the eye from the environment. Opacification of the cornea secondary to inflammatory, degenerative, traumatic, and other causes also lead to blockage of light entering the eye. This can cause a decrease in visual acuity. Additionally, irregularities of the normally smooth, transparent cornea can lead to light scattering with glare symptoms and diminished contrast sensitivity. Treatment of corneal disease usually involves corneal transplantation in which the physician surgically replaces the diseased cornea with a clear donor cornea. This procedure is very successful, with healthy grafts occurring in most cases.

**Cataract.** A cataract is an opacity or discoloration of the normally clear crystalline lens. It may occur as a developmental abnormality, secondary to systemic disease, and as a change due to aging. Cataract is the most common cause of decreased vision in the United States, not correctable with glasses. Patients with cataracts, as with corneal opacification, complain of gradual, painless blurring of vision, glare intolerance, and loss of contrast sensitivity. The location of the cataract and the degree of overall lens opacification determines the severity of visual impairment.

Treatment of a cataract involves the surgical removal of the cloudy lens. This is done when poor visual function caused by the cataract interferes with a patient's ability to lead a normal, productive life. The surgeon and the patient make the decision to operate, with consideration of age, occupation, visual needs, and the status of the other eye. Because cataract surgery is performed on an outpatient basis and is extremely successful in aiding visual rehabilitation, for these and other reasons, indications for surgery have become more liberalized. Thus, lifestyle and quality of vision have become more heavily weighted in the decision-making process.

Present technique in cataract surgery involves extracapsular extraction, in which the surgeon aspirates (removes) the cloudy lens contents from the eye, leaving the lens cover or capsule in place. An intraocular lens implant replaces the missing lens and supplies the lost optical power. Alternative optical rehabilitation, rarely used in modern ophthalmological practice, includes contact lenses and spectacle correction.

Certain systemic diseases lead to the development of cataract. These include diabetes and galactosemia (an inherited metabolic disorder). Frequently, these conditions can be treated directly; often this therapy will prevent cataract from occurring in the first place. Once an opacity has occurred, medical therapy to affect resolution of a cataract does not exist; surgery must be performed to resolve the problem.

**Other forms of ocular media opacification.** Another form of ocular media opacification can occur in the vitreous jell (a clear jelly-like substance that fills the eye ball). Degenerative products, metabolic deposits, blood, traumatic scar tissue, and other opaque material can become suspended in the vitreous jell, impairing light passage.

Depending on the cause of the opacification and the status of the other ocular tissues, surgical removal of the vitreous jell (vitrectomy) will help clear the media and restore visual integrity. Unfortunately, many causes of vitreous opacification are associated with severe problems involving other segments of the eye, making vitrectomy only moderately successful for restoring useful vision.

## Glaucoma

Another common ocular disease is glaucoma. Glaucoma is a disease of the eye characterized by an increase in intraocular pressure, resulting in atrophy of the optic nerve. Impairment of the outflow of aqueous fluid from the eye causes elevated pressure and damage to the optic nerve (see Figure 1).

Two major types of glaucoma are those with open and closed angles. In open angle type glaucoma, the trabecular meshwork (a supporting structure) is clinically open and normal but fails to function properly. In narrow (closed) angle type glaucoma, the anatomy of the affected eye is visibly different, with shallowing of the anterior chamber and a narrow approach to the chamber angle. This very narrow angle, under certain inciting circumstances, can close leading to loss of aqueous outflow and elevation of the intraocular pressure. In glaucoma, the increased ocular pressure causes structural damage to the optic nerve. With loss of nerve tissue, the visual field of the affected eye becomes progressively more constricted. Patients often notice visual symptoms only after marked damage has occurred because the central visual acuity is usually spared until late in the disease.

Patients with severe constriction of the field of vision in both eyes, such as seen in advanced glaucoma, are extremely disabled. Even with 20/20 central vision, these patients appear manifestly blind.

There are various treatment modalities for glaucoma. They include topical and systemic medication, laser therapy to open the chamber angle in narrow angle glaucoma, and laser therapy to enhance outflow function in open angle glaucoma. Also, treatment may involve surgery to affect drainage of aqueous fluid from the eye through surgically created new channels. These procedures are generally successful.

Glaucoma is a chronic disease, which rarely goes into spontaneous remission; as such, patients need daily medication. Compliance with therapy is often a problem because no distinct visual symptoms arise when a patient discontinues medication. Blindness in glaucoma can occur slowly, sometimes taking years. Often the irreversible damage occurs before the patient is aware there is a problem.

## Retinal Diseases

The retina is the film-like nerve layer lining the inside of the eyeball. Diseases that cause atrophy and scarring of the retina are not reversible. Once damage has occurred, as with other parts of the central nervous system, the individual permanently loses function. Medical and surgical therapy primarily provide prevention, not cure.

**Age-related macular degeneration.**In the United States, age-related macular degeneration (ARMD) is a major cause of legal blindness in patients over 65 years of age. Several changes occur in the macula, or central retina, of patients with macular degeneration. These include drusen (pale subretinal deposits), irregularities of the normally smooth retinal light reflex, and the abnormal growth of new blood vessels in the space beneath the retina. When pathological deposits and irregularities of the lining beneath the retina occur alone, we call the degeneration "dry" or atrophic; when subretinal new blood vessels leak and bleed, the degeneration is "wet" or diskiform. Diskiform degeneration can lead to severe, often sudden loss of central vision.

Patients with age-related macular degeneration complain of loss of acuity, loss of contrast sensitivity, blind spots, and distortion. The peripheral vision usually remains normal because the damage seen in macular degeneration occurs primarily in the central retina, sparing the periphery. Affected patients may function adequately in public (walking and interacting with other people) through use of their peripheral visual field; yet, fine tasks (reading, driving, and fine dexterity) that require good central acuity, may be difficult or impossible.

Laser eradication of new blood vessel membranes under the retina is the only treatment option available for age-related macular degeneration. Because of the undetermined cause and relentless degenerative nature of this disease, most research involves attempting to find the cause, rather than a cure. The hope is to stop the disease long before the retina becomes impaired.

**Diabetic retinopathy.** Another major disease affecting the retina is diabetic retinopathy. It is 1 of the 4 most frequent causes of newly diagnosed cases of legal blindness in the United States. Clinically, there are three types of diabetic retinopathy (Duane, 1988):

1. nonproliferative or mild, with scattered hemorrhages in the retina.

2. preproliferative or moderate, with signs of a poor oxygen supply to the retina leading to more pronounced damage.

3. proliferative or severe, with marked lack of oxygen to the retina causing the growth of delicate, easily torn new blood vessels on the optic nerve and retinal surface.

Proliferative retinopathy is the most damaging type, with complications of vitreous hemorrhage, retinal detachment, and secondary glaucoma. Treatment of diabetic retinopathy has improved greatly with the discovery of laser therapy. Ophthalmologists now use laser treatment (total retinal photocoagulation) to destroy damaged peripheral retina tissue in proliferative retinopathy, thus decreasing the tendency toward new blood vessel growth. Focal laser treatment of leaking blood vessels also is useful. Patients with diabetic retinopathy may manifest visual function ranging from normal to lack of light perception. Because some patients with diabetes are young and may have the disease for many years, and because of associated systemic complications of the disease, careful monitoring by physicians of multiple specialties is necessary.

## Heredofamilial Diseases

There are numerous diseases wherein people inherit certain ocular diseases associated with multiple systemic anomalies. These diseases are numerous. Variable genetic signs often accompany inherited ocular diseases.

**Retinitis pigmentosa.** This disease is a bilateral, progressive, hereditary disorder which may be either recessive or dominant. It presents with a gradual loss of function of the peripheral retina. Night blindness and loss of the field of peripheral vision are two common complaints as the disease progresses. Loss of central acuity may not occur until late in the course of the disease.

In severe forms of retinitis pigmentosa, an individual may lose peripheral vision by adulthood, leaving only a small central "island" of vision. These patients, as with patients who have severe glaucoma, are markedly restricted in their ability to move about the environment. From a rehabilitation standpoint, these patients must be made aware their disease is a gradual, progressive process that will eventually lead to blindness. Plans must be made to cope with this eventuality. Because retinitis pigmentosa and other heredofamilial diseases may be associated with systemic problems such a deafness, anomalies of the extremities, and hypogenitalism, a multidisciplinary approach is often necessary in managing the disease.

## Optic Nerve and Central Nervous System Disease

Many diseases that affect the central nervous system can also cause visual problems. Demyelinating processes such as multiple sclerosis can lead to optic neuropathy, double vision, and nystagmus (jerking of the eyes). Vascular and tumor processes also can affect the visual pathway including the optic nerve, the chiasm, the optic tracts, visual radiations, and the visual cortex. Disease of these visual pathways often leads to loss of specific components of the visual field. Because the etiologies of these diseases are diverse, an appropriately qualified medical specialist for the given situation should provide the treatment (neurologist, internist, and neurosurgeon). Depending of the severity of tissue damage, some return of visual function may occur with treatment.

# EXAMINATION OF THE VISUAL SYSTEM

An ophthalmologist performs an evaluation of the visual system for any pathology. It is necessary to establish this foundation before consideration of visual rehabilitation. The disease process must be defined and understood; then the best possible corrected spectacle vision is prescribed.

Ocular examination first includes a thorough history regarding changes in visual acuity, distortion, glare tolerance, pain, prior trauma, and previous surgery. A family history is also important especially concerning such entities as glaucoma, macular degeneration, and retinitis pigmentosa.

The physical examination begins with assessment of visual acuity, both distant and near vision. The ophthalmologist evaluates the ocular adnexa (lids and orbit) and uses a slit lamp microscope to obtain a stereoscopic view of the conjunctiva, cornea, sclera, and vitreous jell. The ophthalmoscope helps evaluate the retina (macula, blood vessels, and peripheral retina) and the optic nerve.

Additional tests include perimetry, color vision assessment, and stereoacuity. Recent advances in electrophysiology now allow testing of retinal (electroretinogram) and optic nerve (visual evoked response) function. These sophisticated tests may be particularly helpful in the diagnosis and monitoring of patients with retinitis pigmentosa and demyelinating diseases.

Once the ophthalmologist completes an accurate ocular examination, therapy can be initiated to give the best possible physical visual function. With the knowledge that the patient is performing at optimal functional visual capacity, the rehabilitation counselor can direct attention to other areas, both physical and psychological. The goal is to help the patient use remaining physical abilities, with other developed competencies, to lead a productive life.

# FUNCTIONAL LIMITATIONS

## Physical

As discussed earlier in this chapter, the actual visual loss is but one component of the whole functioning person. Remaining strengths and competencies help define the person's ability to proceed with a life in healthy fashion.

When a person has a visual disability, increased effort must be used to do even routine tasks. The International Classification of Impairments, Disabilities and Handicaps (Colenbrander, 1977) proposed five parameters to measure the effect of this effort on daily life: physical independence, mobility, economic independence, employment, and social integration. These parameters can impact both the mundane and profound encounters in a person's life. Visual loss, as with other disabilities, can negatively impact any or all activities, stressing the individual's ability to cope.

In defining the specific functional disability caused by visual loss, it is best to approach it in a visual task-related fashion. One needs to determine the individual's capability of performing visual tasks.

Colenbrander (1977) used this approach (see Table 1). His proposed disability spectrum varies from no disability to total disability. The visual tasks a person may complete, such as reading, define the level of function. A person with slight disability can perform visual tasks without special aids, often needing only strong reading glasses. Moderate disability means the individual cannot perform fine tasks without special aids. Severe disability mandates the use of visual aids and, in addition, implies that even with such aids, the person is unable to function without significant difficulty. A person with profound visual disability cannot perform visually close tasks at all and has moderate difficulty with even gross visual tasks. Near total and total disability means the patient must rely on the other senses; vision contributes practically nothing to the person's functional ability.

## Table 1
## LEVELS OF VISUAL DISABILITY

| | |
|---|---|
| Slight visual disability | Can perform visual tasks without special aids (may require reduced reading distance) |
| Moderate visual disability | Can reach near-normal performance with special aids (magnifiers) |
| Severe visual disability | Can perform visual tasks with aids but at reduced level (reading speed, reading endurance reduced) |
| Profound visual disability | Cannot perform most detailed visual tasks (reading), experiences difficulty with gross visual tasks (mobility), increased reliance on other senses |
| Near total visual disability | Vision unreliable; relies mainly on other senses |
| Total visual disability | No vision; relies on other senses entirely |

From "Dimensions of visual performance" by A. Colenbrander, 1977, **Transaction-American Academy of Ophthalmology and Ortolaryngology, 83**, p. 332-337. Reprinted by permission.

Besides actual visual acuity, Colenbrander's classification suggests other factors in defining visual disability. One such additional factor is orientation-mobility, the ability to use vision to recognize correctly one's position with respect to the immediate environment and the ability to travel safely, comfortably, and independently. Orientation-mobility relates directly to functioning in the home and workplace, and plays a vital role in a person's perception of personal freedom and independence.

Factors contributing to orientation-mobility capabilities include residual vision, age at onset of visual loss, posture and balance abilities, intelligence, body image, space orientation, auditory-tactile abilities, and personality. Although each individual is different, with unique capabilities, several comments usually are true for orientation-mobility skills (Marron & Bailey, 1982). Any residual vision, even the ability to perceive only light, is helpful. Substantial loss of the field of vision is more debilitating than loss of central vision. Also, actual skills correlate poorly with visual acuity.

Another factor in the general extent of a disability is the individual's living skills. Every person develops habits that allow smooth physical functioning during daily life. These habits become more important in the individual who has a disability. The person's ability to smoothly handle such tasks as food preparation, bathing, using toilet facilities, grocery shopping, and other activities, plays a major role in life adjustment. The rapidity of onset and duration of visual loss, combined with the general psychological make-up of the individual, define the degree of difficulty with which these skills can be learned or relearned.

Similar to daily living skills, vocational skills are a major component of successful independent functioning. The ability to perform job tasks well and provide for oneself and one's family, greatly enhances self-esteem. It also helps reduce financial worry and family conflict (Brazelton, Stamper, & Stern, 1970).

The physical components of adjustment to visual loss, which include actual physical vision skills, orientation-mobility, daily living, and vocational skills, all interconnect during complex life events. The individual with a visual impairment draws upon all these components to cope with needs. A person with a visual impairment must use many non-visual sources of competence to function independently. Such competencies include physical dexterity, non-visual job skills, natural talents, and refinement of the remaining senses. It is these competencies, besides residual vision, the rehabilitation counselor must help the patient discover and develop.

## Psychological

Another major component of overall adjustment to visual loss is the emotional impact. Blindness or partial loss of vision does not produce mental illness, but can cause intense anxiety. A person's ability to cope with this anxiety determines the extent of healthy behavior (Keegan, Ash, & Greenough, 1976; Mehr, Mehr, & Ault, 1970). In the presence of repressed anger, anxiety, and depression, behavior patterns could follow that are pathological. Underlying psychological strengths help combat such reactive behavior. An individual establishes emotional stability over many years; situational stress, such as loss of sight, challenges these competencies.

The period of greatest stress in visual loss usually occurs at the onset of the loss, when "hope is lost," not at the point of complete, final blindness (Neu, 1975). While sudden loss of vision is extremely traumatic emotionally, it may be easier to cope with ultimately than the uncertain, slow visual loss seen in many chronic ocular diseases.

Certain factors affect the way a person reacts emotionally to the loss of sight. Foremost among these are the basic psychological strengths already in place. Additionally, age plays an important role. Younger individuals tend to be more resilient from the severe psychological sequelae generated by loss of sight. Middle-aged individuals appear to be at greatest risk of having psychological difficulty, perhaps because of other stresses associated with changes occurring during mid-life.

Another variable is the overall degree of visual loss. The more profound the visual loss, the more difficult the adjustment. Reactions of friends and relatives also influence how well an individual copes. Encouragement and caring can supplement the patient's own strengths. Additional factors that impact on a person's ability to adjust emotionally include the patient's physical health, financial status, and vocational situation.

When considering the emotional reaction to visual loss with associated fear and anxiety, one must remember the loss causes a multitude of effects influencing various facets of life. Carroll (1961) outlined many secondary losses that occur with the loss of sight. These include loss of physical integrity, loss of visual contact with the environment, loss of some ability to communicate, and partial loss of mobility.

With some loss of physical integrity, the individual may no longer feel "whole." This may result in feelings of isolation; the person may withdraw from social relationships. Vision is the sense that defines our remote environment. The sighted person easily recognizes remote object characteristics such as size, shape, position, speed, and direction. Persons with visual impairment have lost part or all of this recognition ability. Unless other cues exist, the individual is limited in contact to the immediate environment. This limitation can evoke strong feelings of fear and anxiety. The term "visual background" relates to the whole picture that sighted people constantly absorb. Body language, facial expressions, shadows suggesting time of day - these experiences are missing when a person loses the sense of sight.

In summary, both physical and psychological factors are important in defining the functional status of the visually impaired individual. The term "visual disability" refers to one's ability to perform tasks visually. Visual function involves many factors, both physical and psychological. Awareness by the rehabilitation counselor and the patient of these multiple components will help form a foundation upon which to build new skills. A person may be totally disabled visually but with new acquired competencies in non-visual areas can still achieve physical, psychological, and economic independence, and social integration. In such circumstances, the visual impairment will no longer be a severe, disabling condition.

## *Vocational*

The limitations of visual loss, both physical and psychological, can impact the person's ability to do many work tasks. As noted previously, visual loss and the individual's reaction to this loss, can vary greatly. This makes generalization of employment capabilities difficult. The counselor needs to evaluate each individual's limitations and skills as a unique situation.

Certain considerations are self-evident. For example, the person with severe central and peripheral visual loss, would be incapable of operating heavy equipment or driving a motor vehicle. Central loss of acuity also prevents a person from doing fine tasks such as craftwork, drafting, and standard reading. The total loss of peripheral vision makes it impossible for one to move rapidly around the environment in such job tasks as waiting tables, floor sales, and nursing.

The difficulty with assessing vocational rehabilitation potential is in both obvious areas and "gray zones" in which vision is only partially impaired and job tasks, although difficult, are not insurmountable. In this setting, careful analysis of the situation by the rehabilitation counselor is necessary to determine the level of flexibility of both the visually impaired individual and the employer. The counselor can implement such factors as lighting, seating, visual aids, computer aids, and reasonable accommodation. In the proper context, such assistance in the workplace can transform a previously impossible situation into a productive job setting.

Psychological factors also exist in the visually impaired that influence rehabilitation efforts. Specific fears and concerns may interfere with the ability to make necessary adaptations. Having already lost the ability to function visually, the person may be afraid to "fail again" at a new job task, and not take the risks required for success. The duration of visual disability may be pivotal in this emotional adjustment. A visual deficit acquired early in life may be well compensated for by adulthood, allowing job-related adjustments to progress unimpeded. Recent loss in a young adult can lead to psychological stress that may be more disruptive.

In vocational adjustment, education and the ability and desire to learn new skills are the foundations of career adjustment. With recent advances in audio and visual aids and computer generated resources, the visually impaired individual now has many resources available for improving skills and abilities. A primary consideration in learning is the person's motivation and attitude. Either new skills for the current career situation or skills for a completely new career can be acquired through education, training, assistive devices, residual vision, and existing physical, mental, and emotional competencies.

Most visually impaired individuals can be helped to pursue a satisfying vocation within their capabilities. This can occur when a rehabilitation counselor thoroughly assesses visual requirements of the job and helps provide reasonable accommodation, wherever possible. Education and selection of attainable objectives will supplement nonvisual factors such as level of education, intelligence, interests, technical skills, and aptitudes.

# REHABILITATION POTENTIAL

When considering the rehabilitation potential of the visually impaired person, the counselor must keep in mind that the term disability refers to the person's ability to perform tasks visually, not the level of visual function. Training and assistive devices improve visual task performance without influencing the actual level of vision. This occurs through the fostering of existing competencies in vision and in other areas. Although different types and degrees of vision impairment call for different individualized approaches, the general goal of rehabilitation remains the same - physical and economic independence, and social integration through enhancement of existing skills.

Vision rehabilitation is a joint effort involving many different professionals interacting with the individual. Training, instructing, and counseling are necessary components of the process, as is medical management of the underlying visual problem (Greenblatt, 1988). Members of the rehabilitation team include classroom teachers, orientation-mobility instructors, social workers, rehabilitation counselors, psychologists, and physicians. Each member plays a specific, important role in the rehabilitation process. Good communication between these professionals will enhance coordination of efforts and insure the best possible outcome.

## Figure 2

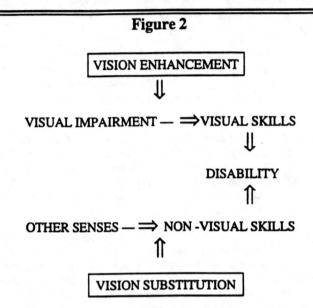

From **Manual for eye examination and diagnosis** (3rd ed.) by M.W. Leitman, 1988, Oradel, NJ: Medical Economics Books. Reprinted by permission of Blackwell Scientific Publications, Inc.

In physical rehabilitation, one makes efforts to obtain the best possible use of residual vision (vision enhancement) and to provide non-visual skills that can substitute for actual visual function (see Figure 2). Vision enhancement involves the use of magnifiers, telescopic aids, colored filters, and computer and video generated magnification screens. These devices generally present the person with an enlarged image that is easier to see. They require a level of fundamental visual function necessary to discriminate such visual objects (Faye, 1984). Most states and large cities have agencies, centers, and institutes that will provide exposure, training, and access to visual aids. Expenses, however, often influence the availability of high-tech instruments (Hollins, 1989).

Non-visual means of decreasing visual disability include visual substitution and orientation-mobility training. Visual substitution involves the use of other modes such as memory, hearing, braille, talking clocks, talking books, guide dogs, and computer generated script readers to perform vision-related tasks. Individuals can often obtain these skills and devices at centers, which deal with vision-enhancing aids. Orientation-mobility training, usually performed by specifically trained and qualified therapists, helps the individual move freely about the environment. Because many factors influence orientation-mobility, people may vary in the potential benefits of this type of therapy. It is the obligation of the counselor to determine status of the auditory system in all clients with severe visual impairment, since it is the auditory system that will be the mainstay for mobility.

Length of disability, severity of disability, nature of personal adjustment, and positive or negative attributes of family and environment complicate vocational rehabilitation of individuals with visual impairment. Besides individual psychological counseling to help the individual cope with stress, anxiety, and fear associated with visual loss, additional adjunct therapy may be helpful. Support groups composed of other individuals with visual impairment have proven a valuable assist in the coping process. The spouse and family of the individual and other individuals with similar disabilities, can often work together in a group to express and deal with feelings of anxiety, frustration, anger, and guilt. Many questions and problems can be resolved through interaction with other group members in similar situations.

Rehabilitation counselors can greatly enhance the status of blind or visually impaired persons. Through careful assessment of the individual's needs and awareness of the level of visual function, and existing non-visual competencies, the counselor can provide appropriate guidance and support. Additionally, the counselor can help the individual select attainable goals and define and outline tasks necessary to reach those goals.

In the community, many resources exist to help visually impaired individuals. Awareness of these resources and a willingness to communicate freely with others providing service to people with visual impairment will strengthen the rehabilitation counselor's own ability to provide a vital, important service.

# CASE STUDY

Ms. Emma Letterman is a 51-year old, married woman with progressive glaucoma. The Letterman's have one grown child who is not dependent on them for support. Emma also has a back injury, which limits her to light work. For the past 10 years, she has been an elementary school teacher, **Dictionary of Occupational Titles** (U.S. Department of Labor, 1977, 1981), # 092.227-010. Before receiving her Master's degree in elementary education, she worked for 5 years as a teacher aide, D.O.T. # 099.327-010. Her first job within the school district was in the cafeteria where she worked as a cashier, D.O.T. # 211.462-010. She became a teacher's aide after working for 1 year as a cashier. The physical exertion of all three of her previous jobs are as described in the **D.O.T.**

Recently, Ms. Letterman went on temporary disability because of deteriorating vision due to glaucoma. She is now considered legally blind. After her condition stabilized, she decided to return to her career as a school teacher. The school district refused to allow her to return, stating they had a medical evaluation concluding she was legally blind. It was their position that a blind person could not do the job of a school teacher. She decided to seek the services of a rehabilitation counselor. Her desire is to return to classroom teaching.

## Questions

1. Describe Emma's three jobs in terms of skill levels and exertional levels. Provide a vocational profile.

2. Do you feel Ms. Letterman can return to any of these jobs, considering both the back problem and the visual limitation? Support your answer with a discussion of occupationally significant characteristics of the three previous jobs.

3. As her counselor, what position will you take regarding the school district's refusal to return her to work as a teacher? Support your opinion.

4. What other possibilities would you recommend?

# REFERENCES

Andreoli, T.E., Carpenter, C.C.J., Plum, F., & Smith, L.H., Jr. (Eds.). (1990). **Cecil essentials of medicine** (2nd ed.). Philadelphia, PA: W.B. Saunders.

Brazelton, F.A., Stamper, B., & Stern, V. (1970). Vocational rehabilitation of the partially sighted. **American Journal of Optometry and Archives of American Academy of Optometry, 47,** 612-618.

Carroll, T.J. (1961). **Blindness: What it is, what it does and how to live with it.** Boston, MA: Little, Brown.

Colenbrander, A. (1977). Dimensions of visual performance. **Transaction-American Academy of Ophthalmology and Otolaryngology, 83,** 332-337.

Duane, T.D. (Ed.). (1988). **Clinical Ophthalmology.** Philadelphia, PA: J.B. Lippincott.

Faye, E.E. (Ed.). (1984). **Clinical low vision,** (2nd ed.). Boston, MA: Little, Brown.

Greenblatt, S.L. (1988). Teaching ophthalmology residents about rehabilitation. **Ophthalmology, 95,** 1468-1472.

Hollins, M. (1989). **Understanding blindness: An integrative approach.** Hillsdale, NJ: Lawrence Erlbaum Associates.

Keegan, D.L., Ash, D.D.G., & Greenough, T. (1976). Blindness: Some psychological and social implications. **Canadian Psychiatric Association Journal, 21,** 333-339.

Leitman, M.W. (1988). **Manual for eye examination and diagnosis** (3rd ed.). Oradell, NJ: Medical Economics Books.

Marron, J.A., & Bailey, I.L. (1982). Visual factors and orientation-mobility performance. **American Journal of Optometry and Physiological Optics, 59,** 413-426.

Mehr, H.M., Mehr, E.B., & Ault, C. (1970). Psychological aspects of low vision rehabilitation. **American Journal of Optometry and Archives of American Academy of Optometry, 47,** 605-611.

Neu, C. (1975). Coping with newly diagnosed blindness. **American Journal of Nursing, 75,** 2161-2163.

Schroeder, S.A., Krupp, M.A., Tierney, L.M., Jr., & McPhee, S.T. (Eds.). (1990). **Current medical diagnosis and treatment.** Norwalk, CT: Appleton & Lange.

U.S. Department of Labor (1977). **Dictionary of occupational titles** (4th ed.). Washington, DC: U.S. Government Printing Office.

U.S. Department of Labor (1981). **Selected characteristics of occupations defined in the Dictionary of Occupational Titles.** Washington, DC: U.S. Government Printing Office.

Vaughan, D., Asbury, T., & Tabbara, K.F. (Eds.). (1989). **General ophthalmology** (12th ed.). Norwalk, CT: Appleton & Lange.

## About the Author

William C. Panek, M.D., is an Assistant Professor of Ophthalmology in the Glaucoma Division of the University of California, Los Angeles, Jules Stein Eye Institute. He is the Associate Chief of Ophthalmology at the Veterans' Hospital, West Los Angeles, California, and Director of the UCLA Mobile Eye Clinic.

# Chapter 16

# CANCER

by
*Mary Margaret Elmayan, M.S., P.T.*

## INTRODUCTION

Cancer is a term that conjures up fears; these include fears of disfigurement, mortality, pain, abandonment, loss of livelihood, fiscal setbacks, helplessness, and the unknown. This chapter provides information to assist rehabilitation counselors who work with clients who currently have or have had cancer. By personally confronting these universal fears, the rehabilitation professional may become more effective in dealing with clients facing this historically dreaded disease.

The word, cancer, describes over 100 different diseases sharing a distinguishing characteristic, the uncontrolled growth and spread of abnormal cells. Cancerous cellular masses comprise "malignant" tumors. This excludes "benign" tumors encompassing abnormal growth of normal cells, which do not spread. Tumor thus refers to both benign and malignant abnormal cellular growths of either normal (i.e., noncancerous) or abnormal (i.e., cancerous) cells. Only a medical pathologist's microscopic examination can definitively diagnose cancer (Cade, 1986; Holleb, 1986). Oncology is the scientific study of the biological, chemical, and physical properties of cancerous tumors.

The disease of cancer has been present throughout the millennia. The ancient Greeks treated cancerous growths with leeches and with balancing the four humors. Some Egyptian mummy remains reveal well preserved tumors. In modern times, cancer remains a disease on the rise only partly due to an aging population; the age-adjusted national cancer death rate is also on the rise. Certain environmental and occupational contributing factors responsible for this increase include excessive radiation exposure, maternal use of diethylstilbestrol (D.E.S.), asbestos contact, and a high fat and nitrate diet. Cigarette smoking accounts for 30-40% of cancer deaths (predominantly, but not limited to, lung cancer) (see Table 1). Tobacco-related cancer deaths may rise even more dramatically during the 1990s. This is partially because of the "Women's Liberation Movement" of the 1960s, which unfortunately condoned smoking in women as socially acceptable (American Cancer Society, 1981, 1991).

The estimated number of new cancer cases in 1991 is 1.1 million (American Cancer Society, 1991). Cancer will strike 1 out of 3 Americans and affect 3 out of 4 families. Cancer is the leading disease-cause of death in children between the ages of 3 and 14; yet, childhood cancer accounts for only 1 in 100 cases. The National Center for Health Statistics noted the fiscal impact of cancer was $104 billion in 1990. This includes $35 billion in direct medical costs, $12 billion for morbidity costs (costs of lost productivity), and $57 billion for mortality costs. Cancer accounts for 10% of all disease-incurred costs in the United States (Brown, 1990).

Of those who were diagnosed with cancer in 1990, 4 out of 10 persons will be considered cancer survivors (i.e., alive 5 years after termination of cancer treatment). If one were to eliminate the non-cancer related causes of death of the cancer patient, the 5-year survival rate approaches nearly half. With advances in early diagnosis and treatment techniques, the 5-year survival rates have dramatically improved (American Cancer Society, 1991).

## Table 1
## CANCER DEATH RATES BY SITE, UNITED STATES, 1930-87

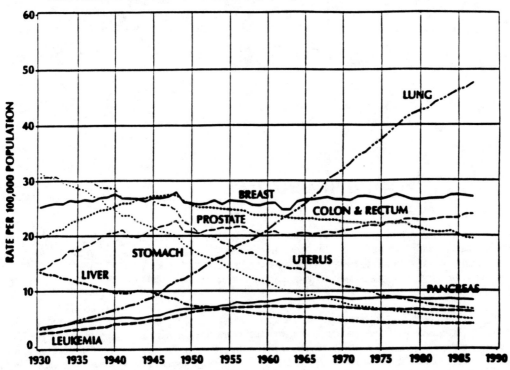

From **Cancer Facts and Figures 1991** (p. 3). By the American Cancer Society, 1991, Atlanta, GA: National Headquarters, American Cancer Society, Inc. Reprinted by permission.

# SYMPTOMATOLOGY

For many years, the American Cancer Society has sought to teach "CANCER'S 7 WARNING SIGNALS" to the public and the health care sectors alike (see Table 2). Unfortunately, some cancers initially lack signs and symptoms. For example, a tumor less than one centimeter in diameter is nearly impossible to feel, yet contains over one hundred million cancer cells. Health care providers may suspect a person as "at risk" for cancer based solely upon a familial history of cancer or based on occupational, environmental, or viral exposure (see Table 3). Routine cancer screening examination schedules should be followed conscientiously by every health care provider. These routine screenings with prompt physician consultation in the presence of any of the "7 Warning Signals" can dramatically improve the outcome of cancer treatment (American Cancer Society, 1991).

There are other signs and symptoms that may suggest the presence of cancer, although generally less indicative of a specific cancer site. These may include an unexplained weight loss of at least 10 pounds, a fever of unknown origin, unexplained fatigue, and pain, especially constant pain that does not ease with rest. The above signs, symptoms, and signals can be caused by any number of disease processes. A cancer diagnosis must be left to the qualified physician. Through expertise and a detailed medical evaluation, the physician uses a process of systematic

## Table 2
## CANCER'S SEVEN WARNING SIGNALS

1. Change in bowel or bladder habits
2. A sore that does not heal
3. Unusual bleeding or discharge
4. Thickening or lump in breast or elsewhere
5. Indigestion or difficulty in swallowing
6. Obvious change in wart or mole
7. Nagging cough or hoarseness

From **Cancer Facts and Figures 1991** (p.27). By the American Cancer Society, 1991, Atlanta, GA: National Headquarters, American Cancer Society, Inc. Reprinted by permission.

elimination to rule out other diseases, forms a tentative diagnosis, and finally confirms the presence of cancer (American Cancer Society, 1981, 1991; Cade, 1986).

# PATHOLOGY AND DIAGNOSIS

## *Pathology*

As previously stated, cancer is a general term given to over 100 different diseases, all characterized by uncontrolled growth and spread of abnormal cells. It is a multi-faceted process, not completely understood by medical science. The theory most often suggested is that an "initiator" factor quickly and irreversibly transforms a previously normal cell into an abnormal state. Secondly, a "promoter" factor more slowly allows for this abnormal growth; in early stages, it may still be reversible (Andreoli, Carpenter, Plum, & Smith, 1990; Rubin, 1983; Wilson, Isselbacker, Petersdorf, Martin, Fanci, & Root, 1991).

This cancerous or malignant growth gradually spreads by direct extension from the original site; it may impinge and invade neighboring tissues and organs. Cancer cells also may spread to distant sites by dislodging, detaching, and gaining access to the circulatory and lymphatic systems. This process is called metastasis. The areas of preferred spread by cancer sites are well established and documented (Ciba Foundation Symposium, 1988; Harris & Liotta, 1990).

## *Diagnosis*

Pathology, the study of disease through microscopic examination of body tissue and organs, is the only medically accepted means to diagnose cancer. A biopsy or removal of tissue for pathological study, is required for a definitive diagnosis. One must consider the general medical status of a patient, size and location of the tumor, and anticipated extent of required tissue sample(s) for biopsy. Biopsy techniques include "closed" approaches,

# Table 3
## ETIOLOGIC AGENTS IN HUMAN NEOPLASMS -
## ENVIRONMENTAL CARCINOGENS

| Causal Factor | Neoplasm | Evidence of Exposure | Occupation and Type of Exposure |
|---|---|---|---|
| **Chemical Agents** | | | |
| Aromatic amines, esp. β-naphthylamine | Papilloma and cancer of bladder, urinary tract | Compounds in urine | Cutaneous, respiratory exposure; chemical workers producing dye stuffs, rodenticdes, lab reagents |
| Benzol | Leukemia, lymphoma | Anemia, bone marrow aplasia | Cutaneous, respiratory exposure; coal tar refiners, solvent manuf., painters, printers, mech. using solvents |
| Coal tar, pitch, creosote, anthracene | Cancer of skin, larynx, bronchus | Chronic dermatitis, warts, photosensitivity of hands, face, exposed areas | Cutaneous, respiratory exposure; coke oven workers, coal tar distillers, lumber indus., chemical workers |
| Petroleum, shale and parrafin oils, waxes, tars | Cancer of skin | Chronic dermatitis, wax boils, warts in exposed areas | Cutaneous exposure; workers in oil refineries, wax and asphalt prod., mechanics |
| Isopropyl oil | Cancer of sinus, larynx, bronchus | | Resp. exposure; producers of isopropyl alcohol |
| Asbestos | Cancer of bronchus, mesothelioma | Pulmonary asbestosis, asbestos bodies in sputum, asbestos warts on fingers | Respiratory exposure generally, >2 yrs; asbestos miners, shippers, millers, pipe fitters, others; generalized pulmonary fibrosis (asbestosis) present |
| Chromium | Cancer of bronchus | Chronic dermatitis, chrome holes in skin, perforated nasal system | Respiratory ( and cutaneous) exposure; workers engaged in chromate ore reduction |
| Nickel | Cancer of nasal cavity, sinus, bronchus | Nasal polyps, chronic bronchitis, dermatitis | Respiratory exposure; nickel miners, shippers, and refiners; nickel carbonyl resp. agent(?) |
| Arsenic | Cancer of skin, bronchus, bladder | Keratoses (esp. palms and soles) | Smelters, pesticide manufacturers |
| Vinyl chloride | Hemangiosarcoma of liver | | Chemical workers |
| **Physical Agents** | | | |
| Ionizing radiation | Cancer of skin, thyroid, tongue, tonsil, sinus, bronchus, osteogenic sarcoma, leukemia | Radiation dermatitis | Percutaneous or systemic exposure for therapeutic purposes (e.g., treatment of spondylitis, polycythemia), or by accident (radium-dial workers); respiratory exposure; pitch-blender miners |
| Ultraviolet radiation | Cancer of skin | Chronic active dermatitis, hyperkeratosis, exposed areas | Cutaneous exposure; farmers, watermen, other outdoor workers; rarely predisposing factors (e.g., xeroderma pigmentosa) |

From **The principles and practice of medicine** (22nd ed., p. 372) by A.M. Harvey, et al., editors, 1988, Norwalk, CT: Appleton and Lange. Reprinted by permission.

encompassing fine needle aspiration, "scrapings" or exfoliative cytology (e.g., Pap smear), and surgical incisional/excisional or "open" approaches.

**The pathologist's role in diagnosis.** The role of the pathologist is to address four major concerns. First, is to determine if the tumor is malignant or benign. Second is to establish, if possible, the primary site for the malignancy. The pathologist histologically classifies the tumor or determines what "normal" tissue has become abnormal and caused the tumor. The four broad cancer classifications are the following (American Cancer Society, 1991):

1. Sarcomas - cancer of bone, muscle, or connective tissue.
2. Carcinomas - cancer of epithelial cells (such as skin), lining of lungs and colon, and breast.
3. Leukemias - cancer of blood-forming organs.
4. Lymphomas - cancer of infection-fighting organs.

Third is to determine how much the cancerous cells resemble the normal cells of origin. Two common differentiation grades to identify the new cancer cells have been established, one numerical and one descriptive:

**Grade 1** = "well-differentiated" and most resembling the tissue cells at its site of origin.

**Grade 2 & 3** = "moderately-differentiated," some semblance to the tissue cells of origin.

**Grade 4** = "poorly-differentiated," bearing least semblance to the tissue cells of origin.

---

## Figure 1
## TYPES OF CANCER

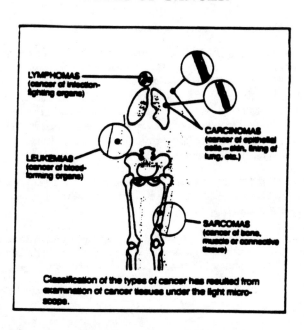

---

From **A cancer source book for nurses** (rev. ed., p. 10) by the American Cancer Society, 1981, New York: American Cancer Society, Professional Education. Reprinted by permission.

The higher grade or the less (i.e., poorly) differentiated cancers hold the worst prognosis.

Lastly, the pathologist needs to determine how far the cancer has spread. This determination, or the "staging" process is a joint effort between the surgeon and pathologist. The staging process seeks to ascertain, micro and macroscopically, the extent or spread of the cancerous tumor growth present.

Oncologists commonly use the letters, T N M with subscript numbers 0-4 (0 = least; 4 = most) as follows:

T = tumor size

N = lymph node involvement

M = extent of metastatic growth

A cancer diagnosis requires the "T" subscript to be at least "1," as "0" denotes no evidence of any tumor or cancer cells. The larger the tumor size respective to its site of origin, the higher the subscript number. Lymph nodes (the "N" subscript) draining the cancer site are subsequently examined, with "0" denoting an absence of any localized cancer spread, to a "4" or extensive lymph node involvement. The "M" refers to how numerous and pervasive the non-contiguous cancer growth(s) (metastases) extend. Thus, a tumor staged $T_2$ $N_1$ $M_0$ is less extensive and potentially more curable than one staged $T_4$ $N_3$ $M_2$.

# EVALUATION AND TREATMENT

## Evaluation

Evaluation of the cancer patient includes a thorough assessment. Typical areas of concern to the diagnostician include: familial history of cancer; concurrent disease processes; occupational and environmental exposures; past medical history; sexual practices; past and current drug use; weight and dietary habits; and onset, progression, and behavior of cancer signs and symptoms. The physical exam generally includes: listening to the lungs, heart, and bowel; observation of the skin and eyes for changes (e.g., rash, dryness, bruising, and discoloration); palpation of the lymph nodes and glands for nodules or swelling; inspection of the reproductive organs, especially for symmetry and possible discharge; and a neurological assessment, including reflex, tone, sensation, and strength testing; and observation of functional ability (Andreoli et al., 1990; Rubin, 1983; Wilson et al., 1991).

A variety of laboratory tests are available to the diagnostician. Laboratory tests help establish baseline studies for vital organ function and capacity. They also serve as milestones against which to gauge treatment results (either tumor regression or possible local or metastatic tumor growth).

The oncologist is a physician who specializes in the medical management of the cancer patient. A precise, accurate, and thorough work-up leading to a specific diagnosis is critical. The diagnosis and evaluation ultimately determine which treatment will be most effective and hold the best promise of a favorable outcome.

## Treatment

The mere mention of cancer treatment regimes available to a newly diagnosed cancer patient may be as traumatic as the initial diagnosis of cancer itself. It seems there is a popularly held belief that cancer treatment is worse than the disease. This erroneous idea is founded largely on ignorance. The following discussion seeks to promote a greater understanding and respect for cancer treatment therapies, with both their positive and negative side effects (Glucksberg & Singer, 1980).

**Surgery.** As previously discussed, surgery plays a key role in establishing a definitive diagnosis. Historically, surgery has been the best hope for a cancer cure by removing the cancerous growth from the body. Cancers treatable by surgery are shown in Table 4. Surgical excision can range from partial excision of small tumors in tissues and organs, to complete removal or amputation of a body part. The inherent danger in surgical management lies in the inadvertent "seeding" or microscopic dispersal of cancerous cells (American Cancer Society, 1981).

Surgery is often the treatment of choice. Frequently, the general nutritional status of the patient before extensive, invasive surgery, is poor. A pre and post-operative nutritional regime is instituted to help the patient build the reserves necessary to ensure adequate healing, prevent unnecessary complications, and shorten recovery time. The relative success of surgical intervention has become more promising, more sophisticated, and less permanently debilitating, both functionally and cosmetically, than in the past. The prominence of surgery in the quest for a "cure" has somewhat diminished, as physicians use surgery more selectively since the advent of chemotherapy and radiation therapy. Non-curative surgical intervention may be effective in the relief of symptoms of pain and discomfort caused by tumor pressure and obstruction on nerves and vital body functions, through partial removal or "debulking" of tumors (American Cancer Society, 1981; Cade, 1986; Rubin, 1983).

## Table 4
## CANCERS TREATABLE BY SURGERY

| | |
|---|---|
| **Laryngeal** | if no metastases |
| **Lung** (localized) | 20% 5-year survival |
| **Kidney** | 30 to 50% 5-year survival if early and localized |
| **Bladder** | superficial, well-differentiated |
| **Breast** | localized, and depends on what kind of surgery and adjunctive therapy |
| **Genital** | |
|   **Penis** | very low survival rate |
|   **Prostate** | 50% 5-year survival if localized |
|   **Testis** | good for certain types, especially if early |
|   **Cervix** | if early |
|   **Ovary** | certain types, if early |
|   **Endometrium** | if low pathology grade |
|   **Vulva** | for stage 1 |
|   **Vagina** | if early, but recurrence rate is 20% |
| **Brain** (some) | depends on type, stage, location |
| **Skin** | other than melanoma |
| **Bone** | only parosteal osteosarcoma |

From **A cancer source book for nurses** (rev. ed., p. 30) by the American Cancer Society, 1981, New York: American Cancer Society, Professional Education. Reprinted by permission.

**Chemotherapy.** Historically, physicians used chemotherapy as a "last-ditch" resort, but it now has come into the forefront in the treatment of cancer. Chemotherapy has been used since World War II, when exposure to nitrogen mustard gas was found to improve symptoms in soldiers with certain blood tumors. Dr. Charles Huggins pioneered the use of the female sex hormone estrogen to cause shrinkage of prostate cancer for which he received the Nobel prize.

Chemotherapeutic agents or drugs destroy those cells that are undergoing or about to undergo mitosis (cell reproduction). Since cancer cells reproduce more quickly then most, but not all, normal cells, the cancer cells are least resistant to destruction by chemotherapy. The side effects of chemotherapy are obvious and understandable. They include hair loss, mouth sores, nausea, vomiting, diarrhea, fatigue, and lethargy caused by decreased blood counts with a loss of infection-fighting ability. The smaller and more rapidly growing tumors are most vulnerable to the effects of chemotherapy. This contrasts and complements surgery, which is more effective against the larger, more slowly growing tumors (Andreoli et al., 1990; Wilson et al., 1991).

Physicians also use chemotherapy when there is a lack of solid tumor (e.g., leukemia and lymphomas) or lack of objective surgical findings (i.e., no primary site can be established with a poorly-differentiated cell). Chemotherapy is also effective in the relief of symptoms caused by tumor growth when a "cure" may no longer be possible. Such symptoms might include pain and decreased mobility.

Chemotherapy agents may be administered orally, intravenously, or intramuscularly. There are instances when chemotherapy may be placed, via surgical techniques, more directly into or near a desired target area. The frequency and duration of chemotherapy varies, depending upon the tolerance of the patient to the side effects, body weight, blood counts, and type and responsiveness of the tumor. The white blood cells, primarily the neutrophils, are most critical in fighting infection. Chemotherapy will be withheld if white blood cell values drop to levels that place the patient at risk of being left without sufficient defenses to fight infection. Such infections may be viral, bacterial, or fungal. Some commonly seen infections in the immunosuppressed chemotherapy recipients include CMV (cytomegalovirus), thrush (yeast infections of the mouth), and shingles (herpes zoster).

There are five major categories of chemotherapeutic agents: alkylating agents, antibiotics, anti-metabolisms, hormones (steroids), and vincalkaloids. Tumor responsiveness is based upon the inherent trait of the tumor itself and the mode and efficacy of the selected chemotherapeutic treatment agent. Tumors are most vulnerable to the first course of chemotherapeutic treatment, as cancer cells can develop resistance to an administered chemotherapeutic agent. Chemotherapy destroys only a set percentage of cancer cells at one time, rather than a set number of cells. In theory, this means it is impossible to destroy all the cancer cells.

Therefore, the first chemotherapy treatment holds the best promise for a patient. The cancer cells have developed no resistance and there are no accumulated toxic side effects. Also, combination chemotherapy, in which more than one agent is used, may improve the outcomes over a single agent use. Indications for combination chemotherapy include: a large tumor burden; the "curative" side effects from a single drug prove too severe; or the tumor cells develop resistance to a given agent. The evaluation of a patient's response to chemotherapy is classified into the following categories (Andreoli et al., 1990; Rubin, 1983; Wilson et al., 1991):

**Complete remission** —complete tumor regression for one month or longer with full functional status;

**Partial remission** —tumor regresses at least 50% with no new tumor growth;

**Improvement** —tumor regresses 25-50%; or

**No response** —the tumor regresses less then 25% with no subjective improvement.

Cancer "cures" (i.e., 5-year survival) are achieved using chemotherapy.

**Radiation therapy.** The history of radiation therapy dates from the turn of the century. Henri Becquerel, Marie and Pierre Curie shared the Nobel prize in physics in 1903 for this discovery. Wilhelm Roentgen pioneered the application of x-rays in the visualization of internal body parts. Radiation therapy employs high-energy, electromagnetic radiation with high-speed, subatomic particles that are absorbed by the body's tissues. Like chemotherapy, this damages the DNA of the fastest growing and replicating cells of cancerous and noncancerous cells alike, (e.g., hair, bone marrow, and oral and gastrointestinal tract lining). Radiation therapy interrupts and blocks the cellular reproductive cycle. Unlike most chemotherapies, radiation therapy is administered to and directed toward a highly localized area (Albert, 1984; American Cancer Society, 1981).

Throughout the years, radiation oncologists have determined the radiosensitivity and tolerance levels of various body tissues and organs. These are recorded in radiation absorbed dosages (RADS). Thus, the tumor sensitivity itself, the location of a tumor, and the tissues through which the external beam must pass contribute toward establishing optimal dosage levels. The goal is to destroy the tumor without permanently harming healthy tissues. The technology for external beam radiation production has improved over the years, from being absorbed at the skin level, to deeper penetration with little skin damage. This is due to the increasing use of higher frequency and shorter wave lengths of the particles. Besides the marked advances in external beam radiation therapy, there is the internal "beam" implant or brachytherapy. The physician inserts implants or "seeds," consisting of rice-shaped pellets, tiny beads, or wires, into special molds that hold them in or near the desired target site. A computer helps determine the precise strength and location of the implants. Since the penetration level is only approximately one-third inch, there are negligible side effects on the surrounding healthy tissues. After a prescribed period of between 1-6 days, the implants are removed. Surgical assistance may be required to penetrate tissue areas and to remove the molds.

In contrast to the internal implants that are performed on an inpatient basis and last less than a week, the external beam radiation therapy sessions may be done on an outpatient basis. This therapy generally takes 2-8 weeks. Radiation goals, like chemotherapy and surgery, may be curative or palliative. A typical curative external beam course lasts 6-8 weeks, with tumor irradiation being the desired outcome. A palliative course generally lasts no longer than 2 weeks. Palliative radiation goals may include shrinkage of the tumor in situations where overlaying structures may not tolerate a curative dose or to minimize cellular spread or tumor seeding. Radiation therapy can be the single most effective agent in the control of bone pain and cessation of bleeding.

Depending upon the site of administration, some side effects of radiation therapy are like those of chemotherapy, as they affect the most rapidly dividing cells. Radiation therapy given to the brain will cause hair loss; radiation to the lower spine may cause nausea, vomiting, and diarrhea. Nearly all radiation therapy causes fatigue due to bone marrow suppression of red blood cell production and dropping blood count. Fatigue is also due to the body's attempts at cellular repair and removal of destroyed cells after each treatment session. For possible future treatment, radiation fields are permanently outlined on the patient with cosmetically invisible tattoos.

Radiation therapy, unlike chemotherapy, may cause problems to a few people not evident during the treatment sessions. The body's "protective" response to radiation exposure proves insidiously harmful to some individuals. Months or years after radiation treatment, the body very slowly thickens tissues, especially the microscopically small blood vessels and lymphatics, ultimately occluding or closing them. A patient may develop massive arm or leg swelling as the draining lymphatic channels become occluded. The joints may become stiff and nonfunctional, and skin ulcers may develop as the oxygen supply so necessary for supple and healthy tissues vanishes. If any portion of the lungs or heart receives radiation exposure, potentially life-threatening pneumonitis and pericarditis (swelling and inflammation) can develop. Moreover, a radiation therapy patient is at much higher risk for developing a secondary or treatment-induced tumor. The overall percentage of patients who eventually develop such radiation-induced tumors is low.

In summary, radiation therapy has much to offer the cancer patient, including high cure rates for certain cancers. Researchers are testing a method involving high heating of the radiation fields by diathermy or other local, comfortable, and deep-warming methods to evaluate if tumors are responsive to radiation at lesser dosage levels. This would reduce the curative RAD levels; results are promising (American Cancer Society, 1981; Andreoli et al., 1990; Holleb, 1986).

Additional areas of research in the treatment of cancer include immunotherapy, hyperthermia, and monoclonal antibodies. These are briefly described below:

**Immunotherapy.** This treats cancer disease by using the body's ability to resist infection. The medical oncologist stimulates a patient's immunosurveillance system in the hopes it will destroy the cancer by antibody production. Results to date have been less promising than those achieved with more conventional methods.

**Hyperthermia.** Hyperthermia raises the temperature of the tumor cells using localized deep heating. Physicians use ultrasound, diathermy, and microwaves as these modalities cause little heat perception at the skin surface and penetrate to destroy the more vulnerable cancer cells, while sparing the healthy cells. Trials have been small, with the most promising results using a combination hyperthermia and radiation therapy treatments.

**Monoclonal Antibodies.** Discovered in 1978, these microscopic cells seek out and destroy only targeted cancer cells. They can be used diagnostically in the visualization of cancer spread by using radio markers. The goal is to have these cells deliver microscopic packets of chemotherapy directly to targeted cancer cells, sparing systemic-wide effects of chemotherapy. Results have been promising.

**Combination therapy.** Generally, the most effective treatments combine the various modalities described above. The combination of one therapy aids and facilitates the function of another. When one therapy promotes the action of another, it is called adjuvant. Thus, the resulting side effects would also be greater, save for the fact guidelines call for therapeutic levels to be dropped because of greater cell destruction. Studies reveal even those individuals with early stage disease and apparent successful surgical intervention, achieve a better "cure" and long-term survival if prophylactically treated with adjuvant therapy (Cade, 1986; Harvey, Johns, McKusick, Owens, & Ross, 1988; Holleb, 1986).

**Non-medical treatment approaches.** Other less medically proven theories, relying more heavily on personal testimony than on scientifically proven and tested methods, include the areas of influence and interaction of the body and mind. Siegel (1988), a physician trained in the traditional medical model, has devoted much of his time and energies to this subject. He believes, with some scientific proof, that positive and negative thoughts of a person with cancer can help release powerful substances in the body. Less scientifically proven, this theory maintains that a patient who visualizes a cure, can achieve destruction of cancer cells. Also, Siegel believes much of Western medicine's healing powers may not be due solely to surgical technique, but also to a patient's belief it will provide a cure.

There are non-medical treatment approaches, commonly known as quackery. These have included Laetrile (ground apricot pits), enemas, potions, and macrobiotics (diets and vitamins). These rely solely on personal testimony and lack scientific rationale. Also, they may be dangerous and hazardous to a person's health. Frequently, though not exclusively, the location of these treatment centers is outside the United States. Nonetheless, they may fill an important psychological need for a cancer patient by surrounding the client with a generally pleasant, optimistic, and supportive environment.

# FUNCTIONAL LIMITATIONS

Functional limitations may be the result of the disease or the treatment. Chart 1 describes possible limitations, the causes and potential implications and strategies. If the limitations are the result of treatment, they may be temporary. If they result from the disease, the limitations may be temporary or permanent. Included in this chapter are two scales that rate various levels of functional limitations (see Tables 5 & 6). It should be noted these are broad, sweeping limitations and should be used carefully when evaluating a particular client. The ratings can be used as supplemental information to a client's total medical condition. Discussed below are some of the more common and specific limitations, their causes, and rehabilitation strategies/implications.

# Chart 1
## SPECIFIC LIMITATIONS, THEIR CAUSE(S), AND
## REHABILITATION IMPLICATIONS

| Specific Limitations | Cause (s) | Rehabilitation Strategies/Implications |
|---|---|---|
| Fatigue | Weight loss due to tumor metabolic consumption;Chemo and radiation side effects due to bone marrow suppression and body's attempt to deal withcellular repair;Poor respiratory patterns due to: lung cancer, lung stiffness due to chemo (i.e., bleomycin), inadvertent radiation therapy field exposure | Extra rest; stress reduction strategies, lessening of work hours, energy conservation techniques, relaxation training; flammable precautions (i.e., no exposure to combustibles) if client using supplemental oxygen; flexible work hours to cope with scheduled chemo or radiation treatment induced fatigue |
| Arm(s) and Leg(s) Swelling | Mechanical obstruction of lymphatic vessels by tumor; Surgical obliteration of lymphatic channels; End-stage cardiac function | Wearing of surgical, heavyweight support garment hose/sleeve/glove decreases fine motor dexterity; keep affected part elevated relative to heart; Avoid potential injury and infection to affected parts (e.g., no gardening, construction, heavy lifting/carrying, heat [including sun and water] exposure, chemical/caustic exposure) |
| Radical Neck Dissection | Surgical excision of oral-facial cancers with loss of the nerve supplying a major shoulder muscle (trapezius) | Client unable to raise arm out from side; forward lifting of 5 lbs. or over on involved side prohibited as there are no muscle substitutes |
| Long Bone Fracture(s) | Cancer metastasis; Radiation damage; Excessive bone loss due to age or medications (osteoporosis) | NO pressure/weight-bearing to all non-united arm/leg fractures; use of crutches/walker/wheelchair for all leg fractures; use of sling/cast for all arm fractures |
| Spinal Fracture(s) | Cancer metastasis; Radiation damage; Excessive bone loss due to age or medications (osteoporosis) | NO lifting/twisting/prolonged sitting or standing postures; "halo" type braces (secured through skull) for neck instability with neurological signs |
| Extremity Paralysis | Tumor invasion of nerves; Side effects of chemotherapy (vinca-alkyloids); Surgical damage; Surgical removal of entire muscle for muscle cancer (i.e., rhabdomyosarcoma) | Extremely light weight bracing to protect joints; limited lifting/carrying; potential for strength loss; functional loss accentuated if dominant arm involved; loss of bilateral coordination |
| Mastectomy | Surgical removal of breast cancer (male and female) | Lifting prohibited for early weeks post-surgery to allow weakened muscles to heal and regain strength; usually only restrictions are same as for swollen arms; full function anticipated within three months |
| Broviac and Hickman Catheters | Necessity/desire for "permanent" and pain-free chemotherapy administration in large vessels | Avoid tugging at line; NO lifting/carrying over ten lbs.; incision site to be kept very clean (antiseptic); avoid electrical exposure as catheter line contains metal, leading towards the heart |
| Cardiac Arrhythmias | Chemotherapy toxicity (Adrianmycin); Anemia due to bone marrow suppression | NO physical work/exertion until medically supervised ECG treadmill and functional activities monitored, and parameters established with appropriate cardiac medication levels established |
| Mentation Changes | Cancer metastatic to brain; Primary cancer origin is brain; Side effects of chemo or radiation therapy; Electrolyte imbalances; Side effects of pain control medications | Evaluate client's safety and judgement for daily living and work (e.g., operation of heavy machinery, driving, reaction times, ability to follow multi-step commands or deal with multiple and simultaneous stimuli) |

| | | |
|---|---|---|
| Laryngectomy | Removal of voice box and normal air flow due to cancer | Avoid irritating airborne substances (e.g., dust, smoke, perfumes, aerosols); avoid direct water contact; gauze cover must be worn to prevent mucus loss or accidental inhalation of substances; inability to lift as cannot hold breath; loss of normal, intelligible speech; alternative communication devices available; surgical puncture of the esophagus can create a "voice" with prosthesis |
| Oral-Facial Defects | Surgical removal of cancerous lesions (including eye, nose, tongue, jaw, palate, chin, ear and/or cheekbone); Hair loss due to chemo and radiation therapy | Cover nose defects with gauze to filter particles; prosthesis to restore cosmesis, palate function, and speech; may have difficulty with public interface/interaction due to disfigurement; hair pieces, scarves, or caps; regrown hair may be different texture or color; adaptive eating utensils, diet modification |
| Skin Sensitivity | Skin cancer; Radiation therapy | Avoid sun and heat exposure; wear protective clothing and maximum sun block |
| Ostomy | Cancers of the gastrointestinal tract removed by rerouting bowel and/or urinary tracts | Generally, no functional or sexual limitation; avoid rubbing/irritating ostomy site as client wears pouch to "catch" waste products |
| Lower Extremity Amputation | Sarcoma or metastatic disease | Ambulation/mobility may be limited, especially on uneven terrain; lifing/carrying may be precluded by upper extremity use of cane or walker; meticulous skin care needed for residual limb if using a prosthesis, due to poor skin healing post chemo and radiation therapy and depleted nutritional stores |

## Table 5
## ECOG* PERFORMANCE STATUS SCALE

| Status | Definition |
|---|---|
| 0 | Normal Activity |
| 1 | Symptoms, but ambulatory |
| 2 | In bed < 50% of the time |
| 3 | In bed > 50% of the time |
| 4 | 100% bedridden |

*ECOG = Eastern Cooperative Oncology Group

From **Clinical oncology: A multi-disciplinary approach** (p. 91) by R. Rubin, 1983, Atlanta, GA: American Cancer Society. Reprinted by permission.

## Table 6
## KARNOFSKY PERFORMANCE STATUS SCALE

| | Percent | |
|---|---|---|
| Able to carry on normal activity; no special care is needed | 100 | Normal; no complaints; no evidence of disease |
| | 90 | Able to carry on normal activity; minor signs or symptoms of disease |
| | 80 | Normal activity with effort; some signs or symptoms of disease |
| Unable to work; able to live at home; cares for most personal needs; a varying amount of assistance is needed | 70 | Cares for self; unable to carry on normal activity or do active work |
| | 60 | Requires occasional assistance but is able to care for most of his needs |
| | 50 | Requires considerable assistance and frequent medical care |
| Unable to care for self; requires equivalent of institutional or hospital care; disease may be progressing rapidly | 40 | Disabled, requires special care and assistance |
| | 30 | Severely disabled; hospitalization is indicated though death not imminent |
| | 20 | Very sick; hospitalization is necessary |
| | 10 | Moribund; fatal processes progressing rapidly |
| | 00 | Dead |

From **Clinical oncology: A multi-disciplinary approach** (p. 91) by R. Rubin, 1983, Atlanta, GA: American Cancer Society. Reprinted by permission.

## Team Approach

The cancer patient presents the rehabilitation counselor with many challenges. A team approach is the most effective way of providing rehabilitation to the patient with cancer (Dietz, 1981; Holleb, 1986). Besides the rehabilitation counselor, possible team members include the patient, physician, nurse, physical therapist, occupational therapist, speech therapist, social worker, pharmacist, dietician, family members, and psychologist. These team members, communicating with one another, maximize the client's potential. For example, the pharmacist can suggest medication changes to achieve adequate pain control with minimal side effects. The dietician can suggest diet modifications and supplements to help offset fatigue. These professionals can be a source of help and inspiration in the management of the oncology patient.

## Advanced Cancer

The patient with advanced cancer often develops multiple areas of metastases involving various organ systems. As the disease progresses, so do the side effects of chemotherapy, radiation therapy, and surgery. These patients have multi-systemic problems. The advanced cancer patient may present with cardiac irregularities, stroke-like hemiplegia (one-sided arm and leg paralysis) or paraplegia-like (lower body) paralysis, orthopedic fractures, vascular swelling of an arm or leg, pain, and immunosuppression, to name but a few. Any one of these, let alone a combination, provides a challenge to the rehabilitation counselor. For a more extensive explanation of treatment problems and resulting functional limitations, refer to the chapters on the respective organ systems. The rehabilitation professional must be able to deal with multi-systemic problems and prioritization of treatment goals. The excitement and reward lies in helping the cancer patient achieve meaning, fulfillment, and a quality of life in light of constantly changing circumstances (Aaronson & Beckman, 1987; Haney, 1984).

## *Counseling*

Individual or group counseling may help alleviate emotional problems associated with either an active disease process or disabilities resulting from cancer (Glucksberg & Singer, 1980; Haney, 1984). Many self-help cancer groups have formed where persons can exchange experiences, disseminate information and resources, and share problems related to their disability.

# REHABILITATION POTENTIAL

The rehabilitation potential for a diagnosed cancer patient depends on many factors. A comprehensive, holistic evaluation and assessment of the individual's support systems, financial and medical resources, age, education, work history, and functional abilities and limitations is important. In addition, any coexisting disease processes coupled with the cancer (stage, grade, and type) and treatment (type, length, and side effects) contribute toward formulation of the rehabilitation plan. The smaller, localized, and more slowly-growing tumors generally have a better prognosis. Individuals with more extensive function and an optional state of health are able to tolerate more aggressive and potentially curable treatment. A person with significant and positive anticipated life events - the birth of a grandchild, marriage of a child, or visit to long-missed relatives abroad - tends to survive longer.

Another factor unique to the cancer patient is that it behooves the rehabilitation practitioner to think of the cancer patient as "recovering" instead of "cured." It takes only one cell in the body, encased and protected in an atherosclerotic plaque, to escape the effects of chemotherapy. Years later, it can break free and cause disease recurrence. Although the incidence for this is very low, it remains documented and does occasionally occur.

The patient with cancer, desiring to maintain gainful employment, faces major obstacles. Given the average length of employment of 2-3 years for all individuals, even the cancer patient with a limited prognosis should be encouraged and supported. Employers and co-workers are fearful of the oncology patient at best, and, at times, illegally discriminatory. Employers and co-workers alike fear excessive absenteeism, rising insurance costs, cosmetic and functional deficits, and fear of "catching" cancer, although all the above are overwhelmingly without foundation. The cosmetic and functional limitations are often largely surmountable.

The cancer patient's employment attendance record is often better than that of workers with other diseases, and compares favorably to the average worker who does not have a disability. Health insurance benefits for a client seeking employment at a company may have an exclusion clause for current or pre-existing diseases. Other employers have a "guaranteed issue" plan in which newly hired workers are eligible for benefits despite past medical history (American Cancer Society, 1984; Stone, 1975; Wheatley, 1974).

Flexibility and close communication with the client, employers, family, and other members of the rehabilitation team remain the key to effective intervention. The November 1983 American Cancer Society's policy statement on disability states the following regarding disability and cancer. "In contrast to many other individuals disabled or handicapped by injury or defects, the cancer patient may have a 'dynamic disability.' The degree of disability in some patients will be affected by exacerbation or remission of the disease and/or its treatment."

The rehabilitation counselor has traditionally been trained to perform well in what J. Herbert Dietz, Jr. has described as the restorative level of rehabilitation; i.e., "goal setting when no major residual limiting disability need be expected and the patient will either be cured or be essentially free of restrictive disease for an appreciable time." Yet, the rehabilitation counselor must be mindful and encompass that other segment of the oncology population addressed by the American Cancer Society's policy statement. J. Herbert Dietz, Jr., has described this population as in need of supportive goals, "when persistent residual disease must be expected although under relative control and where ongoing and residual disability can be minimized." (Dietz, 1981).

Perhaps the greatest challenge for the rehabilitationist is to work with the client who has recurrent disease and acute episodes within the context of a chronic disease. These are not most oncology patients, though they may often comprise the majority of rehabilitation team members' oncology caseload. The rehabilitation counselor should not give false hope, nor take it away, but help the oncology patient find meaning and quality in living.

Discussion of rehabilitation potential is not complete without mentioning prevention. Preventive regular screening, periodic examination especially for "at-risk" persons, and aggressive management of identified cancer can decrease incidence and increase survival rates. The American Cancer Society (1991) estimated that 83% of lung cancer deaths are due to cigarette smoking. Smoking accounts for 30% of all deaths from cancer and is a major cause of other diseases such as heart disease, chronic obstructive pulmonary disease, and cerebrovascular disease. Occupational hazards, especially certain types of radiation and chemicals, increase a person's risk of cancer. These occupational conditions are being studied and are under continued surveillance. Exposure in the workplace, however, accounts for a small percentage of cancer (American Cancer Society, 1991; Shaw, 1981).

# CASE STUDY

Cancer of the testes constitutes only 1% of male cancers but accounts for more deaths in males 15-34 years of age than any other cancer disease. This case study presentation concerns this type of cancer.

Steve is a 22 year-old, married male, with one child. Although he did not complete the 11th grade, he received his G.E.D. (equivalency of a high school diploma). There is no additional school or training. He is co-owner with one other partner, of a small, but highly successful company. By trade, Steve is an electrician and is a member of the local electricians' trade union.

The **Dictionary of Occupational Titles** (U.S. Department of Labor, 1991) classifies this job as: telephone electrician (telephone and telegraph) (D.O.T.# 822.281-018). Steve and his partner install, test, and repair telephone and communication systems. They update and expand old equipment, install new computerized systems, and also wire burglar alarm devices and related equipment. Both partners are involved with repairing and restoring this electrical and electronic equipment. The work involves use of small handtools and testing devices, the ability to read schematics, and knowledge of electrical and electronic principles. Lifting and carrying on the job involves a maximum of 50 pounds, with repetitive lifting of up to 25 pounds.

Steve was in good physical and emotional health until April of 1986, when he noticed a non-tender lump on his right scrotum. Two months later, he underwent a right orchiectomy (testicle removal) and lymph node dissection. The medical diagnosis at that time was embryonic cell carcinoma of testicular origin, well-differentiated, stage $T_2 N_0 M_0$. He also received a complete course of Actinomycin-D and Velban chemotherapy. Three months postoperatively, he returned to work, maintained sexual function, and physicians felt he was disease-free with an excellent prognosis.

Approximately one year later, a routine cancer follow-up visit (including a chest x-ray) revealed a solitary, metastatic right lower lobe pulmonary lesion. His oncologist initiated chemotherapy, using a combination of agents. His lesion disappeared. Again, the oncologist believed him disease-free or in remission.

Steve returned to work after completion of chemotherapy and was fully independent in all activities. His partner had managed to cover necessary work activities in his absences by employing other union members on a temporary basis.

One year later, Steve again had lung nodules. The laboratory results indicated one nodule on both sides of the lung. He underwent an open biopsy (thoracotomy). Only 1 out of the 6 nodules was cancerous. Yet, within one month of open chest surgery, he developed left-sided brain seizures. The new diagnosis was metastatic testicular disease to the brain; he immediately underwent neurosurgery for removal of the brain tumor.

After the craniotomy procedure, he again developed left-sided weakness. Steve had a significant loss of strength in his left arm. His left leg was also affected and he needed to use crutches to ambulate. Steve's balance was poor. He remained bedridden most of the day. There were no speech or visual deficits.

Following radiation therapy, he had a Broviac catheter placed for adjuvant chemotherapy. He received physical and occupational therapy. Symptoms gradually subsided and he was able to return to work on a part-time basis. His functional limitation was for sedentary work. There was a 25% residual deficit in the left upper extremity. In terms of ambulation, he could walk for short distances with the aide of a cane. At the company, his main work responsibilities were now administrative, analyzing work sites, and writing bids and service contracts. He remained asymptomatic and was able to gradually increase his work effort to full-time at the sedentary level of exertion.

## Questions

1. Discuss the staging process and the use of the subscripts TNM. Early in diagnosis, Steve's cancer was thought to be at stage $T_2 N_0 M_0$. From what you know now, was this accurate?

2. Why was radiation therapy not given to his lung nodules?

3. What were some precautions for him to take in returning to work with a Broviac catheter in place?

4. Give a vocational profile including age, educational level, exertional and skill level of any work activity, occupationally significant characteristics, and transferable skills (if any).

5. Was the return to modified work realistic? Were transferable skills used in the return to work? What other possibilities are there using transferable skills?

# REFERENCES

Aaronson, N.K., & Beckmann, J. (Eds.). (1987). Monograph Series of the European Organization on Research and Treatment of Cancer (EORTC). In **The quality of life of cancer patients** (Vol. 17). New York: Raven Press.

Albert, E. (Ed.). (1984). **Cancer rehabilitation**. New York: Raven Press.

American Cancer Society (1981). **A cancer source book for nurses** (rev. ed.). New York: American Cancer Society's Professional Education.

American Cancer Society (1984). **Cancer: Your job, insurance, and the law**. New York: Author

American Cancer Society (1991). **Cancer facts & figures--1991**. Atlanta, GA: Author.

Andreoli, T.E., Carpenter, C.C.J., Plum, F., & Smith, L.H., Jr.(1990). **Cecil essential of medicine** (2nd ed.). Philadelphia, PA: Harcourt Brace Jovanovich.

Brown, M.I. (1990). Special report: The national economic burden of cancer; an update. **Journal of the National Cancer Institute, 82,** 1811-1814.

Cade, B. (Ed.). (1986). **Cancer manual** (7th ed.). Boston, MA: American Cancer Society, Massachusetts Division.

Ciba Foundation Symposium (1988). **Metastasis.** New York: John Wiley & Sons.

**Dietz, J.H., Jr. (1981). Rehabilitation oncology.** New York: John Wiley & Sons.

Glucksberg, H., & Singer, J.W. (1980). **Cancer care: A personal guide.** Baltimore, MD: Johns Hopkins University Press.

Haney, C. (1984). **Psychosocial factors in the management of patients with cancer.** New York: John Wiley & Sons.

Harris, C.C., & Liotta, L.A. (1990). **Genetic mechanisms in carcinogenesis and tumor progression.** New York: Wiley-Liss.

Harvey, A.M., Johns, R.J., McKusick, V.A., Owens, A.H., Jr., & Ross, R.S. (Eds.). (1988). **The principles and practices of medicine** (22nd ed.). Norwalk, CT: Appleton and Lange.

Holleb, A. (Ed.). (1986). **The American Cancer Society cancer book: Prevention, detection, diagnosis, treatment, rehabilitation, cure.** New York: Doubleday.

Rubin, R. (1983). **Clinical oncology: A multi-disciplinary approach.** Atlanta, GA: American Cancer Society.

Shaw, C.R. (1981).**Prevention of occupation cancer.** Boca Raton, FL: CRC Press.

Siegel, G.S. (1988). **Love, medicine & miracles: Lessons learned about self-healing from a surgeon's experience with exceptional patients.** New York: Harper & Row.

Stone, R.W. (1975). Employing the recovered cancer patient. **Cancer, 36,** 1.

U.S. Department of Labor (1991). **Dictionary of occupational titles** (4th ed., revised). Washington, DC: author.

Wheatley, G.M. (1974). The employment of persons with a history of treatment for cancer. **Cancer, 33,** 441.

Wilson, J.D., Isselbacker, K.J., Petersdorf, R.G., Martin, J.B., Fanci, A.S., & Root, R.K. (Eds.). (1991). **Harrison's principles of internal medicine** (12th ed.). New York: McGraw Hill.

## *About the Author*

Mary Margaret Elmayan, M.S., P.T., has been the Clinical Education Coordinator for Physical Therapy at the City of Hope Medical Center, Duarte, California, where she pioneered many innovative rehabilitation treatment approaches for a large oncology service; an Assistant Professor in Physical Therapy at Mount Saint Mary's College, Los Angeles, California; and a member of the American Cancer Society's Professional Education Committee.

# Chapter 17

# HEMOPHILIA

by
*Laurence J. Logan, M.D.*

## INTRODUCTION

To be an effective advocate for individuals with hemophilia, the rehabilitation counselor needs to understand both the clinical behavior of the disorder and its impact on the patient. Contrary to popular misconception, persons with hemophilia are not fragile individuals only suitable for very specialized jobs located in protected environments. Often called "bleeders," many people erroneously believe individuals with hemophilia are vulnerable to rapid blood loss upon exposure to the slightest trauma. In reality, these people bleed no more rapidly or excessively from minor cuts and superficial abrasions than do persons who do not have hemophilia. This is because the earliest phases of clotting are unimpaired in hemophilia. With modern treatment, individuals can work safely and productively in a variety of jobs.

Hemophilia is a hereditary, chronic bleeding disorder resulting from deficient functioning of a factor essential for blood coagulation. Predominantly affected is the musculoskeletal system. If untreated, progressive crippling occurs. Researchers have identified 13 plasma coagulation factors, so far. The term "hemophilia" refers to a clinical disorder that results from a reduced amount or function of either factor VIII or factor IX. Treatment consists of replacing the missing factor.

### Hemostasis

Normal blood clotting occurs in two major overlapping phases: **primary** and **secondary** hemostasis (to stop bleeding). Primary hemostasis consists of formation of a "primary hemostatic plug" that initially stops bleeding after injury. This plug consists of platelets (the clotting cells in the blood stream), which adhere to exposed collagen in the damaged blood vessel wall. Von Willebrand factor (vWF), acting somewhat as a "glue," is essential for effective platelet adhesion to collagen. Attachment to collagen stimulates platelets to release adenosine diphosphate (ADP) causing the platelets to adhere to one another thereby forming the primary plug.

Generation of fibrin from its precursor, fibrinogen, constitutes the secondary phase of hemostasis. The primary platelet plug forms a scaffold (or matrix) upon which the fibrin is deposited. Conversion of fibrinogen to fibrin entails a complex series of biochemical reactions, in which numerous proteins known as "coagulation factors" take part. Factors VIII and IX are particularly critical for generation of an effective fibrin clot. Deficiency of either factor results in hemophilia (Logan, 1988a).

Centuries before we knew about Mendelian genetics or the complexities of blood coagulation, Talmudic scriptures of the second century described the sex-linked transmission of the disorder now known as hemophilia. The genetic defects accounting for deficiency of factor VIII (hemophilia A, "classic" hemophilia) and of factor IX (hemophilia B, "Christmas" disease), both occur on the X chromosome. Males have one X and one Y chromosome (XY), whereas females have two X chromosomes (XX). A mother carrying the defect ($X^h$) on one of her X chromosomes ($X^hX$) may transmit hemophilia to her son ($X^hY$) or pass the defect to a daughter ($X^hX$) who will also be a carrier for the disease. The mother may transmit her normal X chromosome to her son (XY) or daughter (XX). True to Mendelian genetics, sons of a carrier mother and a normal father have a 50% chance of having hemophilia and daughters have a 50% chance of being carriers. Since a father with hemophilia ($X^hY$) contributes only his Y chromosome to his sons, none will have hemophilia. All his daughters will receive his $X^h$ chromosome and will be carriers ($X^hX$) (see Figure 1).

## Figure 1
## THE GENETIC TRANSMISSION OF HEMOPHILIA

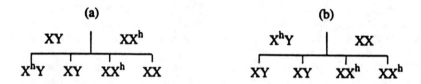

(a)Normal male and female carrier of hemophilia. Each son has a 50% chance of having hemophilia; each daughter has a 50% chance of being a carrier. (b)Male with hemophilia and normal female. All daughters are carriers; all sons are normal.

This explains why hemophilia is almost exclusively a disease of males. Infrequently, this genetic defect ($X^h$) does account for an abnormal bleeding tendency in women. Mating of a male with hemophilia ($X^hY$) and a carrier female ($X^hX$) can result in a truly hemophiliac female ($X^hX^h$), but this is extraordinarily rare. More commonly, a carrier female's level of coagulation factor is reduced enough to result in abnormal bleeding.

How can this be explained? If one considers that the gene which governs production of effective factor VIII or factor IX is located on the X chromosome, one is not surprised that carriers (as a **group**, **not** as individuals) have factor levels about half that of non-carriers (normal factor level activity is 50-170%). But why do non-hemophilic men and women have similarly normal factor levels. That is, why do not "normal" women (XX) who have two X chromosomes, produce twice as much factor as "normal" men (XY) with just one X chromosome?

The answer to this and to why some carriers will be low-factor-level-carriers lies in a complicated fact of biology (called Lyonization), which occurs in very early fetal development. To keep a genetic balance, female embryos "inactivate" one of the two X chromosomes in each cell, and all subsequent cell divisions reflect that "decision." This inactivation is totally random. The random selection of one or the other of the two X chromosomes is purely by chance, much like flipping a coin results in "heads" or "tails." Because the "normal" woman inactivates 50% of her X chromosomes, her level of factor VIII and factor IX is equivalent to a "normal" man's level.

Now, consider what happens when a carrier ($X^hX$) randomly inactivates one or the other of her X chromosomes. The majority will have factor level 50% of normal. Just as when flipping a coin, one may occasionally flip "heads" 10 times in a row, some carrier women will inactivate more of their normal X chromosomes leaving a preponderance of $X^h$ chromosomes. The end result is that as many as 28% of carriers may have factor levels low enough to result in abnormal bleeding under certain circumstances. Of these, some will have levels in the range of moderately severe hemophilia and, therefore, be at risk for various bleeding complications from various medical and dental procedures or after injury (Wincott, 1977).

Often, there may be no family history of hemophilia. The technology of modern molecular biology has confirmed at least 30% of cases of hemophilia arise from mutation. The mutation may appear in the male infant himself, but probably more often arises in his mother or in his maternal grandmother. Genetically governed deficiencies of the other coagulation factors, although rare, do occur and may result in bleeding abnormalities. The genetics, severity, nature of the bleeding, and possible disabilities associated with these disorders usually differ markedly from hemophilia.

Deficiency of factor VIII accounts for approximately 85% of cases of hemophilia; deficiency of factor IX accounts for the remaining 15%. Critical as they are for coagulation, the amounts of factors VIII and IX present in normal plasma are extremely small, and can be measured only in sophisticated research laboratories. For clinical purposes, one measures the level of each of these factors by its **functional** activity. The normal functional level of both factors, based upon a pool of plasma samples from normal persons, is 1.0 unit/ml of plasma. This is expressed as 100% activity. Values for factor VIII and factor IX in normal persons range from 50-170%.

## Severity

Physicians stratify the severity of hemophilia according to levels of factor activity. Factor levels less than 1% constitute **severe** hemophilia; between 1-5% are **moderately severe**, and from 6-30% are **mild**. Important clinical differences exist among these three groups. The minimum amount of each factor necessary for adequate coagulation is approximately 30%. Levels between 30-50% may be seen in extremely mild hemophilia or in some women who are carriers. It is very important to note that the severity of hemophilia **runs true within kindred**, i.e., all affected males within an extended family have equivalent levels of the factor. Clinically notable hemophilia occurs once in about 20,000 births (1 in every 10,000 males). This incidence is remarkably constant in all races, socioeconomic groups, and geographic areas. Presumably, the somewhat high mutation rate accounts for this uniform distribution of the disease.

## Von Willebrand's Disease

Von Willebrand's disease (vWD), a different hereditary bleeding disorder, involves an abnormality of the von Willebrand factor (vWF) and a modest to moderate reduction in factor VIII. Rarely will vWD be mistaken for moderately severe to severe hemophilia because the clinical features of bleeding due to defective primary hemostasis are very different from those of defective secondary hemostasis, including hemophilia. In abnormal primary hemostasis plug formation (as in vWD), we see prolonged bleeding from minor cuts or abrasions and persistent oozing from mucosal surfaces. We do not see the joint bleeds and deep muscle hematomas (collections of blood) that characterize the more severe forms of hemophilia. Mild forms of hemophilia and vWD may be clinically mistaken for each other. The hematologist (an internist or pediatrician who specializes in blood disorders) must define precisely which disorder is the cause for the mildly decreased factor VIII level because the genetics, clinical course, treatment, and disability features are so different.

# PATHOLOGY AND SYMPTOMATOLOGY

## Pathology

The hallmark of the hemostatic defect in **severe hemophilia** involves repeated bleeding into joints (hemarthrosis) and muscles (producing hematomas) either following minimal trauma or apparently "spontaneous." In descending order of frequency, hemarthroses occur in the knees, elbows, ankles, shoulders, hips, and wrists. Without significant trauma, bleeding into the hands is uncommon. Bleeding into the spine almost never occurs. The frequency of hemarthrosis in severe cases varies widely from patient to patient, despite similar levels of coagulation factor activity. Joint bleeds may occur as often as two or three times a week, especially in the younger years. As the person enters adult life, episodes typically become less frequent. Some severely affected persons may not have a significant hemarthrosis for months.

The results of repeated bleeding into joints is hemophilic arthropathy (joint disease). Spontaneous bleeds are uncommon in patients with **moderate hemophilia** but hemarthroses or muscle hematomas may be triggered by mild to moderate trauma. **Mildly affected** patients may show increased amounts of bruising and hematoma formation following significant trauma, but generally, on a daily basis, they have no symptoms.

Frequently, a man with mild hemophilia (or occasionally a carrier with a low factor level) remains unaware of any coagulation abnormality until he encounters unexpected profuse, excessive bleeding. This can occur after a tooth extraction, during major surgery, following injury, or in similar circumstances.

Bleeding into the joint capsule initiates the development of hemophilic arthropathy. The inner surface of the joint capsule is lined by a vascular connective tissue called the synovial membrane. Various blood components together with enzymes released from the synovium cause inflammation of the membrane. Ferritin, a particularly damaging iron material formed from destroyed red blood cells is absorbed by the synovial membrane. The synovial membrane responds to these insults by proliferating a fibrous, highly vascular tissue. Chronic synovitis ensues. Because this abnormal synovium, rich in friable blood vessels, is located near the articulating surfaces, the frequency and severity of hemarthroses further increase (Gill, Thometz, Scott, & Montgomery, 1989).

This vicious cycle leads progressively to degeneration of cartilage, destruction of bone, and replacement of the joint space with fibrous (scar) tissue. The bones may fuse (ankylosis) resulting in deformity and a severely impaired range of motion. The earlier stage of synovial proliferation and joint destruction somewhat resembles the pathological events of rheumatoid arthritis, whereas end-stage hemophilic arthropathy is more similar to severe osteoarthritis.

Pain, limited range of motion, and joint deformity lead to atrophy (wasting) of adjacent supporting muscle groups and weaken the stability of the joint. Instability further enhances a tendency for bleeding into the joint and the surrounding tissues. One can readily see how this self-perpetuating, self-reinforcing pathological process results in inevitable joint damage. Early vigorous medical therapy can interrupt this chain of events. Once hemophilic arthropathy has fully developed, it often progresses, despite medical therapy. Aggressive medical treatment may sometimes slow the pace.

## Symptomatology

The boy with hemophilia discovers early in life that he can tell when a bleed has started, sometimes hours before objective evidence is manifest. The "aura," which signals the start of a joint bleed, is described variably by different individuals. They may describe it as a feeling of warmth, a tingling or bubbling sensation, a "ping," or even a vague feeling of a "restless" discomfort in the joint. Minutes to hours later, the physical findings of hemarthrosis appear.

These include swelling, increased warmth of the joint, and some degree of limitation of motion. Hemarthrosis is often very painful, the severity of the pain reflecting the magnitude of the bleeding.

**Chronic synovitis.** This condition involves persistent or recurrent swelling of a joint, often without marked pain (unless there has been recent hemarthrosis) and a surprisingly mild reduction of joint mobility. Chronic pain with features similar to osteoarthritis occurs with more advanced arthropathy.

**Hematoma.** Bleeding, whether spontaneous or following mild trauma, occurs deep within muscles forming hematomas in severe hemophilia. Although common, hematomas occur less frequently than hemarthroses. The most frequent sites are the large flexor muscle groups in the lower and upper extremities and the "retroperitoneal muscles" (the iliacus and psoas muscles). "Retroperitoneal bleeds" in the large intra-abdominal muscles are debilitating and potentially serious. Even small hematomas in the iliacus muscle, which lies within the interior of the pelvic wall, may produce marked pain in the groin and anterior thigh region. The patient cannot extend his leg fully and maintains his hip in a flexed position. Repeated bleeding into the same site, producing large hematomas, can result in contracture deformities. Proper and timely treatment of muscle bleeding has reduced this complication. Delayed or inadequate treatment of hemarthoses may result in deformity, especially in the ankle, knee, or elbow, but also occasionally in a shoulder or hip.

**Nerve palsies.** Although uncommon, nerve palsy may result from compression of a nerve due to extensive bleeding into the muscle through which the nerve passes. Although generally reversible, the palsy can become permanent.

**Excessive bleeding.** Persons with severe hemophilia, with a virtual absence of factor VIII or factor IX, are more likely to bleed excessively into any traumatized organ. They are also prone to bleed more readily into structures diseased in such a way as to favor bleeding (e.g., stomach ulcer, bladder tumor, inflamed pancreas, kidney). Bleeding from otherwise normal kidneys occurs at least once in 75% of persons with hemophilia and is usually of no consequence.

Intracranial bleeding accounts for about 25% of deaths in hemophilia and usually (but not invariably) follows trauma. Any head injury occurring on the job (or elsewhere) needs immediate evaluation. Early treatment of head injury by replacement of the missing factor may prevent complications. The modestly increased incidence of seizure disorder in people with hemophilia probably stems from previous head injuries where there was intracranial bleeding.

Bleeding into the oral cavity requires prompt attention, particularly if the bleeding occurs in critical areas such as the tonsillar region (e.g., as in a fulminant, exudative tonsillitis), the posterior pharyngeal wall (e.g., trauma from a straw or popsicle stick), or under the tongue (e.g., after biting down "wrong" on a sharp piece of food). Unchecked bleeding from these anatomic sites can, at times, progress rapidly and interfere with breathing. While not excessively common occurrences, these situations require immediate evaluation and treatment.

# DIAGNOSIS AND EVALUATION

## Diagnosis

When there is a known family history of hemophilia on the maternal side of a woman's family, a prospective mother will often have seen a hematologist to clarify whether she is a carrier. If her father has hemophilia, she should know she is a carrier. A carrier has several options:

1. Have no children.

2. Establish the sex of the fetus early in pregnancy, by amniocentesis, and choose to end the pregnancy if the fetus is a male.

3. Establish whether the male fetus has hemophilia by analysis of an intrauterine fetal blood sample. If the male fetus proves to have hemophilia, she may choose to end the pregnancy or she may continue with it, knowing her son will have the substantial benefits of modern therapy.

4. Proceed with the pregnancy without a prenatal diagnosis with the intent of accepting the outcome.

Diagnosis of hemophilia can be made at birth by analysis of umbilical cord blood. When there is no family history of hemophilia, prolonged bleeding will suggest the presence of severe hemophilia. A hematologist establishes the diagnosis of hemophilia, its type (deficiency of factor VIII or of factor IX), and the degree of severity (percent level of factor activity). By the time the person with hemophilia sees a rehabilitation counselor, he will know not only the diagnosis but much more about the disease and its effect upon him.

## Evaluation and Assessment

Hemophilia is presently an incurable but not usually fatal disease. The man with hemophilia must adapt himself effectively to be maximally self-sufficient, socially integrated, productive, and happy. A multidisciplinary health care team is beneficial to address the problems of the person with hemophilia as he progresses from childhood through adolescence and adult life. Nowadays, due to advances in modern medical treatment, many individuals live into old age. The team concept spawned the development of a comprehensive network of hemophilia treatment centers throughout the nation and in many parts of the world (Kasper & Dietrich, 1985).

The treating physician sees the patient, if otherwise in good health, at least yearly for an annual comprehensive evaluation. The hematologist collects a detailed history and performs a complete physical examination. Appropriate laboratory tests and x-rays are ordered. One does an assessment of the patient's immune system and directs special attention to liver function tests for presence or absence of antibodies against hepatitis viruses, and for evidence of a carrier state of hepatitis B virus. The physical therapist and orthopedist establish the patient's baseline level of functioning at this examination, at a time when there is no acute problem occurring. Evaluation of range of joint motion and functional capacity result in an updated orthopedic diagnosis. A treatment plan is then adapted to the needs of the patient.

A nurse specialist or nurse coordinator conducts a nursing assessment. The nurse evaluates the patient's lifestyle, his understanding of the disease, and whether he is a candidate for self-administration (self-infusion) of the missing coagulation factor. If he is already on home treatment, the nurse reviews the patient's ability to self-infuse, his understanding of proper dosage schedules for various types of bleeding events, and his records of self-treatment. The nurse specialist is a major source of ongoing education for the patient.

A social worker assesses the impact of hemophilia on the patient's life, more specifically on family, work, and recreation. Further appointments are scheduled when the social worker sees maladaptive patterns or underdeveloped coping skills.

The data gathered at the annual examination can provide invaluable assistance to the rehabilitation counselor. Information about the overall amount of difficulty a patient is having and the amount of time he is likely to miss from school or work can be estimated. The evaluation can include an index of the patient's reliability, compliance with the medical regimen, general physical condition (including musculoskeletal), emotional stability, and specific complications.

It is important to pay careful attention to proper dental hygiene. The physician will emphasize prompt treatment of dental caries and measures to prevent gum disease. Although these patients are no more susceptible to dental disease than the general population, the restoration or removal of teeth and treatment of periodontal disease require special conditions and treatment methods. Accordingly, each comprehensive center must have dentists and oral surgeons on the team who are familiar with hemophilia.

# TREATMENT

## *Replacement of Missing Factor: Cryoprecipitate*

**Cryoprecipitate.** The person with hemophilia does not bleed more profusely, but he continues bleeding because he cannot make an adequate clot due to deficiency of factor VIII or factor IX. These very crucial coagulation factors are normally present in blood in minuscule amounts. Until about 25 years ago, there was no adequate way to supply amounts of the missing factor sufficient to stop major hemorrhage. In the early 1960s, researchers noted when they thaw plasma slowly, the part that remains frozen longer is especially rich in factor VIII (Pool, Hershgold, & Pappenhagen 1964). This momentous observation lead to more effective management of severe hemophilia. This plasma fraction, called "cryoprecipitate," made possible replacement of factor VIII to levels that could normalize blood coagulation. This capability revolutionized hemophilia care.

**Factor cryoprecipitate.** During the following decade, medical researchers developed concentrate preparations increasingly more abundant in factor VIII. Factor VIII concentrate is prepared and packaged in vials that are stable at room temperature and are reconstituted with a small volume of sterile water, whenever needed for infusion. The quantity of plasma necessary to provide amounts of factor VIII sufficient to manufacture these concentrates requires many donors (between 5,000-25,000). Similar concentrates containing factor IX were developed soon after. These latter preparations contain other vitamin K dependent coagulation factors (prothrombin [factor II], factor VII, and factor X). Until very recently, preparations of "pure" factor IX have not been available.

## *Self-infusion*

The concentrate products make possible a temporary, complete correction of the genetic coagulation defect by normalizing the level of missing factor. The ability to correct the bleeding abnormality, although transiently, inspired physicians caring for people with hemophilia to work toward prevention of the disabling musculoskeletal complications through prompt treatment of bleeding episodes. This objective, formulated by the comprehensive hemophilia treatment centers, led to the home treatment program, now an established part of hemophilia care (Dietrich, 1991). Parents of a child or the older patient may be trained in self-supervised infusion, provided the responsible person(s) exhibits willingness to undertake rigorous instruction encompassing:

1.  How to store and prepare the concentrate for use.

2.  The technique of venipuncture.

3.  Detailed education focused upon the theoretical and medical evaluation of hemorrhages.

The success of self-supervised infusion may be difficult because of several factors. There may be diminished venous access or mechanical difficulties in accessing veins for infusion due to arthropathy of the upper extremities. Also, some people experience a mental block when attempting to puncture their veins.

Prompt self-administration of concentrate at the first symptom of a bleed is often all that is needed. Mild swelling or pain usually responds to a single, timely infusion. Early treatment often makes it possible for the patient to avoid missing school or work. Immediate therapy interrupts the pathological process leading to permanent joint damage. If there is a delay of treatment for an episode of bleeding into a joint (hemarthrosis) or the joint bleed is severe, the individual may need concentrate and a splint. This immobilizes the joint and helps control bleeding. If the bleed occurs in a lower extremity, crutches may be required for a day or two to rest the lower extremities during acute hemorrhage.

## Joint Complications

To preserve joint mobility, progressive physical therapy is begun as soon as possible after control of the bleed. Application of ice to the painful joint early in hemarthrosis very often provides symptomatic relief and might sometimes alter the course of the bleed. Less frequently than in previous years, patients with severe hemarthroses may require hospitalization for a few days to ensure immobility, to confirm adequate concentrate administration, and to provide supervised physical therapy. Acute hemarthroses can be extremely painful; the patient may need analgesic medication, often a narcotic.

If an acute joint bleed is severe and the swollen joint is extremely tender, one can obtain dramatic and immediate relief by aspiration of the joint. Also, if the joint is otherwise healthy, aspiration helps prevent worsening synovitis. Regular, ongoing prophylactic treatment with concentrate is suitable for some patients. Others may administer a prophylactic dose before engaging in activities likely to cause bleeding.

## Chronic Pain

Because hemophilia is a chronic disease often complicated by both acute and chronic pain, use of analgesics must be carefully regulated and monitored to minimize development of narcotic dependence. In a few cases, drug dependence may erupt into clear-cut drug abuse, sometimes in association with excessive alcohol use. These individuals must be identified early and targeted for appropriate counseling or enrollment in a drug abuse rehabilitation program. Individuals with hemophilia pose a real problem for many orthodox drug abuse regimens because they often have had a lifelong experience of real and often very severe pain. Complete elimination of potent analgesic medication, typically the ultimate goal of most drug abuse programs, is usually neither feasible nor attainable.

Drug rehabilitation programs may, however, greatly benefit the person who has begun to abuse pain medication in an attempt at self-medication for symptoms of depression or anxiety. Use of non-pharmacological alternatives in pain control should be maximized. Short-acting non-steroidal anti-inflammatory agents (e.g., ibuprofen) can safely be used in most patients and can provide considerable relief from chronic pain. Aspirin must be strictly avoided because of its long-lasting inhibitory effect on platelet function, which further delays blood clotting.

## Therapeutic Tools

Availability of concentrate preparations has made it possible to perform any invasive diagnostic procedure or surgical operation in a person with hemophilia. Physicians can perform various orthopedic surgical procedures to help patients with advanced cases of arthropathy, including emplacement of artificial joints (endoprostheses). Total knee and hip replacements have dramatically improved the quality of life for many individuals (Logan, 1988b; Luck, 1988).

Other therapeutic tools are available for use in certain circumstances. Desmopressin, a synthetic antidiuretic molecule that releases factor VIII from storage sites in mild, and some moderate cases of hemophilia A, is often used instead of factor VIII concentrate. Antifibrinolytic drugs (e.g., epsilon-amino-caproic acid, tranexamic acid), prevent homeostatic dissolution of clots and are beneficial when used with factor concentrate for dental extractions, gum bleeding, and other oral bleeding problems. Epistaxis (nose bleed) and menorrhagia (heavy menstrual periods in low level carriers) also can be treated with these drugs (Ogston, 1984).

## Epidemiology-Effects of Treatment

Less than two decades after replacement therapy and home treatment became available, data began to accumulate attesting to dramatic improvement in the lives of hemophilia patients. The number and length of hospitalizations decreased. Visits to hospital emergency rooms and hemophilia clinics decreased in inverse relation to the number of infusions given at home. "Home treatment" refers to self-supervised treatment and should be understood to include "office or factory treatment" and "school treatment." Days absent from both school and work decreased. The number of persons employed who have hemophilia increased. Studies from the United States, United Kingdom, Norway, the Netherlands, and other countries reported identical trends (Evensen, Thaul, & Groan, 1979; Marshall, 1977; Stuart et al., 1980; Varekamp et al., 1989).

New concentrates are very expensive. Today, drug companies use newer, more refined technologies in the preparation of concentrates. The result has been further dramatic increases in cost. Nonetheless, recent data suggest that despite the expense of hemophilia care and especially of concentrate, replacement therapy is cost effective when balanced against decreased productivity without the treatment (Etzel, 1981; Schimpf & Niederberger, 1981; Smith, Keyes, & Forman, 1982). The effects of dramatic cost increases of factor derived from newer technology remain to be seen.

By the mid-1980s, persons with hemophilia were entering adulthood with milder or no arthropathy. Prompt self-infusion and judicious prophylactic use of concentrate permitted these people to lead fairly normal, active lives. Fifteen percent of severe hemophilia cases in the Netherlands surveyed in 1985 had no joint damage at all (Smith et al., 1989). These were predominantly younger individuals. Within two decades of replacement treatment, all nations with well organized hemophilia treatment programs reported remarkable increases in life expectancy (Aronson, 1988; Ikkala et al., 1982; Larsson, 1985; Rizza & Spooner, 1983; Rosendaal et al., 1989).

Before 1960, survival beyond young adulthood of those with severe hemophilia was rare. For example, the mean age at death during the decades between 1940-1960 in Sweden was 23 years for severe and 50 years for mild cases. The United States, Denmark, Finland, and the Netherlands reported similar data. By 1985, the mortality rate for severe cases had improved to approximately that of people who smoke (Smith et al., 1989). When we factor in the important decrease in death rate among young adults (previously discerned to be a period of high mortality), the average life span approaches that of the general male population.

Investigations undertaken to assess the impact of replacement therapy on quality of life have revealed enhanced mobility, decreased disability, and increased realization of educational and vocational goals. Decreased pain and discomfort, together with an increased sense of independence favor an improved social life. More individuals with hemophilia have married. They have enhanced self-esteem and improved overall sense of well-being. In one study, 80% of patients 18 years of age and older considered their health "good to excellent," a percentage close to the general male population (Rosendaal et al., 1990).

These subjective assessments correlated poorly with objective measurements such as functional impairment and ability to work. Clearly, measuring "quality of life" is a difficult matter. Still, the observation that persons with hemophilia, despite their chronic illness, were essentially as satisfied with quality of life as were healthy persons demonstrates the capacity for positive adaptation.

Unfortunately, the treatment advances of the past 25 years brought triumph and tragedy. In 1982, the first case of the acquired immune deficiency syndrome (AIDS) in a person with hemophilia was reported (Center for Disease Control, 1982).

# COMPLICATIONS OF THERAPY

Widespread use of factor VIII and factor IX concentrates prepared from very large donor pools has not been without complications. Three major kinds of problems have occurred.

## Development of Inhibitors of the Missing Coagulation Factor

Five to 15% of patients with hemophilia A who receive replacement therapy develop alloantibodies to factor VIII, called factor VIII inhibitors (or antibodies). Inhibitors form in response to "foreign" factor VIII and can result from infusion of any factor VIII-containing product, including plasma and cryoprecipitate. Less common are factor IX inhibitors, which occur in 2-3% of hemophilia B cases. An inhibitor neutralizes the activity of administered factor (i.e., prevents a rise in the level of factor and thus cancels the beneficial effect of the replaced factor on blood coagulation). In addition, most patients with an inhibitor respond to infusion of the missing factor by an anamnestic reaction (i.e., generation of even greater amounts of inhibitor).

Hemophilia patients with inhibitors do not bleed more frequently than those without, but the bleeding can no longer be controlled by supplying the missing factor. Special concentrates of "activated" coagulation factors are moderately helpful in controlling bleeding in many patients with inhibitors of factor VIII or factor IX. Factor VIII concentrate from pig plasma will be at least transiently effective in achieving hemostasis. Patients with inhibitors, despite treatment options, fare distinctly less well than those without. Newer treatment approaches to the inhibitor problem are under investigation. It is not known why the vast majority of hemophilia cases do not develop these antibodies as the result of replacement treatment.

## Viral Contamination of Concentrate Preparations

**Hepatitis B virus (HBV).** Eighty-five percent of hemophilia patients heavily treated before 1984 have antibody to the HBV, and 2-4% are chronic carriers as the result of having received concentrate contaminated with this virus. Currently, all potential donors are screened for presence of the HBV and blood from those who test positive is discarded. Also, since 1984, concentrates have been treated by heating or by other methods known to destroy or inactivate this agent. These efforts appear to have eradicated the HBV from concentrate preparations. In addition, vaccines against HBV have recently become available. All newly diagnosed hemophilia cases and those who do not have antibodies to HBV are routinely vaccinated.

**Non-A, non-B hepatitis (hepatitis C [HCV]).** HCV, also carried in the blood, is somewhat resistant to dry heat treatment and persists in some concentrates that are free of HBV or HIV contamination. A recently introduced test to detect HCV carriers in donors as well as novel virucidal techniques should help eradicate this virus from treatment products.

**Human immunodeficiency virus (HIV).** The most devastating and unexpected negative consequence of widespread concentrate usage was the discovery that these preparations could carry the HIV. Factor concentrates were widely contaminated with the virus between 1979-1984. Heat treatment, directed at killing the HBV, was begun in 1984. It was coincidentally found to have destroyed the HIV. Though all currently marketed concentrates are believed to be free of HIV, most persons with hemophilia who were heavily infused during 1979-1984 were exposed to the HIV. Ninety percent of severe hemophilia patients who are factor VIII deficient and 60% of factor IX deficient patients are HIV antibody positive.

Presently, the progression of HIV infection to AIDS appears to parallel at least roughly that of gay males and intravenous drug abusers. Whether some of the patients with hemophilia will escape this sequence is unknown. Feelings of uncertainty about the future have resurfaced and range from denial in some, to fear, anger, anxiety, and depression in others. Adolescents and young adults who have accepted hemophilia as a manageable, chronic disease compatible with a fairly normal, long life, now face uncertainty about their futures. Reticence, confusion, and a myriad of conflicting emotions concerning development of relationships with women are deeply troublesome for otherwise healthy young men. Patients who are HIV antibody positive fear becoming stigmatized, thereby encountering difficulties in several areas:

1. Employment

2. Health and life insurance

3. Educational opportunities

4. Meaningful personal relationships

As the public has become increasingly aware of "a connection" between hemophilia and AIDS, many persons with hemophilia (including some HIV antibody negative persons) have begun to withhold, from employers and potential employers, the fact that they have hemophilia. Some with obvious arthropathy claim some form of "arthritis" to account for their disability. Concealing the diagnosis from employers can have serious limitations in terms of long-term benefits. Rehabilitation counselors will need to assess carefully the unique and individual ways patients cope with hemophilia and their HIV antibody status.

Most comprehensive hemophilia treatment centers have expanded their total care of hemophilia to include management of those who are seropositive for HIV. Periodic evaluations include surveillance of the person's immune system, guidance to prevent spread of the virus to sexual partners, therapeutic intervention with antiviral therapy, and treatment of the medical complications if AIDS ensues. The traditional core of health care providers working closely with the comprehensive centers now includes experts in pulmonary, infectious disease, immunology, oncology, and other specialties.

## *Thrombosis*

Previously available factor IX concentrates are preparations contaminated with variable amounts of other coagulation factors dependent upon vitamin K for synthesis, besides factor IX. These include prothrombin (factor II), factor VII, and factor X. "Activation" of one (factor VII) or more of these factors can make the product more likely to produce unwanted blood clots, apart from supplying factor IX. Such thrombotic events usually occur to immobile patients who receive large doses. Newer, more "purified" factor IX products now available should eliminate this problem.

# FUNCTIONAL LIMITATIONS

The rehabilitation counselor can expect to encounter widely different degrees of functional limitations among clients with hemophilia. The extent of limitation usually correlates inversely with the individual's level of the deficient coagulation factor. Some older clients, or clients with severe disease who have not had the benefits of modern treatment, may have severe, generalized arthropathy. A few need to use wheelchairs for ambulation. Most younger men have minimal or no joint deformities. The ages in between younger and older, include men with a wide spectrum of limitations. Some men who were previously severely limited due to a deformed joint have had surgical correction of the deformity by insertion of an endo-prosthesis to restore function.

Individuals with hemophilia who grew up during this era of modern treatment have few vocational limitations. Counselors will need to surmount any residual notions that these clients necessarily require sedentary jobs, must be in protected environments, cannot perform manual labor jobs, and will frequently miss work because of disease. In reality, many individuals work successfully as longshoreworkers, housepainters, construction workers, waiters, warehouse workers, barbers, hairdressers, gasoline station attendants, and also in light and sedentary white collar and blue collar vocations. One needs to discourage persons with severe hemophilia, especially those who bleed more frequently, from jobs requiring maneuvers potentially traumatic to joints (e.g., repetitive clutch pedal operation in a man with chronic left knee arthropathy) and occupations clearly dangerous because of a particular person's deformity.

Because the person with hemophilia can normalize his coagulation mechanism within minutes, many potentially hazardous jobs offer little more risk than to other workers. Counselors need to plan vocational rehabilitation efforts according to the specific limitations of the particular client. In terms of environmental factors, there are no specific limitations.

## General Observations

**Intellectual functioning.** These persons have no inherent intellectual limitation. Some studies suggest higher than average intelligence (Taylor, 1976). Data collected during the 1960s and early 1970s showed a notable gap between scores on intelligence tests and achievement tests, the lower achievement attributable to disrupted school attendance. The average educational level attained was considerably less than by men in the general population. Within two decades following the advent and implementation of factor replacement and self-supervised treatment, several countries reported the achievement by people with hemophilia of an educational level at least equivalent to age-matched, unaffected men (Evensen et al., 1979; Stuart et al., 1980; Varekamp et al., 1989).

**Educational and vocational factors.** A recent report of educational and vocational achievement in Pennsylvania showed persons with hemophilia had attained statistically significant higher levels of education than the general male population in Pennsylvania. The study also revealed that significantly fewer individuals with hemophilia were employed. Most other similarly conducted research also shows these results. Failure of employment opportunities to increase to an extent expected by closure of the gap between intellectual capacity and educational achievement can be attributed to discriminatory hiring practices (Nimorwicz & Tannebaum, 1986).

These studies also indicated those employed tended not to be in positions commensurate with their level of education. These findings also suggested continued discrimination by employers. Several explanations for the Pennsylvania study data have been suggested. These include psychosocial dynamics of persons with hemophilia, negative incentives to work created by potential loss of federal assistance and medical coverage, and most important, continued ignorance and fear concerning hiring. The recently enacted 1990 Americans with Disabilities Act may change this situation.

Persons with hemophilia generally show vocational interests similar to the general male population. One study of men with hemophilia between the ages of 16-22 showed no difference in interests by the 19-Field Interest Inventory (Grobler, 1981). Another, using the Strong-Campbell Interest Inventory, demonstrated a slight preference for human service occupations (medicine, social work, and psychology) (Taylor, 1976). This latter finding may reflect an inclination for persons with hemophilia to identify with the professional people who have helped them.

**Psychosocial factors.** Psychosocial dynamics in men with hemophilia have provided focus for considerable investigation. As a group, these individuals display the same range of psychological variation present in non-affected persons. The Minnesota Multiphasic Personality Inventory showed, in two separate studies (Lohmann, Voges, Meuter, Rath, & Thomas, 1979; Taylor, 1976), no increase in major mental disturbances among men with hemophilia. A report which used the South African Personality Questionnaire concluded there were no statistically significant differences between persons with hemophilia and non-affected persons in measured aspects of personality (Grobler, 1981).

These and other observations suggest there seems to be no general personality pattern for persons who have hemophilia. Repeatedly, it is noted that men with hemophilia are optimistic and exhibit strong ego strength. Many of these men believe that coping with their disease has given them a "hardihood" they would not otherwise have developed. Despite these observations, the rehabilitation counselor needs to be aware of specific psychological limitations that sometimes appear (Jonas, 1977).

When a boy with hemophilia is born, the mother, because of the sex-linked mode of transmission of the disorder, often experiences feelings of guilt. Particularly in previous decades before the dramatic therapeutic advances of the past 30 years, the mother's feelings of personal responsibility for the boy's condition commonly led to severe emotional reactions affecting the entire family. On rare occasion, the mother reacted by deserting or rejecting the child.

More commonly, she developed extreme anxiety and a pronounced tendency toward overprotectiveness. Severe curtailment of the child's activities, coupled with excessive attention and indulgence, often leads to development of an overdependent, passive, frightened personality who has feelings of hopelessness, pessimism, and social isolation. By contrast, the boy may respond with denial and behavior leading to reckless, "dare-devil" activities, and pathological risk-taking.

Utilization of comprehensive hemophilia centers has provided the family with opportunities for early counseling, education, and the benefits of modern medical treatment. Better understanding of the disease and its therapy has helped to mitigate unhealthy parental concerns. A tendency toward excessive protectiveness still persists, as does the intense, often ambivalent, mother-son relationship.

As in many chronic illnesses, depression may surface in the young adult, resulting in overly pessimistic expectations about the course of the disease and the potential for future disability. This constellation of depression, pessimism, and pervasive uncertainty has become particularly prevalent in the young men who are HIV antibody positive. Unemployment often diminishes self-esteem and increases passivity, pessimism, and depression. The client's self-concept as "unemployable" may be a key reason for reluctance to seek a job or failure to present oneself in the best possible light. Feelings of despair often associated with "unemployability" may sometimes result in failure to obtain a job, thus leading to reinforcement of initial self-doubts. A psychological vicious cycle then follows.

Examination of the effects of unemployment in persons with hemophilia in Scotland disclosed the following. Those unable to find or maintain employment were less well adjusted, more depressed, and more dependent. They typically failed to plan for the future. Also, they experienced more psychological and psychosomatic symptoms than their employed counterparts (Markova, Lockyer, & Forbes, 1980; Stuart et al., 1980). If the rehabilitation counselor can help the client surmount reticence and negativism regarding employability, the client will be able to take a critical step forward.

## Specific Functional Limitations

Physical limitations vary with the individual. Arthropathy of the lower extremity weight bearing joints is most likely to be physically limiting. For some individuals, elbow or shoulder joint disease may pose the greatest limitation. The client and a member of the hemophilia center team can provide reliable information about which joints are disabling and in what manner. A knee with almost no range of motion due to severe arthropathy, but with only rare hemarthroses may be less disabling for many jobs than a right elbow with severe chronic synovitis and frequent bleeds, in a right-handed person.

## Vocational Limitations

Viewed as a group, persons with hemophilia have few vocational limitations. On an individual basis, the counselor may see a variety of limitations. The magnitude of the disease correlates closely with the presence of vocational limitations. Clients with severe hemophilia who are on self-supervised treatment are best able to cancel the effects of an accident on the job that causes a bleed. There is a strong correlation between successful self-management of the disease and the ability to function in the work place.

Most clients with mild and many clients with moderate disease have almost no vocational limitations. As previously discussed, the frequency of bleeding episodes varies greatly among persons with severe hemophilia, despite equivalent levels of factor VIII or factor IX. A characteristic feature of severe disease, especially among those who bleed more frequently, is **unpredictability**. Joint bleeds and hematomas often appear to be spontaneous. Therefore, persons with hemophilia may not always optimally perform certain jobs in which unbroken continuity of activity is essential. A 15-minute break is generally all the individual needs for adequate treatment of self-infusion, as long as there is a semi-private place on the job where he can do the procedure.

Repeated trauma to joints with chronic synovitis causes pain and may trigger hemarthrosis. Factor administration, even when given prophylactically, may not always prevent bleeding. Vocational limitations depend on the specific joints involved.

By contrast, clients with more advanced arthropathy usually have less frequent bleeding episodes but may have chronic arthritis of one or more joints similar to severe osteoarthritis. A sedentary vocation in which the client sits in one position most of the day can result in severe stiffness of affected joints. These individuals need to move about periodically throughout the day to prevent excessive joint stiffness and pain.

Some persons with hemophilia have residual deformities of joints or muscles that may cause specific vocational limitations. Others have limitations for certain vocations due to special circumstances that arose from indirect complications of the disorder or from complications of therapy. The rehabilitation counselor must evaluate the resultant vocational limitations individually. Members of the comprehensive hemophilia center team can be of great assistance in providing precise assessment of functional limitations.

Most persons with hemophilia can perform equal to their peers who do not have hemophilia in a variety of jobs and professions. Inaccurately perceived limitations by prospective employers because of lack of understanding of this disorder far outweigh actual functional limitations caused by the disorder.

# REHABILITATION POTENTIAL

The potential for rehabilitation of most individuals with hemophilia is excellent. Effective treatment of bleeding episodes, prevention or minimization of the disabling complications of joint bleeds, and the ability to correct deformities by surgery have greatly enhanced employability. Because of modern treatment modalities, many persons who have hemophilia have completed high school; many have additional education.

Some clients developed irreparable deformities before the advent of modern medical therapy and others did not receive adequate medical treatment. Appropriate medical treatment can delay further progression of existing disabilities and help prevent additional complications. The rehabilitation counselor may consider the initial status upon first seeing the client as relatively stable and work with the client toward selecting a vocation in which the disability will not adversely affect functioning on the job.

For clients who bleed frequently, the opportunity to self- infuse at the worksite effectively reduces morbidity and loss of work time. The ability to store concentrate and necessary accessories (needles, syringes, and gauze pads) is very important. Many clients will infuse secretly to disguise their underlying condition. The HIV problems discussed above have enhanced many clients' inclination toward secrecy about their hemophilia. Because the public has "made a connection" between hemophilia and AIDS, even clients who are HIV antibody negative may conceal their hemophilia.

Some employers have a first aid room where an individual can self-infuse at the worksite. Company (industrial) physicians and nurses should be encouraged to avail themselves of the local hemophilia center's assistance and guidance. Rehabilitation counselors can help educate employers by providing current information on modern medical treatment of this disease.

Persons with hemophilia can self-infuse in their offices or in the restroom. Some will self-infuse at a nearby gasoline station or restaurant to conceal their hemophilia. Perhaps we will begin to see a change of this type of behavior with implementation of the 1990 Americans with Disabilities Act.

Although physicians recommend availability of locations at the work site for treatment of bleeds when indicated, systematically collected data reflect a remarkably infrequent need for such treatment. One well designed study from the United Kingdom includes 368 successfully employed individuals (Stuart et al., 1980). Most of these men had moderately severe to severe hemophilia. Ninety percent of this sample reported satisfaction with their employment and had not requested any special considerations.

Despite this, 25% felt their job was somewhat unsuitable for a person with hemophilia because of heavy physical work and risk of cuts and bruises. When the researchers evaluated frequency and cause of bleeding, the data showed most incidents precipitating bleeding were impact injuries totally unrelated to job-related heavy work or operation of dangerous machinery. Instead, injuries in the work place were usually due to accidents, such as falls or bumping into furniture or doors, circumstances not directly related to the work itself.

Persons with hemophilia frequently learn to compensate for their limitations and, therefore, often have fewer injuries than other individuals having similar jobs. Employers need awareness that, in the above-mentioned studies, persons with hemophilia had on the average less than one bleed a month at work. Also, only a small minority of these episodes occurred because of travel to or from work.

Seventy-five percent of employees studied had less than one bleed a month while at work. Within a year's time, 70% reported no bleeds at work requiring urgent treatment. Seventy-six percent of approximately 400 clients remained in the same job for more than 3 years. Other studies described similar successful work performance by persons with hemophilia (Evensen et al., 1979; Markova et al., 1980; Marshall, 1977; Nimorwicz & Tannebaum, 1986; Stuart, 1980; Varekamp et al., 1989).

In some respects, people with hemophilia may be optimal clients for vocational rehabilitation because, although there is presently no cure, the disease itself is not fatal and can be effectively controlled. If unexpected deterioration of joint status or other unforeseen medical factors alter the client's physical abilities, he may again become a candidate for vocational guidance and rehabilitation.

Many of the current generation of persons with hemophilia will have far greater vocational difficulties because of HIV-related health problems than from hemophilia. There is also the problem of societal and employer discrimination against persons with hemophilia, further complicated by the AIDS epidemic.

The rehabilitation counselor needs to be knowledgeable in the modern methods of hemophilia treatment. Most employers are unfamiliar with recent medical advances that allows persons with hemophilia to live near-normal lives. Self-supervised infusion, although commonplace, is not understood by most employers. The counselor will need to educate employers in this and other areas of treatment to maximize potential employment opportunities for these clients.

# CASE STUDY

Joseph Hanson is 18 years of age, single, and living with his parents in a small Midwestern town. He recently graduated from high school, receiving average grades throughout his educational experience.

Described as a "loner," Joseph has one or two close friends and avoids large gatherings and most social events. Besides having hemophilia, Joseph is in good health and has no major complications of the disease. Occasionally, he will need to self-infuse, but has no problem doing this.

You have been assigned as his rehabilitation counselor. For the initial interview, his mother accompanied him and insisted on sitting in on the interview. Although she provided useful information, she did most of the talking and stated she would attend all future appointments, as it is her opinion that, by attending these meetings, it will be in her son's best interest.

Joseph was hesitant about discussing his interests, although her appeared to enjoy repairing the family cars and doing minor mechanical and electrical repairs around the home. His mother was of the opinion these activities were potentially dangerous and need to be avoided. She believes Joseph should attend the local community college and pursue a career in accounting, as her husband is an accountant. Joseph could "follow in his father's footsteps," in her opinion. Also, she believes Joseph should do sedentary work, needs to be in a protected environment, should not perform manual jobs, and may need time off work because of occasional "bleeds."

Joseph was of the opinion that this goal would be "O.K." as he did not have any other ideas as to what to pursue. His mother insisted he be enrolled in the accounting program next week as the next semester was starting in 6 weeks.

## *Questions*

1. Discuss hemophilia in terms of Ms. Hanson's opinion that Joseph needs to do sedentary work, stay away from manual jobs, be in a protected work environment, and will need time off for occasional bleeding episodes.

2. How will you deal with Ms. Hanson's insistence on sitting in on all counseling appointments and her desire to have Joseph immediately enroll at the community college?

3. How will you proceed with vocational rehabilitation services?

4. Explain self-infusion and other aspects of hemophilia as if you were speaking to a potential employer.

5. If Joseph were to marry, what are the chances of any male offspring having hemophilia and a female child being a carrier? Discuss this both from the standpoint of his marrying a "non-carrier" woman and a woman that "carries" the hemophilia trait.

6. As Joseph gets older, will he have a tendency to develop limited range of motion in some of his joints? Discuss.

7. Joseph is HIV antibody negative. How and when will you discuss this and the fact that he has hemophilia with a potential employer? The employer will ask if Joseph is at risk to become HIV positive from his factor concentrate.

## REFERENCES

Aronson, D.L. (1988). Cause of death in hemophilia A patients in the United States from 1968 to 1979. **American Journal of Hematology, 27,** 7-12.

Dietrich, S. L. (1991). **Comprehensive care for people with hemophilia.** New York, NY: National Hemophilia Foundation.

Etzel, F. (1981). The cost of haemophilia treatment and the cost of the lack of treatment. **Haemostasis, 10**(Suppl. 1), 65-68.

Evensen, S.A., Thaule, R., & Gran, K. (1979). Self-therapy for haemophilia in Norway. **Acta Medica Scandinavica, 205**, 395-399.

Gill, J.C., Thometz, J., Scott, J.P., & Montgomery, R.R. (1989). Musculoskeletal problems in hemophilia. In M.W. Hilgartner & C. Pochedly (Eds.), **Hemophilia in the child and adult** (3rd. ed., pp. 28-30). New York, NY: Raven Press.

Grobler, T. (1981). Personality, self-concept and vocational interest of a group of adolescent haemophiliacs. **Haemostasis, 10**(Suppl. 1), 259-261.

Ikkala, E., Helske, T., Myllylä, G., Nevanlinna, H.R., Pitkänen, P, & Rasi, V. (1982). Changes in the life expectancy of patients with severe haemophilia A in Finland in 1930-79. **British Journal of Haematology, 53**, 7-12.

Jonas, D.L. (1977). Psychiatric aspects of hemophilia. **Mount Sinai Journal of Medicine, 44**(3), 457-463.

Kasper, C.K., & Dietrich, S.L. (1985). Comprehensive management of haemophilia. **Clinics in Haematology, 14**(2), 489-512.

Larsson, S.A. (1985). Life expectancy of Swedish haemophiliacs, 1831-1980. **British Journal of Haematology, 59**, 593-602.

Logan, L.J. (1988a). Hemostasis and bleeding disorders. In J.J. Mazza (Ed.), **Manual of clinical hematology** (pp. 288- 294). Boston, MA: Little, Brown.

Logan, L.J. (1988b). Pre and post operative aspects of endoprosthesis in hemophilia. In E.P. Mauser-Bunschoten & P.J. Van Duke (Eds.), **IIIrd van Creveld Symposium on Hemophilia** (pp. 37-43). The Netherlands: Bilthoven.

Lohmann, R, Voges, B., Meuter, F., Rath, K.U., & Thomas, W. (1979). Psychopathology and psychotherapy in chronic physically ill patients. **Proceedings of the 4th Congressional International College of Psychosomatic Medicine, 31**, 267-276.

Luck, J.V. (1988). Surgical management of advanced hemophilic arthropathy. In E.P. Mauser & P.J. van Duke (Eds.), **IIIrd van Crevald Symposium on Hemophilia** (pp. 21-36). The Netherlands: Bilthoven.

Markova, I., Lockyer, R., & Forbes, C. (1980). Self-perception of employed and unemployed haemophiliacs. **Psychological Medicine, 10**, 559-565.

Marshall, F.N. (1977). Vocational rehabilitation and the hemophiliac. **The Mount Sinai Journal of Medicine, 44**(3), 464-469.

Nimorwicz, P., & Tannebaum, J. (1986). Educational and vocational achievement among hemophiliacs: The Pennsylvania experience. **Journal of Chronic Diseases, 39**(9), 743-750.

Ogston, D. (1984). **Antifibrinolytic drugs**. New York: John Wiley & Sons, Ltd.

Pool, J.G., Hershgold, E.J., & Pappenhagen, A.R. (1964). High potency anti-haemophilic factor concentrate prepared from cryo-globulin precipitate. **Nature, 203**, 312.

Rizza, C.R., & Spooner, R.J.D. (1983). Treatment of haemophilia and related disorders in Britain and Northern Ireland during 1976-80: Report on behalf of the directors of haemophilia centres in the United Kingdom. **British Medical Journal, 286**, 929-933.

Rosendaal, F.R., Smith, C., Varekamp, I., Bröcker-Vriends, A.H.J.T., van Dijck, H., Suurmeijer, T.P.B.M., Vandenbroucke, J.P., & Briët, E. (1990). Modern hemophilia treatment: Medical improvements and the quality of life. **Journal of Internal Medicine, 228**(6), 633-640.

Rosendaal, F.R., Varekamp, I., Smit, C., Bröcker-Vriends, A.H.J.T., van Dijck, H., Vandenbroucke, J.P., Hermans, J., Suurmeijer, T.P.B.M., & Briët, E. (1989). Mortality and causes of death in Dutch haemophiliacs, 1973-86. **British Journal of Haematology, 71,** 71-76.

Schimpf, K., & Niederberger, M. (1981). Cost effectiveness in treatment of severe hemophilia. **Haemostasis, 10**(Suppl. 1), 185-187.

Smith, C., Rosendaal, F.R, Varekamp, I., Bröcker-Vriends, A., Van Kijek, H., Suurmeijer, Th.P.B.M., & Briët, E. (1989). Physical condition, longevity, and social performance of Dutch haemophiliacs, 1972-85. **British Medical Journal, 298,** 235-238.

Smith, P.S., Keyes, N.C., & Forman, E.N. (1982). Socioeconomic evaluation of a state-funded comprehensive hemophilia-care program. **New England Journal of Medicine, 306**(10), 575- 579.

Stuart, J., Forbes, C.D., Jones, P., Lane, G., Rizza, C.R., & Wilkes, S. (1980). Improving prospects for employment of the haemophiliac. **British Medical Journal, 280,** 1169-1172.

Taylor, C. (1976). Rehabilitation counseling. In D.C. Boone (Ed.), **Comprehensive management of hemophilia** (pp. 128-130). Philadelphia, PA: F.A. Davis.

Varekamp, I., Smit, C., Rosendaal, F.R., Bröcker-Vriends, A., Briët, E., van Duck, H., & Suurmeijer, T.P.B.M. (1989). Employment of individuals with haemophilia in the Netherlands. **Social Science Medicine, 28**(3), 261-270.

Wincott, E. (1977). Psychosocial aspects of hemophilia: Problems, prevention, treatment modalities, research, and future directions. **Mount Sinai Journal of Medicine, 44**(3), 438-455.

## About the Author

Laurence J. Logan, M.D., F.A.C.P., is an Associate Clinical Professor of Medicine in the Section of Hematology, University of Southern California School of Medicine in Los Angeles, California. He has been co-director of the Hemophilia Center at Orthopaedic Hospital in Los Angeles and is currently co-director of the Huntington Hospital Hemophilia Center in Pasadena, California.

# Chapter 18

# SICKLE CELL DISEASE

by
*Cage S. Johnson, M.D.*
*and*
*Robert B. Francis, Jr., M.D.*

## INTRODUCTION

Sickle cell disease is a multisystem disorder in which the abnormal shape and physical characteristics of the red blood cell (rbc) cause secondary manifestations throughout the body as a result of intermittent microvascular obstruction, ischemia (reduced blood flow), and infarction (cell death). Nearly any body system may be affected by the disease process leading to a wide variety of single or combination disabilities. Sickle cell disease gets its name from the half-moon (crescent) shape that the sickle rbc assumes in the circulation. For the rehabilitation counselor, some knowledge of the disease process is essential for adequate evaluation of the rehabilitation potential for persons with sickle cell disease. A brief description of the structure and function of both the normal and sickle hemoglobin (Hb) molecules and their respective rbc follows (Johnson, 1981; Serjeant, 1985; Williams, Beutler, Erslev, & Lichtman, 1990).

## HEMATOLOGY

### The Red Blood Cell (RBC)

The purpose of the red blood cell (rbc) is the uptake of oxygen in the lungs and the release of that oxygen in the tissues. As the rbc passes through the lungs, oxygen binds to the Hb molecule. In the tissues, oxygen is exchanged for carbon dioxide, which is carried back to the lungs by the hemoglobin (Hb). The individual exhales carbon dioxide and inhales fresh oxygen.

There are two special characteristics of the rbc involved in this process. One is that the rbc is very pliable and hence can squeeze through the terminal capillaries of the blood vessels. These terminal capillaries are the link between the arteries and the veins and form an extensive network throughout each organ in the body so that nutrients and waste products can easily diffuse from the cells into the bloodstream.

The second characteristic is that the rbc has a biconcave (round) shape that allows gases to pass easily into the rbc at the lung capillaries. Figure 1 is a scanning electron microphotograph of normal disk-shaped rbcs (magnified x 6,000). Inside these cells are the millions of hemoglobin molecules. The bone marrow produces the rbcs; these blood cells remain in circulation for 120 days. The bone marrow constantly makes new rbcs to replace old ones. Each day, the body destroys about 1% of the total rbcs that are replaced by an equal number of new cells (Williams et al., 1990).

## Figure 1
## NORMAL RED BLOOD CELL

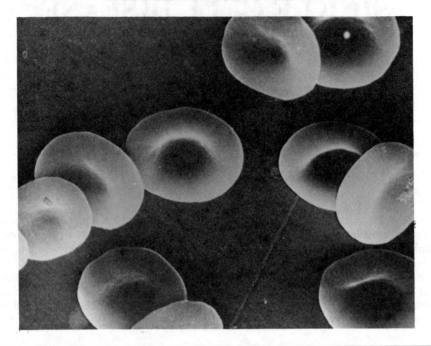

Courtesy of Richard F. Baker, Ph.D., University of Southern California School of Medicine, Los Angeles, California.

### The Three Types of Hemoglobin

Inside each rbc are millions of molecules of Hb. Four protein chains called globin and four iron-binding molecules called protoporphyrin make up each Hb molecule. The protoporphyrin-iron complex is called heme, and the molecule is identified by the term hemoglobin. The globin chains stabilize and solubilize the heme and facilitate oxygen binding and release in the lungs and tissues. Each globin chain wraps tightly around a heme, forming the "pocket" that protects the heme from destruction by the oxygen. When Hb picks up oxygen, the heme pockets open slightly and the oxygen molecules enter. After the blood releases oxygen at the tissue level, the heme pockets close. When rbcs are destroyed, the globins break down into their individual amino acids and are used again. The remaining iron recycles to make new Hb. The protoporphyrin does not recycle, but breaks down into bilirubin, and the liver excretes it into the gut as part of the bile.

There are three types of **normal** hemoglobin, each made up of different combinations of the four normal globin chains ($\alpha$, $\beta$, $\gamma$ and $\delta$ globins). Ninety-six percent of the normal hemoglobin composition is HbA (two $\alpha$ and two $\beta$ chains). Of the remaining hemoglobin, 3% is type $A_2$ (two $\alpha$ and two $\delta$ globins) and 1% is type F or fetal hemoglobin (two $\alpha$ and two $\gamma$ globins). When a person is 3 months of age, beta chain production replaces gamma chain production, so that Hb A gradually replaces Hb F (Williams et al., 1990).

Our parents pass on certain features to us; the unit that determines which physical features we inherit is called the gene. Genes are contained within the chromosomes. An individual inherits one chromosome from the mother and one from the father. The genes for alpha chains that help make up hemoglobin are on one pair of chromosomes, while the beta, gamma, and delta chain genes are on another pair of chromosomes. Therefore, each chromosome in a pair controls half the total globin chain production. Each globin chain gene guides the rbc to make a specific globin chain; the globin chains match with a heme and then assemble into a complete Hb molecule.

# ETIOLOGY

## *Sickle Cell Disease and Abnormal Hemoglobin*

There are various types of hemoglobin. Sickle cell disease is a genetic disorder in which a mutation in the gene for a globin chain leads to production of an abnormal hemoglobin that alters the structure or function of the red blood cell. Most cases of sickle cell disease occur among people of African and Mediterranean ancestry. About 8% of Black persons in this country carry one abnormal beta globin gene for Hb S (sickle cell trait), about 2% carry one abnormal beta globin gene for Hb C, and another 2% carry one abnormal gene for beta thalassemia. About 1 in every 500 Black children has inherited two abnormal beta globin genes and has a sickle cell disease. Considerable scientific evidence indicates that these abnormal Hb genes arose in African, the Mediterranean area, and some Southeast Asian countries as partial protection against malaria.

## *Sickle Cells and Obstruction of Blood Flow*

As previously mentioned, sickle cell disease is named for the characteristic half-moon (crescent) shape that rbcs containing Hb S develop when the cells release oxygen. On deoxygenation, the presence of valine (Hb S) instead of glutamic acid allows adjacent Hb molecules to bind to each other. As additional binding occurs, a tubular crystal is formed as seen in Figure 2. In this transmission electron microphotograph (magnified x43,000) of a section through a sickled cell, the tubular crystals are seen across the length of the cell. The presence of hemoglobin S in the rbcs allows the formation of tubular crystals. These tubular crystals distort the cell into the characteristic sickled shape, as seen in Figure 3.

Compare the appearance of this cell with Figure 1. This scanning electron microphotograph (magnified x 4,000) shows cells from a person with sickle cell anemia which have been deoxygenated. The cell shows the classical "sickled" shape for which the disease was named. Because of the result of the "sickle-unsickle" cycle, the red cell membrane becomes damaged, leading to the consequences of sickle cell disease. When the cell is reoxygenated, the Hb S crystals disperse and the cell returns to the biconcave (round) shape.

After several cycles of crystal formation and dissolution, the rbc becomes permanently sickled and much more rigid than the normal rbc. One calls this rigid, fragile cell the irreversibly sickled cell. The fragile, irreversibly sickled cell is destroyed easily as it passes through the blood vessels, shortening its lifespan to 15 days, rather than the normal 120 days. Bone marrow production of rbcs increases to keep up with the rate of destruction. Even at maximum output, the marrow is unable to manufacture enough cells to maintain a normal Hb level and a severe anemia (hemolytic anemia) occurs (Williams et al., 1990).

These rigid irreversibly sickled cells can become wedged in a capillary and obstruct blood flow, a condition called ischemia (Stuart & Johnson, 1987). Consequences of this vascular occlusion include pain from lack of oxygen, cell necrosis (infarction), and healing by scar tissue formation (fibrosis). The size of the obstructed vascular area and the amount and duration of the ischemia determine the degree of pain or organ damage. Although vascular occlusion can affect any of the body organs, certain vascular beds are particularly susceptible; these include the bone marrow,

# Figure 2
## SICKLED CELL

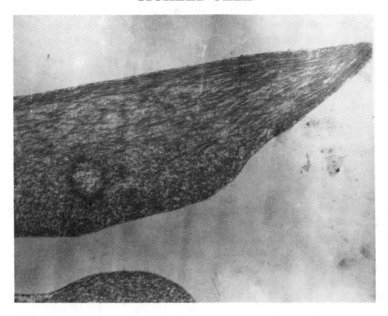

Courtesy of Richard F. Baker, Ph.D., University of Southern California School of Medicine, Los Angeles, California.

# Figure 3
## DEOXYGENATED SICKLED CELL

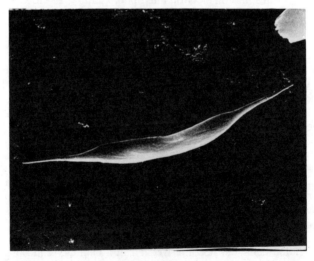

Courtesy of Richard F. Baker, Ph.D., Unversity of Southern California School of Medicine, Los Angeles, California.

spleen, lung, kidney, and bones. One calls these episodes of vascular obstruction sickle cell crises when they produce acute symptoms. The factors that precipitate "crises" are not completely understood, but infection, dehydration, or exposure to extremes of temperature appear to play a role, as may mental or physical stress.

# TYPES OF SICKLE CELL DISEASE

There are three major types of sickle cell disease. In sickle cell anemia (1), the person inherits the Hb S gene from both parents. Hemoglobinopathy SC (2) describes the inheritance of the gene for Hb S from one parent and the gene for Hb C from the other parent. The sickle thalassemias (3) involve the inheritance of one gene for Hb S and one gene for beta thalassemia from each parent (Table 1). Other abnormal Hbs can be inherited with Hb S and cause disease but are infrequent. Table 1 summarizes the hemoglobin compositions in the three main types of sickle cell disease, in sickle cell trait, and in normal persons.

## Table 1
### HEMOGLOBIN COMPOSITION IN VARIOUS CONDITIONS

| Condition | Hb A | Hb A$_2$ | Hb F | Hb S | Hb C |
|---|---|---|---|---|---|
| Normal | 96% | 3% | < 2% | — | — |
| Sickle cell anemia | — | 3% | 2-15% | 80-95% | — |
| Hemoglobinopathy SC | — | — | 2% | 49% | 49% |
| Sickle $\beta^0$ thalassemia, (severe type) | — | 5% | 5-20% | 70-85% | — |
| Sickle $\beta^+$ thalassemia, (mild type) | 10-30% | 5% | 5-20% | 50-70% | — |
| Sickle cell trait | 58% | 3% | 1% | 38% | — |

## Sickle Cell Anemia (SCA)

The most common and most severe form of sickle cell disease is SCA (Serjeant, 1985). Hemolytic anemia is present in an individual by the age of 6 months, although vascular occlusion symptoms may not appear until 1 year of age. Persons with SCA have severe anemia. They have frequent painful crises during childhood, and loss of function of the spleen (an organ with multiple blood-cleaning functions) predisposes them to severe infections. Until recently, bacterial infections were the most common cause of death in children. Now, prophylactic treatment with penicillin has nearly eradicated this problem (Gaston et al., 1986). During the adolescent years, there is often a lessening in the occurrences of crises, as viral infections decline and as these individuals learn to avoid other precipitating factors.

Children with sickle cell anemia frequently have delayed growth. They also have a delay in the growth spurt and in puberty. About half of the persons with SCA are tall and thin with abnormally long limbs. Delayed growth and sexual maturation appear to be related to nutritional factors, although the exact mechanism is still not clear. Researchers have not determined a specific treatment for this (Wethers, 1989).

As adults, there is wide variation in disease manifestations and severity. Approximately 10% of individuals have extremely benign disease, whereas only 25% have a severe form with frequent hospitalizations for pain control. Most persons have symptoms requiring hospitalization only once a year or less (Platt et al., 1991). The long-term effects of recurrent vascular occlusion, ischemia, infarction, and fibrosis may cause one or more types of chronic organ damage, and management of organ complications may become a major issue. The most common causes of death in these individuals are infections, stroke, lung disease, and chronic renal failure. Many people with this condition now survive into middle age and beyond, as the result of advanced technology and modern medical treatment. For any particular individual with this disease, one cannot predict with certainty the ultimate prognosis (Murthy & Haywood, 1981).

## Hemoglobinopathy SC

In hemoglobinopathy SC, Hb S and Hb C each make up half the hemoglobin (Hb) within the red blood cell. In this type of anemia, the person inherits hemoglobin S from one parent and hemoglobin C from the other parent. Hemoglobinopathy SC is not as common as SCA (about one-third less common). By the time an infant is 6 months old, hemolytic anemia will be evident; vaso-occlusive symptoms often will become evident in early adulthood. The anemia is less severe than that of SCA. Crises and infections are less frequent than in SCA, although occasional patients have severe disease. Bone disease (aseptic necrosis) and retinal vessel involvement (sickle retinopathy) are more common than in SCA, whereas other types of organ damage are less common (Sergeant, 1985, Williams et al., 1990).

## Sickle Thalassemia

Sickle thalassemia results when an individual inherits the genes for both Hb S and beta thalassemia. In the severe form of thalassemia, there is a complete suppression of beta globin production so that virtually all of the Hb is Hb S. Persons with the mild form of thalassemia produce some Hb A, as there is only a partial suppression of beta chain production. The severe form of sickle thalassemia is similar to sickle cell anemia in its blood chemistry, onset, course, and prognosis. The mild form of sickle thalassemia has minimal to moderate anemia. Its onset, course, and prognosis is similar to that of hemoglobinopathy SC (Serjeant 1985, Williams et al., 1990).

## Sickle Cell Trait

There is no disease associated with sickle cell trait. Those people with sickle cell trait have received one gene for Hb S from one parent and one for Hb A from the other parent. Since Hb A is somewhat more stable than Hb S, more than half the Hb is A, and Hb S is less than half. Although the rbcs of these individuals do not normally sickle, they can be induced to do so in the laboratory under extreme deoxygenation. The presence of hemoglobin A protects these individuals. Therefore, the rbc survival is normal, and there is no anemia. These individuals do not have crises, frequent infections, nor chronic organ damage.

Despite the lack of evidence for any complications related to sickle cell trait, there is some concern about the risk of extreme hypoxia (deficiency of oxygen) in certain environments for those with Hb S trait. Consequently, in the past, employers have denied individuals with sickle cell trait participation in high-altitude aviation and deep-sea diving occupations. The evidence justifying such policies is circumstantial at best. The most convincing evidence, based on large population studies and on controlled experimental observations, fails to support any restriction on occupational goals for individuals with sickle cell trait (McKenzie, 1982). This knowledge is important for vocational rehabilitation planning.

# SPECIFIC COMPLICATIONS OF SICKLE CELL DISEASE

Sickle cell crises, chronic hemolytic anemia, recurrent infections, acute and chronic organ damage, lower extremity ulceration, bone disease, and chronic central nervous system damage are complications of sickle cell disease. Persons with sickle cell anemia are affected by these complications more often and with greater severity than those with either hemoglobinopathy SC or sickle thalassemia. Yet, some persons with SCA have rare crises and function very well (Diggs, 1965; Sergeant, 1985).

## Sickle Cell Crises

There are four types of sickle cell crises. These are (1) vaso-occlusive, (2) aplastic, (3) splenic sequestration, and (4) hyperhemolytic. The most common is the vaso-occlusive ("painful") crisis. Vaso-occlusive crisis (1) has a sudden onset, usually lasts 5 to 6 days, and may be localized in one area of the body or generalized. The pain is deep and has an aching quality. A precipitating event is not always identified, but infections, dehydration, and exposure to cold or wet conditions can precipitate a crisis. While these crises cause substantial pain, they do not cause death unless accompanied by other complications.

Worsening anemia characterizes the three other kinds of crises. In the aplastic crisis (2), there is a temporary suppression of the rbc precursor cells in the marrow, usually by a viral infection. Splenic sequestration crisis (3) is characterized by a bacterial infection that causes the spleen to enlarge rapidly, trapping rbcs and preventing them from reentering the bloodstream. Hyperhemolytic crisis (4) occurs due to infections, certain drugs or toxins, and results in an acute worsening of the chronic hemolytic (the breaking down of red blood cells) anemia. In these types of crises, hemoglobin levels fall faster than the bone marrow can manufacture red blood cells, and the anemia becomes life-threatening. The person may require blood transfusion. Aplastic, splenic sequestration, and hyperhemolytic crises are common only in SCA.

## Chronic Hemolytic Anemia

Anemia is more severe in sickle cell anemia than in the other forms of the disease because in SCA, the rbcs are destroyed more rapidly. Due to the need for increased rbc production, the bone marrow space enlarges to accommodate the increase in rbc production; consequently, the bones become thinner. Reshaping of bone by this process may produce prognathism (obvious jaw protrusion) and other bony deformities. As these deformities of bone may produce malocclusion of the teeth with accompanying tooth and gum disease, proper dental management is important in the rehabilitation of these persons.

The rapid rbc destruction produces large amounts of bilirubin. This may produce jaundice and the individual may have a yellow color in the eyes and skin. Gallstones may form in the gallbladder. Nearly all patients will eventually develop gallstones; some will need surgical removal of the gallbladder. Anemia will cause the heart to pump harder and faster than normal to deliver adequate amounts of oxygen to the tissues. The increased workload on the heart and lungs causes fatigability, exertional dyspnea (difficult breathing on exertion), and dizziness or a feeling of disorientation. There will also be a tendency to have a decreased tolerance for physical activity.

## Recurrent Infections

A major cause of morbidity (illness) and mortality (death) in sickle cell disease, especially in children, is bacterial infection. The frequency of these infections is many times that of the normal population. Although physicians do not understand the exact reasons for the increased susceptibility to infection, one factor is the damage to the spleen caused by sickled cells.

As persons with sickle cell disease age, ongoing exposure to bacteria and viruses allows the development of natural antibodies, which can help contain infections. Septicemia (infection in the blood) and meningitis (infection of the membranes of the spinal cord or brain) are life-threatening infections that commonly occur in sickle cell disease. Prophylactic treatment with penicillin has substantially reduced the risks of these infections and markedly improved childhood mortality (Gaston et al., 1986). After the age of 10, the occurrence of septicemia and meningitis declines, but high incidences of localized infections, such as pneumonia, pyelonephritis, and osteomyelitis, persist (Serjeant, 1985, Williams et al., 1990).

## Chronic Kidney Disease

Infarcts (tissue necrosis) due to sickling occur in the kidneys of adults with SCA; this leads to renal dysfunction. Multiple infarcts and frequent infections involving the kidneys lead to progressive uremia, and the need for kidney dialysis may occur. One particular aspect of the renal lesion in sickle cell disease is loss of the ability to conserve water; this complication is nearly universal, so that persons with any one of the sickling diseases need to continuously drink large amounts of fluid to prevent dehydration and its exacerbation of sickling. The rehabilitation counselor must note the importance of the client having free access to water at the workplace. Pyelonephritis (bacterial infection) is common in all forms of sickle cell disease.

## Acute and Chronic Lung Disease

Pulmonary complications occur frequently in people with sickle cell disease. The most common lung complication is pneumonia. Many people with sickle cell disease require hospitalization for this complication. Despite adequate antibiotic therapy, the pneumonia typically takes 10-14 days to resolve. Obstruction of pulmonary blood vessels by sickled cells may result in pulmonary infarction. Frequent pulmonary insults result in scarring of the lungs, which impairs gas exchange. Pulmonary insufficiency and pulmonary hypertension can occur. The reduced pulmonary function tends to exacerbate the sickling process.

## Chronic Eye Disease

Individuals with hemoglobinopathy SC or sickle thalassemia may have sickle cell retinopathy; it is less common in people with SCA. An infarction of the retina stimulates new blood vessel growth into the vitreous cavity of the eye, similar to the neovascularization that occurs in diabetes mellitus. These abnormal vessels bleed or cause retinal detachment, resulting in diminished vision.

## Lower Extremity Ulceration

During adulthood, leg ulcers are common in those with sickle cell anemia, but less common in hemoglobinopathy SC and sickle thalassemia. Due to infarcts in the skin around the ankles, these ulcers gradually become larger and are difficult to heal. Prolonged standing in one position makes these ulcers worse. The wearing of fitted elastic stockings may decrease recurrences of leg ulcers.

## Acute and Chronic Bone Disease

Vaso-occlusion of the bones and joints may lead to severe physical limitations. Bone infarcts (aseptic necrosis) in the lower extremities and the vertebrae of the spinal cord can precipitate fragmentation and collapse of the involved bone and degenerative osteoarthritis in older individuals. This condition can result in severe limitations of function (Johnson, 1981).

Acute arthritis may occur due to infarcts in a joint capsule. This condition is characterized by redness, swelling, and intense pain around the affected joint. Further, since infarcted bone is an excellent culture medium for supporting bacterial growth, osteomyelitis (infection of a bone), or pyoarthrosis (infection of a joint) is a frequent complication of sickle cell disease.

## Chronic Heart Disease

Because of the anemia, cardiomegaly (an enlarged heart) and heart murmurs are typical for the person with sickle cell disease. The cardiac output is higher than normal, as expected for the degree of anemia. Occasionally, individuals have non-related congenital valvular heart disease and other forms of heart disease. It is unknown whether sickling causes any direct cardiac dysfunction.

## Chronic Central Nervous System Damage

If an individual contracts meningitis, it must be promptly treated as permanent central nervous system damage can result. Occlusion of the intracerebral arteries results in thrombosis and cerebral vascular accident (stroke); cerebral hemorrhage can occur.

# FUNCTIONAL LIMITATIONS

This section discusses both the physical and psychological functional limitations for persons with sickle cell disease. Social and vocational limitations also are described.

## Physical Limitations

Physical limitations are present primarily in the areas of fatigue and weakness associated with anemia or with sickle cell crises (Sinnette & Gillman, 1974). The average occurrence of these events is 1-2 a year, although there is great individual variation. Not all episodes are severe enough to require hospitalization. The crisis usually resolves within a week. Yet, there may be an additional period of 5-10 days where the individual may have some residual symptoms. Some persons can maintain work activity throughout sickle cell crises; others need to take time off work. For individuals needing time off work, this varies from 1 day to several days and, sometimes, 1 or 2 weeks. This is dependent not only on the individual, but also on the exertional level of work activity. This is one reason it is important to consider the exertional level of work activity when providing vocational rehabilitation (Farber, Koshy, Kinney, & the Cooperative Study of Sickle Cell Disease, 1985).

Persons with sedentary or light work are able to continue working through the sickle cell crises more often than persons who have more physically demanding jobs. When providing vocational rehabilitation for individuals who are changing jobs or are entering the labor force for the first time, the counselor needs to consider this carefully with the client that has occasional sickle cell crises.

Chronic hemolytic anemia, a deficiency of red blood cells, causes increased fatigue and loss of strength. This is the reason most persons with sickle cell disease need to avoid work that is heavier than the medium level of exertion;

many will be limited to a maximum of sedentary or light work activity. Keeping in mind that additional complications may occur as the individual ages, a maximum of medium work is typically advisable.

## Environmental Factors

There are some environmental conditions that may exacerbate symptoms. One should avoid conditions of extreme cold or intense heat. Jobs involving exposure to cold and damp conditions need to be avoided; these environmental factors precipitate sickling of the red blood cells. Exposure to employment environments with noxious fumes, high levels of dust, or poor ventilation may not be tolerated well by these individuals, especially those with a history of pulmonary problems.

Such situations may aggravate the risk of pulmonary infections because of irritation of lung tissue, and could cause hypoxia (deficiency of oxygen). Hot and humid conditions add stress on the heart and may precipitate dehydration if the individual does not consume sufficient amounts of water. On all jobs, it is important for persons with sickle cell disease to have easy availability to water or other fluids to prevent the possibility of dehydration. Physicians advise persons with sickle cell disease to remember to drink water as much as possible throughout the day.

## Psychological Factors

Sickle cell disease is a chronic condition that requires careful attention throughout an individual's lifetime. Emotional stress can exacerbate symptoms and make management of the overall disease more difficult.

The disease itself, with its inherent uncertainty, causes emotional upheaval. An inability to predict or control symptoms can lead to heightened anxiety and increased frustration. Recurrent painful episodes of sickle cell crises add to the emotional lability of the condition. These episodes can occur spontaneously or be provoked by infection, dehydration, or hypoxia. Understandably, emotional difficulties are common in persons with sickle cell disease.

These factors may contribute to poor self-esteem, depression, and anxiety. Self-concept and self-image are formed early in childhood; with recurrent episodes of sickle cell crises and repeated hospitalizations, children with sickle cell disease often develop dependent personalities and passive-aggressive characteristics (Falvo, 1991; Kumar, Powars, Allen, & Haywood, 1976).

The amount of emotional stress at work also may play a part in producing symptoms. This issue is controversial as people react differently to perceived stress. Some persons "thrive on stress" on the job and do fine when confronted with stressful events. For most individuals, however, emotional stress causes negative physiological and psychological reactions. These responses can cause sickle cell crises in persons with sickle cell disease.

## Social and Vocational Limitations

The person growing up with sickle cell disease may have problems in school because of excessive absenteeism due to recurrent sickle cell crises. Chronic complications of the disease, such as leg ulcers, also may impact on school attendance and performance (Alleyne, Wint, & Serjeant, 1977). Poor educational achievement because of repeated absences will make vocational rehabilitation more difficult (Damlouji et al., 1982; Farber et al., 1985). In adult life, work history may also be affected. The vocational background may contain gaps in employment and a history of jobs held for only short periods of time.

**Chronic kidney disease.** With renal failure, anemia worsens, and signs and symptoms related to anemia increase. This exacerbates fatigue and causes reduced exercise tolerance. Physicians can readily treat anemia by transfusion or, more recently, with replacement of the hormone, erythropoietin. In addition, uremia may affect intellectual functioning, including concentration ability and prolonged mental effort. These symptoms generally respond to dialysis.

**Chronic lung disease**. In lung disease, dyspnea (shortness of breath) becomes the limiting factor for exertional level. With sickle cell disease, there is the added complication of the effect of hypoxia (deficiency of oxygen) on the sickling process. Persons with this complication tend to have more frequent, acute symptoms and develop associated complications of sickling such as bone disease, which further limit their activities. Arterial blood gas and pulmonary function testing results can help the counselor determine exercise capacity and the appropriate vocational goals. Analysis of the physical demands, both usual and occasional, for a particular vocation is required. Job restructuring can be helpful when a possible position has occasional physical demands beyond the person's capability. As functioning is likely to deteriorate further over time, during rehabilitation assessment it is useful to consider future progression of the disease.

**Chronic eye disease**. This functional limitation is dependent on the extent of visual loss and the improvement that can be gained from visual aids. One can find visual field defects and visual loss in one or both eyes in sickle cell disease. The rehabilitation counselor needs a current visual evaluation to help determine the actual loss and limitations associated with that loss.

**Chronic leg ulceration**. Leg ulcers produce pain and limitation of motion of the affected extremity. This may affect activities such as walking, standing, climbing, and balancing. Prolonged standing is one possible cause of these ulcers. The counselor needs to assess these possible complications and the resulting functional limitations for clients considering return to gainful employment.

**Chronic bone disease**. Bone and joint disease interfere with activity because of pain, deformity, and loss of strength. The nature of the impairment depends upon which joints are involved. Walking, standing, bending, climbing, or balancing may be affected. Some degree of disability can be overcome by learning new techniques for physical activities through physical therapy. Prosthetic implant surgery may be successful for such patients. Although some loss of dexterity following surgery is to be expected, the relief of pain and recovery of strength more than compensate for the loss of motion.

**Chronic heart disease**. Exercise capacity is the major limiting factor in those rare individuals with cardiac disorders. Heart failure produces fatigue, dyspnea, and weakness. Cardiac rhythm disturbances typically can cause dizziness, weakness, or fainting. In addition, cardiac disease carries the risk of sudden death. This possibility increases emotional disability. Exercise stress testing can help delineate the degree of disability and indicate vocational limitations.

**Chronic central nervous system damage**. The functional limitations following stroke or brain hemorrhage relate to the area of the brain damaged and the extent of damage. Physical disability that results can be extensive. Emotional and intellectual disabilities also occur. The damage produced by brain injury is not progressive, and adaptation to the resulting disabilities allows for improvement in function. The rehabilitation counselor needs a careful evaluation of the individual with respect to current job or school setting, the type and degree of functional impairment, and the physical and intellectual demands of potential employment or school possibilities. Besides physical disability, loss of ability to do activities at a rapid pace is an important vocational factor for such persons, as are impairments in speech, hearing, and vision. These latter impairments are often more limiting in the workplace than the physical impairments.

# REHABILITATION POTENTIAL

Persons with sickle cell disease have a wide range of potential for rehabilitation. Most have mild disease and will not need vocational rehabilitation services. Those with moderate or severe disease may have chronic complications and organ damage and be candidates for vocational rehabilitation. An individual with recurrent sickle cell crises may benefit from the services of a rehabilitation counselor.

Sickle cell disease is unpredictable and the course of the condition uncertain. Rehabilitation counselors need to be able to interact with employers to explain the symptoms of the illness. A person with an otherwise good employment record may be able to use sick leave time for occasional sickle cell crises. The counselor may want to look into reasonable accommodation when facilitating a return to work for someone with moderate to severe sickle cell symptoms.

The 1973 Rehabilitation Act and the 1990 Americans with Disabilities Act provided legislation to help individuals who have disabilities obtain equal access in several crucial areas, including employment. The Americans with Disabilities Act was instrumental in requiring that employers consider reasonable accommodation for people with disabilities. Employers are not allowed to question if a prospective employee has a disability, but instead may only inquire as to whether that individual can perform the essential functions of the job in question. A pre-employment physical examination can be given only after a conditional offer of employment is made.

There are different methods and techniques of providing reasonable accommodation, as described by King and Backer (1989) and Lotito and Pimentel (1990). Employers can usually provide reasonable accommodation at minimal cost. West (1991) pointed out that 50% of reasonable accommodation cost employers $50 or less and 70% cost $500 or less.

One example of reasonable accommodation for persons with sickle cell anemia is an informal agreement with the employer that the individual will attempt to work through minor illnesses and save or accumulate sick days to be used for the occasional sickle cell crisis. Another accommodation is to have the worker put in non-paid overtime between crises to be used when work is missed during a crisis.

On-site observation of the job may help the counselor in efforts to modify physical aspects of the job. When an individual is having difficulty with physical exertion on the job, the counselor should consider attempting to assist the client in modifying the amount of lifting and carrying required. Sometimes, one can break down the amount lifted and carried into lighter loads; if this is not possible, the counselor may want to assist the client and employer in job restructuring.

An important factor for the counselor to consider is the mental stress on the job and its affect on the potential development of a sickle cell crisis (Falvo, 1991). Modification of emotional stressors is more difficult than modification of physical activities. Often, it is impossible to modify emotional stress factors. At times, positive facilitation by the counselor can be effective and result in decreasing emotional stress components of the job. Employer education may create a more thorough understanding of the disease and help in diminishing work-related stress for the employee.

Before determining rehabilitation potential, it is important for the counselor to understand any individual complications and whether time off work is necessary when a sickle cell crisis occurs. With this information, appropriate medical consultation, and an understanding of the provisions of the Americans with Disabilities Act, the rehabilitation counselor will be equipped to provide rehabilitation for individuals with sickle cell disease.

# CASE STUDY

Mr. Leo Jones is a 53 year-old college-educated (B.A. degree), self-employed machinist with hemoglobinopathy S beta thalassemia. He developed bacterial septicemia (infection in the blood) and multiple complications of sickle cell disease, requiring hospitalization for 6 months. Because of this illness, both his marriage and his machinist business failed. His wife left him, taking their two children, ages 7 and 10, with her. The marriage problems and failed business contributed to his anxiety and depression. The treating physician noted Mr. Jones had severe depression and referred him for psychological counseling.

The job of a machinist (D.O.T.# 600.280-022) (U.S. Department of Labor, 1991) involves setting-up and operating machine tools, and fitting and assembling parts to make or repair metal parts, mechanisms, tools, or machines. A machinist applies knowledge of mechanics, shop mathematics, metal properties, and layout and machining procedures in daily work activity. One reads blueprints, diagrams, and mechanical drawings, and uses precision-measuring tools and devices. The machinist uses handtools and power tools throughout the work shift. Mr. Jones had been self-employed for 30 years.

Due to physical limitations related to bone destruction (avascular necrosis) in both hips, Mr. Jones was unable to return to his machinist business, which often required 10-hour days, 6 days a week. Besides himself, he had two helpers in the business. The work involved occasional lifting up to 80 pounds when shipment orders arrived. Besides these shipment orders, the work demanded lifting up to 45 pounds with repetitive lifting of 20-25 pounds. Mr. Jones stood or walked 50% of the work day.

For the next few years, after the acute episode of septicemia, Mr. Jones' physician hospitalized him 6-8 times a year for acute pain crises and for recurrent bone infections (osteomyelitis). Eventually, Mr. Jones began to see his children again and his depression cleared. He requested vocational rehabilitation; a counselor from the State Department of Rehabilitation provided counseling, guidance, and job placement. These services successfully resulted in placing him as a reader and driver, providing services for the blind.

Since taking on these work responsibilities, Mr. Jones has had a remarkable decrease in frequency of hospital admissions, which he relates to improved self-care. Proper rest, careful attention to fluid intake, and monitoring of physical activity have contributed to the improved clinical course of the disease. With this medical improvement, Mr. Jones and his family reunited. He has been able to maintain a home for his family and continue work.

This case points out an important aspect of chronic illness management, self-care, and its influence on the course of chronic disease. Careful attention to these aspects allowed this individual to reduce the frequency of exacerbations of sickle cell disease through prevention and self-management.

## Questions

1. Outline a vocational profile for Mr. Jones including age category, educational level, work history (exertion and skill levels), occupationally significant characteristics, and transferable skills, if any.

2. If Mr. Jones had decided to remain in his machinist business, how would you as his rehabilitation counselor approach this decision? Provide supporting arguments.

3. Can you recommend use of transferable skills as another viable vocational rehabilitation option for Mr. Jones? If so, describe what skills are transferable and to what skilled or semiskilled jobs.

4. Discuss the rehabilitation goal pursued in this case and why the counselor may have recommended it. Do you agree with this rehabilitation plan? Explain.

5. Speculate how Mr. Jones was able to achieve this vocational goal.

# REFERENCES

Alleyne, S.I., Wint, E., & Serjeant, G.R. (1977). Social effects of leg ulceration in sickle cell anemia. **Southern Medical Journal, 70,** 213-214.

Barrett, D.H., Wistozek, I.E., Abel, G.G., Rouleau, J.L., Platt, A.F., Jr., Pollard, W.E., & Eckman, J.R. (1988). Assessment of psychosocial functioning of patients with sickle cell disease. **Southern Medical Journal, 81,** 745-750.

Damlouji, N.F., Kevess-Cohen, R., Charaches, F., Georgopoulos, A., Folstein, M.R. (1982). Social disability and psychiatric morbidity in sickle cell anemia and diabetes patients. **Psychosomatics, 23,** 925-931.

Diggs, L.W. (1965). Sickle cell crisis. **American Journal of Clinical Pathology, 44,** 1-19.

Falvo, D.R. (1991). **Medical and psychosocial aspects of chronic illness and disability.** Gaithersburg, MD: Aspen.

Farber, M.D., Koshy, M., Kinney, T.R., & the Cooperative Study of Sickle Cell Disease (1985). Cooperative study of sickle cell disease: Demographic and socioeconomic characteristics of patients and families with sickle cell disease. **Journal of Chronic Diseases, 38,** 495-505.

Gaston, M.H., Verter, J.I., Woods, G., Diamond, S., Holbrook, T., Gill, F.M., Ritchey, K., Follette, J.M., & the Prophylactic Penicillin Study Group (1986). Prophylaxis with oral penicillin in children with sickle cell anemia. **New England Journal of Medicine, 314,** 1593-1599.

Johnson, C.S. (1981). Sickle cell disease. In W.C. Stolov & M.R. Clowers (Eds.), **Handbook of severe disability** (pp. 349-362). Washington, DC: U.S. Government Printing Office.

King, R.B., & Backer, T.E. (1989). **Overcoming challenges: A guide to selective job placement of workers with disabilities.** Los Angeles, CA: National Medical Enterprises.

Kumar, S., Powars, D., Allen, J., & Haywood, L.J. (1976). Anxiety, self-concept and personal and social adjustments in children with sickle cell disease. **Journal of Pediatrics, 88,** 859-863.

Lotito, M.J., & Pimentel, R. (1990). **The American with Disabilities Act: Making the ADA work for you.** Northridge, CA: Milt Wright and Associates.

McKenzie, J.M. (1982). Vocational options for those with sickle cell trait. **American Journal of Hematology/ Oncology, 4,** 172-178.

Murthy, V.K., & Haywood, L.J. (1981). Survival analysis by sex, age group and hemotype in sickle cell disease. **Journal of Chronic Diseases, 34,** 313-319.

Platt, O.S., Thorington, B.D., Brambilla, D.J., Milner, P.F, Rosse, W.F., Vichinsky, E., & Kinney, T.R. (1991). Pain in sickle cell disease. **New England Journal of Medicine, 325,** 11-16.

Serjeant, G.R. (1985). **Sickle cell disease.** Oxford, England: Oxford University.

Sinnette, C.H., & Gillman, R.A. (1974). Vocational rehabilitation and sickle cell anemia. **Urban Health, 3,** 38-41.

Stuart, J., & Johnson, C.S. (1987). Rheology of the sickle cell disorders. **Balliere's Clinical Hematology, 1,** 747-775.

U.S. Department of Labor (1991). **Dictionary of occupational titles** (4th ed., revised). Washington, DC: Author.

West, J.(Ed.).(1991). **The Americans with Disabilities Act: From policy to practice**. New York, NY: Milbank Memorial Fund.

Wethers, D.L. (1989). Delayed growth and sexual maturation in sickle cell disease. **Annals of the New York Academy of Science, 565**, 137-142.

Whitten, C.F., & Fischoff, J. (1974). Psychological effects of sickle cell disease. **Archives of Internal Medicine, 133**, 681-689.

Williams, W.J., Beutler, E., Erslev, A.J., & Lichtman, M.A. (Eds.). (1990). **Hematology** (4th ed.). New York, NY: McGraw-Hill.

## About the Authors

Cage S. Johnson, M.D., is a Professor of Medicine in the Division of Hematology at the University of Southern California School of Medicine, in Los Angeles, California. An internationally known authority in the field, he is currently Director of the Adult Sickle Cell Program at the Los Angeles County-University of Southern California Medical Center. Dr. Johnson is a consultant to the National Institutes of Health and the California Department of Health Services and serves on the Board of Directors for the Sickle Cell Self-Help Association and the Sickle Cell Disease Research Foundation.

Robert B. Francis, Jr., M.D., is an Associate Professor of Medicine in the Division of Hematology at the University of Southern California, School of Medicine. A nationally known authority in the field of coagulation protein physiology and their role in the problems of sickle cell disease, he is Director of the Coagulation Laboratory at the University of Southern California, Los Angeles, California.

# Chapter 19

# DIABETES MELLITUS

by
*Richard D. Hornichter, M.D.*

## INTRODUCTION

Diabetes mellitus (referred to as diabetes throughout this chapter) is a chronic disorder of carbohydrate metabolism characterized by abnormal elevations in blood glucose (sugar). Type I diabetes is due to a deficiency of insulin, which is normally produced by the beta cells of the Islets of Langerhans situated in the pancreas. Type II diabetes may involve inadequate insulin production, in some cases, but may also be associated with insulin resistance, especially in the obese individual.

In the uncontrolled state, the individual with diabetes will often exhibit the three classical symptoms (commonly called the three "polys"): polyuria (increased urination), polydipsia (increased thirst), and polyphagia (increased hunger). Other symptoms may include fatigue, weakness, and weight loss. With adequate regulation of blood glucose, reversal of these symptoms will occur.

The rehabilitation counselor will provide rehabilitation services to individuals with diabetes when complications of diabetes develop and interfere with workplace, school, or home performance. If a person with diabetes is under good control and free of complications, it is unlikely that contact with a rehabilitation counselor will be initiated, unless diabetes is a secondary condition. Rehabilitation professionals may see persons with poorly controlled diabetes and those with serious associated complications, such as visual loss, amputation of a lower extremity, or renal failure. The counselor also may see younger individuals with insulin dependent diabetes, Type I, who are having difficulty achieving adequate control of blood sugar levels.

### Epidemiology: Prevalence, Incidence, and Statistics

Due to the number of persons with diabetes in the United States and worldwide, and the frequency and spectrum of associated medical conditions, any discussion of diabetes assumes enormous importance from medical, human, rehabilitation, and economic aspects. Prevalence is the total number of persons known to have a disorder or disease at a particular time. Between 3.1% and 3.4% of the United States population between the ages of 20 and 74 years have the diagnosis of diabetes (Kovar, Harris, & Hadden, 1987). In 1987, the latest statistics available, 6.8 million persons in the United States had diagnosed diabetes (DeStefano et al., 1990). It is assumed the prevalence of undiagnosed diabetes is equal in number to diagnosed cases (Harris, Hadden, Knowler, & Bennett, 1987). This is partially due to the minimal symptoms or asymptomatic status of patients with mild diabetes. Also, many people with diabetes have symptoms but do not seek medical help.

Impaired glucose tolerance refers to an individual who has blood glucose abnormalities, discovered on glucose testing, that is not severe enough to warrant a full diagnosis of diabetes. This condition was formerly labeled "borderline diabetes" or "chemical diabetes." Kovar, Harris, and Hadden (1987) estimated that in 1980, 4.6% of individuals in this country between the ages of 20 and 74 had impaired glucose tolerance. More recently, Harris (1989) estimated this figure at 11.2%. Impaired glucose tolerance constitutes two-thirds of all glucose intolerance in the United States (Harris, 1989). The remaining one-third of glucose intolerance are actual diagnosed cases of diabetes.

Another study cited the prevalence rate of diabetes at approximately 2.5/100 population (Drury & Powell, 1986). Incidence is the number of persons diagnosed with a particular medical condition for the first time during the preceding year. From 1982 to 1987, the incidence rate of diabetes in the United States has been approximately 2.8 to 2.98/1000 population per year (DeStefano et al., 1990).

The prevalence of both diagnosed and undiagnosed diabetes increases with advancing age. Between the ages of 65 to 74, the prevalence of diabetes is about 41.5% (Kovar, Harris, & Hadden, 1987). A positive relationship exists between the incidence of diabetes and being overweight (Hadden & Harris, 1987). Individuals who are 50% or more above the desirable body weight are five times as likely to have diabetes as people within the normal weight range (Kovar, Harris, & Hadden, 1987). Overt diabetes is four times more likely to develop in those with impaired glucose tolerance than in individuals with normal ability to process carbohydrates (Hadden & Harris, 1987). Besides these influences, a positive genetic factor is also operative in inheritance of diabetes (Harris, Hadden, Knowler, & Bennett, 1987). Diabetes tends to occur more commonly in families, but inheritance does not strictly follow the classic laws of genetics.

Diabetes occurs throughout the world and in all ethnic groups. In some ethnic groups, the prevalence of diabetes is much higher. In the United States, about 15% of patients with diabetes are Black (Drury & Powell, 1986); the prevalence of diabetes, both diagnosed and undiagnosed, is higher among Black people (Drury & Powell, 1987). A recent study pointed out this is not due to a possible increased incidence of obesity (O'Brien et al., 1989). About 6% of patients with diabetes in the United States are of Hispanic origin (Drury & Powell, 1986).

## Mortality and Morbidity

Diabetes is the seventh leading cause of death in the United States (DeStefano et al., 1990; Hadden & Harris, 1987). Death from diabetes-related conditions is under-reported, since diabetes is recorded on the death certificate of only about 40% of the people who have had the disorder (DeStefano et al., 1990). Among adults, diabetes is the leading cause of new cases of blindness (Hadden & Harris, 1987). Twenty-five percent of kidney failure in this country is due to diabetes (Hadden & Harris, 1987). These staggering figures emphasize the impact of diabetes upon the health and rehabilitation resources of this nation and the world.

# MEDICAL ASPECTS

## Clinical Spectrum

From the clinical standpoint, diabetes has two major aspects. The most prominent is blood glucose abnormality. If an individual has an abnormally elevated level of glucose (sugar) in the blood, diabetes is present. The individual also may have glycosuria (sugar in the urine) as an additional abnormal finding.

Diabetes may occur as a component of other medical conditions, but in the vast majority of cases this is not the situation, and the diagnosis is apparent and straightforward. Associated factors may involve genetic influences and overweight. Besides the abnormal blood glucose levels, diabetes is also viewed from a vascular (blood vessel) standpoint. Most of the serious complications associated with diabetes are vascular in origin. Only 7-10% of deaths due to diabetes result directly from the disease itself (Olson, 1988); complications are responsible for the majority of morbidity and mortality associated with diabetes.

## Complications

**Vascular disease.** Vascular disease of the larger arteries, called macrovascular disease, is common among persons with diabetes. This involves narrowing and occlusion of arteries at various locations in the body. There is a decrease in blood supply to tissues beyond the narrowed or occluded areas of involved arteries. This condition is clinically found in the arteries of the retina of the eyes, coronary arteries of the heart, cerebral arteries supplying the brain, arteries of the kidneys, and the arteries of the lower extremities. Microvascular disease, occlusions of the smaller arteries, may occur independently or in association with larger arterial disease. Peripheral vascular disease, involving variable contributions from macrovascular (large blood vessel) and microvascular (small blood vessel) components, is a leading cause of foot infections and subsequent amputation in patients with diabetes.

**Neuropathy.** Persons with diabetes often have abnormal nerve function resulting in diabetic neuropathy, especially in the lower extremities. This condition may manifest itself as painful sensations, parasthesias (abnormal sensation), and numbness (loss of sensation); in the later stages one may experience total loss of sensation in the feet. There also may be interference with muscular function at various locations in the body since the motor nerves supplying those muscles may be abnormal. The exact cause of diabetic neuropathy is not fully understood. Involvement of the microvasculature of the nerves may play a role; abnormal metabolism within the nerves also may be a causative factor (Ellenberg, 1981).

**Combined peripheral vascular disease and peripheral neuropathy.** When the lower extremities of a person with diabetes are affected by a combination of peripheral vascular disease and peripheral neuropathy, a special vulnerability to trauma and infection exists. In the presence of diabetic neuropathy, including decreased sensation, trauma may occur without the individual being aware of it. This can lead to the development of breaks in the skin or foot ulcers. Such ulcers frequently become infected. Foot infections in the presence of vascular insufficiency are extremely difficult to treat and may lead to the development of non-healing infected foot ulcers. These may develop into gangrene. This cycle of events frequently leads to lower extremity amputation. This scenario all too often occurs among individuals with diabetes.

**Visual complications.** Diabetic retinopathy (pathology of the retina) is a leading cause of blindness. Physicians can see specific abnormalities known as microaneurysms, abnormal weakening of the retinal arteries. These microaneurysms are prone to bleeding in the retina, which can interfere with vision.

**Renal failure.** The kidneys of patients with diabetic nephropathy (kidney pathology) have a specific microscopic pattern known as nephrosclerosis. This abnormality, found only in the kidneys of persons with diabetes, affects the ability of the kidneys to function effectively. This causes loss of protein in the urine and abnormal build up of body waste products in the blood, since the kidneys are unable to eliminate them normally. Diabetic renal disease is usually progressive and responsible for significant morbidity. Patients with end-stage renal disease often need dialysis.

**Arteriosclerosis.** Generalized arteriosclerosis or "hardening of the arteries," involving narrowing and occlusion of arteries throughout the body, may be more advanced at an earlier age among persons with diabetes than among the general population. Diabetes is frequently associated with abnormally elevated blood lipids (fats), such as cholesterol and triglyceride, that also can contribute to arteriosclerosis (Olson, 1988). This is especially true for the coronary arteries.

## Type I versus Type II Diabetes

Currently, two major types of diabetes represent two ends of a clinical spectrum. At first glance, these appear to be two different diseases. Type I diabetes, also known as "insulin dependent diabetes mellitus" (IDDM), was formerly called "juvenile onset type" or "labile diabetes." This condition is characterized by absolute insulin insufficiency. The pancreas loses its capacity to produce insulin and the individual needs to take insulin injections daily. Without insulin, the person is unable to metabolize glucose, with resultant elevations in blood glucose concentrations.

In extreme circumstances, such patients may develop diabetic ketoacidosis, a severe metabolic disturbance characterized by accumulation of abnormal substances in the blood and urine. This condition may lead to diabetic coma and possible death. Even with daily insulin therapy, blood glucose regulation often is erratic and difficult to control. Approximately 7% of individuals with diabetes have Type I. Type I diabetes usually occurs in younger patients.

Type II diabetes, also known as "non-insulin dependent diabetes mellitus" (NIDDM), was formerly called "maturity onset type" or "non-ketosis prone diabetes." In response to a meal, the pancreas normally secretes insulin. With respect to Type II diabetes, there may occur an initial delay in insulin secretion followed by over-secretion. With time, patients may develop deficient insulin secretion.

Several factors contribute to the abnormal blood sugar levels in Type II diabetes. Insulin resistance, which is a common feature of obesity, is a significant factor, since most patients with Type II diabetes are obese. The cellular sites of insulin action, known as insulin receptors, may be defective. Abnormalities in other hormones involved in glucose level regulation or factors yet unknown may play significant roles. The vast majority of patients with diabetes (93%) have Type II (Davidson, 1986). Patients with Type II diabetes tend to be older than those with Type I, hence, the former nomenclature.

Despite the differences noted, both Type I and Type II diabetes show abnormal elevations in blood glucose. Additionally, patients with each type of diabetes tend to develop the same kind of complications.

## Blood Glucose Control and Development of Complications

Before the discovery of insulin in 1922, patients with Type I diabetes had very short life spans. With insulin therapy, patients have lived longer and the complications associated with diabetes have became more apparent. A critical question has been the relationship of blood glucose control to the development of complications. Physicians previously believed there was little relationship between blood glucose control and the development of complications. They prescribed a "free diet" which allowed patients a less restrictive diet.

Current thinking, supported by overwhelming evidence in the medical literature, strongly favors the concept that there is a relationship between control of blood glucose and development of complications of diabetes (American Diabetes Association, 1990b; Olson, 1988). This being the case, it is worth the great expenditure of effort and resources to treat and educate patients so they may attempt to maintain their blood glucose as normal as possible.

## Therapy of Diabetes

Although there is no cure for diabetes, modern therapy offers management designed to control blood glucose levels and thus attempt to prevent complications. Treatment of diabetes is simple in theory but difficult in practice, since it involves the balancing of at least four important variables. The variability of dietary intake, medications (insulin or oral hypoglycemic agents), exercise, and emotional factors are involved on a daily basis. The patient is committed to continuous involvement in the daily management of this condition. The following quotation is appropriate, "Patient education and knowledge is important because, aside from contacts with a physician or other health care practitioner, health care of diabetics is primarily self-care." (Drury & Shannon, 1987, p. 1). Since the rehabilitation counselor will have professional interaction with persons with diabetes, it will be useful to be familiar with the principles of therapy for diabetes.

**Diet.** Diet is the mainstay of therapy; it is the most difficult aspect to teach and to learn. Sometimes, dietary regulation may be the only therapy required for NIDDM. Each patient with diabetes should have a specific dietary program prescribed by a knowledgeable professional. The total number of calories per day; the percentages of carbohydrate, protein, and fat that make up those calories; and the distribution of allowed food per meal are important. The ability to teach dietary principles is limited by the individual's capability and desire to understand and follow through appropriately.

**Insulin.** Insulin can only be administered by injection. It is the required therapy for Type I diabetes and is also necessary for some Type II patients. Available insulins vary in their onset and duration of action. Rapid onset, short-acting insulins include Regular and Semilente. Intermediate acting insulins, with approximately 24-hour duration, include NPH and Lente. Long-acting insulins, of up to 36-hour duration, are Ultralente and protamine zinc insulin (PZI) (Olson, 1989). Most insulin-dependent patients use mixtures combining short-acting with an intermediate or a long-acting insulin. Many patients require two or more daily insulin injections. The availability of different insulin types allows for greater individualization of the therapeutic regimen. Commercially, insulin is extracted from beef or pork pancreas. Human insulin manufactured by recombinant DNA technology or by chemical alteration of pork insulin, is now widely available.

Patients using insulin therapy are at risk for developing "insulin reactions" or low blood sugar (hypoglycemia). This will occur more frequently when the person misses a meal or suddenly increases the amount of exercise. Insulin-dependent patients can be educated to recognize and treat this common situation. Immediate ingestion of carbohydrates (i.e., sugar) will usually raise blood sugar levels and relieve the hypoglycemic situation. Prolonged hypoglycemia can lead to brain dysfunction and coma.

**Testing.** Patients with diabetes can test their urine and blood sugar levels at home. The procedures are simple and easily done by placing a drop of urine or blood on a testing tape. The results allow the person to estimate the urine or blood sugar. Urine sugar generally reflects blood sugar, but is much less accurate. These procedures allow for better control of diabetes.

**Oral hypoglycemic agents.** The sulfonylurea class of drugs are oral hypoglycemic agents. These agents stimulate the pancreas to release previously manufactured and stored insulin and may have a beneficial effect upon the insulin receptor level (Whitehouse & Kahkonen, 1981). Patients take them orally. Since Type I diabetes is characterized by absolute insulin deficiency, these drugs are useless in this group of patients. Sulfonylurea drugs are only of benefit for patients with Type II diabetes, who are unable or unwilling to maintain adequate blood sugar control with dietary therapy alone. Currently, six different oral hypoglycemic agents are available in this country. These vary in their duration of action. Patients with Type II diabetes may take single or multiple doses per day, as prescribed by the treating physician.

**Exercise.** Exercise has a beneficial effect in lowering blood glucose, may be of benefit for the peripheral arterial circulation, and is recommended for patients with diabetes. Additionally, exercise lowers blood lipids and increases insulin sensitivity in diabetes (Olson, 1988). Yet, the variability of physical exercise on a daily basis may contribute to blood glucose lability and insulin reactions, especially in the Type I patient. Patients with Type II diabetes, who tend to be older, may be limited in their exercise tolerance due to cardiovascular problems, peripheral vascular conditions, or other medical complications.

**Emotional factors.** The emotional status of the person probably plays a role in the daily regulation of blood glucose. A particular individual's adaptation to environmental stresses may influence blood sugar fluctuations. Patient education has an important function in contributing to the emotional well-being of the individual, especially in diabetes management. The rehabilitation counselor, when interacting with patients who have diabetes, should attempt to emphasize positive aspects of lifestyle.

## Control

Blood glucose control is a therapeutic objective. The term "control" lacks precise definition. Control of diabetes must be defined within the context of each individual and the ability to learn and understand the principles of management. Most physicians would agree that "tight control" of blood glucose is desirable, but universal agreement on a definition is lacking. The parameters marking control are different for children with diabetes than for elderly patients.

Glycosylated hemoglobin is a laboratory measurement that provides an estimate of the average blood sugar over the preceding 3 months from the date obtained. Since it measures a broader time span than individual blood glucose determinations, glycosylated hemoglobin is the best evidence of diabetic control. This being the case, maintenance of glycosylated hemoglobin values at as near normal as possible is the desirable standard of "control" in diabetes.

# REHABILITATION ASPECTS

## Statistics

Persons with diabetes often have significant disabilities and may require services of a rehabilitation counselor. About 15% of the general population of the United States is limited in their activities due to one or more chronic conditions or impairments; over 50% of persons with diabetes are so limited (Drury & Powell, 1986). A history of heart attack or stroke is more than twice as frequent, while blindness is roughly five times more prevalent (Huse, Oster, Killen, Lacey, & Colditz, 1989). Among individuals with non-insulin-dependent diabetes, in 1986, 951,000 individuals were totally disabled. This study estimated the real cost to society as $19.8 billion; $11.6 billion in health care costs, $2.6 billion in lost productivity related to disability, and $5.6 billion related to non-productivity due to premature mortality (Huse, Oster, Killen, Lacey, & Colditz, 1989).

## Special Considerations

Besides the specific requirements made necessary by diabetes itself, multiple complications may coexist producing an imposing array of physical and emotional disabilities in the same individual. This situation may present practical limitations in relation to the rehabilitation potential of patients. The rehabilitation counselor is an important source of patient education for prevention and limitation of progression of physical disabilities. The counselor also can provide practical information on dealing with the functional limitations and associated emotional aspects.

Complications of diabetes are manifestations of end-organ damage. These associated conditions are not reversible, yet may be delayed in appearance or progression by adequate diabetes therapy. The following discussion will be limited to the more common and specific examples of complications in diabetes.

## Lower Extremity Amputation

A frequent common occurrence in association with diabetes is lower extremity amputation, which is about 15 times as common among individuals with diabetes. In 1985, over 50,000 persons with diabetes in the United States had these amputations (Bild et al., 1989). This represents the result of a combination of vascular insufficiency, both macrovascular and microvascular, and peripheral neuropathy.

Due to absent or decreased sensitivity, persons with diabetes may not be aware of trauma occurring to their feet. When the feet are numb, it is difficult to perceive pain. Localized areas of trauma or breaks in the skin of the feet may develop into ulcers. The ulcers are slow to heal or do not heal at all due to decreased blood supply in the area. Bacterial infection is likely to follow. Due to vascular insufficiency, delivery of effective antibiotic treatment becomes difficult in an infected foot ulcer. The infection may spread locally and become deeper. Gangrene is a frequent consequence. Further spread of the infection via the blood may occur and is life threatening. Amputation becomes the only possible alternative.

Due to insufficient blood supply, the surgeon may need to amputate at a higher level than might be required in a non-diabetic, to provide adequate blood supply for post-operative healing. Below the knee (BK) amputation is a common consequence of the scenario noted above; occasionally, the amputation needs to be above the knee (AK). The assistance of the rehabilitation counselor to help plan for future employment within new physical limitations becomes crucial at this point.

A foot care program is important for patients with diabetes (American Diabetes Association, 1990a). They should not walk barefoot; nail care can be provided by a qualified podiatrist. Feet should be bathed in warm water and lubricating lotion applied before bedtime to keep the skin soft and prevent drying and cracking. New shoes need to fit properly and have a break-in period to prevent blister formation. Even minor skin breaks should be reported to the patient's physician for evaluation.

## Visual Loss

Loss of vision, partial or complete, due to diabetic retinopathy is another frequent complication. Microaneurysms are the specific lesions found only in the retinal blood vessels of patients with diabetes. A microaneurysm is a weakened bulging of the involved retinal vessel. These microaneurysms are prone to rupture and bleed, causing retinal hemorrhages and interference with vision. The body attempts to form new blood vessels to circumvent the involved areas. These new vessels, called "neo-vascularization," are themselves weak and subject to further bleeding. Laser photocoagulation is a modern treatment of this condition. Damage may be minimized by early treatment.

From a rehabilitation standpoint, individuals with diabetes may find it more difficult to master Braille due to poor two-point discriminations if numbness is present in the fingers (Olson, 1988). Failing vision imposes a new set of limitations. Blind persons with diabetes often need much psychological support. Individuals who go through a rehabilitation program early in the course of vision loss show improved psychosocial functioning (Bernbaum, Albert, & Duckro, 1988).

## Neuropathy

Diabetic peripheral neuropathy involving the lower extremities often causes a lack of sensation and perception, numbness, and parasthesias. The role of numbness and decreased pain perception of diabetic neuropathy in the development of lower extremity amputation has been mentioned. The parasthesias of diabetic neuropathy typically manifest as burning, feelings of coldness, or other painful sensations of the feet, often becoming worse at night.

Besides lower extremity involvement by peripheral neuropathy, there are other specific syndromes of abnormal nerve function in diabetes. These may involve both peripheral nerves and autonomic nerves and may feature associated vascular abnormalities. Treatment of these conditions is very difficult, especially since the exact etiology is unknown. The neuropathies occurring in persons with diabetes are responsible for significant morbidity and often require extensive rehabilitation interaction.

## Renal Failure

Diabetic nephropathy is progressive and may lead to chronic renal failure with dialysis as the only therapeutic option. Although the rehabilitation potential of these patients may be limited, special programs have achieved some success. Psychological help and daily living support may be two rehabilitation interventions required.

# FUNCTIONAL LIMITATIONS

If a person with diabetes is under good control and lacks complications, there will be few work restrictions. Individuals taking insulin or oral hypoglycemic agents should try to avoid irregular hours or rotating work shifts, but this sometimes cannot be avoided. It is desirable for persons with diabetes to have work schedules that remains as consistent as possible for optimum control of blood glucose. Variations in exercise will predispose these individuals to variations in blood glucose levels. An occupation that requires consistent amounts of physical activity throughout the workday is preferred to one in which the physical demands vary greatly. Of course, jobs often require a variety of work duties with differing physical demands. A knowledgeable individual can adjust medication therapy and diet.

The individual taking insulin will need a readily available source of sugar to combat insulin reactions. All insulin-dependent individuals should carry hard candy or another source of sugar to alleviate insulin reactions if they occur. Persons who are in good control can manage occasional hypoglycemic reactions so that they go unnoticed by others at the workplace.

The longer diabetes has been present, the greater the potential for complications. This is at least partially dependent on the degree of control an individual has maintained, how quickly a physician is consulted for treatment, as well as adherence to the physician's recommendations. Although some individuals remain relatively free of complications, the rehabilitation professional will see those persons with complications that interfere with work functions.

An individual with decreased vision may need job accommodation. The degree of visual loss and the prognosis for further loss are crucial factors. The greater the amount of visual loss, the more important it is for the counselor to consider occupations requiring less reliance on the eyes for primary work functions. Secondary job duties may be modified or eliminated through provision of reasonable accommodation.

Lower extremity complications may require job modification involving less ambulation, lifting, carrying, and standing. The degree of lower extremity involvement will determine the amount of work restrictions required. If a lower extremity amputation has occurred, sedentary work will be realistic. Exercise is important for good blood glucose control and general health; individuals should exercise within realistic limits. The level of amputation and the individual's adaptation must be considered before restricting an individual to sedentary work only. Above-the-knee (AK) amputations are rarely necessary for persons with diabetes (Burgess & Romano, 1968).

Mild to moderate neuropathy of the lower extremities may not preclude heavier types of work, whereas moderately severe or severe neuropathy may preclude all but sedentary work activity. The individual and the treating physician can offer advice on the appropriateness of certain physical activities at the workplace and at home.

Limitations of function may occur when there are skin problems at an amputation site. Proper hygiene of the amputation site must occur continuously. The skin of the stump needs daily inspection and care. Small skin problems can quickly develop into ulcerations, which impede proper fit of the prosthesis, limit ambulation activity, and require medical consultation.

Individuals who have neuropathy that involves the hands may have a problem with fine finger dexterity and discrimination of small objects. A person with visual loss and this type of neuropathy will have difficulty reading Braille because of the sensitive touch needed for this activity.

Complications involving the circulatory system may significantly limit physical activity. The counselor can be guided by the restriction of physical activity noted by the treating physician.

Persons with renal failure usually have multiple complications. Depending on the multiplicity of complications and the degree of renal failure, work activity may be restricted to part-time, at best. The counselor may want to consider homebound work for certain individuals. Careful medical assessment will be helpful to the rehabilitation counselor.

Emotional factors play a role in control of diabetes. Emotional instability complicates treatment. An emotionally stressful event may result in a rise in blood glucose levels. If an occupation is stressful and affects good blood glucose control, intervention by a rehabilitationist is appropriate. The counselor also needs to consider the stress component of work when developing potential rehabilitation plans. It should be kept in mind that some individuals may handle emotional stress very well and may almost "thrive on stress." For these persons, occupational stress may not be a significant factor for the counselor to consider.

# REHABILITATION POTENTIAL

Individuals with diabetes under good control and with no complications will not need the services of a rehabilitation counselor. If the diabetes is a secondary condition, the counselor needs to consider it as an important factor. Attitude is crucial in this and other disabilities. The person with diabetes who has a positive attitude and outlook will probably have good potential for rehabilitation.

For individuals dependent on insulin, proper insulin therapy and adaptation to medical recommendations will increase chances of successful rehabilitation planning. Poor control and failure to follow medical advise will impede chances for a successful outcome.

Visual loss, if significant, will impact the ability to perform many jobs. This is dependent on the amount and type of visual acuity necessary to conduct the various job duties and whether these are primary or secondary job functions. It may be possible to assign secondary functions to another worker through the provision of reasonable accommodation. The worker with visual loss can be assigned portions of other workers' activities in trade for functions the person cannot perform. Visual loss will affect rehabilitation potential but to a varying extent, depending on the factors discussed above.

Although not all patients with lower extremity amputation are good candidates for wearing an artificial limb, many of working age are candidates for fitting and use of a prosthesis. The purposes of a prosthesis are to restore mobility and increase independence (Steinberg, 1991). Most amputations will be below-the-knee (BK), as discussed previously. For amputations that are above-the-knee (AK), ambulation will be more difficult and will consume additional energy. If the prosthesis fits well and is used properly and regularly, rehabilitation potential will remain.

Bilateral lower extremity amputation usually results in the person ambulating with use of a wheelchair. On occasion, an individual can learn to use two lower extremity prostheses for ambulation. This depends on the age and general medical health of the individual (Steinberg, 1991). Potential for rehabilitation will depend on general health, as other medical complications probably exist.

All persons using a lower extremity prosthesis must learn a new technique of walking. Walking with a prosthesis requires mental concentration as this type of activity is not part of the normal mode of ambulation that a person acquired early in life. Gait training by a physical therapist will help an individual become proficient at this new means of ambulation. The therapist needs to become familiar with the person's home and work activities to provide the most useful gait training possible.

# CASE STUDY

You are employed at a community college as a counselor specializing in providing academic and career counseling for students with disabilities. One of your clients is a 20-year old female student who wants to take vocational interest tests to confirm her occupational objective.

Jeannie has Type I diabetes and takes insulin twice a day. She has no complications or other health problems.

Her college major is police science and she wants to become a police officer (Police Officer I, [government service], D.O.T.# 375-263-014). The interest testing confirms her vocational goal. Other interests, according to the testing results are nursing and teaching. In discussing this with Jeannie, she stated her primary interest is police work and she sees no reason why she cannot pursue this as a career. The job description of a police officer follows.

A Police Officer I (government service) patrols an assigned beat on foot, using a motorcycle, or in a patrol car, to prevent crime or disturbances, and is responsible for arresting law offenders. Also, the officer is involved in controlling crowds and dispersing gatherings that become unruly or dangerous. Rendering first aid at accidents and investigating causes and results of accidents are part of the job duties. The officer will direct and reroute traffic around emergency situations. Part of the job involves issuing warnings and tickets to traffic violators and inspecting public establishments requiring licenses to insure compliance with rules and regulations.

The work of a police officer involves medium level exertion and rotating shifts. Job demands vary daily and change continuously throughout any particular day. Environmental conditions include extremes of temperature, noise, and hazardous occurences.

## Questions

1. Specify the skill level and the physical activity requirements (lifting, carrying, walking, and so forth) of a Police Officer I.

2. Identify the occupationally significant characteristics (worker traits) and transferable skills of a Police Officer I (government service).

3. Is Jeannie's occupational goal realistic? Discuss.

4. Describe what further counseling services, if any, you plan to offer Jeannie.

5. Jeannie wants to know more about diabetes and the possible future of the disease for her. How would you respond to these questions?

6. What are the implications of diabetes in regard to future functional limitations?

# REFERENCES

American Diabetes Association (1990a). Standards of medical care for patients with diabetes mellitus. **Diabetes Care, 13**(Suppl. 1), 10-13.

American Diabetes Association (1990b). Blood glucose control in diabetes: Position statement. **Diabetes Care, 13**(Suppl. 1), 16-17.

Bernbaum, M., Albert, S.G., & Duckro, P.N. (1988). Psychosocial profiles in patients with visual impairment due to diabetic retinopathy. **Diabetes Care, 11**, 551-557.

Bild, D.E., Selby, J.V., Sinnock, P., Browner, W.S., Braveman, P., & Showstack, J.A. (1989). Lower-extremity amputation in people with diabetes. **Diabetes Care, 12**, 24-31.

Burgess, E.M., & Romano, R.L. (1968). The management of lower extremity amputees using immediate postsurgical prosthetic fitting. **Clinical Orthopedics, 57**, 137.

Davidson, J.K. (1986). **Clinical diabetes mellitus**. New York: Thieme.

DeStefano, F., Dougherty, B.L., Ford, E.S., German, R.R., Newman, J.M., Olson, D.R., Sepe, S.J., Stevenson, J.M., Vinicor, F., Wetterhall, S.F., & Will, J.C. (1990). **Diabetes surveillance, 1980-1987**. Washington, DC: U.S. Department of Health and Human Services.

Drury, T.F., & Powell, A.L. (1986). Prevalence, impact and demography of known diabetes in the U.S. In the **1985 National Health Interview Survey of Health Promotion and Disease Prevention**. National Center for Health Statistics: Advance Data From Vital and Health Statistics. Public. #114. (U.S. Department of Health and Human Services Publication No. PHS 86-1250). Hyattsville, MD: Public Health Service.

Drury, T.F., & Powell, A.L. (1987). Prevalence of known diabetes among Black Americans. In the **1985 National Health Interview Survey of Health Promotion and Disease Prevention**. National Center for Health Statistics: Advance Data From Vital and Health Statistics. Public. #130. (U.S. Department of Health and Human Services Publication No. PHS 87-1250). Hyattsville, MD: Public Health Service.

Drury, T.F., & Shannon, I.I. (1987). Perceptions of U.S. adults with non-insulin-dependent diabetes. In the **1985 National Health Interview Survey of Health Promotion and Disease Prevention Disease Prevention**. National Center for Health Statistics: Advance Data From Vital and Health Statistics. Public. #141. (U.S. Department of Health and Human Services Publication No. PHS 87-1250). Hyattsville, MD: Public Health Service.

Ellenberg, M. (1981). Diabetic neuropathy. In H. Rafkin & P. Raskim (Eds.), **Diabetes mellitus** (Vol. 5, pp. 259-263). Bowie, MD: Robert J. Brady.

Hadden, W.C., & Harris, M.I. (1987). Prevalence of diagnosed diabetes, undiagnosed diabetes, and impaired glucose tolerance in adults 20-74 years of age: United States 1976-1980. **National Center for Health Statistics: Advance Data From Vital and Health Statistics, Series 11, # 237**. (U.S. Department of Health and Human Services Publication No. PHS 87-1687). Washington, DC: U.S. Government Printing Office.

Harris, M.I. (1989). Impaired glucose tolerance in the U.S. population. **Diabetes Care, 13**, 464-474.

Harris, M.I., Hadden, W.C., Knowler, W.C., & Bennett, P.H. (1987). Prevalence of diabetes and impaired glucose tolerance and plasma glucose levels in U.S. population aged 20-74 years. **Diabetes, 36**, 523-534.

Huse, D.M., Oster, G., Killen, A.R., Lacey, M.J., & Colditz, G.A. (1989). The economic costs of non-insulin-dependent diabetes mellitus. **Journal of the American Medical Association, 262,** 2708-2713.

Kovar, M.G., Harris, M.I., & Hadden, W.C. (1987). The scope of diabetes in the United States population. **American Journal of Public Health, 77,** 1549-1550.

O'Brien, T.R., Flanders, W.D., Decoufle, P., Boyle, C.A., DeStefano, F., & Teutsch, S. (1989). Are racial differences in the prevalence of diabetes in adults explained by differences in obesity? **Journal of the American Medical Association, 262,** 1485-1488.

Olson, O.C. (1988). **Diagnosis and management of diabetes mellitus** (2nd ed.). New York: Raven.

Steinberg, F.U. (1991). Rehabilitation after amputation: Restoring mobility and independence. **Diabetes Spectrum, 4,** 5-9.

Whitehouse, F.W., & Kahkonen, D.M. (1981). Oral hypoglycemic agents. In H. Rafkin & P. Raskim (Eds.). **Diabetes mellitus** (Vol. 5, pp. 129-136). Bowie, MD: Robert J. Brady.

### *About the Author*

Richard D. Hornichter, M.D., is a Clinical Associate Professor of Medicine at the University of California, Los Angeles, School of Medicine in Los Angeles, California. He is also in private practice in Beverly Hills, California, specializing in diabetes.

# *Chapter 20*

# RESPIRATORY DYSFUNCTION

## Chronic Obstructive Pulmonary Disease
## and
## Neuromuscular Disorders

by
*Ahmet Baydur, M.D.*

## INTRODUCTION

Chronic respiratory disorders are the third leading cause of death in the United States. The decline in cardiovascular deaths in recent years is in contrast to the surge in respiratory diseases related to smoking and other environmental pollutants. In addition, neuromuscular diseases, while less common in prevalence than the chronic obstructive airway disorders, comprise a major cause of respiratory impairment and failure. They also account for a significant source of disability and prolonged respiratory care in this country. With knowledge and appropriate selection, both categories of respiratory disability are amenable to rehabilitation from a respiratory perspective.

The basic premise of rehabilitation is to attempt to return the patient with chronic respiratory problems to as self-sufficient and useful a role in society as feasible. The following factors impact rehabilitation: the patient's age, the nature and stage of the illness, the person's overall health, the existence of medical complications, the possibilities for retraining and return to work, and the job market.

The purpose of this chapter is to provide an overview of the common chronic obstructive respiratory disorders, as well as respiratory impairments encountered in patients with neuromuscular diseases. This will include definitions, diagnostic features, treatment, limitations, and rehabilitation potential for these conditions.

## CHRONIC OBSTRUCTIVE PULMONARY DISEASE (COPD)

### Introduction

Chronic obstructive pulmonary disease (COPD) is a disorder characterized by abnormal tests of expiratory flow from the lungs that do not change markedly over periods of several months' observation (American Thoracic

Society, 1987). Emphysema and chronic bronchitis are the two major disorders usually included in the definition of COPD. Asthma is also a type of COPD, characterized by reversible airway hyperreactivity. There occurs improvement in airflow following inhalation with a bronchodilator.

## Pathology and Symptomatology

**Chronic bronchitis.** Chronic bronchitis is the result of excessive secretion of mucus and airway inflammation. There is a strong association with inhalation of irritants, by far the most common of which is cigarette smoke. Certain occupational irritants are also important, such as dusts from cotton or mining, and fumes from paints, plastics, and various solvents.

**Emphysema.** Emphysema is caused through destruction of lung tissue by enzymes released by white blood cells that collect in lung tissue. The lungs tend to remain in an expanded position and do not collapse in the normal manner to allow for full expiration of air. Cigarette smoking leads to an influx of massive numbers of different forms of white blood cells and macrophages (cells that defend against bacteria and particulate matter) into the lungs. A rare genetic condition, $\alpha_1$ - antitrypsin deficiency, increases the potential for attack by enzymes in the body. Since only a small percentage of cigarette smokers develop symptomatic COPD, other factors must contribute to lung damage. Frequent bronchial problems in childhood and occurrence of bronchitis in infancy lead to bronchial disturbance many years later. Allergies are associated with an unusually high frequency of upper respiratory infections and decrease in lung function.

**Asthma.** Asthma is an episodic, inflammatory disease characterized by airway hyperreactivity, reversible bronchospasm (spasmodic contraction of the bronchial muscle) with thickening of the muscular wall, mucus membrane edema, and sputum overproduction. While asthma itself causes no permanent structural damage in the lungs, mucus plugging of airways may lead to atelectasis (collapse of the lung) or pneumonia. Most exacerbations do not have a specific identifiable cause; careful investigation may reveal one or more triggering allergic causes, such as molds (e.g., Penicillium), pollen, or tree resins (e.g., Western red cedar). Some persons who are otherwise without symptoms develop bronchospasm following exercise or exposure to cold air. When tested by inhaling a precise dose of bronchoconstrictor substance, these patients often show evidence of bronchial hyperreactivity.

## Diagnostic Evaluation

**Clinical assessment.** The symptoms of COPD are variable, according to the specific disease entity that predominates and additional modifying factors. The clinical symptoms include cough, sputum production, sneezing, and dyspnea (shortness of breath). Generally, chronic cough and sputum production suggest the presence of bronchitis. Dyspnea indicates fatigue of the breathing muscles and causes increased difficulty in respiration. Occasionally in COPD, particularly in patients with emphysema, dyspnea is the only symptom. In this situation, emphysema is subtle in onset and slowly progressive. Any of these symptoms may appear by themselves, depending on which particular type of abnormal physiology predominates.

The physical findings associated with COPD also tend to reflect the site and extent of predominating underlying structural abnormalities. Hyperinflated obstructed lungs empty relatively slowly. By contrast, patients with small, fibrotic, restricted lungs (such as seen in asbestos workers) have a shortened, rapid expiratory time.

Wheezing usually indicates bronchospasm and airway hyperreactivity, and often suggests airway obstruction that is reversible. Decreased breath sounds reflect reduced peripheral airflow due to destruction (as in emphysema). Tachypnea (rapid breathing), use of accessory respiratory muscles, and intercostal retraction (muscles between ribs suck in) indicate excessive work of breathing and respiratory distress.

Patients with emphysema who are in bronchospasm frequently want to sit up and lean forward to help in breathing. This position relaxes the accessory neck muscles and causes the diaphragm to be pushed upward and operate in a mechanically more efficient manner. Paradoxical breathing (loss of coordination between movements of the rib cage and abdomen, which normally rise and fall together during breathing) is a sign of impending respiratory failure. Severe hyperinflation forces the diaphragm to work under adverse conditions. The goal of therapy is to release the trapped air and prevent ventilatory failure due to inspiratory muscle fatigue.

**Assessment of pulmonary function.** Following the medical history and physical examination, the next step in diagnosis consists of objective measurements of air flow and lung volume. Spirometry testing is the most important way to measure the breathing capacity of the lungs. In this test, the patient blows into a machine (called a spirometer) as hard and as fast as possible. The machine measures both the expelled amount of air (called the vital capacity, VC) and the speed of expiration of the air (the forced expiratory volume in one second, $FEV_1$). Graphs based on age, sex, and height provide the most ideal comparisons between the patient and the normal population. All patients who have COPD should have spirometry testing on a regular basis.

It would be beneficial to screen all persons at risk for developing COPD (e.g., habitual cigarette smokers) by regular spirometric testing to detect mild abnormalities. The rationale is that severe disease might be prevented by smoking cessation and early treatment measures. Repeated spirometric testing following a bronchodilator should be obtained to determine presence of reversibility of airway obstruction and to provide guidance for rational therapy. An improvement in the $FEV_1$ following bronchodilator, suggests the presence of an asthmatic component in the COPD.

COPD is characteristically associated with hypoxemia (lack of oxygen in the blood) of varying severity and, in advanced stages, with hypercapnia (increased amount of carbon dioxide in the blood). Arterial blood oxygenation should be assessed in all patients with moderately severe airflow limitations at the time of initial evaluation and, subsequently, at appropriate intervals. A high blood count of red cells (secondary erythrocytosis) suggests low levels of oxygen in the blood and a need to evaluate the need for oxygen therapy. Electrocardiographic evidence of right ventricular enlargement of the heart suggests the presence of pulmonary hypertension and a need for measuring blood oxygen levels and possibly providing supplemental oxygen. An exercise test may be indicated when considering the need for oxygen therapy or when seeking other causes of disability in patients whose exercise tolerance seems out of proportion to the limitation of airflow.

## Management of Chronic Obstructive Pulmonary Disease

**Prevention.** Of primary importance is the avoidance of bronchial irritants, such as cigarette smoke and other environmental pollutants. Physicians recommend immunization against influenza and pneumococcus (a common bacterium causative of many exacerbations in patients with COPD) in all individuals with chronic respiratory disorders, particularly if they are over 60 years of age.

**Treatment.** The principle treatment for patients with COPD is the bronchodilators. These medications both decrease airway reactivity and reverse bronchospasm. They are given orally, by injection, or by aerosol inhalation. Used in recommended doses, these medications are relatively safe, although particular care should be used in elderly patients who have cardiovascular illness.

Physicians prescribe oxygen therapy in all patients who have documented low blood oxygen levels or clinical or electrocardiographic evidence of pulmonary hypertension and cor pulmonale (right heart enlargement and failure) or secondary erythrocytosis. Prognosis for patients with COPD with chronic hypoxemia (deficiency of oxygen) improves with an increase in the length of time oxygen is administered. One achieves the best results when oxygen is used 24 hours a day. Ambulatory patients can be provided with portable oxygen delivery systems (liquid or compressed gas). These devices also provide for home oxygen use.

## Home Care for COPD Patients

Health services should be provided to individuals and families in their homes for promoting, maintaining, and restoring health, or minimizing the effects of illness and disability. Home care includes medical and dental care, nursing, respiratory care, physical therapy, speech therapy, occupational therapy, social work, nutrition, homemaker services, home health assistance (aides), transportation, laboratory services, and medical equipment and supplies (American Thoracic Society, 1987).

The goals of home care are to:

1. Improve the quality of life by allowing patients with advanced disease to remain in their environment and be with family and friends.

2. Minimize or prevent complications that would require hospitalization.

3. Detect changes in physical and psychosocial status that indicate the need for changes in management.

4. Provide treatment for the patient's primary diagnosis and foster adherence to the therapeutic program.

5. Foster a positive and independent attitude.

Referral to an organized home health program is necessary for patients when there is doubt the medical care program can be carried out in the home. Reasons for this are a patient's lack of knowledge, motivation, adequate family caregivers, and severity of illness. The latter situation includes patients with repeated hospitalizations who need regular supervision for an indefinite period.

## Home Mechanical Ventilation

Patients with complex treatment programs, such as home ventilator care, also need supervision by a home health care agency. The care of tracheostomy ventilator-assisted patients in the hospital setting is extremely expensive; some of these patients can be managed safely in the home. Most prefer the home environment to living in a hospital. Now, the principle role for mechanical ventilation in the home is in the management of patients with respiratory failure in neuromuscular disease. Patients with severe COPD are rarely suitable candidates for mechanical ventilation at home because of complicated and frequently unstable medical problems. Management of these patients in the home is usually considered impractical and unsafe.

A very select group of patients with severe, stable COPD, who cannot maintain adequate gas exchange on their own may be candidates for home ventilation (American Thoracic Society, 1987). When ventilator support is discontinued, patients may experience increased dyspnea (shortness of breath). The quality of life and physical well-being of such patients may be improved with intermittent mechanical ventilatory support, rather than with continuous ventilation. These patients can use negative pressure ventilation at night. The long-term efficacy of this modality of ventilation has not been proven. More recently, intermittent positive pressure ventilation applied through a nasal mask or adaptors has been used with limited success in patients with COPD (Carrey, Gottfried, & Levy, 1990).

## Functional Limitations of Patients with COPD

**Respiratory impairment and disability.** Gaensler and Wright (1966) distinguished between the terms "impairment" and "disability" as these terms apply to a particular function. **Disability determination** consists of assessing a person's **capacity to function** in a specific manner and comparing this to the required level for a specific performance. Evaluation of "capacity" in this sense requires consideration of factors other than health, such as education and age. Failure to recognize that "capacity" involves more than just the person's medical impairment or physical abilities, can lead to misunderstanding between physicians and administrative agencies making decisions on disability.

By contrast, **impairment** implies that the capacity for a specific function has become less than the person previously possessed. Since the physician usually does not know the person's prior capacities to perform, comparisons are made to normal statistical figures. Due to the wide variation of capacities for most specific functions, lung function testing has greater accuracy for depicting **capacity** than for determining presence or absence of a precise degree of impairment (Gaensler & Wright, 1966). The rating of respiratory impairment falls within the province of a physician's expertise to quantitate. Determination of disability is an administrative and medical decision that requires consideration of many nonmedical as well as medical variables (American Thoracic Society, 1986).

## Rehabilitation of Patients with COPD

**Comprehensive care programs.** In chronic, progressive respiratory disorders, comprehensive care programs that use multidisciplinary treatment approaches to the various aspects of the disease achieve greater success (Belman, 1989). Comprehensive care programs believe their approach is more likely to be successful than intermittent and occasional patient-physician contact. Ample evidence shows patients participating in such programs experience improved well-being and a decrease in the number of subsequent hospitalizations. Several authors have described the key components of comprehensive care programs (Hodgkin, 1979; Hudson & Pierson, 1981; Lertzman & Cherniack, 1976; Petty, Nett & Fenegan, 1969):

1. Patient and family education.

2. Treatment of bronchospasm by bronchodilators or reduction in bronchial secretions.

3. Treatment of bronchial infections.

4. Treatment of right heart failure.

5. Oxygen therapy.

6. Chest physical therapy, including breathing technique training.

7. Exercise reconditioning.

8. Psychosocial management, including vocational rehabilitation.

The American College of Chest Physicians' Committee on Pulmonary Rehabilitation (Petty et al., 1969) defines pulmonary rehabilitation as follows: "An art of medical practice in which an individually tailored, multidisciplinary program is formulated, which through accurate diagnosis, therapy, emotional support, and education stabilizes or reverses both the physiopathology and psychopathology of pulmonary disease." Pulmonary rehabilitation attempts to return the patient to the highest possible functioning allowed by the pulmonary disability and overall life situation.

Based on the aforementioned description of COPD, the emphasis of the program is on setting realistic goals based on knowledge of the effect of impaired pulmonary function on exercise performance. Accurate assessment of the patient's capacity to improve is important both for the patient and for members of the rehabilitation team. This information is required for the rehabilitation program to succeed. Exercise training is the mainstay treatment in pulmonary rehabilitation, but there is no agreement on the best methods of exercise or the mechanisms by which patients can achieve improvements (Belman, 1989). Commonly used methods include use of a treadmill or stationary bicycle. Oxygen supplementation should be used by patients who become oxygen deficient with exercise. Patients sufficiently motivated to continue exercise programs over time usually show objective evidence of increased exercise tolerance.

**Breathing exercises.** These exercises improve respiratory muscle efficiency by increasing a patient's control of expiratory flow and respiratory rate. Improved respiratory efficiency decreases shortness of breath and occasionally improves exercise tolerance. Inspiratory resistance loading may improve tolerance to dyspnea and physical stress (Pardy & Leith, 1985). This is done by asking the patient to inhale several times during the day through a device which has an opening that can be progressively decreased in size. These exercises require motivation and cooperation by the patient. When performed regularly over several months, one usually can see evidence of increased inspiratory muscle endurance.

**Education.** The rehabilitation process includes a continuing program of education. Whenever possible, the patient must know the schedule of each medication and understand its purpose. Guidelines for clinical response in the hospital include improvements in signs, symptoms, lung function tests, and arterial blood gases. Criteria for hospital discharge depends on the patient's ability to improve functional work capacity and activities of daily living, and maintain self-care as much as possible.

**Pulmonary disability.** The antecedents of pulmonary disability due to COPD may be based either on reversible or reactive changes in the pulmonary system (as in asthma or bronchitis) or on nonreversible, anatomic, structural changes (as in emphysema). The consequences of these alternatives are dependent on three basic systems (Plummer, 1984):

1. The interaction of the patient and the physical environment.

2. Social interaction with those significant others and treating personnel in contact with the patient.

3. The transactional results of the varied interactions involved in the disability and the therapeutic interventions developed to help the patient and family cope.

Rehabilitation professionals are in a position to make a significant impact on the psychosocial aspects of pulmonary rehabilitation.

## Vocational and Rehabilitation Aspects of COPD

**Team approach.** Vocational rehabilitation of patients with COPD can be achieved through the effective participation of all members of a rehabilitation team. The character of the disease is such that some patients are subject to severe respiratory infections, frequently requiring hospitalization. This may result in a patient's inability to cope with regular employment. It causes a disruption of socioeconomic status that imposes a great psychological impact on the individual and the family, often leading to feelings of despair and uselessness. In many communities, these patients are not considered trainable for any vocation. Yet, a 5-year study at the Pulmonary Department at the Institute of Rehabilitation Medicine of New York University Medical Center, indicated a large number of individuals with COPD can be rehabilitated to self-care and some for work (Rusk, Haas, & Castillo, 1968).

The purpose of the medical rehabilitation program is to increase the patient's activity level to the optimum within physiological capabilities. Along with the medical team members are the occupational therapist, social worker, rehabilitation counselor, and job placement specialist. They are necessary for the complex task of restoring the patient to the fullest physical, emotional, social, economic, and vocational potential. There will be a better prognosis for a return to work if the rehabilitation counselor intervenes early. The ideal time to begin vocational exploration is when the physician is taking the psychosocial history, at a time when the patient is not in a respiratory crisis, and may still be able to return to previous employment.

At the inception of the total rehabilitation program, a patient is referred to the rehabilitation counselor for an interview and evaluation. The director of the chest rehabilitation service will recommend the physical activity that will be most suitable for the patient. The rehabilitation counselor is thus made aware of the patient's clinical status and work tolerance.

**Vocational factors.** Information is obtained from the patient regarding personal-social background and educational-vocational history. The vocational background is an important primary area of concentration; the counselor should detail it and include a transferable skills analysis, whenever appropriate. Vocational data to be explored in detail include: job titles of previous employment, dates of employment, salary, job duties, job satisfaction, and reason for termination of employment. The counselor also obtains information about military service and present means of support. An important factor is use of illegal drugs and alcohol. In addition, to help assess the degree of physical impairment and its relationship to daily activities and functional work capacity, the physician may ask the patient to answer a questionnaire, such as the one shown below.

## PATIENT QUESTIONNAIRE

*Please read the following statements carefully and then check all of the items that describe your condition best. Note: "Shortness of breath" refers to breathing trouble, difficulty in breathing, or trouble in catching your breath.*

a. ____ *Pretty much restricted to home; spend considerable time in bed or sitting in chair, and almost never go out because of shortness of breath.*

b. ____ *Shortness of breath during normal activities such as showering or dressing.*

c. ____ *Can do only certain kinds of work which do not require physical exertion (desk work, checker, time-keeper, etc.).*

d. ____ *No significant trouble or restriction because of shortness of breath in my normal every day activities.*

e. ____ *Do not require help from others for any of my normal activities, such as dressing, bathing, etc.*

f. ____ *Am short of breath even at rest.*

g. ____ *Probably am not capable of working in any regular employment because of my shortness of breath.*

h. ____ *Shortness of breath occurs only with severe exertion, such as running.*

i. ____ *Can walk several blocks at my own pace without shortness of breath, but cannot keep up with others my age.*

j. ____ *Need help from others in some of my normal daily activities such dressing, bathing, etc.*

k. ____ *Am employable in my regular job.*

l. ____ *Am pretty much restricted to home, but get out fairly frequently if someone takes me.*

m. ____ *Need help because of shortness of breath with almost all of my essential activities, such as dressing, bathing, preparing meals, etc.*

n. ____ *Have shortness of breath on almost any exertion, have to pause in climbing a flight of stairs, or walking a block or so, to catch my breath.*

o. ____ *Can take care of my personal needs such as dressing or bathing, but I have too much shortness of breath to participate in other activities such as going to church or synagogue, social activities, hobbies, working around the house, etc.*

p. ____ *Get short of breath on climbing one flight of stairs or walking up a hill, but not while walking on level ground.*

q. ____ *Do not require any help from others in any of the normal daily activities which I usually must carry out.*

The rehabilitation counselor is the coordinator between the different members of the rehabilitation team and serves as a liaison with community agencies. After discussion with the team, the counselor refers the patient to the appropriate professionals and agencies.

One may classify patients into four clinical and vocational rehabilitation groups (Hodgkin, 1979):

1. Those who can return to their previous work activity.

2. Those who should and can be retrained for more suitable work.

3. Those who can work only in sheltered employment.

4. Those who can only be trained for self-care.

Proper evaluation and categorization of the patient's capacities are essential to successful vocational rehabilitation (Gordon & Haas, 1955; Kass, Dyksterhuis, Rubin, & Patil, 1975; Lustig, Haas & Castillo, 1972; Miller, Taylor, & Pierce, 1963). Care should be exercised in selecting patients for vocational rehabilitation. Factors to consider include recent significant changes in lifestyle and evidence of rapid clinical deterioration, personality change, substance abuse, and psychological or social dysfunction. Whether a patient's cardiorespiratory reserve will enable a return to a previous job, on a full or part-time basis, is an important factor. If the patient's tolerance to work will require job modification, the rehabilitation counselor can help facilitate this process. Once a patient is physically rehabilitated, training in new vocational areas commensurate with educational level and decreased respiratory capacity may be needed. The training for a new job should take into account the current and future labor market.

**Sheltered or home employment.** Some patients can function only in sheltered employment or at home where special respiratory equipment is available. Occupational therapists, rehabilitation counselors, and job placement specialists can help find suitable settings for productive work. The occupational therapist can train those who are unable to care for their households or themselves in energy-saving methods. This will enable the patient to do some tasks, including housekeeping, shopping, and other activities of daily living with less dependence on others. These methods include (Hodgkin, 1981):

1. Perform activities slowly.

2. Avoid noxious fumes.

3. Avoid areas of excessive heat, cold, and humidity.

4. Plan ahead to decrease ambulation and minimize body movements.

5. Change activities frequently.

6. Spread activities that promote fatigue or dyspnea throughout the day.

7. Transport heavy objects using carts or tables with wheels.

8. Perform most work activities while sitting with a work surface (table) at hip level to minimize flexion and abduction.

9. Perform work activities while standing with the work surface (table) at a body level, minimizing trunk flexion or hyperextension.

10. Store utensils, tools, and similar devices in cabinets whose height minimizes active trunk flexion, hyperextension, and active flexion of the shoulder girdle.

11. Use electric appliances (can opener, mixer, electric knife) to eliminate or minimize manual performance of daily activities.

Several factors impede vocational rehabilitation. These may include age, psychosocial problems, severity of respiratory impairment, progression of disease, limitations in skills and abilities, and poor labor markets in certain fields.

## Case Study #1

Ms. Ann Jones, a 49 year-old married policewoman, was referred because of a persistent complaint of exertional dyspnea. Prior to becoming a policewoman, she received her Associate of Science degree in police science at a local community collge. She and her husband have raised two daughters, both of whom are currently attending a local state university. Her husband is also a police officer and is currently employed. The medical history of this condition began 7 years ago following an episode of pneumonia, which was treated with antibiotics. Ms. Jones complained of productive cough, fever, and rapid breathing at that time; subsequently, she noted exertional dyspnea while walking on level ground. She smoked cigarettes (1 pack per day for 25 years) until last year, stopped, and subsequently gained 25 pounds. Past medical history includes several previous episodes of bronchitis, pneumonia, and the flu. She denies allergies and cardiac disease. She has been a police officer for 17 years.

Physical examination revealed limited chest expansion and marked decrease in expiratory sounds throughout. Her resting pulse rate was 92 beats per minute. The rest of the examination was unremarkable.

Spirometry showed a forced vital capacity of 3.2L (90% predicted) and forced expiratory volume in one second for 2.3L (72% of the FVC). Lung volume subdivisions were slightly decreased. Arterial blood gases on room air showed a slightly reduced oxygen tension. During an exercise test, she was found to be inappropriately dyspneic on exertion, just as she stated. She hyperventilated inappropriately for the stress. The gas collection analysis during the exercise test also indicated a large dead space in the lungs, both during rest and exercise suggesting mismatching of ventilation and blood supply to the lungs (ventilation - perfusion mismatch), accounting for the decreased oxygen tension. In normal individuals, there should be little or no mismatching.

## Questions

1. Does this person have an identifiable medical condition?

2. Assign Ms. Jones a vocational profile, including age category, educational level, exertional and skill levels of work, occupationally significant characteristics, and skills.

3. Describe Ms. Jones' possible functional limitations as related to her job.

4. Should she attempt to continue working as a police officer?

5. If you recommend she continue her employment, what advice would you give her and her employer regarding reasonable accommodation, if any?

6. What alternative rehabilitation possibilities can be considered in her case? Pay attention to the use of transferable skills, if she has any.

# NEUROMUSCULAR DISEASES

## Introduction

Pulmonary complications occur commonly in patients with neuromuscular diseases. One may see respiratory failure or aspiration pneumonia. The end-stage neuromuscular patient is unable to adequately ventilate the lungs, made vulnerable not only by weakened muscles of respiration, but also by other recurrent respiratory complications. Less commonly, a patient with mild neuromuscular disease may suddenly deteriorate and have an acute respiratory crisis not associated with pneumonia, or have a sudden decline in strength. This event can be produced by relatively isolated diaphragmatic weakness or by a blunted central respiratory drive in association with weakening respiratory muscles.

Neuromuscular diseases are conveniently described depending on the part of the motor unit they affect. They can be categorized as (Ringel & Carrol, 1980):

1. Diseases of the anterior horn cell (neuronal disorders), such as spinal muscular atrophies, amyotrophic lateral sclerosis (Lou Gehrig's disease), and poliomyelitis.

2. Neuropathies due to metabolic, endocrine, toxic, hereditary, immunologic causes, and vitamin deficiency.

3. Diseases of the neuromuscular junction such as myasthenia gravis and botulism.

4. Muscle diseases (myopathies) such as muscular dystrophy, myotonic disorders, inflammatory myopathies (polymyositis, dermatomyositis), metabolic myopathies, and toxic myopathies (caused by alcohol and certain drugs).

## Clinical Features of Neuromuscular Disease

The following describes clinical and laboratory features of some representative conditions commonly associated with respiratory complications. Spinal cord injuries are discussed elsewhere in this book.

**Amyotrophic lateral sclerosis (ALS).** Amyotrophic lateral sclerosis is a progressive adult form of motor neuron disease. It is sporadic, with an annual incidence of 1-2 per 100,000 population and a 2:1 male predominance (Bobowick & Brody, 1973). Peak incidence occurs in the sixth decade of life. Amyotrophic lateral sclerosis usually begins with insidious wasting and weakness of one hand or leg. It typically involves muscles of the thumb or anterior tibial muscles, producing footdrop. Patients frequently note painful cramps as an early complaint, and fasciculations (synchronous contraction of muscle groups innervated by a single axon). Atrophy and weakness progress proximally, without sensory loss, involving the shoulder or hip girdle and the contralateral arm or leg. Difficulty in swallowing and aspiration pneumonia are frequent complications.

Despite profound involvement of cranial and spinal innervated muscles, respiratory symptoms are uncommon in ALS until very late in the progression of the disease. Patients and health care workers are frequently unaware of respiratory problems despite relatively severe ventilatory impairment. Occasionally, ALS patients initially seek medical attention due to respiratory insufficiency or even respiratory failure. Some patients develop coexistent aspiration, pulmonary emboli, or superimposed obstructive pulmonary disease. The cause of ALS remains unknown.

Treatment of ALS at this time is palliative. This includes measures of providing nutrition and prevention of aspiration. Vigorous chest physiotherapy is essential to prevent respiratory complications. For patients who desire, assisted ventilation can be provided, first at night, then on a full-time basis. All efforts should be made for psychosocial evaluation of the patient, significant others, and discharge resources; eventually, complete dependence on life support becomes the rule.

**Diseases of muscle (myopathies).** Myopathies are disorders of muscles in which there is no evidence of neural abnormality. They include the genetic dystrophies, congenital myopathies, myotonic disorders, periodic paralyses, glycogen and lipid storage diseases, inflammatory myopathies, and several endocrine or toxic disorders. In a myopathy, weakness is usually symmetrical, involves all four limbs, and is more prominent proximally (closer to the trunk rather than the distal parts of the extremities). Patients will have difficulty in raising their arms over their heads, climbing stairs, and getting out of seated positions.

Characteristic of the genetic dystrophies is progressive muscle weakness. The most common varieties include Duchenne's dystrophy, myotonic dystrophy, limb girdle dystrophy, fascioscapulohumeral dystrophy, and the progressive external ophthalmoplegias. Duchenne's dystrophy is a sex-linked recessive disease that begins in males between the ages of 3-5 years and is progressive, with death occurring before the age of 20. Proximal weakness, enlarged limb muscles (particularly in the lower extremities), tight heel cords, and marked elevation of serum enzymes occur. A deficiency of the protein, dystrophin, has recently been shown to be the probable cause of Duchenne's muscular dystrophy.

Myotonic dystrophy is a dominant, non-sex linked inherited disease. Symptoms include varying degrees of diffuse facial and extremity weakness, delayed relaxation of muscles (myotonia), cataracts, gonadal atrophy, ptosis (drooping eyelids), and frontal balding. Limb girdle dystrophy is recessively inherited and characterized by the slow development of proximal weakness of the shoulders and hips. It usually begins in the first two decades of life. In fascioscapulohumoral dystrophy, one sees slowly progressive weakness of the face, shoulders, and upper arms. As with other autosomal dominant disorders, there is considerable variability in the degree of impairment of patients; minimally affected family members often go undetected for years.

Studies of pulmonary function in myopathies are similar to other "restrictive" respiratory disorders. Rideau, Jankowski, and Grellet (1981) found vital capacity (VC) underwent characteristic ascending, plateau, and descending phases. VC during the plateau phase was the best prognosticator of life-span. Baydur, Gilgoff, Prentice, Carlson, and Fischer (1990) reported similar findings. Cough will be impaired if the expiratory muscles are weakened. Patients dependent on the use of wheelchairs for ambulation, regardless of diagnosis, develop serious postural problems, skeletal distortion, and general muscular atrophy. The progressive muscular weakness often involves the heart muscle, a problem which can lead to heart failure and rhythm disturbances.

**Poliomyelitis.** Poliomyelitis is an acute infectious viral disease. During the first half of the twentieth century, poliomyelitis was the major neuromuscular disease causing respiratory dysfunction in the Western world. In most patients, the acute polio infection does not cause paralysis. The end stage of the disease is characterized by paralysis and atrophy of muscles. The extent of muscle paralysis may range from minimal to widespread, involving muscles of the trunk and extremities.

Worldwide immunization with the Salk (1955) and Sabin (1960) vaccines, has made acute poliomyelitis a rare disease; epidemics of "infantile paralysis" will recur if the population at risk does not continue immunization. As many as 25% of cases of paralysis involved paralysis of respiratory muscles, requiring temporary use of assisted ventilation. Infrequently, patients would require permanent assisted ventilation if the damage to respiratory muscles was widespread.

While polio has declined rapidly, there remains a significant population of polio survivors capable of a full life span. Epidemiologists estimate there are 300,000 survivors of the disease. Approximately 40% of these survivors have experienced a reduction in function beyond the simple aging process, called post-polio syndrome (Speier, Owen, Knapp, & Canine, 1987). These patients experience significant difficulty with clinical and vocational management. The predicament of the post-polio survivor can serve as a rehabilitation model for other disabling conditions with similar pathology. The major examples are incomplete spinal cord injury (particularly quadriplegia), myelodysplasia, Guillain-Barré syndrome, and spinal muscle atrophy. Symptoms similar to those occurring in post-polio syndrome are occurring in these patients, including those of respiratory impairment and sleep apnea syndrome.

There are two dominant theories on the etiology of post-polio syndrome: (1) late failure of the motor neuron system due to the initial illness formed during the acute healing process (Wiechers, 1985); (2) muscle damage from accumulated strain by chronic overuse of a system previously weakened by the initial polio. The latter is a more likely etiology for the late effects of poliomyelitis. Bennett and Knowlton (1958) termed this "overworked weakness." The cause is imbalance between the available muscle force of the post-polio muscle and the functional demands of a normal life style. Clinical reports correlate strength loss with vigorous activity and weight gain (Perry, 1985). Chronic low grade pain, with periodic acute exacerbations, occurs as the result of the initial infection. These patients typically need to overextend themselves to accomplish activities of daily living and vocational duties.

The diagnosis of post-polio impairment depends on clinical findings. These include weakness, atrophy, and a limp. All are difficult to define in most of today's symptomatic polio survivors. Postural adaptations obscure potential limps. Having normal motor control, the polio survivor can gain function by substituting one muscle group for another. These substitutions are so subtle they escape all but the most experienced observer. As a result, post-polio patients often appear far less disabled than they are, having significant, but undetected functional limitations, including loss of respiratory function.

**Guillain-Barré syndrome.** Acute Guillain-Barré syndrome, or acute inflammatory radiculopathy, is a relatively symmetrical paralytic disease of unknown cause. It is the most common form of acquired demyelinating neuropathy encountered by pulmonologists, having an annual incidence of about one case per 100,000 (Schonberg, Hurwitz, Katona, Holman, & Bregman, 1981). Risk factors for Guillain-Barré syndrome include prior infections with certain viral agents and mycoplasma (a primitive microorganism without a cell wall). Other factors have included surgery and neoplasia, particularly Hodgkin's disease and lymphoma. The onset is subacute, with progression to maximum weakness within 2 weeks in over 50% of cases and within 4 weeks in over 90% (Asbury, 1981). Weakness is the major complaint, usually beginning symmetrically in the legs. Paralysis or weakness of the facial and extraocular muscles may develop. There may be variable sensory symptoms with numbness and tingling in a stocking-glove distribution.

Autonomic nervous system dysfunction is frequent, and may involve sympathetic and parasympathetic nervous system symptoms (bouts of hypertension, loss of sweating, arrhythmias, and loss of normal blood pressure response). Respiratory insufficiency requiring assisted ventilation occurs in 20-50% of cases (Kennedy, Danielson, Mulder, & Kurland, 1978). Early detection of respiratory impairment is important. The need for assisted ventilation is variable, with durations of up to 30 months reported. The average time on a respirator is approximately 2 months (Moore & Owen, 1981).

## Pathophysiology of Respiratory Muscle Weakness

The severe poliomyelitis epidemics of the early 1940s and 1950s made it necessary to have objective criteria for starting treatment with a respiratory aid and guiding subsequent weaning from the respirator (Dail & Affeldt, 1957; Ferris, Warren, & Beals, 1955). Vital capacity is reduced and it decreases regularly with progression of the disease. The decrease in vital capacity is attributed to weakness of respiratory muscles, decreased pulmonary and chest wall compliance, and patchy microatelectasis (micro-pulmonary tissue collapse). Such changes may explain why reductions in vital capacity are greater than anticipated for the degree of respiratory muscle weakness.

## Therapeutic Approaches to Respiratory Failure in Patients with Neuromuscular Disease

**Resting the respiratory muscles: assisted ventilation.** Currently, this is the best method to allow respiratory muscles to recover normal function. While this is a logical approach in acute respiratory failure, intermittent rest therapy with ventilation in patients with chronic respiratory failure has only recently regenerated interest, especially for use with people with neuromuscular disorders. This form of therapy was popular during the polio epidemics of the 1940s and 1950s. Mechanical ventilation dramatically reduces the oxygen cost of breathing in acutely fatiguing muscles. Assisted ventilation almost immediately and dramatically decreases perfusion to the respiratory muscles, allowing blood and energy supplies to be redirected to other vital tissues, which desperately need them.

Intermittent rest therapy in patients with chronic respiratory insufficiency has been successful when measured in terms of patient well-being. Patients note improved sleep, waking up refreshed and without morning headaches. They feel more alert during the day and can complete daytime tasks with less fatigue.

It is important for the rehabilitation counselor to be familiar with home care ventilation since thousands of patients with chronic respiratory failure return to the community. Some of these individuals seek re-entry into the job market.

Rochester and Martin (1985) have outlined the criteria for chronic respiratory muscle rest therapy; they and Hill (1986) have outlined types of ventilators used in rest therapy. These devices include:

1. Body (negative-pressure) ventilator
   a. Drinker tank respirator
   b. Cuirass (shell)
   c. Body wrap (fits like a poncho over the body with holes for the neck and wrists).

These devices are usually used at night or intermittently in patients with a variety of neuromuscular and chest wall disorders. Occasionally, they may be useful in patients with far-advanced chronic obstructive pulmonary disease. They have the advantage of not necessitating a tracheostomy and its attendant disadvantages. Muscles can rest enough to allow the patient to perform daytime activities of living.

2. Positive-pressure ventilation

This form of ventilation is recommended for patients who cannot be maintained on body ventilators (Rochester & Martin, 1985). The condition can be due to end-stage weakness, recurrent aspirations, sleep-disordered breathing, or severely abnormal respiratory mechanics, which cannot be overcome by negative-pressure ventilation. Positive-pressure ventilation is usually delivered through a tracheostomy. More recently, physicians have used a nasally applied device with some success to provide intermittent positive-pressure ventilation (Ellis, Bye, Bruderer, & Sullivan, 1987).

Because of potential complications of tracheostomies and the special care required to maintain them, a multidisciplinary approach is required to teach the patient and family management of the tracheostomy and the ventilator (Fischer & Prentice, 1982; O'Donohue et al., 1986). Those patients who choose this modality can maintain more independence and an improved quality of life at home. It is cost-effective compared to continuous hospitalization. Home care ventilation costs about 30% of hospitalization in a critical care unit (Fischer & Prentice, 1982).

**Ventilatory muscle training.** The inspiratory muscles can be trained to increase their endurance and strength. While promising in some areas, it remains limited in its success rate for two reasons. One is because of the need for persistent patient compliance; the second is because for a given disease, it is not clear whether respiratory muscle strength or endurance should be enhanced (Pardy & Leith, 1985).

1. Strength training - consists of repetitive daily maximum inspiratory and expiratory efforts held for several seconds. It can be effectively used in quadriplegia, COPD, cystic fibrosis, and tuberculosis. Some patients with muscular dystrophy and spinal muscular atrophy can use this methodology.

2. Endurance training - consists of maximum voluntary ventilation (MVV) or maximum sustained ventilation (MSV) maneuvers. Increasing MSV is its own measure of success. It has been used effectively in cystic fibrosis and COPD. Inspiratory resistive loading also increases endurance in patients with cystic fibrosis and quadriplegia.

3. Limb or whole body exercise - limited reports are available but these exercises appear to be effective in increasing the maximum voluntary ventilation (MVV) in COPD.

Cessation of respiratory training programs results in a return to pretraining testing values within about one week. Physicians generally do not recommend exercise of respiratory muscles in degenerative neuromuscular conditions such as polio, Guillain-Barré syndrome, and amyotrophic lateral sclerosis.

**Oxygen therapy in respiratory muscle fatigue.** Oxygen improves exercise performance by reversing or preventing the adverse effects of hypoxia on muscle energy metabolism. It reverses hypoxic pulmonary vasoconstriction and heart failure, in turn improving blood supply to the respiratory muscles (Rochester & Martin, 1985).

**Diaphragm pacing.** Physicians have used diaphragm pacing on a limited basis. It is used primarily in those conditions where conventional forms of respiratory support are undesirable or inadequate (Glenn & Sairenji, 1985).

**The role of nutrition in respiratory muscle fatigue.** The increased work of breathing associated with respiratory failure increases caloric demands that cannot be met, leading in turn to loss of muscle mass, strength, and endurance (Askanazi et al., 1982; Rochester, 1986). While refeeding is an important factor in the recovery of respiratory failure and muscle fatigue, consideration must be given to proper ratios of carbohydrate, protein, and fat. Several studies suggest appropriate nutritional support can successfully phase (wean) some patients from mechanical ventilation. In some studies, as many as 80% of patients on assisted ventilation were successfully phased when they received adequate nutritional support (Askanazi et al., 1982; Fraser, 1986; Kelsen, 1986; Rochester, 1986).

## Functional Limitations in Neuromuscular Disease

There are two levels of concern regarding disability in neuromuscular disease. First is the functional limitations imposed by the physical impairment and the substitutions required. The second concern is the discrepancy between functional ability and the functional demands of work. As defined earlier in the section on chronic obstructive pulmonary disease, the capacity to function requires consideration of multiple factors, including respiratory impairment, education, age, gender, economic circumstances, social environment, and energy requirements of a given occupation (American Thoracic Society, 1986; Gaensler & Wright, 1966). Two people with an identical respiratory impairment (based on lung function) will be differently affected in their life situations.

Breathing involves repetitive contraction of the diaphragm and accessory respiratory muscles. Fatigue and muscle pain in some neuromuscular disorders, such as in older poliomyelitis patients, are common symptoms cited by patients. Dyspnea (difficulty in breathing) is often a manifestation of respiratory muscle fatigue. Other physical problems of neuromuscular patients include progressive impairment of speech, scoliosis of the spine, and respiratory failure.

The question of the "quality of life" for ventilator-dependent patients has often been raised, usually by those with little or no direct experience with their long-term care (Fischer & Prentice, 1982). This problem is most often encountered with parents of the Duchenne's muscular dystrophy patient who is approaching respiratory decompensation (Gilgoff, Prentice, & Baydur, 1989). Yet, these young men adapt to a respirator and wheelchair more readily than most older patients.

By contrast, older patients with long-standing respiratory impairment, who are slowly developing respiratory failure and a need for assisted ventilation, require special delicacy and tact. For example, post-polio survivors have managed their care over the past 40 years with independence from health professionals, except in acute crises. When their margin of reserve has decreased, the specter of a tracheostomy recalls the dark days of the 1950s, when many of these people experienced emergency tracheostomies in iron lungs. Seeing many others around them dying, it is understandable when they resist the recommendation for a tracheostomy 30 years later, a recommendation that causes them to relive the experience. Many will accept a tank respirator to tide them through their illness. Nasally applied intermittent positive pressure ventilation is a more recent modality available to provide a noninvasive means of assisted ventilation in those patients with marginal respiratory function. Such modalities also can be helpful in patients with sleep apnea syndrome.

Sleep-disordered breathing often occurs in patients with symptoms of nocturnal insomnia, daytime somnolence, and elevated daytime arterial carbon dioxide tension levels. Sleep-disordered breathing also can be associated with psychological disturbances, such as anxiety, irritability, loss of concentration, and depression.

## Vocational Limitations in Neuromuscular Disease

Depending on the nature and extent of the paralysis, respiratory and global muscle involvement may result in an entire spectrum of vocational limitations. For patients with physical impairment, activities such as ambulation and employment present major challenges. Disability is reflected by fatigue from muscular overuse, a visible limp, slowness of gait or inability to walk, or dyspnea.

As with chronic obstructive pulmonary disease, shortness of breath can be assessed by a careful history. Such a history should include documentation of specific activities leading to shortness of breath, intensity, type, and duration of exercise causing these episodes, and time required for recovery. The physician should note the influence of circumstance and emotion, posture, unusual sensations, and variations of daily weather and seasonal changes. Other influencing factors should be recorded, such as the degree to which shortness of breath interferes with work or recreation, approximate date of onset, progression or regression in severity since onset, and whether shortness of breath occurs during rest (Gaensler & Wright, 1966).

Tests designed for direct measurement of "work capacity" are desirable in the evaluation of impairment or disability. Therapists use several graded exercise tests involving a treadmill or stationary bicycle. Gaensler and Wright (1966) have emphasized two problems in this regard. First, it is not usually possible to reproduce in the laboratory specific types of exertion required for various occupations, nor is it possible to mimic the duration of effort required for regular employment. The distress associated with work experienced by most patients with severe pulmonary impairment, including those with neuromuscular disorders, is related to several activities. These include prolonged duration of low level activity, no facilities for rest on the job, and the exertion, frustration, and discomfort experienced in travel to and from the job.

A second problem is motivation. Those persons desiring rehabilitation tend to perform to the best of their ability when asked to do graded exercise tests. By contrast, individuals claiming total disability or financial compensation may be less motivated to exercise to maximum potentials.

Among patient populations studied, polio survivors have the highest rate of employment (Danchin, 1989; De Vivo, Rutt, Stover, & Rine, 1987; Deyoe, 1972; El Ghatit, 1978; Hayward & Seaton, 1979). They are highly motivated to raise families and maintain full-time gainful employment. Many have attended college and received advanced degrees. Because of their personal experience, they often function as counselors, sometimes for other patients with neuromuscular diseases. Yet, because of the muscle overuse syndrome, they have had to curtail their daily activities and reduce employment hours, much to their distress. The situation in patients with more progressive neuromuscular disorders is usually more devastating because of near complete loss of muscle function and various other disturbances, resulting in severe limitations of function.

## Rehabilitation Potential in Neuromuscular Disease

Chest rehabilitation in neuromuscular disorders is basically geared to reduce or relieve hypoxemia (lack of oxygen in the blood) and hypercapnia (increased carbon dioxide in the blood), and to cope effectively with respiratory infection. Patients use their own resources as much as possible to achieve these goals. In all conditions, after hospital discharge, the patient practices the procedures and techniques adopted in the hospital.

All patients are prescribed thoracic expansion breathing exercises. Deep breathing exercises encourage inspiration of air and lung expansion. Patients who are hyperventilating require breathing exercises, such as diaphragmatic breathing and pursed lip breathing to help them achieve a slower and deeper breathing pattern. Since this breathing technique may increase the work of breathing, the goal is to balance the improvement in alveolar (pertaining to air cells of the lungs) ventilation against the patient's discomfort.

Reconditioning exercises, while important in patients with spinal cord injury, may present a problem in patients with motoneuron diseases and myopathies. Many feel muscle fatigue exacerbates further muscle tissue destruction and should be avoided. There is no effective method for determining the point at which fatigue from exercise is reached. Patients with progressively debilitating muscle disorders, such as poliomyelitis, need to limit their daily activities to what is most comfortable. They should not push themselves beyond their tolerance limits when conducting their occupations, leisure activities, or home life. If they already receive assisted ventilation, particularly at night, they need to add time on ventilation during the day.

Buchanan, LaBarbera, Roelofs, and Olson (1979) found 76% of families with children with Duchenne's muscular dystrophy identified psychological issues to be the major problem confronting them. In 1984, Madorsky, Radford, and Neumann highlighted psychosocial issues surrounding death and dying in this population. They found discrepancies in perceived services and needs in this area. The families and patients overwhelmingly desired more training, education, and support when approaching terminal issues. While only 22% of patients and 17% of parents reported having been offered counseling services, 74% of the clinic staff regarded these services as readily available.

To address these issues, Gilgoff, Prentice, and Baydur (1989) described the establishment of a special clinic to work with patients and families at the time of impending respiratory failure. This clinic combines the skills of a pulmonologist, a pediatrician, and a respiratory nurse specialist, with the support of physical, occupational, speech, and respiratory therapists, and a psychologist. The clinic has three objectives:

1. Educate the patient and the family.

2. Institute elective ventilation before the onset of acute respiratory failure to those patients who select this option, and provide ongoing support for these patients and their families.

3. Provide psychological support to those patients and family members when the wish is not to receive assisted ventilation.

For patients desiring mechanical ventilation, sequential following of the vital capacity and carbon dioxide levels provides a useful guide in predicting the need for mechanical ventilation before acute respiratory failure occurs. This allows respiratory support to be started early, making the transition to a respirator less stressful and preventing the occurrence of an emergency situation and lengthy hospitalization. Sharing information with patients and families allows them to formulate constructive life plans. In this way, the patient and family can become active members of the health care team, rather than solely relying on a medical bureaucracy.

## Case Study #2

Mr. Bernard Wexler is a 53 year-old pharmaceutical sales representative who has experienced progressively increasing fatigue and inappropriate dyspnea on exertion over the past 3-4 years. His wife works as a pharmacy technician. They require both incomes to support themselves and their three children. He has been able to continue his work as a sales representative for a pharmaceutical company, but is having trouble with the extensive driving on his sales route due to increasing fatigue and muscle aches, especially near the end of the work day. Prior to his work at the pharmaceutical company, he was an assistant manager in a retail store for 3 years. Before becoming an assistant manager, he was a men's clothing salesperson in the same store for several years.

According to his family, he has been hospitalized four times over the past two years for "breathing problems." One episode of respiratory failure required mechanical ventilation. Mr. Wexler has been on supplemental ventilation at home for two brief periods of time. Thus far, he has been able to take sick leave and use vacation time for the time off work due to illness.

This individual suffered poliomyelitis at the age of fourteen, when he required an iron lung for assisted ventilation. Subsequently, the ventilator was discontinued. Mr. Wexler has experienced some weakness of his arms and shoulders since then.

## Questions

1. What is the major symptom of an individual with post-polio syndrome? Does Mr. Wexler have just this symptom or does he also demonstrate symptoms present in other neuromuscular diseases?

2. Assign this person a vocational profile paying particular attention to the exertional levels and skill levels of present and former work.

3. Describe this individual's functional limitations.

4. Can Mr. Wexler attempt to continue working at his present job?

5. If you recommend continued employment, what advice would you give him and his employer regarding reasonable accommodation?

6. Suggest rehabilitation possibilities if Mr. Wexler cannot continue work in his former occupation. If possible, use transferable skills.

# REFERENCES

American Thoracic Society (1986). Evaluation of impairment/disability secondary to respiratory disorders. **American Review of Respiratory Diseases, 133**, 1205-1209.

American Thoracic Society (1987). Standards for the diagnosis and care of patients with chronic obstructive pulmonary disease (COPD) and asthma. **American Review of Respiratory Disease, 136**, 225-244.

Asbury, A.K. (1981). Diagnostic considerations in Guillain-Barré syndrome. **Annals of Neurology, 9**(suppl.), 1-5.

Askanazi, J., Weissman, C., Rosenbaum, C., Hyman, A.I., Milic-Emili, J., & Kinney, H.M. (1982). Nutrition and the respiratory system. **Critical Care Medicine, 10**, 163-172.

Baydur, A., Gilgoff, I., Prentice, W., Carlson, M., & Fischer, D.A. (1990). Decline in respiratory function and experience with long-term assisted ventilation in advanced Duchenne's muscular dystrophy. **Chest, 97**, 884-889.

Belman, M.J. (1989). Pulmonary rehabilitation. In G.L. Baum & E. Wolinsky (Eds.), **Textbook of pulmonary diseases** (4th ed., Vol. 2, pp. 1107-1121). Boston, MA: Little Brown.

Bennett, R.L., & Knowlton, G.C. (1958). Overwork weakness in partially denervated skeletal muscle. **Clinical Orthopaedics, 12**, 22-29.

Bobowick, A.R., & Brody, J.A. (1973). Epidemiology of motorneuron diseases. **New England Journal of Medicine, 288**, 1047-1055.

Buchanan, D., LaBarbera, C., Roelofs, R., & Olson, W. (1979). Reactions of families to children with Duchenne muscular dystrophy. **General Hospital Psychiatry, 1**, 262-268.

Carrey, Z., Gottfried, S., & Levy, R.D. (1990). Ventilatory muscle support in respiratory failure: Nasal positive pressure ventilation. **Chest, 97,** 150-158.

Dail, C.W., & Affeldt, J.E. (1957). Vital capacity as an index of respiratory muscle function. **Archives of Physical Medicine and Rehabilitation, 38,** 383-391.

Danchin, N. (1989). Work capacity after myocardial revascularization: Factors related to work resumption. **European Heart Journal, 9,** 44-47.

De Vivo, M.J., Rutt, R.D., Stover, S.T., & Rine, P.R. (1987). Employment after spinal cord injury. **Archives of Physical Medicine and Rehabilitation, 68,** 494-498.

Deyoe, F.S. (1972). Spinal cord injury: Long term follow-up of veterans. **Archives of Physical Medicine and Rehabilitation, 53,** 523-529.

El Ghatit, A.Z. (1978). Variables associated with obtaining and sustaining employment among spinal cord injured males: A follow-up of 760 veterans. **Journal of Chronic Disease, 31,** 363-369.

Ellis, E.R., Bye, P.T.P., Bruderer, J.W., & Sullivan, C. (1987). Treatment of respiratory failure during sleep in patients with neuromuscular disease: Positive-pressure ventilation through a nose mask. **American Review of Respiratory Disease, 135,** 148-152.

Ferris, B.G., Warren, A., & Beals, C.A. (1955). The vital capacity as a measure of the spontaneous breathing ability in poliomyelitis. **New England Journal of Medicine, 252,** 618-621.

Fischer, D.A., & Prentice, W.S. (1982). Feasibility of home care for certain respiratory-dependent restrictive or obstructive lung disease patients. **Chest, 82,** 739-743.

Fraser, I.M. (1986). Effects of refeeding on respiration and skeletal muscle function. In Nutrition and Respiratory Disease. **Clinics in Chest Medicine, 7,** 131-139.

Gaensler, E.A., & Wright, G.W. (1966). Evaluation of respiratory impairment. **Archives of Environmental Health, 12,** 146-189.

Gilgoff, I., Prentice, W. & Baydur, A. (1989). Patient and family participation in the management of respiratory failure in Duchenne's muscular dystrophy. **Chest, 95,** 519- 524.

Glenn, W.W.L., & Sairenji, H. (1985). Diaphragm pacing in the treatment of chronic ventilatory insufficiency. In C. Roussos & P.T. Macklem, **The thorax, part B, lung biology in health and disease** (Vol. 29, pp. 1407-1440). New York, NY: Marcel Dekker.

Gordon, E.E., & Haas, A. (1955). Energy cost during various physical activities in convalescing tuberculosis patients. **American Review of Tuberculosis, 71,** 722-731.

Hayward, M., & Seaton, D. (1979). Late sequlae of paralytic poliomyelitis: A clinical and electromyographic study. **Journal of Neurology, Neurosurgery, and Psychiatry, 42,** 117-122.

Hill, N.S. (1986). Clinical application of body ventilators. **Chest, 90,** 897-905.

Hodgkin, E. (1979). Chronic obstructive pulmonary disease. **Current concepts in diagnosis and comprehensive care.** Park Ridge, IL: American College of Chest Physicians.

Hodgkin, J.E. (1981). Pulmonary rehabilitation. In D.H. Simmons (Ed.), **Current pulmonology** (Vol. 3, pp. 361-380). New York, NY: Wiley.

Hudson, L.D., & Pierson, D.J. (1981). Comprehensive respiratory care for patients with chronic obstructive pulmonary disease. **Medical Clinics of North America, 65**, 629-645.

Kass, I., Dyksterhuis, J.E., Rubin, H., & Patil, K.D. (1975). Correlation of psycho-physiological variables with vocational rehabilitation; outcome in chronic obstructive pulmonary disease patients. **Chest, 67**, 433-440.

Kelsen, S.G. (1986). The effects of undernutrition on the respiratory muscles. In **Nutrition and Respiratory Disease: Clinics in Chest Medicine, 7**, 101-110.

Kennedy, R.H., Danielson, M.A., Mulder, D.W., & Kurland, L.T. (1978). Guillain-Barré syndrome: A 42-year epidemiologic and clinical study. **Mayo Clinic Proceedings, 53**, 93-99.

Lertzman, M.M., & Cherniack, R.M. (1976). Rehabilitation of patients with chronic obstructive pulmonary disease. **American Review of Respiratory Disease, 114**, 1145-1165.

Lustig, F., Haas, A., & Castillo, R. (1972). Clinical and rehabilitation regimen in patients with chronic obstructive pulmonary disease. **Archives of Physical Medicine and Rehabilitation, 53**, 315-322.

Madorsky, J.G.B., Radford, L.M., & Neumann, E.M. (1984). Psychosocial aspects of death and dying in Duchenne muscular dystrophy. **Archives of Physical Medicine and Rehabilitation, 65**, 79-82.

Miller, W.F., Taylor, H.F., & Pierce, A.K. (1963). Rehabilitation of the disabled patient with chronic obstructive pulmonary disease. **American Journal of Public Health, 53**(suppl), 18-24.

Moore, P., & Owen, J. (1981). Guillain-Barré syndrome: Incidence, management, and outcome of major complications. **Critical Care Medicine, 9**, 549-555.

O'Donohue, W.H., Giovannoni, R.M., Goldberg, A.I., Keens, T.G., Make, B.J., Plummer, A.L., & Prentice, W.S. (1986). Long-term mechanical ventilation. Guidelines for management in the home and at alternate community sites. Report of the Ad Hoc Committee, Respiratory Care Section, American College of Chest Physicians. **Chest, 90**, 1S-37S.

Pardy, R.L., & Leith, D.E. (1985). Ventilatory muscle training. In C.H. Roussos & P.T. Macklem (Eds.), **The thorax, part B, lung biology in health and disease** (Vol. 2, pp. 1353-1371). New York, NY: Marcel Dekker.

Perry, J. (1985). Normal and pathological gait. In **Atlas of orthotics: Biomechanical principles and applications** (2nd ed., pp. 76-111). St. Louis, MO: C.V. Mosby.

Petty, T.L., Nett, L.M., & Fenegan, M.M. (1969). A comprehensive care program for chronic airway obstruction: Methods and preliminary evaluation of symptomatic and functional improvement. **Annual Review of Internal Medicine, 70**, 1109-1120.

Plummer, J.K. (1984). Psychosocial factors in pulmonary rehabilitation. In J.A. O'Ryan & D.G. Burns (Eds.), **Pulmonary rehabilitation** (pp. 146-172). Chicago, IL: Year Book Medical Publishers.

Rideau, Y., Jankowski, L.W., & Grellet, I. (1981). Respiratory function in muscular dystrophy. **Muscle and Nerve, 4**, 155-164.

Ringel, S.R., & Carrol, J.E. (1980). Respiratory complications of neuromuscular disease. In W.J. Weiner (Ed.), **Respiratory dysfunction in neurologic disease** (pp. 113-156). Mt. Kisco, NY: Futura.

Rochester, D.F. (1986). Malnutrition and the respiratory muscles. In **Nutrition and Respiratory Disease: Clinics in Chest Medicine, 7**, 91-99.

Rochester, D.F., & Martin, L.L. (1985). Respiratory muscle rest. In C.H. Roussos & P.T. Macklem (Eds.), **The thorax, part B, lung biology in health and disease** (pp. 1303-1328). New York, NY: Marcel Dekker.

Rusk, H.A., Haas, A., & Castillo, R.M. (1968). Department of Pulmonary Services, Institute of Rehabilitation Medicine, New York University Medical Center. In **A pilot study to determine the feasibility of promoting the use of a systematized care program for patients with chronic obstructive pulmonary disease.** Social and Rehabilitation Services, Department of Health, Education and Welfare. Project RD-2571-G-67. Human Interaction Research Institute, Los Angeles, CA.

Schonberg, L.B., Hurwitz, E.S., Katona, P., Holman, R.C., & Bregman, D.J. (1981). Guillain-Barré syndrome: Its epidemiology and association with influenza vaccination. **Annals of Neurology, 9**(suppl), 31-38.

Speier, J.L., Owen, R.R., Knapp, M., & Canine, J.K. (1987). Occurrence of post-polio sequelae in an epidemic population. In L.S. Halstead & D.O. Weichers (Eds.), **Research and clinical aspects of the late effects of poliomyelitis** (pp. 39-48). White Plains, NY: March of Dimes Defects Foundation.

Wiechers, D.O. (1985). Pathophysiology and late changes of the motor unit after poliomyelitis. In L.S. Halstead & D.O. Wiechers (Eds.), **Late effects of poliomyelitis** (pp. 91-94). Miami, FL: Symposia Foundation.

## *About the Author*

Ahmet Baydur, M.D., F.A.C.P, F.C.C.P., is an Associate Professor of Clinical Medicine at the University of Southern California, School of Medicine in Los Angeles, California, and Director of the Chest Medicine Service at Rancho Los Amigos Medical Center, Downey, California.

# Chapter 21

# CARDIOVASCULAR DISEASE

by
*John Johnson, M.D.*
*and*
*James Getzen, M.D.*

## INTRODUCTION

The purpose of this chapter is to assist the rehabilitation counselor to understand medical evaluations regarding the degree of impairment to the cardiovascular system. This is viewed in relationship to an individual's ability to perform activities of daily living, particularly in reference to independence and employment. This chapter reviews the major causes of heart disease, with particular attention to the incidence affecting various age groups, and the functional limitations and rehabilitation potential resulting from cardiovascular disease.

Several main categories of commonly encountered heart abnormalities and diseases, their causes, and the resulting complications are discussed. Reference is made to the methods of evaluating the severity of these problems. The authors discuss various levels of cardiac performance and their relationship to respective types of employment. A principle direction of this chapter is a discussion of the cause, symptomatology, pathology, and evaluation of physical abilities of persons with coronary disease. Increasingly, the direction of medical studies and treatment focus is on determining the principle course of coronary artery disease in the employed population. Modern research is directed toward preventing and decreasing the progression of this disease, with the goal of increasing longevity and improving the quality of life.

With the application of this knowledge, the survival time of persons with cardiovascular disease continues to increase. Thus, it is likely the need for vocational rehabilitation intervention will increase yearly to keep up with medical advances and prolonged life expectancy. The rehabilitation counselor's challenge is to assist this growing population to remain vocationally competitive and productive.

Heart disease is a leading cause of death in the United States. Approximately 1.5 million heart attacks occur in the United States each year; about 50% of these individuals survive. One-third of the 1.5 million are under 65 years of age and are potential recipients of vocational rehabilitation (Braunwald, 1988).

This chapter reviews the following general types of heart conditions:

1)      congenital heart disease in the adult
2)      valvular heart disease
3)      mitral valve prolapse
4)      myocardiopathies

5)      hypertension and hypertensive heart disease
6)      coronary artery disease
7)      congestive heart failure

In the first five groups (i.e., congenital, valvular, mitral valve prolapse, myocardiopathies, and hypertensive heart disease), there is heart strain or progressive heart muscle failure that eventually may develop into congestive heart failure. In all groups, employability is dependent on a timely diagnosis, the potential of correcting or improving the disease process, anatomical abnormalities, and the provision of rehabilitation services.

In coronary artery disease, which represents the largest category, there is progressive inability of the heart muscle to function properly, primarily due to decreased blood flow. As coronary artery disease progresses, it affects other areas of the heart as well (i.e., neurological control of the heart beat). After a given quantity of muscle mass has been destroyed, the heart may develop pump failure or congestive heart failure, resulting in an inability of function. There are many ways of evaluating and testing for coronary artery disease; these methods are discussed in this chapter. Not all the medical and laboratory tests discussed are necessary to determine work capability of an individual; the physician estimates functional ability through an evaluation of test results and clinical judgment (Andredoli, Carpenter, Plum, & Smith, 1990; Braunwald, 1988).

# FUNCTIONAL AND THERAPEUTIC CLASSIFICATIONS OF HEART DISEASE

The following discussion refers to the functional capacity of the heart and is adapted from criteria described by the New York Heart Association (see Figure 1). Physicians and researchers accept this protocol nationally as the standard for classification of cardiac conditions. Described in two sections, both classifications are evaluated concurrently in order to derive a cardiac status determination (Criteria Committee of the New York Heart Association, 1964, 1973).

## Functional Classification

The "Functional Classification" is an estimate of a person's symptoms. It is described in four classes, I through IV (see Figure 1). Class I represents a person with no symptoms, while class IV represents a person who develops discomfort with any physical activity and has symptoms even at rest. Classes II and III describe symptoms in between these two extremes.

## Therapeutic Classification

The "Therapeutic Classification" reflects the amount of physical activity recommended. There are five classes describing extremes from Class A, representing those individuals with no physical activity restriction to those in Class E whose physical activity is almost totally restricted. Clearly, this information has serious and important implications for the rehabilitation counselor.

# Figure 1
## NEW YORK HEART ASSOCIATION CLASSIFICATIONS OF PATIENTS WITH HEART DISEASE

**Functional Class**

| | |
|---|---|
| Class I | Patients with heart disease who have no symptoms of any kind. Ordinary physical activity does not cause fatigue, palpitation, dyspnea, or anginal pain. |
| Class II | Patients who are comfortable at rest but have symptoms with ordinary physical activity. |
| Class III | Patients who are comfortable at rest but have symptoms with less than ordinary effort. |
| Class IV | Patients who have symptoms at rest. |

**Therapeutic Class**

The functional capacity of a patient does not always determine the optimal amount of physical activity. Accordingly, the therapeutic classification is a prescription for the amount of activity the physician believes wise in the individual case, considering all factors.

| | |
|---|---|
| Class A | Patients whose physical activity need not be restricted. |
| Class B | Patients whose ordinary activity need not be restricted, but who should be advised against severe activity. |
| Class C | Patients whose ordinary activity should be restricted. |
| Class D | Patients whose ordinary activity should be markedly restricted. |
| Class E | Patients who should be at complete rest in bed or in a chair. |

Adapted from **Diseases of the heart and blood vessels: Nomenclature and criteria for diagnosis (1973), (7th ed.)** by the Criteria Committee of the New York Heart Association, Boston, MA: Little, Brown. Reproduced with permission, copyright American Heart Association.

## Subclassifications

In addition, there are two subclassifications that counselors may encounter in medical records. Subclassification One, "potential heart disease," includes individuals who have no evident cardiac disease, but should be followed by periodic examinations because of the presence or history of an etiological factor that might cause heart disease. An example is diabetes mellitus.

Subclassification Two is termed "possible heart disease;" it applies to persons with symptoms or signs involving the heart but in whom diagnosis of cardiac disease is uncertain. This subclassification involves conditions such as mitral valve prolapse. There are many other specific subclassifications that researchers have developed including those for valvular heart disease, hypertensive heart disease, cardiomyopathies, and coronary artery disease. These classifications, although helpful, are highly technical and specifically directed for the physician's use in the respective required therapeutic regimes and evaluation of permanent impairment (Engelbert, 1989).

## Documentation of Heart Problem

Common to all the classifications and subclassifications is the documentation of the type of heart problem, including date of onset, severity, causation, and rate of progress of the specific disease process. Direct medical intervention and treatment of the primary condition, such as diabetes or hypertension, is designed to prevent or minimize the secondary cardiac disease process. In general, medical treatment of the specific heart problem attempts to reduce abnormal heart beats, control heart rate, improve the strength and quality of the heart beat, and reduce blood pressure. These measures will result in maintaining the stabilization of the person's condition, improvement of well being, and ultimately in increased work capacity (DeBusk, 1982).

# CONGENITAL HEART DISEASE IN ADULT LIFE

Congenital heart disease is a condition caused by various malformations of the heart, which develop during gestation, and become apparent during infancy or childhood. Many congenital heart problems are of such a critical nature that they require varying types of surgical or manipulative procedures to improve the cardiovascular anatomy and function. Not all untreated individuals have residual problems; however, many who live into adulthood will develop serious problems that may require intervention to improve or correct the abnormalities. Early adult heart failure is a common and major problem in this group and necessitates aggressive treatment and evaluation to determine the functional limitations and work restrictions. The rehabilitation counselor needs to have knowledge of these limitations when attempting to return someone to employment.

# VALVULAR HEART DISEASE

In the adult population under 65 years of age, valvular heart disease is usually a result of rheumatic fever that typically occurred in childhood. Rheumatic fever in the United States, once a devastating disease, has become rare, especially in warmer climates. It was more common in the early part of the twentieth century. Improved understanding in prevention and antibiotic treatment has reduced not only the incidence and recurrence rate, but the severity and frequency of this disease. The importance of rheumatic heart disease as a cause of permanent disability has markedly lessened in the past 30 years.

Rheumatic valvular disease, one of the chief complications of this disease process, may become symptomatic between the middle teens and mid-30s, depending, in large part, on the severity of the original acute process. Although acute rheumatic fever also leads to acute myocardiopathy (abnormal changes in the heart muscle), the disease causes damage to the heart valves, including the mitral valve, the aortic valve, and the tricuspid valve, in this order (see Figure 2). The mitral and aortic valves may become stenotic (constricted or narrowed), insufficient (the valve leafs do not come together, thus allowing leakage), or a combination of both. The tricuspid valve is not subject to stenosis, yet, it can become insufficient. The greater the number of valves affected, the sooner the individual will develop heart failure, and the more severe the failure (Braunwald, 1988; Schroeder, Krupp, Tierney, & McPhee, 1990).

In recent years, surgical replacement of diseased valves has improved to such a degree that most individuals with rheumatic valvular disease can hold jobs not requiring heavy work or exposure to trauma. Many individuals have had prosthetic heart valve replacement. Individuals with valve replacement require medication to prevent abnormal blood clotting. One commonly prescribed preparation for this condition is Coumadin (warfarin sodium). Individuals on this and similar medications may bruise easily and should not work in areas where physical trauma may occur.

Today, there are an increasing variety of types of valve prostheses available. Surgery, performed early in the disease process, often enables the person to lead a near normal life.

# MITRAL VALVE PROLAPSE

In recent years, there has been an increase in the diagnosis of mitral valve prolapse and mucous degeneration of either the mitral or tricuspid valve. Neither of these conditions are related to rheumatic fever; researchers have not determined the exact cause. Possible causes are an undetected congenital defect or a viral infection with inflammation of the heart that historically occurred without symptoms at some time in the individual's life.

## Figure 2
## THE HUMAN HEART

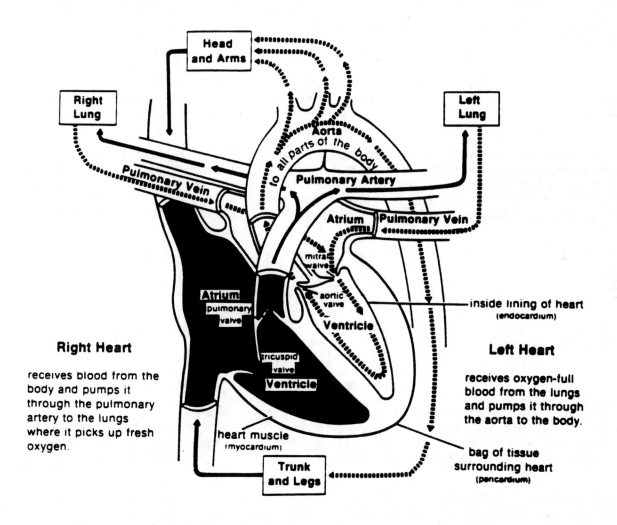

**Right Heart**

receives blood from the body and pumps it through the pulmonary artery to the lungs where it picks up fresh oxygen.

**Left Heart**

receives oxygen-full blood from the lungs and pumps it through the aorta to the body.

The symptoms of mitral valve prolapse may present in various ways. Frequently, the finding of a simple asymptomatic extra heart sound may arouse the suspicion of the examining physician. This condition is also known as the systolic click murmur syndrome, because the physician frequently hears a clicking sound on the chest wall over the mitral valve area of the heart. It may also be accompanied by a degeneration of the valve musculature known as mucous degeneration. In some cases, this mucous degeneration also may affect the tricuspid valve. When both mitral and tricuspid valves are diseased, the person will develop cardiac insufficiency, which progresses into heart failure. The mitral valve is the valve between the left atrium and left ventricle; the tricuspid valve rests between the right atrium and the right ventricle (see Figure 2).

An important symptom and complication of mitral valve prolapse is the occurrence of arrhythmias (abnormal rhythms of the heart). The arrhythmias may vary from occasional extra heart beats to episodes of ventricular tachycardia (rapid heart beat), or in rare cases, complete heart block. Although mitral valve prolapse occurs in both men and women, it is more frequently diagnosed in 20-30 year-old women. Neither mitral valve prolapse nor mucous degeneration of the mitral or tricuspid valve have a definite etiology (cause). Congenital weakness of the supporting tissues in the heart is one theory, especially for mitral valve prolapse, and virus myocarditis (inflammation of the heart musculature) has been suspected for mucous degeneration.

In individuals with mitral valve insufficiency without a definite history of rheumatic fever, one must suspect the presence of mitral valve prolapse and mucous degeneration. The sudden appearance of arrhythmias and mitral valve prolapse seen on echocardiography easily establishes such a diagnosis. Mitral valve prolapse is treated symptomatically for the arrhythmias and for congestive heart failure, if it should occur. Valvular replacement is usually not indicated, but in the occasional case of severe insufficiency with heart failure, this procedure may be life saving.

Most individuals with mitral valve prolapse under control, have no difficulty in carrying out normal physical work requirements, except heavy lifting and carrying of heavy objects. Mucous degeneration of the mitral valve, and possibly the tricuspid valve, is a more progressive disease than mitral valve prolapse. In this disease, valvular replacement is the rule for both the mitral or tricuspid valve; unfortunately, the long term results of surgery have been disappointing. These individuals are restricted to light or sedentary work (Andredoli et al., 1990; Schroeder et al., 1990).


# MYOCARDIOPATHIES


## *Medical Implications*


This group of diseases involves an inflammation and resulting weakness within the heart muscle. Myocardiopathies are secondary to infectious processes or chemical toxic exposure, as well as part of the disease process of diabetes mellitus. Virus myocardiopathies are more frequently found in younger persons. The virus causes inflammation and weakness of the heart muscle and sometimes interferes with normal nerve conduction throughout the heart. During the acute phase, individuals may need hospitalization and intensive care for stabilization. They may also require short-term medication or, in the more serious cases, a pacemaker for cardiac irregularities.

Some of these individuals, even after the acute phase has passed, experience arrhythmias in the form of extra heart beats and require medication for control. Others may require medication to support the myocardium (the muscle layer of the heart). For this purpose, the physician often prescribes a digitalis preparation. In most cases, after the acute stage has passed, the person can continue in customary work requirements, with the exception of heavy lifting and arduous labor.

**Diphtheria and typhoid fever.** Diphtheria and typhoid epidemics occur throughout the world and both diseases may cause severe myocarditis. In these cases, some individuals may have arrhythmias and develop symptoms of congestive heart failure. Diphtheria is a preventable disease that rarely occurs in the United States, due to wide spread immunization programs. Typhoid fever is not common in the United States except in some southern states; there are immunizing preparations available if disease outbreaks occur.

Large numbers of non-immunized persons facilitate the spread of these diseases, especially of diphtheria, and increase the severity and the propensity of complications, such as myocarditis. Contamination of water and food may lead to multiple or widespread numbers of typhoid cases. Most cases of myocarditis caused by either diphtheria or typhoid fever are severe and require prolonged periods of recovery and reconditioning. After recovery, these individuals are usually limited to light and sedentary work activity.

**Diabetes mellitus.** If less than optimally controlled, diabetes may cause complications resulting in poor function of one or more organs of the body. Poorly controlled diabetes may directly bring about cardiac muscle disease resulting in progressive, congestive heart failure. The individual with diabetes needs regular medical supervision and should maintain as normal a blood glucose and body weight as possible. Maintaining a proper diet is essential. Although diabetic myocardiopathy is not 100% preventable, the probability and severity can be favorably modified by proper medical care. The diagnosis of a myocardiopathy usually requires restriction to light or sedentary work.

**Alcoholic myocarditis.** Alcoholic myocardiopathy (cardiac muscle inflammation and weakness) is brought about by the toxic effects of alcohol and partially by poor nutrition. Proper medical care for the alcoholic and complete abstinence from alcohol is mandatory in order to reduce the severity of the myocarditis (inflammation of the myocardium). Once developed, the pathology of alcoholic myocarditis cannot be improved by treatment and is not curable. General improvement in body health and functioning is the goal of alcohol rehabilitation programs. This requires abstinence from alcohol, good nutrition, and treatment of secondary complications. Every effort should be made to provide and maintain an ongoing therapeutic prevention program, such as Alcoholics Anonymous (AA).

Medical care of myocarditis due to alcoholism is of limited success; therefore, treatment is directed toward secondary problems, including any presenting arrhythmias. In this condition, the alcohol directly affects the heart muscle. The physical level of exertion on the job is critical and requires ongoing monitoring by a physician.

**Surgery.** Surgical intervention, especially if valvular heart disease is present, may improve residual work capacity. However, when an individual has had prolonged strain on the heart muscle, valvular replacement may serve to improve cardiac function, but not necessarily improve the condition of the deteriorated myocardium.

## Psychological Implications

The psychological status of the person with heart disease must always be taken into account (Moss, 1980; Siegrist, 1985; Steptoe, 1981). Individuals may experience a sudden emotional shock when they find themselves restricted and unable to carry out their usual and customary activities.

Emotional complications and stress apply particularly to the individual who develops an infectious-type myocardiopathy or develops congestive heart failure following valvular heart disease and, of course, to those individuals who experience an acute myocardial infarction. Various symptoms of a psychological nature may occur, but the most frequently encountered are fear, anxiety, and depression. The reason for these symptoms is understandable since not only has the individual lost the ability to perform physical tasks, but also the ability to care for family. Obviously, if the acute process is short-lived and recovery is rapid and complete, psychological symptoms tend to dissipate. However, in complicated cases requiring prolonged care due to difficult recovery, the depression is intensified, and the individual may require psychiatric consultation and care.

Another major psychological manifestation is the fear of dying from complications because of a previous or an anticipated future heart attack. This fear may be the result of individuals not realizing their potential capabilities once the acute process has subsided. When this fear becomes immobilizing, it is called "cardiac neurosis"; psychological counseling may help resolve fears and diminish anxiety. Cardiac rehabilitation programs are available in most medical institutions. These programs focus on the preventon of this type of immobilizing reaction.

Today, treatment emphasizes early ambulation and involvement of the individual in a cardiac rehabilitation program as a preventive measure to help avoid this type of immobilizing reaction. With modern advances in technology and medical treatment along with rehabilitation intervention, one can often prevent symptoms of psychological distress. As a result of this treatment approach, most clients regain their strength and functional capacity to return to gainful employment (DeBusk, 1975, 1982; Ellestad, 1986).

# HYPERTENSION

During the normal heart cycle, the action of the heart may be compared to that of a hydraulic pump. When the heart muscle contracts, it propels blood out of the heart chambers. This forceful action is called systole. The pressure is high during the expulsive phase as compared to the phase immediately following, when the heart muscle is at rest. Physicians call this phase diastole. Blood pressure is usually expressed as a fraction, with the systolic pressure written on top and the diastolic pressure written on the bottom (Example, $^{120}/_{80}$ = $^{systolic}/_{diastolic}$). Diastolic pressure represents blood pressure when the heart is at rest. Elevated diastolic blood pressure usually indicates a more serious condition than elevated systolic pressure.

## Definitions

A systolic pressure greater than 140 mm Hg (mercury) and a diastolic pressure greater than 90 mm Hg is usually considered hypertension. There are three classifications of hypertension:

1) Mild hypertension is based on a diastolic blood pressure reading between 90-104 mm of Hg.

2) Moderate hypertension involves a diastolic pressure between 105-114 mm of Hg.

3) Severe hypertension is present when diastolic pressure is greater than 114 mm of Hg.

## Causes of Hypertension

There is no known cause for hypertension in 95% of people that have it. When there is no known specific cause for hypertension, it is called "essential" hypertension. A definite cause of hypertension can be ascertained in only 5% of the hypertensive population and is termed "secondary" hypertension. Secondary hypertension may be related to kidney disease, endocrine abnormalities, increased cardiac output, or vascular abnormalities. Many "secondary" cases of hypertension benefit from surgical intervention or specific medical regimens.

In addition, the factor of heredity has been an important one in hypertension. There has also been familial correlations to blood pressure levels which researchers believe are related to a genetic factor.

## Detection of Hypertension

A person's medical history may be entirely uneventful (no symptoms or complaints) until symptoms of a complication develop. These may represent complications of the specific areas of the system involved and may include coronary artery disease, cardiovascular renal failure, cerebral vascular accident, or peripheral vascular disease. In some cases, commonly encountered nonspecific complaints such as fatigue, headache, nosebleed, change in vision, or muscle weakness may be present.

Physical examination includes functional assessment for any abnormality of the hypertensive person's kidneys, heart, and cerebral vascular system. Physicians evaluate kidney function by urinalysis and blood laboratory studies. Chest x-ray, electrocardiogram, and echocardiogram are used in the assessment of cardiac status. If hypertension is thought to be associated with coronary artery disease, the physician may conduct cardiac stress testing to clarify the diagnosis.

The funduscopic examination (examination of the retina of both eyes) may give clues as to any cerebral vascular changes, which usually denote the severity of the hypertension. In conjunction with the eye examination, the person needs a complete neurological evaluation to determine the functional status of the central nervous system.

## Complications

When complications of hypertension develop, the arterial vessels supplying the brain, heart, kidneys, and general vascular circulation may be involved. In the central nervous system, these complications manifest themselves with symptoms characteristic of strokes or transient ischemic attacks (TIAs) due to lack of blood supply to the brain. Persons with long-standing hypertension may develop symptoms of heart disease due to coronary artery disease or congestive heart failure.

Hypertension may cause significant renal damage leading to renal failure; this damage contributes to the further perpetuation of the hypertensive problems. Peripheral vascular disease is frequently associated with hypertension and is a major cause of disability requiring ongoing treatment. This complication causes pain in the lower extremities, brought on by exercise, such as walking (referred to as claudication) due to diminished blood flow in the legs (Braunwald, 1988).

**Assessment for physical activity in persons with hypertension.** The diagnosis of hypertension dictates a clinical assessment to detect the presence of any other systemic complications. Individuals with uncontrolled hypertension need to reduce physical activity until the blood pressure is brought down to safe levels. The physician will evaluate physical activity levels and suggest modifications, depending on the presence of complications (DeBusk, 1975). The physical limitations experienced with hypertension are primarily the symptoms resulting from coronary artery disease, stroke, and renal failure. Each of these conditions has specific guidelines as to physical disability and resulting levels of activity. Most of the physical limitations are associated with complications of hypertension, rather than the hypertension itself.

In persons with hypertension who do not have subjective complaints or physical limitations, appropriate restrictions related to diet and activity are preventive measures to avoid future complications. The physician will prescribe medication for persons with persistent hypertension to control the elevated blood pressure.

The diet should emphasize both salt restriction and weight reduction. The results of exercise stress testing will help the physician recommend appropriate physical activity. With mild to moderate hypertension, customary work conditions may be adequately tolerated, but must be modified for those persons who have severe hypertension (Goldman, Hashimoto, Cook, & Loscalzo, 1981).

The level of disability of individuals with hypertension is related to the presence and severity of complications. Persons responsive to treatment may be able to continue usual and customary work activities. Vocational retraining is of utmost importance in patients with hypertension who are under adequate medical control and without major systemic complications, but are unable to perform their usual and customary job. In spite of the diagnosis of hypertension, most patients continue leading productive lives with no serious limitations in work activity, recreation, or life style.

# CORONARY ARTERY DISEASE

Coronary artery disease is the leading cause of death in the United States. Approximately 1.5 million heart attacks occur per year in the United States with more than 700,000 resulting in death (Braunwald, 1988). In addition, many people have coronary artery disease not associated with myocardial infarction; yet, these conditions still lead to major problems and disability, causing restriction in occupational activities. These problems are important to rehabilitation counselors since they are occurring with greater frequency in people under 65 years of age.

## *Etiology*

Risk factors for coronary artery disease include a high blood cholesterol level, hypertension, diabetes, emotional stress, obesity, and cigarette smoking. However, these risk factors do not imply a direct causal relationship. Of the risk factors mentioned above, the most significant are plasma cholesterol elevation, cigarette smoking, and elevated blood pressure. High blood cholesterol eventually leads to an accumulation of plaque in the coronary vessels, restricting blood flow. Nicotine from cigarette smoking also restricts blood flow by constricting the vessel walls during smoking.

## *Manifestations of Coronary Artery Disease*

Coronary artery disease leads to myocardial anoxia (lack of oxygen to the heart muscle), due to diminished or absent blood flow. When this occurs, the person may experience chest pain (angina pectoris). This disease may affect the myocardium and the nerve conducting pathways, causing abnormal nerve conduction resulting in irregular heart beats (arrhythmias) or ventricular fibrillation (rapid ineffective pulsations of the heart). When this occurs, the heart muscle suffers a lack of oxygen; if the condition persists, the affected myocardium will die (myocardial infarction).

Persistent arrhythmias may lead to an inefficient pumping function of the heart. When this happens, fluids in the body do not flow properly, thus leading to congestion. This condition is known as congestive heart failure and constitutes a medical emergency.

The four major clinical signs and effects of coronary artery disease are angina pectoris, myocardial infarction, associated arrhythmias, and congestive heart failure. Angina pectoris is a symptom consisting of chest pain, pressure, or vague aching sensations that usually radiate into the neck, jaw, shoulders, or arms. This is usually precipitated by physical activity and often relieved by rest or cessation of the specific physical activity. The discomfort may last from a few seconds to several minutes, but also may be a forerunner of a myocardial infarction (Braunwald, 1988; Schroeder et al., 1990).

## *Myocardial Infarction*

A heart attack occurs when a coronary artery becomes partially or completely occluded by an accumulation of cholesterol, usually associated with a clot in the area of vessel narrowing. This clot develops suddenly at the site of narrowing in the artery. Arterial narrowing also may occur as the result of spasm of the involved artery. The same mechanism may account for an occlusion by any foreign substance circulating in the blood.

Symptoms of a myocardial infarction usually begin with discomfort in the chest similar to angina pectoris. It is more severe and lasts longer than angina. Associated symptoms may include sweating, nausea, vomiting, weakness, shortness of breath, or unconsciousness. Unfortunately, in some cases, there are no warning signs, such as described above, and sudden death may be the only sign of the presence of coronary artery disease.

## Complications

Complications will develop in those who survive myocardial infarction. These include alterations in heart rhythm, incompetent heart valves, and defects in the heart muscle of the ventricles. When severe, these conditions lead to congestive heart failure.

## Treatment

Ideally, the patient is hospitalized as soon as possible when symptoms of myocardial infarction are suspected. When paramedics are called, most are instructed to initiate treatment with the administration of pain relieving medication, oxygen, and supportive measures. In the emergency room, a physician may administer a thrombolytic agent. These clot-dissolving medications are started as soon as possible after the heart attack is suspected, with the goal of improving blood flow in the affected artery. From the emergency room, the patient is admitted to the cardiac intensive care unit for observation. This level of treatment is required for monitoring purposes and to detect any complications of the myocardial infarction so that the hospital staff can initiate immediate and direct medical care.

After stabilization of the acute event and observation in a critical care hospital unit, the patient begins a program involving gradual increase in physical activity. This is started in the hospital and continued on an outpatient basis, often in a cardiac rehabilitation program. The program provides information on coronary artery disease to the patient including dietary management, proper exercise programs, information on medications, and assistance with stress reduction and smoking cessation (Fox & Naughton, 1970).

On-going treatment may involve a medical regimen and possible surgery. Medications are prescribed to control angina pectoris and arrhythmias. Nitroglycerine is a short-acting medication to relieve angina. A person also may take this medication before an activity, if it is assumed that the activity will cause chest pain. The treating physician will prescribe other medication to relieve arrhythmias and also help the body eliminate excess fluid.

Several surgical procedures are currently being used to correct narrowing or blockage of the coronary arteries. One of these, coronary angioplasty, involves the surgical insertion of a balloon-type device into a narrowed artery to flatten the occlusion and allow blood to flow more freely.

Today, the medical evaluation of coronary artery disease includes a coronary arteriogram. This procedure uses a radiopaque substance which is sensitive to x-ray. The cardiologist injects this substance by means of a catheter directly into the coronary vessels. By this means, the cardiologist is able to visualize blood flow restrictions, called stenosis. Stenosis is brought about by the deposition of cholesterol plaques within the coronary vessel walls. This condition is treatable today by means of bypass surgery. The procedure has been made possible as the result of modern technology. In this procedure, the surgeon removes a vein usually from the leg, and uses it to bypass the restricted (stenotic) coronary vessel. This procedure has been perfected to the point that persons do extremely well and are relatively pain free following surgery.

## Disability

The treating physician determines the extent of disability resulting from coronary artery disease by examination, carefully evaluating the data obtained from the medical history, objective testing, documentation, and the person's response to treatment. The historical information is correlated with the New York Heart Association (NYHA) Classifications (see Figure 1). This is helpful in determining the symptomatic as well as therapeutic classification of the person's status and in assessing ability to perform various activities.

The NYHA classification system has been used for the past 25 years and remains among the most helpful clinical determinants in establishing levels of cardiac disability. The physician utilizes these guidelines to classify the patient on both a functional and therapeutic level (see Figure 1).

The factors relating to disability are correlated with objective evaluations. These objective findings are related to the results of exercise testing on a treadmill and designed by several well-accepted scientific protocols. All protocols are presented in relationship to heart rate and blood pressure and are expressed in metabolic requirements. It is customary to estimate the energy cost of physical activity in terms of oxygen consumption required to accomplish a task. The basic metabolic unit for this estimation is called the MET. Studies have established the MET requirements for various activities, both occupational and recreational. All activities require a workload on the body. This workload is expressed in METS, which corresponds to the amount of oxygen required to perform the given task or activity.

The METS of achieved activity are correlated with each individual's level of activity. For example, a patient performs a Bruce Protocol exercise level of 9 minutes (on a treadmill). This individual could be expected to perform up to 10 METS activity, indicating the ability to perform mid-heavy to heavy activity by the New York Heart Association, Functional Class I and Therapeutic Class A.

The documentation MET requirement of coronary artery disease has been derived by subjecting the person to various levels of testing on a treadmill. Stress testing is the primary and the most informative test to determine functional capacity of the heart. There have been various programs to produce a level of stress on the cardiovascular system to establish a specific level of performance. The Bruce or Naughton treadmill tests are most often used to determine functional classification. Various test levels of performance have been correlated with levels of physical activity that relate to a variety of job performance (Braunwald, 1988).

The information obtained from the patient's history and objective data from stress treadmill testing and other laboratory and physical findings, are used to establish a classification of impairment and the patient's optimal level of activity. The extensive evaluations following the diagnosis of coronary artery disease are designed to help the individual establish a more meaningful and better quality of life. The goal of treatment is to decrease any existing impairment and improve functional capacity. Long-term therapy includes a well planned exercise and diet program.

The overall outlook on coronary artery disease is not only the immediate diagnosis and treatment of the person with cardiac disease. It is also to help the person establish a meaningful and productive life, understanding the cause, prevention, and corrective measures that will help attain a high quality of life and employment. This involves a lifelong commitment to the appropriate exercise and dietary program. The encouragement gained from an active exercise program and continuation of productive activity will help establish a secure self-esteem and a healthy psychological outlook.

# CONGESTIVE HEART FAILURE

Congestive heart failure is a term used to describe the end stage symptoms of deteriorated heart function occurring from various causes. It occurs as a result of cardiovascular disease. Because of impaired function, the heart must work harder to deliver a sufficient supply of blood to the body. The heart chambers enlarge (cardiac hypertrophy) and the muscle walls become thicker in an attempt to pump the needed blood. Symptoms include shortness of breath (dyspnea), edema (swelling) in the lower extremities, fatigue, weakness, and abdominal discomfort.

This disorder can occur suddenly due to a heart attack or over a period of years from one of the diseases previously discussed. With treatment of the underlying problem, improvement can occur. Medication relieves some of the symptoms.

Limitations of function depend on the severity of the condition and whether medical treatment alleviates the symptoms. Those individuals with mild congestive heart failure controlled by medication may be capable of their usual work, with some minimal modifications. Workers employed in physically arduous activity may need a change of employment. Counselors will most likely see individuals with moderate heart failure who will be limited to light or sedentary work. Those persons with severe conditions will have an extremely limited capacity for physical exertion and be poor candidates for most employment situations.

# FUNCTIONAL LIMITATIONS

## *Physical Limitations*

Most individuals, depending on the extent of their cardiovascular disease, can perform at least light work. Many will be able to engage in medium level work activity. Heavy lifting and carrying is usually contraindicated for persons with cardiovascular disease. The treating physician is the best resource for determination of physical exertion capacities. Activities such as standing and walking are usually beneficial for the individual with a cardiac condition. The physician will typically recommend physical exercise as part of the conditioning process.

Chest pain (angina pectoris) occurs in some persons who have cardiac disease. This may involve severe pain and constriction about the heart area and radiation of pain down the left arm. Angina is caused by an insufficient supply of blood to a portion of the heart and may be produced by physical overexertion. The pain is usually transitory and relieved by medication (nitroglycerine), taken orally, which dilates the arteries. The person may resume work activity, usually in a few minutes, but is cautioned to avoid the activity that precipitated the angina. Counseling an individual to avoid activities that lead to angina should help remind the person to eliminate the potential complication. The rehabilitation counselor needs to provide vocational guidance in accordance with the person's physical capabilities.

Some persons have arrhythmias and feel palpitations (throbbing sensations) in the chest area. These sensations may occur because of excessive physical activity; work that is within physical abilities may help minimize the occurrence of arrhythmias. In all cases, the counselor needs to discuss the client's compliance with prescribed medication.

The cardiovascular system is affected by extremes of temperature; this environmental factor needs to be avoided. Poor air quality also may adversely affect the person with cardiovascular disease. The counselor's awareness of this and other factors in the work environment can help promote success of the rehabilitation program.

## *Psychosocial Limitations*

The person that has had a heart attack and been hospitalized can benefit from early intervention by a rehabilitation counselor. The total experience of hospitalization, coupled with the separation from home and family, causes a high degree of emotional stress. Early intervention can decrease this stress, by helping the person cope and understand the condition in a more realistic manner. Early contact with the present employer may help facilitate a return to work (Streater & Erlandson, 1984). Socio-emotional support is a crucial resource in working effectively with persons who have had stressful experiences, such as heart attack (Siegrist, 1985). De Wolff (1985) discussed stress intervention at work at the organizational level and the importance of learning coping skills to deal effectively with work stressors.

As previously noted, fear, anxiety, and depression are common emotions felt by persons with cardiovascular disease. The impact can range from minimal to devastating. Thoughts of sudden death can debilitate a person, both socially and vocationally. Most persons have problems adjusting to chronic, serious medical conditions. Individuals who have not adjusted to disability may need emotional support and counseling to help them cope with anxiety and depression. Denial is a normal psychological defense often expressed as part of adjustment to disability. If denial causes the person to ignore symptoms, it may be dysfunctional and lead to the selection of an inappropriate rehabilitation plan.

Some persons do not comply with their medication regimen. Compliance may depend both on willingness and understanding to accurately take medications. Financial problems and attitudinal barriers may contribute to non-compliance; the counselor may need to intervene in this area (Falvo, 1991).

Discrimination in the workplace impedes return to work of some persons with cardiovascular disease. Education of employers concerning this and other disabling conditions helps reduce attitudinal barriers to employment of persons with disabilities. Recent legislation is intended to remove these attitudinal barriers and discriminatory practices.

# REHABILITATION POTENTIAL

Cardiac rehabilitation programs, through their multidisciplinary approach, have helped persons with cardiovascular problems increase performance in work and leisure activities. Improved functioning occurs not only in physical abilities, but also in the mental and social areas, and aids in producing an active and productive life. This treatment approach allow persons with cardiovascular problems to achieve increased awareness of the underlying condition, and to participate in exercise as a preventive and therapeutic measure. With the cardiac rehabilitation programs now available, individuals are able to increase strength and endurance and improve overall functioning. These treatment programs are designed to maximize improvement in physical and psychosocial functioning. The result is greater return of work potential and improved enjoyment of lifestyle.

Through an understanding of the various manifestations of cardiovascular disease, the counselor can enhance the rehabilitation potential of these clients. Many persons with cardiac problems do not understand their condition, its severity, or the functional limitations. Some refuse to regularly and consistently take prescribed medications. Denial may play a part in this, along with the misconception that a lack of symptoms means medications are no longer necessary.

The rehabilitation potential for persons with Functional Class I and Therapeutic Class A and B (see Figure 1) is excellent; these individuals should have no more than slight restrictions on physical exertion and activity. Most will not require rehabilitation counseling services. Rehabilitation counselors will most likely see persons with Functional Class II and III and Therapeutic Class C and D (occasionally Class B), who need modification of work activity. The degree of work adjustment needed will depend on the extent of cardiovascular disease and the physical and emotional components of the person's work activity. Individuals with Functional Class IV and Therapeutic Class E will, in all probability, lack potential for vocational rehabilitation.

Development of appropriate educational and vocational goals, consistent with the client's physical and emotional restrictions, is essential when working with persons who have cardiovascular conditions. Vocational rehabilitation may range from returning a person to the usual and customary job with the same employer, with little modification, to providing a new vocational objective with a different employer. The counselor familiar with the 1973 Rehabilitation Act and the 1990 Americans with Disabilities Act can help maximize a client's work potential.

Investigation of job modification through reasonable accommodation may help both employee and employer maintain a productive work situation. One needs to consider both physical and emotional stress factors of the employment situation. Physical factors are more easily defined than emotional components of a job. Counselors must make sure not to impose their personal assessment of emotional stress; each client will perceive stress in a different way. What is considered stressful for one individual may not be for another.

For persons disabled due to excessive fear, anxiety, or depression, psychological intervention may be needed. Without this treatment, potential for rehabilitation will be minimal. Other factors affecting rehabilitation potential include compliance to a medication regimen, appropriate diet, suitable exercise, and knowledge of the disease state.

Early rehabilitation intervention can help maintain motivation for return to work. The sooner the person receives vocational rehabilitation, the greater the chances for a successful outcome. Since there are frequently emotional factors associated with cardiovascular disease, early vocational intervention can help minimize negative reactions to this chronic disease. Once undue fear, anxiety, and depression develop, the rehabilitation counselor will have additional factors to surmount.

A final dimension to rehabilitation of persons with cardiovascular disease is employer discrimination. Rehabilitation counselors can help educate employers and dispel some of the negative stereotypes employers may have toward persons with cardiovascular problems. As stated by Yuker (1992), "employers value employees who have job skills, social skills, and dependability" (p. 17). Employers who have experience with employees who have disabilities usually have positive attitudes toward them. As more people with disabilities enter the labor force and prove to be good productive employees, we can expect positive attitude change on the part of the employers of these individuals. Counselors can play a crucial role in this process.

# CASE STUDY

Ms. Joyce Albert is 52 years old and currently married. Shortly after receiving her Master of Social Work (M.S.W.) degree, she became employed as a children's social services worker.

This client has multiple disabilities. One year ago, after being diagnosed with coronary artery disease, she had heart bypass surgery, which was considered successful. Joyce is not taking any cardiac medication. Also, she has been taking insulin for the past 10 years to control diabetes. The diabetes is under good control. Ms. Albert has mild to moderate anxiety and depression.

For the previous 9 years, Ms. Albert had been working as a self-employed photographer. Her work involves lifting and carrying up to 40 pounds of equipment. Much of her work involved traveling to different locations for special assignments.

Before becoming self-employed, Ms. Albert worked for various photographic studios, starting out as a photography assistant and working her way up to the level of photographer. She left each job within one year because she felt the manager was not satisfied with her work, although, on each occasion, the manager noted satisfaction with her abilities.

The first major job Ms. Albert had was as a children's social worker. After 2 years, she left the position believing the clients were never satisfied with her work. Yet, her supervisors rated her work as excellent. She then obtained employment as an eligibility worker, but resigned after one year because of a client's complaints. The supervisor told her complaints happened to all eligibility workers and unsuccessfully encouraged her to remain on the job. Following these 2 social work positions, she decided to leave the field and secured employment as a photography assistant.

Joyce Albert's medical restrictions include a maximum of light work, and maintaining good control of her diabetes. She needs to avoid excessive emotional stress.

## Questions

1. Provide a vocational profile for Ms. Albert, including age category, educational level, and work history (skill and exertional levels).

2. Briefly describe several types of cardiovascular disease as discussed in the chapter.

3. What are Ms. Albert's functional limitations that may affect employment?

4. Outline three possible rehabilitation plans for this client.

5. Are there any additional services that may help this individual return to work? Explain.

6. If a client has difficulty breathing and has swelling in the legs, what cardiovascular condition may be present? Identify possible implications.

## REFERENCES

American Heart Association (1979). **Your heart and how it works**. Dallas, TX: Author.

Andredoli, T.E., Carpenter, C.C.J., Plum, F., & Smith, L.H., Jr. (1990). **Cecil essential of medicine** (2nd ed.). Philadelphia, PA: Harcourt Brace Jovanovich.

Braunwald, E. (1988). **Heart disease: A textbook of cardiovascular medicine** (3rd ed.). Philadelphia, PA: W.B. Saunders.

Criteria Committee of the New York Heart Association (1964). **The diseases of the heart and blood vessels: Nomenclature and criteria for diagnosis** (6th ed.). Boston, MA: Little, Brown.

Criteria Committee of the New York Heart Association (1973). **Nomenclature and criteria for diagnosis of diseases of the heart and great vessels** (7th ed.). New York: Little, Brown.

DeBusk, R.F. (1975). The value of exercise stress testing. **Journal of the American Medical Association, 232**, 959.

DeBusk, R.F. (1982). Occupational work evaluation of patients with cardiac disease. A guide for physicians. **Western Journal of Medicine, 137**, 515.

de Wolff, C.J. (1985). Stress intervention at the organizational level. In W.D. Gentry, H. Benson, & C.J. de Wolff (Eds.), **Behavioral medicine: Work, stress, and health** (pp. 241-252). Dordrecht, The Netherlands: Martinus Nijhoff Publishers.

Ellestad, M.H. (1986). **Stress testing: Principles and practices** (3rd ed.). Philadelphia, PA: F.A. Davis.

Engelbert, A.L. (Ed.). (1989). **Guides to the evaluation of permanent impairment**. Chicago, IL: American Medical Association.

Falvo, D.R. (1991). **Medical and psychosocial aspects of chronic illness and disability**. Gaithersburg, MD: Aspen.

Fox, Sam, III, & Naughton, J.P.H. (1970). Physical activity and the prevention of coronary heart disease. **Annals of Clinical Research, 3**, 404-432.

Goldman, L., Hashimoto, B., Cook, F., & Loscalzo, A. (1981). Comparative reproducibility and validity of systems for assessing cardiovascular functional class: Advantages of a new specific activity scale. **Circulation, 64**, 1227.

Moss, S.A. (1980). The psychosocial needs of the cardiovascular patient. In J. Reiffel, R. DeBellis, L.C. Mark, A.H. Kutscher, P.R. Patterson, & B. Schoenberg (Eds.), **Psychosocial aspects of cardiovascular disease** (pp. 39-43) New York: Columbia University Press.

Schroeder, S.A., Krupp, M.A., Tierney, L.M., Jr., & McPhee, S.J. (1990). **Current medical diagnosis and treatment**. Norwalk, CT: Appleton and Lange.

Siegrist, J. (1985). Psychosocial coronary risk constellations in the work setting. In W.D. Gentry, H. Benson, & C.J. de Wolff (Eds.), **Behavioral medicine: Work, stress, and health** (pp. 45-79). Dordrecht, The Netherlands: Martinus Nijhoff Publishers.

Steptoe, A. (1981). **Psychological factors in cardiovascular disorders**. New York: Academic Press.

Streater, S.E., & Erlandson, R.J. (1984). Social and vocational considerations in cardiac rehabilitation. In L.K. Hall, G.C., Meyer, & H.K. Hellerstein (Eds.), **Cardiac rehabilitation: Exercise testing and prescription** (pp. 367-389). Champaign, IL: Life Enhancement Publications.

Yuker, H.E. (1992). Attitudes toward persons with disabilities: Conclusions from the data. **Rehabilitation Psychology News, 19**(2), 17-18.

## *About the Authors*

John Johnson, M.D., is a past Director of the Cardiac Laboratory at the University of Southern California-Los Angeles County Medical Center in Los Angeles, California and at Huntington Memorial Hospital in Pasadena, California. At the present time, he is in private practice in Pasadena and serves as a medical consultant for the California State Department of Rehabilitation.

James Getzen, M.D., is in private practice in cardiology in Pasadena, California and is on the teaching staff of Huntington Memorial Hospital in Pasadena. He is the Director of Cardiac Services and the Cardiac Rehabilitation Unit at Methodist Hospital of Southern California in Arcadia, California.

*Chapter 22*

# BACK AND NECK PAIN IN INDUSTRIAL INJURIES

by
*Emery Hopp, M.D.*

## INTRODUCTION

Neck and back pain are common human conditions. They must be considered normal consequences of aging. For purposes of discussion in this chapter, it is helpful to think of the body as a complex machine with a 30-year warranty.

Why only 30 years? A child born today can expect to live 75 or 80 years as a result of modern medicine and vast improvements in public health. Yet, the life expectancy in ancient times was probably about 30 years. Childbearing began in the early teens. By age 30, an individual was a grandparent, if lucky enough to survive the miserable conditions of disease, exposure to the environment, and the threat of wild animals. After 30 years of age, when the body slowed — combat, carnivores, disease, or the environment called in the expired warranties. Thirty years was enough time to replace a generation; no longer warranty was needed.

The first 20 years of a person's life involves growth. Typically, there is little that goes wrong, and to some extent, automatic repairs occur. When the person completes growth, the human machine should be at peak condition. It then takes about 10 years to run down. This, of course, is when the warranty expires. Take an automobile as an example. If the vehicle is not a lemon (good genetic background) and has proper maintenance (good physical conditioning, no bad habits) - it will last beyond the warranty period. Conversely, if abused or neglected, the automobile will wear out much sooner. Continuing our analogy, the alcoholic, the addict, the smoker, and the "couch potato" will pay a price for their abuse.

As an automobile ages, different systems wear out independently. Also, human body systems wear out. There is an accumulation of functional loss in strength, vision, hearing, reflexes, and cardiopulmonary systems with aging. With the rare exceptions of organ transplants, one cannot replace worn body systems or parts of systems. We must live with them and make the best of it. Modern medicine has extended life, but not youth.

The human spine, though a remarkable compromise between strength and mobility, eventually suffers the effects of constant exposure to gravity, wear, and accumulated trauma. These changes occur in everyone to some extent and can be the cause of much misery and suffering. According to Cailliet (1981), in a discussion about low back pain syndrome, "chronic pain is the most disabling disease of humans" (p. 206).

The social consequences of spinal pain are tremendous. Backache is the major cause of absenteeism at work in employed individuals between 18 and 45 years of age. Every year, there are 10 million people in this country with backache who have more than a quarter million operations on the spine. The cost in medical bills, absenteeism at work and school, lost wages and productivity, is estimated to be between $10 and $50 billion every year (Macnab, 1987).

To some extent, social changes in "advanced" countries are to blame. There is less physical work and less physical conditioning from daily routines. With the softening of our interaction with the environment, there has evolved increased expectations from society in other areas.

# THE BACK

## Anatomy/Pathology/Symptomatology

The human spine has three functions (Crenshaw, 1992; Rockwood, Green, & Bucholz, 1991). It (1) protects the nervous system, (2) supports the body, and (3) allows for movement. Its anatomy reflects these functions. The parts of the spine consist of strong vertebral bodies, separated by clastic discs, which act as shock absorbers and allow limited motion in all planes. The vertebral bodies and discs help form and support the spinal canal, which is the conduit through which the nervous system traverses the body. In addition, portions of the vertebral bodies form a posterior set of joints, the facet joints, that bear some of the weight of the body and guide and restrict motion (see Figure 1) (Longman & Woerdeman, 1978).

Within the lumbar spine, the posterior facet joints and discs form a three joint complex that allows and restricts motion. The spinal cord and nerves pass through the vertebral (spinal) canal. The roof is formed by the lamina and facet joints (superior and inferior articular processes). The walls are the pedicles and the floor is the disc. Short pedicles will significantly reduce the volume of the canal, as will a bulging disc or thickened articular process.

In the cervical spine, the same elements are present but they are smaller and more delicate. The transverse foramen surrounds the vertebral arteries as they ascend to supply the brain with blood.

Figure 2 illustrates the spinal nerves as they exit the spinal cord. They are named for the level of the vertebrae where they exit.

## Discs

The disc has an outer covering (the annulus fibrosis) that surrounds the inner cartilaginous center. The center blends imperceptibly into the outer fibrous layer. In childhood, the center is a soft, cartilaginous gel. With aging, a change in structure occurs; the water content decreases and the gel become thicker and more fibrous. By middle age, the center of the disc is fibrous and subject to cracking. Because of loss of water and microscopic breakdown, the disc loses height and settles. By middle age, the disc loses much of its elasticity and the individual is less flexible and a bit shorter. Since the disc makes up 25% of the spine's height, with advanced age the combined loss of many discs can produce significant shortening (Crenshaw, 1992; Rockwood et al., 1991).

In the average person, after the growth cycle ends (roughly age 20), the discs are fresh and at peak condition. This peak health slowly deteriorates over several decades to produce measurable degeneration. Usually the fourth or fifth lumbar and cervical discs show the first signs of wear, as they bear the most physical stress. Aggressive sports and other strenuous physical activities accelerate wear. Yet, wear is not lessened by inactivity. Being in good physical condition seems to protect the body from symptoms. The body does best when maintained in top physical condition.

# Figure 1
## THE HUMAN SPINE

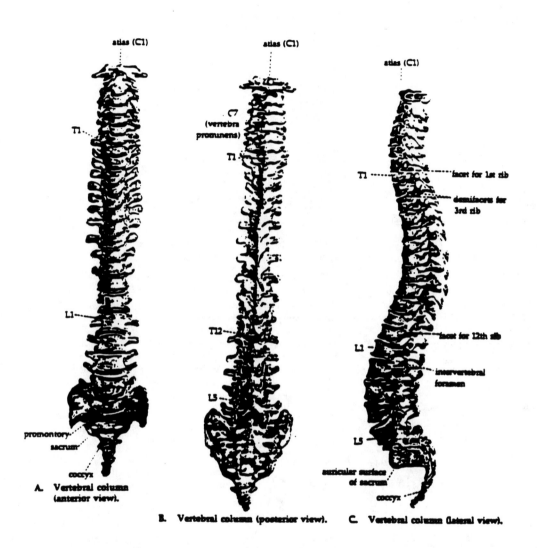

A. Vertebral column (anterior view).

B. Vertebral column (posterior view).

C. Vertebral column (lateral view).

From the **Atlas of Medical Anatomy** (p. 477) by J. Langman and M.W. Woerdeman, 1978, Philadelphia, PA: W.B. Saunders. Reprinted by permission.

It is important to remember that changes on x-rays and other laboratory results do not show pain. They only show the effects of aging or trauma and serve as a record for past changes. Often, a person without any symptoms possesses an extremely worn spine. When one factors in individual variation in response to wear and symptoms, there is little correlation between disease and test results. In one study, 40% of the **asymptomatic** (without symptoms) patients had significant pathological changes in their myelograms. With more sensitive tests such as the MRI (magnetic resonance imaging) and CT (computerized axial tomography) scan, the presence of **asymptomatic** changes is even higher.

# Figure 2
## THE SPINAL NERVES

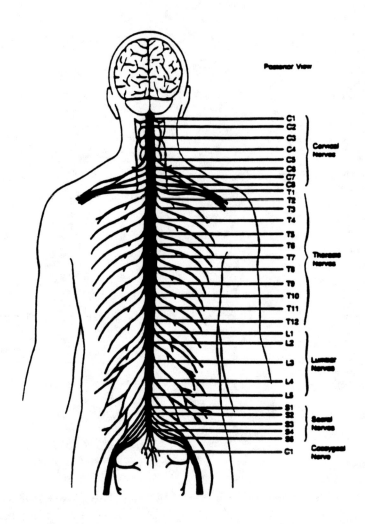

Posterior View

C1
C2
C3
C4      Cervical
C5      Nerves
C6
C7
C8
T1
T2
T3
T4

T5
T6
T7      Thoracic
T8      Nerves
T9
T10
T11
T12

L1
L2
L3      Lumbar
        Nerves
L4
L5

S1
S2      Sacral
S3      Nerves
S4
S5
C1      Coccygeal
        Nerve

From **Pathology: Principles of Disease** by M.J. Miller, 1983, Philadelphia, PA: W.B. Saunders, p. 380. Reprinted by permission.

Pathology increases with age. Roughly 40% of 40 year-olds have demonstrable pathological changes, 60% of 60 year-olds, 70% of 70 year-olds, and so forth. The diagnostic implications are obvious. Nearly all elderly people have changes and many have symptoms. The problem is, which changes, if any, are responsible for the symptoms? Assuming the changes are long-standing, why should the patient be having problems now? Often, finding the answer to that question and the elimination of a certain physical activity or postural problem will return the person to an asymptomatic state (Crenshaw, 1992; Mooney, 1981).

Each patient must be evaluated and treated individually. The goal of treatment is different from one patient to the next. There is an effect on the entire back with aging and settling of the vertebral discs. If a disc does not absorb stress, the stress is transferred to the facet joints. If a disc settles, so does the facet joint; the entire unit fails together. Loss of spacing and shock-absorbent function allows bone-on-bone contact. This contact causes spurring (bone growth) at the corners of vertebral bodies, which may further compromise the bony canal and nerves (DePalma & Rothman, 1970; Finneson, 1973).

Finally, settling of a complex system may not be in line with gravity but may allow the vertebral bodies to slip forward or backward on each other (spondylolisthesis). Such a state, like staggered blocks in a pile, is unstable and prone to painful movements with activity (Finneson, 1973).

## The Facet Joints

These joints guide, protect, and limit motion. This is necessary since the disc allows movement in all directions. The facets also bear some weight and are subject to degenerative arthritis (wear). Degenerative changes in the facets are often the cause of vague aches and pains in the back with radiation to the posterior pelvis and buttocks. They may cause stiffness and restricted movement (Rockwood et al., 1991; White & Punjab, 1978).

**The bony spinal canal.** The remainder of the bony canal acts as a conduit that affords protection to the spinal cord and nerves; the bony spine also supplies windows (foramena) for nerves. The general structure of the spine protects the vulnerable elements of the nervous system, while the associated joint and ligamentous structures allow a high degree of motion. The spinal canal in the lumbar region must be strong enough to support the entire body. The bony lumbar spine with attached discs and ligaments is a segmented, linked system and has little stability by itself. It is strengthened by a complex system of muscle attachments and the hydraulic effects of the abdominal contents.

Muscles provide support to the spine. The muscles on the left side of the spine balance the right side, while the muscles on the right balance the left side. Likewise, the front muscles balance the back, and the back muscles provide balance for the front. The role of the abdominal musculature is critical. The muscles exert inward (hydraulic) pressure similar to squeezing a toothpaste tube in the middle. This inward force results in a large upward force. In toothpaste, something comes out the top. In our body, the torso is raised up, negating the force of gravity and adding structural stiffness to the back. Thus, abdominal muscles and the abdominal cavity contents function as major distractors against the pull of gravity. Very few people maintain good abdominal muscle tone after the age of 20, which puts an added burden on the spine.

How could we have such an imperfect system? Remember the concept of a 30-year warranty. From an engineering stand point, it makes little sense to over-build a structure, having parts last much longer than the design life of the whole product. One might say we now live too long.

It is difficult to define the normal spine. Normal depends on age, genetics, use, abuse, and many other factors. There is a high degree of genetic variation in the spine. Changes occurring from trauma, degeneration, and disease are revealed on diagnostic tests. These effects of aging and of an active life are normal. A normal spine at age 60 will have accumulated many degenerative changes (narrowed disc spaces, arthritis of facet joints, and spurs). These changes usually do not create symptoms.

## Source of Pain

There are several structures that may be sources of pain. Back pain may come from structures other than the spine. This will not be discussed here, other than to say that diseases of the kidney, bowel, and the vascular system may refer pain to the back, and must be considered as sources of symptoms.

Within the spine, pain can arise from the musculoligamentous system (muscles, tendons, and ligaments), the nervous system, and the skeletal system (bones and joints). The skeletal system is subject to degenerative changes, fractures, tumors, and infections. The vertebral discs are the major source of pain in people over 30 years of age. Disc material in the canal elicits an inflammatory reaction from the nerves. Whether this is from mechanical or chemical irritation or an immunological response is uncertain (Frymoyer & Gordon, 1989; Waddell, McCulloch, Kummel, & Venner, 1980).

Often, the physician does not know the precise source of back pain. Eighty to 90% of back pain is nonspecific, making an anatomical diagnosis impossible. Any of the many structures capable of causing pain have the same pain response. Pain results in muscle spasm, which protects injured structures from movement. This spreads or refers the pain upward and downward through the muscles into their attachment points on the skeleton and occurs whether the pain source is the annulus, ligaments, facets, joints, capsule, or muscles. The cause may be due to strains, sprains, tears, arthritis, or irritation from constant tension on a sensitive structure. Local structures cause local pain and radiation of pain into the pelvis or buttocks.

**Radiation of pain.** Pain traveling down the leg and below the knee is indicative of nerve root involvement. Each specific nerve has its own territory, which includes muscle innervation, skin sensation, and reflexes. A specific reflex loss, skin numbness, pain distribution, or weakness is characteristic of each nerve and serves to localize the site of disease. The addition of nerve symptoms is called radiculitis and is the result of inflammation of the nerve (sciatica when the leg is involved). Nerve symptoms are more serious than back pain alone and add to the problem. Pain from nerve inflammation is often more severe than simple back ache. Damage to nerves is hard to ignore; symptoms such as loss of feeling, muscle weakness, or paralysis are of serious concern.

**Disease processes.** Disease processes that may cause nerve symptoms include herniated discs, degenerative spurs, and instability of the back. A herniated disc involves a rupture or herniation of the nucleus pulposus into the spinal canal, often occurring in the lumbar region (see Figure 3). Instability occurs as discs and facets settle; settling

## Figure 3
## NORMAL AND HERNIATED NUCLEUS PULPOSUS (DISC)

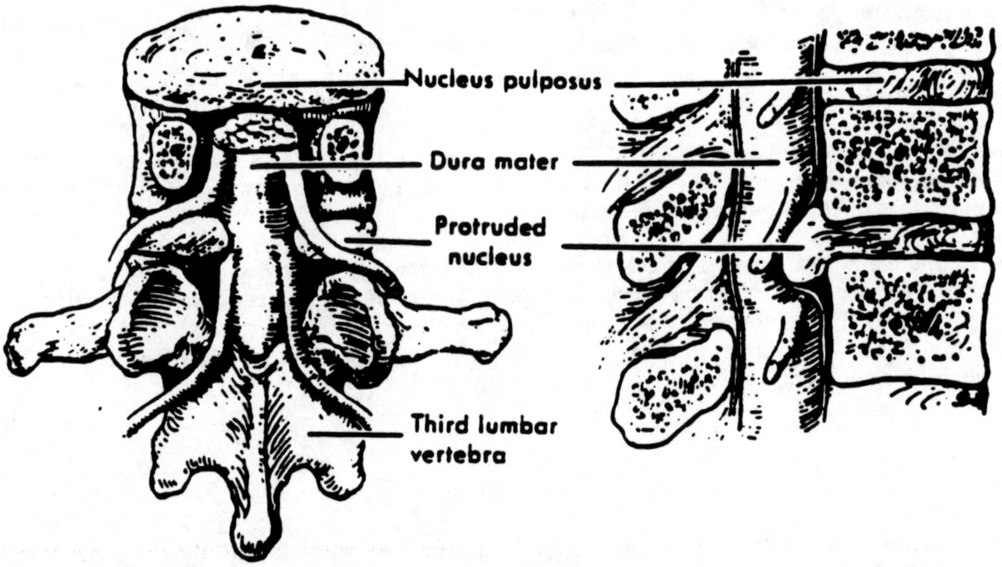

From **Carini and Owens' Neurological and Neurosurgical Nursing** by B. L. Conway, 1978, St. Louis, MO: C.V. Mosby. Reprinted by permission.

causes the bones to slide on each other. Such loss of restraint, allowing motion beyond physiological limits, can cause direct pressure on nerves or stretch them. Permanent weakness, paralysis, and loss of bowel and bladder function may persist after damage to the nervous system.

## Cause of Pain

Pain is a complex perception of the human brain, which interprets messages from nerves located throughout the body. The brain evaluates the information, compares it to past experience, and modifies the messages according to operating psychological factors and the needs of the body at the time (e.g., there is often no pain associated with severe wounds in combat and competitive sports).

**Pain factors.** Nerve impulses within the soft tissues of the spine are activated by conditions that can cause potential or real damage. The function of pain is to alert the body that something is wrong. The response is evaluated by the person according to the situation at the time. A toothache or a bee sting may cause much pain, but past experience dictates a moderate response.

**Age as a factor.** The addition of anxiety or fear of possible consequences may greatly magnify the pain and incapacitate the injured person. Stress, fatigue, and cultural and psychological circumstances greatly affect the reaction to pain. Past history is important in how one reacts. In societies or groups that consider reaction to pain a human weakness, there is very little emotional response to pain.

Causes of spinal pain differ in accordance with the age of the individual. It is rare for children and adolescents to complain of back pain. Their spines are tough and flexible; typically, only severe trauma causes injury.

From 30-50 years of age, the back still possesses a fair amount of youthful vigor and strength. At this stage of life, various parts begin to wear out and cause symptoms. Discs degenerate and frequently cause pain from loss of shock absorbent function or actual protrusion of the disc. Degenerating facet joints, or a combination of disc and facets settling, are other common reasons for pain.

In people 50 years of age and older, as aging progresses, the preponderance of symptoms is caused by degenerative disease. Wear (degeneration) causes permanent anatomical changes and loss of function. As the discs age, they are less able to perform their functions of shock absorption and smooth motion. The older fibrous disc is subject to microscopic tears, which further adversely affect function. Stiffening occurs as the result of calcification of ligaments, spur formation, and inflammatory changes, which take up some soft tissue laxity through scarring and contracture. The result is a stiffer, less mobile, shorter disc segment. The elderly back is shorter, stiffer, weaker, and subject to discomfort. Once one level is affected, the area cannot absorb shock and movement as before. Consequently, stress is transferred to adjacent levels causing them to absorb added stress which results in accelerated wear.

Changes due to advanced age may be asymptomatic, but often cause symptoms from degenerative joints, the compromised spinal canal, or less commonly, disc protrusions (rupture). The discs at this stage are often too fibrotic to herniate. On the rare occasion that they do, they occupy space in a spinal canal already narrowed by degenerative changes. This may cause unrelenting symptoms, including pain, that are not prone to spontaneous resolution.

**Spinal stenosis.** If the canal is compromised by multiple changes, a condition called spinal stenosis occurs. This is analogous to putting size 12 feet into size 10 shoes. Once the back is upright and the effects of gravity shorten the spinal column, back pain, radiating leg pain, and weakness may occur as the result of the squeezing of nerves in the spinal canal. The person is forced to stop and rest to eliminate the effect of gravity on the spinal contents. The symptoms are termed "intermittent claudication", and are similar to vascular disease changes that occur in the lower extremities. Vascular disease changes must be ruled out in establishing the diagnosis. Fractures, arthritic flare-ups, symptomatic spinal stenosis, and disc herniation can all occur in this age group (White, Rothman, & Ray, 1987).

**Compression fractures**. These fractures are very common in the elderly. They occur in vertebral bodies that are so weakened by osteoporosis (loss of bone tissue) that minimal trauma may cause fracture. Lifting a package, bending, falling, or coughing may be sufficient to fracture a susceptible spine. By the time an x-ray shows evidence of osteoporosis, the person may have lost 75% or more of the bone. This bone for all practical purposes is irreplaceable. Women suffer from this disease more often than men. The numbers of osteoporotic compression fractures in the spine increases in older individuals. Compression fractures from osteoporosis rarely, if ever, cause neurological symptoms. They do cause widespread suffering and deformity among the elderly.

# THE NECK

The cervical portion (neck region) of the spine is subject to the same 30-year warranty as the lumbar area. It also shows signs of wear and may become symptomatic in mid-life. The cervical spine is affected to a greater extent by stresses and tension and is more complex and fragile than the lumbar portion of the spine. The muscles that support and move the neck are shared with the shoulders and upper back. This complex arrangement requires a sophisticated coordination system, a system that is easily disturbed.

## Anatomy

**Cervical region**. The two upper cervical vertebrae are highly modified to form the connection to the skull and to allow rotation of the head. The remainder of the vertebrae are more traditional, but still differ from their lumbar cousins. The bones and discs are smaller (there is less weight to support) and the facet orientation is more horizontal, allowing greater freedom of motion.

A significant difference between the two levels in the vertebrae (lumbar and cervical) is the contents of the spinal canal. In the lumbar canal there are spinal nerves. The cervical spine contains the portion of the spinal cord that is an extension of the brain. This area is extremely delicate and does not tolerate more than the slightest trauma without permanent loss of function.

**Degenerative changes**. Age-related changes (degeneration) occur in the discs and facets causing settling of discs and spur formation similar to what occurs in the lumbar spine. Neck pain may come from many sources including musculoligamentous strain, disc degeneration, degeneration of facet joints, or a combination of these. Muscle strain can arise from strenuous activity or injury, fatigue from prolonged driving or clerical work, or the effects of tension and anxiety. Muscle injuries are similar to those in other areas of the body, but may take much longer to recover. Recuperation takes longer because of the complexity and interactions among the muscles of the neck, shoulder, and upper back.

Disc degeneration frequently affects the function of the neck. Common symptoms are neck pain and stiffness referred to the back of the head, shoulders, and interscapular area. A damaged disc causes increased muscular tension and spasm. This serves a protective function initially, by increasing support and aiding the compromised disc. After a period of time, the muscles become sore and irritated at their attachment points to the bones. These points are typically on the back of the skull and tips of the shoulder blades, as well as other bony attachments; they become what is commonly referred to as "trigger points."

## Trauma

The neck is susceptible to trauma from sports, falls, motor vehicle accidents, and similar trauma. Damage is usually caused indirectly from leverage forces applied to the head. These forces push the neck beyond its physiological range of movement and can cause tears of muscles, disruption of discs, fractures, and dislocations of bone. Muscle injuries may be insignificant, or substantial and take months to heal. Skeletal damage may lead to permanent paralysis or death. Severe damage to part of the spinal cord may cause paraplegia or quadriplegia.

The medical history and physical examination are the main sources of information for medical diagnosis of neck problems. If there are only nonspecific symptoms without evidence of nerve root involvement, no further testing is necessary. As in the lumbar spine, many patients have an incidentally abnormal finding revealed by testing, such as a myelogram, CT scan (computerized tomography), or MRI (magnetic resonance imaging). All x-ray results will show some signs of aging and degeneration (Crenshaw, 1992; Rockwood et al., 1991).

Stable fractures result in protective muscle spasm and local pain, but are not serious medical emergencies. Unstable fractures, since they have the potential of causing additional damage to the spinal cord, are medical emergencies.

All neck injuries demand a careful neurological examination of the entire body for clues that document nerve or spinal cord injury. The absence of neurological findings, a full range of motion of the neck, and a lack of significant spasm, rule out significant injury or potential future problems.

# DIAGNOSIS, EVALUATION, AND ASSESSMENT

Most people with neck and back pain do not seek or need medical help. A reduction of activity, rest, and home remedies usually suffice to assist the natural healing process. Most people compensate by slowing down and delaying tasks at home and work. More than 80% of the population has back pain at some time in their lives.

Diagnosing the cause of back and neck pain requires an in-depth medical history and physical examination. The type and progression of symptoms will often fit a pattern for a specific diagnosis of fracture, bursitis, disc herniation, torn muscle, damaged ligament, or arthritic joints, to name but a few ailments commonly encountered. The amount of trauma or disease the human body absorbs before becoming incapacitated is highly variable and modified by lifestyle, peer pressure, emotional state, and physical conditioning.

The physical examination seeks to find deficits in function or deviation from the norm. Severe pain, paralysis, reflex, or sensory losses are serious findings that may fit a pattern of disc herniation, tumor, infection, or systemic disease. Further examination and a focused, more detailed history will usually limit the diagnosis to one or perhaps two possibilities. At this point, laboratory tests including x-rays, magnetic resonance imaging (MRI), computerized tomography (CT scans), and electromyography (EMG) may help in formulating a diagnosis.

A careful physical examination and history establishes the diagnosis, and if surgery is contemplated, the physician can confirm the precise anatomical cause with proper tests. Most cases will respond to time and conservative treatment, saving the inconvenience and expense of tests or the need for surgery.

# TREATMENT

Medical treatment varies from emergency surgery to skillful, conservative medical treatment and psychological support. Treatment of the organic or physical components of injury or disease is somewhat straightforward. Treatment of pain introduces us to complex psychological and social components (Cailliet, 1984). Since 80-90% of the symptoms are nonspecific back pain, treatment is often nonspecific. Most all soft tissue injuries, and many bony injuries respond well to the same basic modalities of treatment. Treatment of the underlying cause is the key in bringing about relief of pain in a short time (Kirkaldy-Willis, 1983; Sternbach, 1974).

There are two types of pain, acute and chronic. They are different in their presentation, treatment, and emotional components.

## Acute Pain

Acute pain is often severe and frightening. The amount of pain may bear no relationship to the significance of the injury. Untreated, severe pain should abate by itself in a short time, generally measured in hours. The natural response to avoid pain is to rest. Rest can involve simple avoidance of the activity that is causing the pain. In some, it may require elimination of many necessary functional activities. The person may need complete bed rest for several days.

There is a continually functioning feedback mechanism that informs the individual, by means of pain, if an activity is suitable or should be temporarily avoided. For instance, if there is very little pain or no pain with walking, it is not harmful to walk. If walking for more than a certain distance or amount of time increases the pain, the body has set temporary limits that the individual should observe. If there is no pain until the person returns to the sport or other physical activity, the sport or other activity needs to be avoided.

In the acute phase, the physician will prescribe treatment to relieve the pain. Treatment consists of any specific procedure used for the amelioration of a disease or pathological condition. Traditional medical treatment includes medication for pain and muscle relaxation, physiotherapy, and traction. Treatment is not intended to eliminate or mask pain in order that the individual can perform tasks or activities that are to be avoided. In most situations, acute pain, characterized by its sharp, severe, localized nature, soon gives way to a more diffuse, vague, and generalized discomfort. Pain medication, used during the acute phase, should be withdrawn as quickly as possible. Whereas narcotics may be appropriate for the acute phase, they are not appropriate for the chronic stages. Their prolonged use often leads to drug abuse and dependency. The physician can prescribe non-narcotic medications after the acute pain resides.

## Chronic Pain

The chronic phase of pain is less severe and poorly localized. It may last several days, weeks, or even months. As with acute pain, if a period of activity does not cause or increase pain, it is not harmful to do that activity. If an activity causes or increases pain, the individual needs to avoid it. Limitations usually decrease as one improves. Generally, back injuries tolerate walking better than standing, and standing better than sitting. As healing progresses, walking tolerance will increase first, than standing. Sitting tolerance is usually the last of these activities to increase, while getting in and out of a chair is often the last painful activity to subside. A person can return to work when there is a tolerance suitable for the activities required of the particular job.

To evaluate the effects of treatment, one must first be familiar with the natural course of disease or injury. While it is true most people have back pain, most back and disc problems disappear spontaneously. About half of the people with back pain get better in the first week. Seventy-five to 80% resolve within two weeks. By two months, 90% are resolved. By four months, 95% are free of major symptoms. The remainder may take longer or require more aggressive treatment. Musculoligamentous conditions usually heal faster than disc problems (Frymoyer & Gordon, 1989; Sternbach, 1974).

## Acute and Chronic Neck Pain

Treatment of neck injuries differs in acute and chronic symptoms. In an acute traumatic injury, rest, heat, and a neck collar support are helpful. Medication for pain control is often necessary. Activity limitation is the best way to relieve symptoms and help recovery. Driving and clerical work are common causes of irritation and should be limited. Stress, anxiety, and fatigue will magnify and prolong the effects of disease or injury. Neck pain is frequently referred to the shoulder and interscapular areas. Reassurance and local treatment (heat or cold) may be helpful. The most important factors to reduce symptoms are rest and limitation of activity.

Radicular (arising from a nerve root) pain from disc pressure on cervical nerves requires stronger medication, greater activity restrictions, and longer term treatment. Allowable activity depends on the severity of local, referred, and radicular symptoms.

Chronic symptoms may evolve several months after an acute injury or gradually arise from situational stress. Less severe chronic symptoms may be interspersed with flare-ups of acute pain. The ability to work is greatly affected and adds to stress, which aggravates symptoms. An individual program of rest, activity modification, medication, and therapy must be found for each person. Physiotherapy of the neck is more effective than in the back region. After the acute pain subsides, traction, together with heat or other modalities to relax sore muscles, may be helpful.

Radicular symptoms of pain, numbness, reflex loss, and weakness usually subside within a month. If the symptoms remain severe or prolonged and if there are frequent recurrences, the treating physician may consider surgery. Surgery is not needed for non-specific (non-radicular) pain.

Chronic neck pain is a common result of exposure to a stressful environment. Symptoms of neck pain and referred pain become a barometer of an individual's response to stress in family life, on the job, and from society. The neck is a target organ for psychosomatic pain resulting in tight, painful, and stiff muscles.

Surgery is less of an option in chronic pain than in traumatic disc ruptures. The problem is not the discs, but a response to a stressful environment. One cannot operate on all degenerated discs; everyone eventually has them. When a degenerative disc ruptures and causes pressure on nerves, surgery may be considered after an appropriate conservative trial, usually consisting of several months. If symptoms are severe and progressive, one may not be able to delay surgery. Yet, since the natural history of cervical disc disease is cyclical, surgery may coincide with the transition into the asymptomatic phase of the cycle.

## Factors Modifying Recovery

Personal injury cases that are litigated and workers' compensation cases take twice as long to get half as well as non-litigated cases. Stress and anxiety may prolong the natural course of the injury indefinitely. One cannot overlook psychological effects; secondary gain also needs to be considered (Deneen & Hessellund, 1986; Matkin, 1985). Secondary gain is more apparent in industrial accidents and personal injury cases. For example, a worker injured on the job, may not want to return to work because of a dislike for the employment situation or a particular supervisor. The litigant in a personal injury case may be hoping for a large financial settlement (Cailliet, 1984). These factors may negate the possibility of a quick return to work.

Other physical factors that predispose people to back problems and delayed recovery are poor physical conditioning, smoking, and driving. Lifting and carrying of heavy weights or repetitive lifting of moderate weights are associated with increased back pain. Nurses and truck drivers have the highest incidence of back problems (Deyo, 1987; Pope, Frymoyer, & Andersson, 1984).

The figures for successful recovery are the same for medically treated and untreated back problems, with two treatment exceptions: surgery and epidural steroid injections. Corsets, physiotherapy, and medication may reduce pain and make the person feel better but do not affect the healing time. Stress and fatigue will increase pain and prolong healing.

Traditional medical treatment includes medication for pain and muscle relaxation, physiotherapy, and traction. There is no scientific proof that any of these modalities affect the outcome of back problems. Temporarily, they may reduce the amount of pain.

Once healing occurs, the patient is at risk of reinjury. Usually, there is a period of several weeks of back pain or referred leg pain that gradually subsides. Avoiding recurrence requires common sense and possibly modified physical activity. A clerical job can be resumed when the patient's sitting tolerance allows. Jobs involving heavier exertion will require more time off work. The average person is better off working part-time or on light duty than sitting at home worrying about health, finances, and personal problems. Being able to do part-time or light duty work builds confidence and prevents deconditioning. It also allows for positive reinforcement from co-workers.

## Spinal Stenosis

This is a condition where the spinal canal becomes too small for its contents. Since the contents are the spinal cord and spinal nerves, the consequences are serious. There are two reasons for degenerative spinal stenosis. First, the settling of the discs with age reduces the height and total volume of the spinal canal. The reduction in height allows the ligament flavum (a ligament that runs longitudinally along the spinal column) to buckle inward and the disc to bulge outward, taking up more space.

Next, the facet joints become arthritic and grow in size, taking up space in the critical area of the nerve root canal. Finally, the vertebral bodies also thicken and form spurs at the level of the exiting nerves. Added to all this is the potential instability of the settled disc and facets. Widespread and often bizarre symptoms can occur with activity and being in the upright position, affecting multiple levels of the spine. The symptoms usually disappear with rest. Most people with spinal stenosis are able to walk less than a block by the time they agree to surgery (Hopp, 1987; Rockwood et al., 1991).

Treatment for spinal stenosis includes physical conditioning, weight loss, medications, epidural steroid injections, and modification of physical activity. If these treatments fail, the physician may recommend surgery. Surgery involves removing much of the bony elements of the affected area of the posterior spine. While relieving pressure on nerves, surgery results in loss of stability. If too much bone is removed, weakness and instability may result; this can lead to subsequent fractures and spondylolisthesis.

To prevent instability, the surgeon may perform a spinal fusion to stiffen the spine. It is not always surgically possible to stabilize an old, osteoporotic, worn spine. This fact and the realization that all disease is not curable is a serious consideration in surgical planning. In spinal stenosis, relief of leg pain and symptoms occurs in 75-80% of patients; back pain is relieved in only 50%. Since the physician performs surgery to relieve leg symptoms, any relief of back pain is an added bonus (Crenshaw, 1992; Hopp, 1987).

# FUNCTIONAL LIMITATIONS

Disability has two components. The first is functional loss from disease or injury. The second is the attitude of the person, which is modified by environmental (home and work) and psychological health.

There are 50 million people with disabilities in the United States, a significant portion of the population. To return them to functional roles in society benefits everyone.

In the back pain patient, return to work may result in recurrent symptoms if preventive measures are not taken. Repetitive lifting, carrying, bending, driving, and heavy equipment operating are difficult physical activities on the back. The person risks a recurrence of injury if allowed to return to work without physical reconditioning and education on care of the spine. The more physically arduous and unskilled the employment, the more difficult it is to alter the job duties and the easier it is for the employer to replace the worker. With more skilled and trained workers, it is less difficult to modify or accommodate aspects of the job duties. There are usually more possibilities for reasonable accommodation in positions of responsibility, such as allowing an injured employee to take more frequent rest breaks, work irregular hours, or delegate some job duties.

Injuries resulting in radiculitis normally recover fully. Occasionally, a nerve sustains permanent damage. In the lumbar spine, the most common loss of function affects the calf. Difficulty in raising up on one's toes or heels can occur, causing the person to have frequent missed steps and falls. A simple brace will allow normal walking. Many occupations will be unaffected, unless strength, speed, agility, or balance are important occupational characteristics of the job. Heavy laborers may be affected, as may heavy equipment operators who require use of the foot for pedal pressure. Highly competitive sports may be impossible, though the person could still do many recreational activities.

Weakness at a level higher than the calf is rare. This is because most disc herniations occur at the last two levels of the lumbar spine. The rare disc injury that affects a higher level may cause temporary weakness of the thigh, and still more rarely, leave residual weakness.

Degenerative changes and spinal stenosis can cause widespread weakness from disease changes occurring in multiple areas of the lumbar spine. Symptoms typically occur with activity and resolve with rest. The person affected is often elderly and no longer employed. Treatment in these cases is directed toward improvement in the quality of life.

Disc herniation in the neck can cause nerve damage, as do herniations in the lumbar region. Movements of the arm and hand are more skilled and delicate as compared with the foot; therefore, any neurological defects of the upper extremities have more profound effects. An accompanying loss of manual dexterity is often evident. This occurs not only from the weakness or sensory loss, but from loss of precise and complex coordination responses in the hand. Such loss makes skilled tasks such as typing (keyboard operations) difficult, as well as activities involving use of hand and power tools. The individual may also experience easy fatigability.

Advanced degenerative changes and spinal stenosis of the neck are much less common than in the lower back. This is fortunate because pressure on the spinal cord causes symptoms in both the arms and legs. Spasticity and weakness of the lower and upper extremities make any activity difficult. Surgery is risky in the neck area and results are less successful than surgical procedures in the lumbar area. Full neurological recovery is uncommon. Individuals diagnosed with advanced degenerative changes and spinal stenosis of the neck are usually elderly; their disabilities are compounded by loss of strength and balance seen with elderly people.

Deconditioning is common from injury and inactivity (Cailliet, 1984). It can prevent return to work and contribute to repeat injuries. Smoking is associated with an increased incidence of back problems, although the mechanism for this is unclear.

Alcohol and drug abuse are a two-fold problem. They are a major cause of injury in that they reduce reaction time, alertness, and concentration. The second aspect is motivational. The role of substance abuse as a cause of work injuries is unknown. However, one-fourth of all workers surveyed had used drugs within the past month prior to injury. The percent of workers abusing alcohol is even higher. Recovery from a work injury as in recovery from a sports injury presupposes the desire to return to work.

If the individual is not motivated, all efforts at rehabilitation are useless. A positive attitude is crucial; there must be motivation to get well, return to work, and function effectively at work. Industry has recently established employee assistance programs (EAPs) to provide professional service for employees that have substance abuse problems and other personal difficulties. The primary purpose of an EAP is to intervene in problems that may lead to work impairment, absenteeism, injury, and even job termination. These programs have both enhanced employees' well-being and increased productivity (Lewis & Lewis, 1986).

Recovery is more often dependent on the emotional component of spinal disease. Many workers have a chaotic family life, no savings, poor coping mechanisms, and limited imagination. When an injury occurs to a person such as this, there is little or no support system available, and recovery becomes difficult or impossible.

# REHABILITATION POTENTIAL

A clear and sharp mind, an inquiring intellect, and a desire to overcome challenges cannot be thwarted by physical disability or pain. Important as well are a sense of pride, a feeling of being needed, and a desire to take responsibility. This is similar to the team spirit in sports.

A very important factor in returning to work is education. A lack of educational experience limits the ability of an injured worker to compensate for limitations or retrain. An older worker in a menial job is usually trapped by lack of education, no transferable skills, lack of advancement possibilities, and physically demanding work. Many union jobs pay well and require little education. They may offer the older worker with seniority the ability to obtain less physically demanding jobs. If not, the individual may have few, if any, options.

Return to work after an injury depends more on how much the worker likes the job and the employer than the injury itself. In the final analysis, it is job satisfaction, not type or extent of injury, that influences a return to work. An additional factor is age. As the person becomes older, jobs become more difficult to obtain and more difficult to perform.

Self-employed persons lose very little time from back injuries; individuals in the professions likewise return to work quickly. This may be explained by their feelings of high job satisfaction. They also receive no income if they do not work, a very powerful incentive to return to work. Farmers, doctors, lawyers, sports professionals, and the like are the most motivated patients. They want to return to the activities that give them satisfaction and to environments where they feel needed.

Experience, talent, adaptability, prior skills, past work history, and reasonable expectations are also important to a successful return to employment. Motivation may be the most important characteristic in a successful transition from injured worker to employed worker.

To treat physical deconditioning, general exercises such as walking, swimming, or bicycling should be combined with specific exercises for each job. "Work hardening" is the term used for physically retraining a person to return to a specific job. Through work hardening, a person gradually increases work tolerances over a specified time.

"Back schools" were begun several years ago to educate injured individuals in the mechanics of back injury. People with back injuries were taught exercises and the proper way to use and stabilize the back at work and in daily activities. It was noted the number of people returning to work after completion of back school was very small. We are not sure if those motivated to return to work would not have returned without the back school.

"Pain clinics" were created in an attempt to address the symptoms that prevent return to work. Their goal was to eliminate dependence on medical treatment, including medication, need for therapy, and visits to physicians. This multidisciplinary approach continues and utilizes the services of social workers, psychologists, occupational and physical therapists, rehabilitation counselors, and physicians. The results from pain clinics are not encouraging. Although there is less dependence on medication and physicians, little improvement on the rate of return to gainful employment occurs. The longer the delay in return to work, the less likely the individual will ever return to productive employment. Once an injured person has been out of work for 2 years, there is less likelihood the person will ever return to work. It seems that an alternative mode of existence without work—supported by others—becomes acceptable. People become conditioned to be non-workers.

Deneen and Hessellund (1986) and Matkin (1985) discussed rehabilitation counseling from the perspective of working in the private sector. Rehabilitation in the public sector was described by Parker (1987) and Rubin and Roessler (1987). Several kinds of vocational rehabilitation services are available through both public and private sector rehabilitation to help injured workers and persons with disabilities return to work. Rehabilitation counselors provide a variety of services including vocational assessment and evaluation, counseling and guidance, rehabilitation plan development, and job placement services. "Job club" (part of job placement services) helps workers with injuries and disabilities share job finding experiences and builds self-esteem (Mayer & Gatchel, 1988). The goal of the counselor in this setting is to facilitate a return to productivity at the highest level possible.

The Americans with Disabilities Act (West, 1991) passed in 1990 and effective as of 1992, encourages use of reasonable accommodation for both current and perspective employees. The counselor can assist employers in providing accommodation through various means, including job modification and job restructuring.

# CASE STUDY

Mr. Joel Binder is a 45 year-old construction worker. The **Dictionary of Occupational Titles** (U.S. Department of Labor, 1991) classifies his job as follows: **D.O.T. 869.687-026 - Construction Worker II** (construction industry). This job is heavy, and typically considered unskilled work activity. Mr. Binder was a laborer and helper at various construction sites for the past 15 years. His primary job duties involved lifting and carrying of equipment and supplies, loading and unloading trucks, and assisting skilled construction workers. In helping the skilled construction workers (especially the carpenters), he acquired many of their skills. One could classify the last seven years of his work as a combination of unskilled and semiskilled work.

This worker is divorced and has two children, both living with their mother in the local area. He pays monthly child support. Joel completed the 10th grade; he received poor grades throughout school.

The injury occurred on the job while Mr. Binder was lifting heavy bags of cement. His diagnosis was a herniated disc in the lower lumbar region between L4 (fourth lumbar vertebrae) and L5 (fifth lumbar vertebrae) and between L5 and the sacrum. Two laminectomies were performed over a 2-year period. It has been one year since the last surgical procedure.

Joel was drinking moderately at the time of the industrial injury. Since the injury, he has continued drinking and, in addition, is taking prescribed as well as non-prescribed pain medication, including Valium.

The worker's treating physician restricts him to light work, including no repetitive bending, stooping, or kneeling. He should alternate sitting and standing/walking throughout the work shift. Standing is limited to 30-minute increments and sitting to a maximum of one hour at a time. He is able to alternate these activities throughout the day.

The previous employer is willing to take Mr. Binder back to modified work, but needs help from a rehabilitation counselor. Concerns of the employer involve Joel's physical limitations, attitude, motivation, and possible substance abuse.

Mr. Binder is willing to see a vocational rehabilitation counselor, but feels he can do only sedentary work activity. He states he no longer drinks and takes only medically prescribed drugs. It is his opinion that the employer may be suggesting a return to work to harass him.

## Questions

1.  Would you, as the rehabilitation counselor, attempt to return Mr. Binder to work with the previous employer? Justify your response in detail.

2.  During the last seven years of work, Joel acquired work skills. Describe what these skills might be and whether they would be transferable to other kinds of work within his medical restrictions.

3.  Describe three alternative rehabilitation plans you can provide for this injured worker.

4.  Identify the positive and negative aspects of this case.

5.  If your state has mandatory workers' compensation vocational rehabilitation, describe the process from the time of injury to possible resolution of the case.

6.  During rehabilitation planning, it becomes evident Mr. Binder does have a substance abuse problem. Identify the actions you may take.

# REFERENCES

Cailliet, R. (1981). **Low back pain syndrome** (3rd ed.). Philadelphia, PA: F.A. Davis.

Cailliet, R. (1984). **Understanding your backache: A guide to prevention, treatment, and relief**. Philadelphia, PA: F.A. Davis.

Conway, B.L. (1978). **Carini and Owens' neurological and neurosurgical nursing** (7th ed.). St. Louis, MO: C.V. Mosby.

Crenshaw, A.H. (Ed.). (1992). **Campbell's operative orthopaedics** (8th ed.). St. Louis, MO: Mosby-Yearbook.

Deneen, L., & Hessellund, T. (1986). **Counseling the able disabled**. San Francisco, CA: Rehab Publications.

DePalma, A.F., & Rothman, R.H. (1970). **The intervertebral disc**. Philadelphia, PA: W.B. Saunders.

Deyo, R. (Ed.). (1987). Occupational back pain. **State of the Art Reviews, 2, 1**.

Frymoyer, J.W., & Gordon S.L. (Eds). (1989). **New perspectives on low back pain**. American Academy of Orthopedic Surgeons Symposium. Park Ridge, IL: American Academy of Orthopedic Surgeons.

Finneson, B.E. (1973). **Low back pain**. Philadelphia, PA: J.B. Lippincott.

Hopp, E. (Ed.). (1987). Spinal stenosis. **Spine: State of the Art Reviews** (No. 3). Philadelphia, PA: Hanley & Belfus.

Kirkaldy-Willis, W.H. (Ed.). (1983). **Managing low back pain**. New York: Churchill Livingstone.

Langman, J., & Woerdeman, M.W. (1978). **Atlas of medical anatomy**. Philadelphia, PA: W.B. Saunders.

Lewis, J.A., & Lewis, M.D. (1986). **Counseling programs for employees in the workplace**. Monterey, CA: Brooks/Cole.

Matkin, R.E. (1985). **Insurance rehabilitation: Service applications in disability compensation systems.** Austin, TX: Pro-ed.

Mayer, T.G., & Gatchel, R.J. (1988). **Functional restoration of spinal disorders: The sports medicine approach.** Philadelphia, PA: Lea & Febiger.

Macnab, I. (1987). **Backache.** Baltimore, MD: Williams & Wilkins.

Miller, M.J. (1983). **Pathophysiology: Principles of disease.** Philadelphia, PA: W.B. Saunders.

Mooney, V. (1983). Evaluation and care of lumbar spine problems. **The Orthopedic Clinics of North America, 14,** 3.

Parker, R.M. (1987). **Rehabilitation counseling: Basics & Beyond.** Austin, TX: Pro-ed.

Pope, M.H., Frymoyer, J.W., & Andersson, G. (Eds.). (1984). **Occupational low back pain.** New York: Praeger.

Rockwood, C.A., Jr., Green, D.P., & Bucholz, R.W. (1991). **Rockwood and Green's fractures** (3rd ed.). Philadelphia, PA: J.B. Lippincott.

Rubin, S.E., & Roessler, R.T. (1987). **Foundations of the vocational rehabilitation process** (3rd ed.). Austin, TX: Pro-ed.

Sternback, R. (1974). **Pain patients - traits and treatment.** Orlando, FL: Academic Press.

U.S. Department of Labor (1991). **Dictionary of occupational titles** (4th ed., revised). Washington, DC: Author.

Waddell, G., McCulloch, J.A., Kummel, E., & Venner, R.M. (1980). Nonorganic physical signs in low back pain. **Spine, 5**(2), 117-125.

West, J. (1991). **The American with Disabilities Act: From policy to practice.** New York: Milbank Memorial Fund.

White, A.H., & Punjab, M.M. (1978). **Clinical biomechanics of the spine.** Philadelphia, PA: J.B. Lippencott.

White, A.H., Rothman, R.H., & Ray, C.D. (Eds). (1987). **Lumbar spine surgery: Techniques and complications.** St. Louis, MO: C.V. Mosby.

## *About the Author*

Emery Hopp, M.D., has practiced medicine in Beverly Hills, California for 20 years. He is an Assistant Clinical Professor of Medicine at the University of California, Los Angeles and created and runs the Spine Clinic at Wadsworth V.A. Hospital in Los Angeles. During the Vietnam conflict, he ran an air force hospital in Da Nang, Vietnam.

# Chapter 23

# RHEUMATIC DISEASES

by
*Thomas D. Beardmore, M.D.*

## INTRODUCTION

### *Definition*

Rheumatic diseases are a group of diseases that affect the supporting structures of the body, including the joints and periarticular tissues (see Figure 1), connective tissues of the skin, bones, muscles, and diseases of the immune system. They encompass a group of inflammatory diseases affecting connective tissue that are insidious in onset, characterized by exacerbations and remissions, and resistant to medical therapy (in that there are no cures, only palliative treatments). Included are arthritis and diseases that cause pain, stiffness, and abnormalities of locomotion. The cardinal features of the rheumatic diseases are the signs of inflammation: warmth, swelling, redness, pain, and loss of motion. Patients with rheumatic disease will have complaints of pain, decreased energy, easy fatigability, stiffness, and loss of motion of their joints. Work endurance and capacity will be affected by these symptoms and with severe involvement, activities of daily living, and locomotion are impaired.

Arthritis is the commonly used term for rheumatic disease that affects the joints; when muscle tissue is inflamed, it is called myositis. Soft tissue rheumatism involves tendons, ligaments, bursa, or muscle, and causes associated stiffness and pain. There are more than 100 rheumatic diseases that result in pain, stiffness, and functional impairment. Some of the common diseases are osteoarthritis (the most common rheumatic disease), rheumatoid arthritis (the highest disability rate), gout, bursitis, tendonitis, fibrositis, systemic lupus erythematosus, ankylosing spondylitis, and osteoporosis. Less common types of rheumatic diseases include myositis, scleroderma, and arteritis (Kelley, Harris, Ruddy, & Sledge, 1985; McCarty, 1985; Schumacher, 1988).

The rheumatic diseases are the leading cause of disability and absence from work in the United States (Colvez & Blenchet, 1981) (see Table 1). They are also the second most common reason why patients visit doctors. These diseases are difficult to diagnose due to the subtlety of symptoms, the fact they have overlapping symptoms with other medical problems, and that they often show a paucity of clinical and laboratory signs and symptoms. Rheumatic diseases tend to develop slowly, respond slowly to treatment, and most require long term care.

### *Rheumatology - A Medical Specialty*

**Rheumatology.** The scientific study and care of the rheumatic diseases is called rheumatology and the medical specialist who deals with the rheumatic diseases is a rheumatologist. This specialty developed within the last 50 years in the United States. The American College of Rheumatology and the Arthritis Foundation are two national organizations interested in promoting research and public education of rheumatic diseases. Both organizations are in

## Figure 1
## THE KNEE JOINT AND THE ADJACENT SUPPORTING STRUCTURES

### Knee Joint

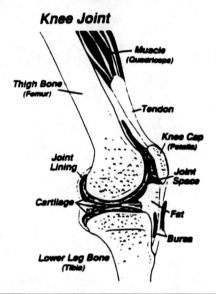

Schematic representation of a normal synovial joint and surrounding soft tissue. Inflammation of these tissues can result in pain. These structures are sites of rheumatic diseases.

## Table 1
## COMMON RHEUMATIC DISEASES AND THEIR IMPACT ON
## THE WORK FORCE IN THE U.S.

| DISORDER | INCIDENCE | IMPACT (LOST WORK DAYS) |
|---|---|---|
| Rheumatiod Arthritis | 2 million | 2.2 million |
| Osteoarthritis | > 16 million | 66 million |

Atlanta, Georgia and are good national reference sources for the rehabilitation counselor seeking disease and resource information concerning the rheumatic disorders.

All urban areas in the United States have practicing rheumatologists and major urban centers have rheumatology training programs at medical schools and large hospitals. These should be the primary referral source of clients for vocational rehabilitation and the main reference source for counselors to solve patient problems. The American College of Rheumatology is the professional organization for rheumatologists in the United States; the Arthritis Foundation is the main organization that raises funds for arthritis research and education in the United States (Kelley et al., 1985; Schumacher, 1988).

**Impact.** The impact of arthritis in the United States is extensive. There are about 37 million people who have arthritis including 200,000 who are under the age of 18. Included are 16 million patients with osteoarthritis between the ages of 25-74, 2 million patients with rheumatoid arthritis, 1 million patients with gout, 250,000 children with rheumatoid arthritis, 300,000 patients with ankylosing spondylitis, and 131,000 patients with system lupus erythematosus. Currently there are over 7 million Americans disabled by arthritis. Arthritis accounts for 500 million days of restricted activities and 68 million days lost from work. It is the leading cause of industrial absenteeism after heart disease and is the second leading cause of disability payments. Rheumatoid arthritis accounts for 2.2 million lost days from work while osteoarthritis accounts for 66 million days lost from work (see Table 1). In the United States, 1 in every 7 people or 14.6% of the population has an arthritic condition. This turns out to be about 12.7% who say they have arthritis, 1% gout, and .9% bursitis (Centers for Disease Control, 1989, 1990).

**Categories of rheumatic disease.** Rheumatic diseases discussed here include three categories. The first (1) involves the diffuse connective tissue diseases, including rheumatoid arthritis, systemic lupus erythematosus, scleroderma, and polymyositis. This category has the highest incidence of and the most severe disability. The second (2) is osteoarthritis, the most common form of arthritis, which accounts for the largest number of lost work days. The last category (3) is ankylosing spondylitis, which causes severe back pain and can be confused with other causes of back pain.

# RHEUMATOID ARTHRITIS

## *Explanation of Disease State*

**Etiology.** Rheumatoid arthritis (RA) is a disorder of unknown etiology. It has an insidious onset and a slow progression. Many physicians feel that rheumatoid arthritis may be a disease of modern times. There are no descriptions of RA in ancient writings and no evidence in ancient skeletons. Only in the last century have researchers clearly separated it from other forms of arthritis. It is a disorder of the connective tissues of the body with exacerbations and remissions. The primary target of this disease is the joint and adjacent supporting structures (see Figure 1). The lining of the joint (synovium) is the site of chronic inflammation. This inflammatory process will produce pain, heat, swelling, and loss of joint motion. The process is locally invasive and the rheumatoid tissue can erode cartilage, bone, and support tissues. Additionally, the body produces enzymes harmful to tissue that can degrade the articular (joint) cartilage (Hochberg, Chang, Swosh, Lindsey, Pincus, & Wolfe, 1990).

**Incidence.** Rheumatoid arthritis is a common disorder affecting approximately 1% of the adult population in the United States. It has a high disability rate, estimated at 21 per 1000 affected people. This disability rate is higher than the next three most common conditions: heart disease, back impairment, and hypertension. In addition, RA patients use more medical services (physician and hospital) than patients with osteoarthritis, back pain, or tendonitis (Kramer, Yelin, & Kelsey, 1984). Rheumatoid arthritis affects women 3 times more often than men and has its peak onset for people in their 20s and 30s. Because of its chronicity and severe consequences, it is a primary focus of arthritis research in the United States (Kelley et al., 1985; Meenan et al., 1981).

**Effects.** The primary effects on the patient are pain, swelling, loss of joint motion, joint deformities, and subsequent loss of function. The disease is one of exacerbations and remissions (alternating periods of worsening and improving); yet, the course is frequently progressive. Pincus et al. (1984) analyzed a group of RA patients followed for 9 years and found declines of function in most measurements; 92% had significantly lower overall function. Of those under 65 years of age who had been working on entrance to the study, 85% showed significant work disability. Meenan, Yelin, Nevitt, and Epstein (1981) studied the financial impact of RA on wage earners and found that patients were earning 50% of their potential. The average individual income dropped, accounting for a 32% decrease in family income. Most patients did not have adequate disability insurance to cover loss of earnings, but did have

## Figure 2
# EXAMPLES OF CHARACTERISTIC DEFORMITIES OF RHEUMATOID ARTHRITIS

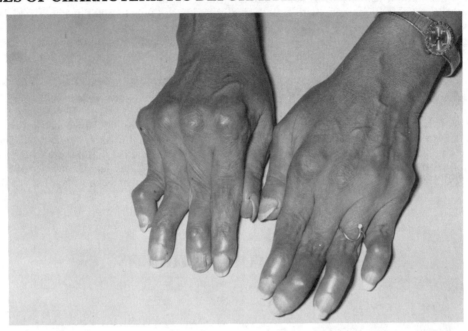

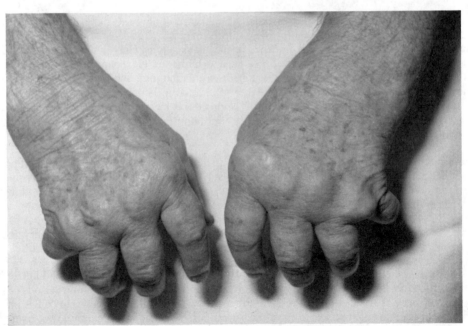

Common hand deformities seen in two patients with rheumatoid arthritis.

medical coverage. Of those with adequate coverage for earnings loss, 59% would only be covered for 6 months or less.

Patients with rheumatoid arthritis have a symmetrical arthritis affecting multiple joints. Initially, it affects the small joints of the body, but eventually may affect all joints of the body. The initial symptoms are in the small joints of the hands and feet where there will be pain, swelling, and loss of motion. Patients also will experience fatigue, morning stiffness, and possibly weight loss.

As the disease progresses, more and more joints are affected and additional disability occurs. The development of characteristic deformities (see Figure 2) of the hands is characteristic. Figure 2 illustrates two examples of common hand deformities seen in patients with rheumatoid arthritis. Represented are flexion deformities and malalignment of the fingers. Pinch, grasp, closure, strength, and fine motor activities may be affected. These deformities are limiting in performance of both work and leisure activities (Makisara & Makisara, 1982). Marked restriction of range of joint motion frequently accompanies these deformities. In addition, some patients may become self-conscious concerning the appearance of their hands or feet and restrict their activities or wear concealing clothing.

Diagnosis. The physician establishes a diagnosis through clinical observation and laboratory tests. Arthritis must be polyarticular and of at least 6 weeks duration before the physician can make the diagnosis. It involves the synovial joints symmetrically. Initially involved are the small joints of the hands and feet; however, any synovial joint may be involved. Although the joints are the main problem, RA is a systemic (occurring throughout the body) disease. Weight loss, fatigue, morning stiffness, occasional fevers, and anemia are common. The development of subcutaneous nodules at pressure points occurs. These soft, non-tender nodules are from a few millimeters to several centimeters in size and are most common at the elbow. Joints are swollen, tender, and show increased synovial fluid. Patients with more severe disease may have inflammation of the lining of the lungs and heart, lung involvement with fibrosis and nodules, or inflammatory vessel disease of the skin and other organs. Dryness of the eyes and mouth is common, as is compression of peripheral nerves adjacent to joints (e.g., carpal tunnel syndrome).

The laboratory features are sparse but patients may have mild anemia and elevation of acute phase reactants (such as the erythrocyte sedimentation rate). A certain percentage will have a serological abnormality called rheumatoid factor. Rheumatoid factor is a true autoantibody and is present in 75% of patients. Some patients will have associated extra articular disease and a more severe prognosis. In early disease, x-rays will show loss of bone density (osteoporosis) and soft tissue swelling about the joints. More advanced disease will show loss of articular cartilage and erosion of bone adjacent to joints and associated malalignment and deformities (McCarty, 1985).

Treatment. Currently, there is no curative treatment. There is good palliative treatment that results in amelioration of symptoms for most patients and long remissions for many. First line treatment involves medications directed at the inflammatory process, which results in decreased inflammation and subsequent decreased pain, decreased swelling, and improved range of motion. The commonly used anti-inflammatory drugs are aspirin (acetylsalicylic acid - ASA) and the nonsteroidal anti-inflammatory drugs (e.g., ibuprofen, indomethacin, naproxen). Many patients will continue to have symptoms in spite of daily nonsteroidal anti-inflammatory drugs and will require second line treatment.

These treatments involve slow acting drugs which have no anti-inflammatory action; the body responds to them in weeks to months after the onset of treatment. The effect of the second line drugs will slowly reduce the inflammatory hyperplastic synovium and may reverse erosions of bone and nodules. Included in these treatments are gold salts, penicillamine, and the cytotoxic drugs, methotrexate and azathioprine. These drugs require several weeks or months to show their effect and require frequent medical visits for administration and toxicity monitoring.

The second line treatments result in a decrease of symptoms and disease progression. Despite these treatments, many patients continue to have progressive disease and have the functional consequences of severe involvement of the joints. This may affect activities of daily living and ability to ambulate.

Total joint replacement has become a standard treatment for advanced joint disease that is progressive, symptomatic, and unresponsive to treatment. Joint replacement (arthroplasty) relieves pain and increases range of motion. Resumption of work and recreational activities may occur after joint replacement (Yelin, Meenan, Nevitt, & Epstein, 1980). Surgeons have achieved successful joint replacement in the hand, wrist, shoulder, hip, and knee, with best patient satisfaction for hip and knee arthroplasties (Kelley et al., 1985).

## Functional Limitations

**Functional status.** Functional limitation in patients with rheumatoid arthritis is of primary concern (Makisara & Makisara, 1982; Yelin, Meenan, Nevitt, & Epstein, 1980). As the disease progresses and the person ages, functional loss becomes progressive. Because of the importance of functional disability, the American College of Rheumatology has established criteria which physicians use to describe the functional state of their patients. Table 2 illustrates these functional classes. Included are normally functioning patients (class I) through functional class IV in which patients are unable to do the usual self-care activities of daily life. Medical reports from physicians include this functional classification. By definition, those referred for vocational rehabilitation primarily will be functional classes II and III. Functional limitations that the patients have are related to the stage of the disease and the body areas involved.

---

### Table 2

### FUNCTIONAL STATUS IN RHEUMATOID ARTHRITIS

| | |
|---|---|
| CLASS I | Able to perform usual activities of daily living. |
| CLASS II | Able to perform all usual self care and vocational activities. Limited in avocational activities. |
| CLASS III | Able to perform all usual self care activities. Limited in vocational and avocational activities. |
| CLASS IV | Unable to perform usual self care activities. |

---

**Chronic pain.** All patients have pain that is chronic in nature and exacerbated by activities of affected joints. In addition, many patients have stiffness of the whole body, primarily a morning phenomenon that may last from several minutes to a few hours. Specific functional disability will occur in each individual, dependent upon the stage of disease and the part of the body involved. This disorder typically causes loss of motion, pain with motion and consequent weakness, decreased strength, and decreased endurance. Involvement of the hands and upper extremities causes pain and loss of motion. This results in decreased ability to do fine dextrous hand activity and reaching activities. With lower extremity involvement, such as the feet, ankles, knees, and hips, the individual will show a decreased ability to stand and walk for long distances (Yelin, Nevitt, & Epstein, 1980).

**Emotional and intellectual factors.** These patients have no emotional limitations except those imposed by a chronic disorder associated with pain and loss of motion. There is an increased incidence of depression; however, it is not greater than would be expected in any progressive chronic disorder. RA does not affect intellectual capacity or the patient's ability to interact on a social level. Occasionally, because of the deforming nature of the disease, patients may experience embarrassment concerning the deformities of their hands. Some may require ambulatory aids such as canes, walkers, or even wheelchairs. Still, these factors in no way influence intellectual function (Meenan et al., 1981).

## Vocational Limitations

**Strength factors.** If the patient's rheumatoid arthritis is not well controlled (i.e., the medical treatment is not optimal), patients may have chronic pain, stiffness, fatigue, and weakness. All these factors have an influence on the ability to work. Most patients, however, will have good control with the first and second line drugs and their vocational limitations will be a consequence of the affected areas of the body. Because of the patient's reduction in strength and the involvement of articulations (joints) that affect movement, most patients will need to be employed in the exertional categories of light or sedentary work. If a patient, before having rheumatoid arthritis, was doing medium work, the limitation may be to light work. Most patients with rheumatoid arthritis will be unable to do heavy and very heavy work. Activities of sedentary and light exertion can be performed without problem for most patients with rheumatoid arthritis (Makisara & Makisara, 1982; Yelin, Meenan, Nevitt, & Epstein, 1980; Yelin, Nevitt & Epstein, 1980).

**Upper extremity involvement.** Hand involvement will result in decreased grip strength and most patients with rheumatoid arthritis will fall below the 5th percentile of a normal population for grip strength. In addition, pinch grip and manual dexterity are affected. All activities involving reaching and quickness of the upper extremities and manual dexterity may be compromised if there is involvement of the hand, wrist, elbow, and shoulder.

**Lower extremity involvement.** This may result in an impaired ability to stand, walk for long periods of time, and walk long distances. Work should be accommodated for the specific deformities. Some patients with rheumatoid arthritis will require special considerations because of their deformities and self-consciousness regarding the deformities.

**Other factors.** There is no impairment in intellectual functioning. Patients will have no more problems with communication, behavior, social interaction, learning, or comprehension than other people. Occasionally, patients will have other health problems related to rheumatoid arthritis. If they have multisystem involvement, this will usually result in decreased strength and endurance.

## Rehabilitation Potential

Patients with rheumatoid arthritis do not have intellectual impairment. Although there is a somewhat shortened life expectancy, this is only a few years less than normal. If the patient needs retraining, counselors can consider a few years rather than a few months when planning the program. The disease is slowly progressive and functional impairment, although usually inevitable, occurs at a slow rate. Most patients need to be trained for a job that requires less exertion and will need to decrease by one or two exertional levels. Therefore, patients able to do very heavy work before will likely need to be retrained for a job that involves medium or light work; those doing light work, typically will need to be retrained for sedentary work (Makisara & Makisara, 1982; Yelin, Nevitt & Epstein, 1980).

There are few studies on the rate of return to work for patients with arthritis. Straaton, Maisiak, Dortch, and Lopez-Mendez (1990), in a report from Alabama, stated that restoration of physical health, finances spent by rehabilitation agencies, and duration the case was open were positively correlated with return to work. Educational level, severity of disability, and financial status had no association with outcome. This is encouraging for the rehabilitation counselor when considering retraining and re-education for patients with rheumatoid arthritis who are unable to do their previous work (Potts & Brandt, 1984; Yelin, Meenan, Nevitt, & Epstein, 1980).

Continued consultation with the patient's physician, allied health professionals (such as occupational and physical therapists), and a work environment specialist can be employed to accommodate the patient's needs in the work environment. The prognosis for work is better for those who are more highly educated because the work skills require less exertion, motor dexterity, and physical exertion. The rehabilitation counselor needs to consider this when retraining patients with rheumatoid arthritis.

# SYSTEMIC LUPUS ERYTHEMATOSUS

## Explanation of Disease State

**Etiology**. Systemic lupus erythematosus (SLE) is a disorder of the immune system, which results in inflammation of the connective tissues and affects multiple organs of the body, commonly the skin, joints, kidneys, and blood. There is no known etiology (cause) for SLE. It is a disorder primarily of women and has an increased incidence in American Blacks, Hispanics, and Asians. The prevalence rate varies, dependent upon the population, from 3-400 per 100,000 population and there are approximately 30 new cases each year per million population. Ninety percent of patients with SLE are women and the peak onset is during the most productive part of life, during the 20s and 30s (Stein, Walters, Dilloon, & Schulzer, 1986).

**Disease features**. The disease has characteristic systemic features, including fatigue, fever, weight loss, and joint pain. All patients have joint pain as a predominant symptom; however, major disability is not related to the joints, but to the systemic involvement. The characteristic clinical course is one of exacerbation and remission that may last for many years. Typically, the disease affects multiple organ systems, but not simultaneously. Joint pain is the most common symptom with involvement of small joints of the body. There is no morning stiffness and deformity is rare when compared to rheumatoid arthritis. Some patients have skin rashes, particularly in sun-exposed areas. There is occasional inflammation of the lining of the heart and lungs, and acute and chronic renal disease, which can progress to renal failure. Some patients have central nervous system involvement that may manifest itself as stroke, psychosis, or depression. Anemia is also a common problem (Hochberg, Engle, Pruitt, & Petri, 1990; Kelley et al., 1985).

**Diagnosis**. This is based on clinical and laboratory features including specific laboratory tests such as the fluorescent antinuclear antibody test. Prognosis for patients with SLE is dependant upon the organs involved and is most severe for those who have renal and central nervous system involvement. Treatment is dependent on the organ system involved. Salicylates (ASA - aspirin) and nonsteroidal anti-inflammatory drugs are used for the joint symptoms. Physicians prescribe corticosteroids for other system involvement, low doses for minor problems and higher doses for more severe problems. Some patients require immune system modulating drugs such as azathioprine and cyclophosphamide, especially those patients with major organ involvement. A few patients will have chronic renal failure and will require dialysis or kidney transplantation. Because of the variable nature of this disease, some patients have only minor problems and others have major problems with increased morbidity (complications) and even early death; these patients require careful clinical follow-up (McCarty, 1985; Schumacher, 1988).

## Functional Limitations

Fatigue is a major problem for patients with SLE; this needs to be considered in the job placement phase of rehabilitation. Although particularly apparent during periods of exacerbation, fatigue is not apparent during remissions. There are no problems with locomotion, motor strength, or control as in other forms of inflammatory arthritis, such as rheumatoid arthritis. A patient's limitations will be dependent upon the organ system involved. Those with pulmonary and cardiac involvement may have shortness of breath and limitations in exertional activities. Patients who have central nervous system symptoms may be limited either by emotional problems or chronic depression. Individuals who have had stroke may have residual problems of hemiparesis that will interfere with locomotion and motor skills in the involved extremities.

## Vocational Limitations

Prognosis for life in patients with SLE is good unless there is involvement of the central nervous system or the kidneys. Educational and training programs that are long in duration can be considered. These clients will not require special environments except they should avoid cold environments, since 25% of these patients will have vasospasm in the extremities when exposed to cold. Fatigue is also a component of the illness. Because of sun intolerance (excessive ultraviolet light exposure can worsen the illness), jobs with excessive exposure to the sun are not advised and should not be considered in job placement. Most patients with SLE will be restricted to exertional categories of medium or less exertion because of the fatigue component (Yelin, Nevitt, & Epstein, 1980; Zelle & Taranto, 1976).

## Rehabilitation Potential

SLE, when in remission, either naturally occurring or medication-induced, will have little or no physical or emotional impairments. This disorder may remain in remission for years. Because of this, these patients are good candidates for retraining and educational programs. In addition, motor and physical limitations are not a common consequence of this disease.

# SYSTEMIC SCLEROSIS

## Explanation of Disease State

**Etiology and effects.** Systemic sclerosis is a chronic disorder of the connective tissue in which there is inflammation of multiple organs of the body, resulting in increased deposits of collagen. The primary target organs are the skin, joints, lungs, gastrointestinal tract, and the heart. There may be extensive fibrosis and tightening, particularly of the hands, face, chest, and feet. Also, there may be inflammation and sclerosis (scarring) of the periarticular structures, the lining of the lungs and heart, lung parenchyma, gastrointestinal tract, and the heart. These patients have great intolerance to cold with spasm of peripheral vessels which may result in gangrene of the tips of the fingers and toes, and even loss of the entire digit. Deformities are not a part of this disease. However, general fatigue, weakness, and loss of motion related to the fibrosis about the joints and skin are common consequences of the disorder (Kelley et al., 1985; Schumacher, 1988).

**Treatment.** Treatment is only palliative and symptomatic. There is no known etiology for systemic sclerosis. Nonsteroidal and other anti-inflammatory drugs may be given for inflammation and pain. Second line drugs, such as penicillamine, if given for long periods, may have beneficial effects on fibrosis. Other treatment is directed at the symptoms related to the affected organs.

## Vocational Considerations

Patients with scleroderma will have impairment in fine motor activities of the hands and activities involving strength of the hands. Grip and pinch will be markedly reduced and range of motion of the wrists, elbows, and shoulders will be mildly decreased. There is no intellectual impairment and ambulation is usually not a problem. Some patients with pulmonary involvement will have fatigue and restricted activity because of shortness of breath upon exertion. Most patients with scleroderma will be confined to jobs at the medium exertional level or below. Those with pulmonary and cardiac involvement will be limited to sedentary activity.

It is important in the vocational rehabilitation of these patients that they work in an environment that is warm and is not subject to extremes of temperature or sudden temperature changes. In addition, they should not have job activities that cause repeated trauma to the hands. Trauma and cold temperatures can result in vasospasm, gangrene, and even loss of fingers. Still, prognosis for life and work is good; the longevity of patients with scleroderma is only a few years shorter than normal. In most patients, this is a slowly progressive disease and, therefore, there is opportunity for vocational training and education (Yelin, Nevitt, & Epstein, 1980; Zelle & Taranto, 1976).

# POLYMYOSITIS

## *Explanation of Disease State*

**Etiology and effects.** Polymyositis and dermatomyositis are uncommon conditions, having an incidence of about 10 new cases a year per million population. This is a disorder of skeletal muscles involving inflammation of the muscles and a gradual loss of strength. Most involved are the proximal muscles of the extremities. Patients have involvement of the shoulder and pelvic girdle muscles. This symptomatically results in difficulty in raising the arms above the head, and in arising from the sitting position.

**Treatment.** Most patients will be treated with corticosteroids and have good response. Those who do not respond well will be treated with second line drugs, such as azathioprine or methotrexate. Most patients with polymyositis have full return of motor strength. Those who do not may have minor degrees of motor weakness. Patients with severe major limitations may have functional capacity similar to individuals with paraplegia for those with lower extremity involvement. For those with both severe lower and upper extremity involvement, functional capacity may be similar to persons with quadriplegia. Fortunately, this complication affects only a few patients.

**Symptoms.** The usual course of polymyositis is a sudden onset of severe weakness and then recovery. For those who do not have return of full strength, usually there is partial return of strength that the person can maintain for years. Only a small number will have continued loss of strength. Remissions may last for many years with few exacerbations.

## *Rehabilitation and Vocational Considerations*

Patients with polymyositis who have significant weakness of the lower or upper extremities will require jobs that have minimal exertional activity. Most will require some Type A walking aids, and ultimately perhaps a wheelchair; work stations will require modification. Once the physician establishes the disability, it is usually static so there is an opportunity for educational training and retraining programs. There is no impairment of intellect, comprehension, and ability to learn.

# OSTEOARTHRITIS

## *Explanation of Disease State*

**Definition and incidence.** Osteoarthritis (degenerative joint disease - DJD) is a disease, degenerative in nature, that affects the articular cartilage lining the surfaces of joints (see Figure 1). The articular cartilage is responsible for the smooth gliding action of joint motion and for a shock absorbing function the body needs for impact loading associated with walking and other force-generating activities. Osteoarthritis is an ancient disease and there is anthropological evidence of osteoarthritis involving the weight bearing joints in fossil skeletons of ancient man. It affects a specific body site and does not have systemic manifestations.

There are two forms of osteoarthritis, primary (etiology unknown) and secondary (due to an underlying cause). Secondary osteoarthritis may follow extensive trauma to a joint, a congenital dislocation, a joint malformation, and other arthritic conditions such as rheumatoid arthritis and gout.

Osteoarthritis is the most common arthritis in this nation and virtually everyone above 65 years of age will have x- ray evidence of osteoarthritis. Most people will not have symptoms. It commonly affects women more than men. This disease involves the wearing away of the surface cartilage at the joint, resulting in pain, swelling, stiffness (particularly with activities), and loss of motion.

The disorder is primarily one of the joint cartilage. Secondary inflammation involving the joint lining is common. One makes a diagnosis based primarily on a patient's symptoms and characteristic x-ray changes that include: loss of cartilage, increased bone density, and bone overgrowth at the joint margin.

**Treatment.** Treatment is symptomatic involving strengthening of muscles around affected joints, analgesics and anti-inflammatory drugs, walking devices, and, if severe, surgery. The use of joint prostheses (total artificial joints) is very effective in advanced osteoarthritis when other treatments are ineffective.

## Functional Limitations

These patients have no systemic features, no other organ system involvement, and no emotional or intellectual consequences from osteoarthritis. This disorder is localized and may be symptomatic with severe functional problems, but more commonly is without problems. Most patients with osteoarthritis are older and many will no longer be working and will not be candidates for vocational rehabilitation. Functional limitations of a patient will be specific for the areas of the body involved.

If there is involvement of the small digits of the hands, individuals will have problems with stiffness and loss of motion that will interfere with finger dexterity and similar activities. Pinch and grip also may be decreased. Common areas involved by osteoarthritis include the cervical and lumbar spine. If these are involved, there will be pain and loss of motion, particularly with rotation and bending. The weight-bearing joints of the lower extremities, particularly the hips and knees, are also commonly involved and have the highest incidence of disability. With hip or knee disease, patients will have pain, particularly with standing and walking. Besides pain, there will be a loss of range of motion and stiffness, especially with the initiation of activities. Other joints are not commonly involved, unless there is secondary osteoarthritis because of previous trauma or joint disease in those areas.

## Vocational Limitations

Since osteoarthritis is a local disease, emotional, intellectual, and other organ systems and health factors are not limitations in the vocational rehabilitation process. If patients have osteoarthritis of the lumbar spine, their ability to bend and lift will be reduced; most of these patients will be reduced by one or more exertional levels. This is also true for the knees and hips. If there is involvement of the knees and hips, activities such as bending, squatting, stair or ladder climbing, long distance ambulation, and long periods of standing may be affected.

## Rehabilitation Potential

The local nature of osteoarthritis and the lack of systemic features makes patients with degenerative joint disease (DJD) good candidates for training and education. The arthritis does not interfere with longevity and educational programs, if needed, can last for years rather than months. Movement is affected, but strength is preserved. Communication, social, and behavioral abilities are unchanged by osteoarthritis, as are learning comprehension and other intellectual skills. Because of the increased age of onset of osteoarthritis, some patients will have other health problems associated with aging.

# ANKYLOSING SPONDYLITIS

## Explanation of Disease State

**Definition and effects.** Ankylosing spondylitis is an inflammatory disorder of the synovial joints and entheses (ligament-bone junction) of the spine. This is a disorder primarily affecting men, with an incidence of men over women of 9 to 1. Initial onset is in the second and third decade of life and presents with pain, stiffness, and loss of motion of the lower back. Frequently, the disorder is mistaken for low back pain of a mechanical or degenerative nature. This disorder is slowly progressive and in its full expression may involve the entire spine from the pelvis to the skull. Initial involvement occurs in the sacroiliac joints (posterior pelvic joints). Also affected are the synovial joints of the back and the ligamentous insertions that join the vertebral bodies. These areas will become inflamed, resulting in pain, swelling, and loss of motion. Approximately 20% of patients with ankylosing spondylitis will have involvement of peripheral joints, primarily in the hips and shoulders. To a lesser extent, there may be involvement of more peripheral joints of the lower extremities and hands (Guillemin, Briancon, Pourel, & Gaucher, 1990).

Ankylosing spondylitis is the most common inflammatory arthritis of the back; however, there are others, including Reiter's syndrome, psoriatic arthritis, and bowel-associated arthritis. These disorders are less common but have similar symptomatology and disability patterns.

**Symptoms.** The pathology of ankylosing spondylitis involves inflammation of the lining of the posterior joints of the back and the ligamentous connections between the vertebral bodies. With progression of the disease, there is fibrous ankylosis (fusion) and later bony ankylosis of these joints with consequent entire loss of motion. Pain is the main symptom of patients with ankylosing spondylitis, which is confined to the back. There is accompanying stiffness and loss of motion. As the disease progresses, stiffness increases; once ankylosis is complete, the pain stops.

**Diagnosis and treatment.** The physician makes a diagnosis by the combination of clinical features, absence of the rheumatoid factor, elevated sedimentation rate, and characteristic x-ray changes, which show involvement of the spinal joints and bony fusion. There is no known etiology for ankylosing spondylitis; treatment will provide temporary relief of symptoms. Treatment involves prescription of anti-inflammatory drugs, particularly indomethacin, and in some patients, phenylbutazone. Other nonsteroidal anti-inflammatory drugs are also effective. In addition, physical therapy with maintenance of proper posture helps prevent development of a fixed flexion posture of the spine.

## Functional Limitations

Ankylosing spondylitis does not usually have systemic features. Occasionally, patients will have involvement of the aortic valve of the heart and some pulmonary fibrosis with resultant symptoms. However, most patients only have the functional limitations related to loss of motion of the spine. Thus, there is impairment with bending, twisting, and rotational motions of the lumbar and cervical spine. If there is involvement of the hips and shoulders, there will be pain, loss of motion, and development of flexion contractures (shortening of tissues surrounding a joint) in those areas.

## Vocational Limitations

There is no impairment of intellectual functioning. Aptitudes, interests, and communication skills are no different from the population and there is no change in life expectancy, unless there is cardiac or pulmonary involvement. These individuals may have environmental restrictions due to limited mobility of the spine.

## Rehabilitation Potential

Most patients with ankylosing spondylitis early in the disease will have little impairment in the range of cervical or lumbar spine, but will have chronic pain. This is controlled by anti-inflammatory drugs or analgesics; hence, the person needs little or no modification of the work environment, except that most patients will require less exertion in their work (Yelin, Nevitt, & Epstein, 1980). As the disease progresses, more patients will be unable to do work that is within the higher exertional categories. This is because of the loss of mobility of the lumbar spine and the loss of the ability to bend forward. Patients with severe involvement will have no motion of the cervical or lumbar spine and must bend from the hips. These persons will need to move their entire body to see to the right or left (Lihtinen, 1981). Life expectancy is normal and most patients can expect to have full, productive lives. There is no impairment in social and behavioral skills. Learning comprehension is unchanged and, except for the few individuals who have cardiac involvement, there are no other health problems associated with ankylosing spondylitis.

# CASE STUDY

Susan Valdez is a 19-year old woman who has had rheumatoid arthritis for 14 years. During this time, she has had long periods of illness when she was confined to her home and, as a result, is still in her last year of high school. The rheumatoid arthritis is currently well controlled and Susan has missed no school for the past six months. This individual takes medication on a regular basis and must visit her physician weekly to receive injections of gold to maintain her disease in remission.

Through the years, Ms. Valdez has required surgery for her arthritis to maintain ambulation. There have been two hip replacements and a knee replacement. Currently, she is able to walk about the house unassisted but uses a motorized wheel chair for ambulating in the community, except for very short distances. Susan has morning stiffness and has arranged to take classes that start at 10 a.m. or later. There is occasional pain in multiple joints including the feet, shoulders, wrists, and small joints of the hands. The physician has prescribed pool exercise. Occasionally, when her wrist (of the non-dominant hand) flares up, Susan wears a wrist splint. In addition to limited ambulation, she requires assistance from her mother to shampoo her hair. Grip strength is 20 pounds, while pinch strength is 5 pounds.

Ms. Valdez is the eighth child of a second generation Hispanic family. She is bilingual, as are all the children. The father passed away several years ago and the mother is currently supported by general relief and contributions from her adult children. Susan's mother does not speak English and has never worked outside the home; she currently sees her life's role as caretaker and aide for her daughter, and assists her in activities of daily living. The relationship between Susan and her mother is close and has been criticized by the health care team as one that promotes dependence rather than independence.

Testing has shown that the client has high average intelligence, social immaturity, and a lack of depression. The health care team feels that the client has been an underachiever in school and at home, relying on her mother and siblings rather than on her own skills. Susan currently does not drive and has not started dating; emotional support is provided by her large family and one girlfriend from school.

The client was referred for vocational rehabilitation counseling at the insistence of the high school principal; she will graduate in six months and has made no plans for the future, following graduation. Susan has done well in school, and has particularly enjoyed the sciences, receiving a senior prize for her achievement in biology. Ms. Valdez is unsure about attending college. There is no family tradition of education (she will be the second in her family to complete high school) and no finances to support a college education. Lupe, one of her sisters, is currently the head cashier at a grocery store and has assured Susan that she can get her a similar job. The mother is against Susan working and feels she should stay home, and if she wishes to work, she should baby sit for her nieces, nephews, and the neighborhood children.

## *Questions*

1. Is this client a suitable candidate for vocational rehabilitation? What additional medical information is needed from her health care team?

2. If you feel she is a suitable candidate for counseling and rehabilitation, what programs would give her the greatest opportunities for long-term employment? Would additional education be indicated?

3. Discuss whether a job as a grocery cashier is a good choice for employment?

4. How do you handle Susan's inability to drive and her dependence upon her mother? Discuss her use of an electric wheel chair to ambulate outside the home. Is reliance upon public transportation an option?

5. What physical problems are to be considered if immediate placement is the rehabilitation goal? List them and indicate the impact on Susan finding and maintaining work.

6. List Ms. Valdez' strengths and problems, both physical and psychosocial, that need to be considered when formulating a vocational rehabilitation program.

# REFERENCES

Centers for Disease Control (February, 1990). National Health Interview Survey, 1987. **Morbidity and Mortality Weekly Report, 39**(6), 99-102.

Centers for Disease Control (November, 1989). National Health Interview Survey, 1987. **Morbidity and Mortality Weekly Report, 38**(46), 788-791.

Colvez, A., & Blenchet, M. (1981). Disability trends in the United States population 1966-76: Analysis of reported causes. **American Journal of Public Health, 71**(5), 464-471.

Guillemin, F., Briancon, S., Pourel, J., & Gaucher, A. (1990). Long-term disability and prolonged sick leaves as outcome measurements in ankylosing spondylitis. **Arthritis and Rheumatism, 33**(7), 1001-1006.

Hochberg, M., Chang, R., Swosh, S., Lindsey, T., Pincus, T., & Wolfe, F. (1990). Preliminary revised ACR criteria for functional status in rheumatoid arthritis. **Arthritis and Rheumatism, 33**, S15.

Hochberg, M.C., Engle, E., Pruitt, A., & Petri, M. (1990). Correlation of disease activity with physical disability in systemic lupus erythematosus. **Arthritis and Rheumatism, 33,** R22.

Kelley, W.N., Harris, E.D., Ruddy, S., & Sledge, C.N. (Eds.). (1985). **Textbook of rheumatology.** Philadelphia, PA: W.B. Saunders.

Kramer, J., Yelin, E., & Kelsey, J. (1984). Social and economic impacts of four musculoskeletal conditions: A study using national community-based data. **Arthritis and Rheumatism, 26,** 901.

Lihtinen, K. (1981). Working ability of 76 patients with ankylosing spondylitis. **Scandinavian Journal of Rheumatology, 10,** 263-265.

Makisara, G., & Makisara, P. (1982). Prognosis of functional capacity and work capacity in rheumatoid arthritis. **Clinical Rheumatology, 1**(2), 117-125.

McCarty, D.J. (Ed.). (1985). **Arthritis and allied conditions.** Philadelphia, PA: Lea and Febiger.

Meenan, R., Yelin, E., Nevitt, M., & Epstein, W. (1981). The impact of chronic disease: A sociomedical profile of rheumatoid arthritis. **Arthritis and Rheumatism, 24**(3), 533-549.

Pincus, T., Callahan, L.F., Sale, W.G., Brooks, A.L., Paynbe, L.E., Vaughn, W.K. (1984). Severe functional declines, work disability, and increased mortality in seventy-five rheumatoid arthritis patients studied over nine years. **Arthritis and Rheumatism, 27**(8), 864-872.

Potts, M., & Brandt, K. (1984). Educational needs of vocational rehabilitation counselors working with clients who have arthritis. **Journal of Applied Rehabilitation Counseling, 15**(2), 22-25.

Schumacher, H.R. (Ed.). (1988). **Primer on the rheumatic diseases.** Atlanta, GA: The Arthritis Foundation.

Stein, H., Walters, K., Dilloon, A., & Schulzer, M. (1986). Systemic lupus erythematosis - A medical and social profile. **The Journal of Rheumatology, 13**(3), 570-576.

Steinbrocker, F. (1990). Functional status in rheumatoid arthritis: American College of Rheumatology Revised Criteria. **Arthritis and Rheumatism, 33,** 15-20.

Straaton, K.V., Maisiak, R., Dortch, M., & Lopez-Mendez, A. (1990). Factors associated with continued employment among arthritis clients served by a State-Federal rehabilitation agency. **Arthritis and Rheumatism, 33**(9) Supplement, S123.

Yelin, E., Meenan, R., Nevitt, M., & Epstein, W. (1980). Work disability in rheumatoid arthritis: Effects of disease, social and work factors. **Annals of Internal Medicine, 95,** 551-556.

Yelin, E., Nevitt, M., & Epstein, W. (1980). Toward an epidemiology of work disability. **Health and Society, 58**(3), 386-415.

Zelle, J.A., & Taranto, K.F. (1976). Health care utilization by persons with chronic disabilities who have been vocationally rehabilitated. **Archives of Physical Medicine and Rehabilitation, 57**(6), 282-290.

## About the Author

Thomas D. Beardmore, M.D., is an Associate Professor of Medicine at the University of Southern California School of Medicine in Los Angeles, California. He is the Chief of Rheumatology and Co-Chief of the Arthritis Service at Rancho Los Amigos Medical Center in Downey, California, and is involved in the rehabilitation of patients who have disabilities as a result of arthritis.

# Chapter 24

# PARAPLEGIA AND QUADRIPLEGIA

by
*Serena S. Hu, M.D.*
*and*
*Jeffrey M. Cressy*

## INTRODUCTION

The catastrophic effects of spinal cord injury (SCI) can be emotionally and physically devastating. Perhaps more so than many other patient groups seen by rehabilitation counselors, patients with spinal cord injuries have several unique characteristics. First, although the most basic physical functions may be drastically affected, the cognitive faculties are usually intact. Second, with proper medical care, the person with a spinal cord injury can be expected to have a near-normal life expectancy. These facts, coupled with the realization that half of all spinal cord injuries occur to persons under the age of 25, underscore the need for appropriate intervention by a rehabilitation counselor.

Spinal cord injury generally occurs as the result of an acute traumatic event, although conditions such as spinal column abnormalities or spinal cord tumors, or injury to the blood supply of the spinal cord can have equivalent effects. Motor vehicle accidents are the leading cause of spinal cord injury, followed by falls and gunshot injuries. Males outnumber females by 4:1 for all spinal cord injuries. The incidence in the general population is between 25-35 per million per year.

## ANATOMY

### Level of Injury

It is appropriate at this point to define several terms used to describe spinal cord injury. The spinal column has bony and ligamentous elements, which surround the spinal cord and its nerve roots. The nerve roots exit the spinal column to supply the muscles, skin, and internal organs. The spine can be divided into several regions. At the highest level in the spine, the neck region, is the cervical spine, consisting of 7 vertebrae and 8 nerve roots. The thoracic spine, at the level of the chest or thorax, has 12 vertebrae and nerve roots. Below the thoracic spine is the lumbar spine, the low back region, consisting of 5 vertebrae and nerve roots. The sacrum also has 5 vertebrae and nerve roots; and the coccyx, or tailbone, has one vertebra and nerve root. A physician describes a patient as having a certain "level" injury by naming the region affected and the level within that region (i.e., cervical level 4 or C4). Corresponding nerve root levels enervate different muscles in the arms, trunk, and legs.

The patient's condition also can be evaluated according to sensory level affected, as there are characteristic patterns of supply to the skin, called dermatomes (Figure 1). The motor and sensory levels may or may not correspond to each other, as the nerve supply, or tracts, within the spinal cord travel in different areas of the cord. Pinprick, light touch sensation, and the ability to perceive one's body part in space (proprioception) also can be differently affected as each of these nerve pathways travels in different tracts. By convention, a patient's neurological level is that which corresponds to the lowest level where the patient has strength against gravity (American Spinal Injury Association Standards, 1990).

## Figure 1
## DERMATOMAL PATTERNS OF SPINAL CORD INJURY

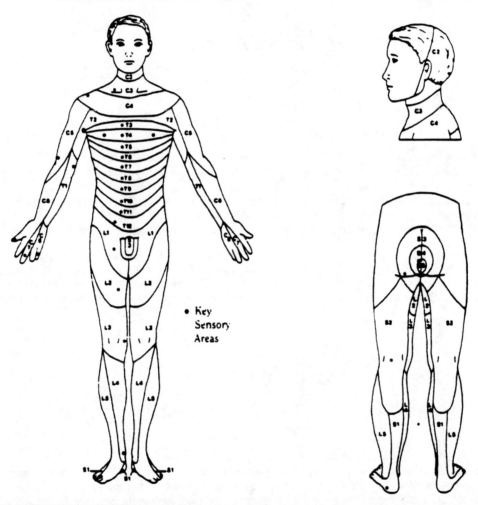

• Key
  Sensory
  Areas

This information was obtained from the "Publication Standards for Neurologic Classification of Spinal Injury Patients," American Spinal Injury Association, pp. 6-7. Reprinted with permission.

In general, the higher the level of injury, the greater the functional loss. Patients experiencing cord injuries at the cervical spine level will have quadriplegia and have involvement of upper and lower extremities; patients with thoracic and lumbar injuries will have paraplegia, involvement of the lower extremities. Areas below the level of injury are affected. At the junction of the thoracic and lumbar regions lies the conus medullaris where multiple nerve roots exit the cord. Below the end of the spinal cord, generally L1, is the cauda equina, where the lumbar and sacral nerve roots travel prior to exiting the spinal column at the appropriate level.

## Complete and Incomplete Spinal Cord Injury

A spinal cord injury can be described as either complete or incomplete. A complete injury means a patient has no functioning motor or sensory nerves below the level of injury. An incomplete injury means there is evidence of preservation of some motor or sensory function below this level (Benson & Keene, 1990). In the first few days after a spinal cord injury, one cannot be certain of the completeness of the injury because of a condition referred to as spinal shock. By the time patients are ready for vocational rehabilitation counseling, the completeness of injury is well established. Complete injuries have no expectation of distal recovery, although they may gain some function of motor or sensory nerves in the zone immediately around the level of injury (sometimes called root recovery).

In contrast, incomplete injuries may have additional recovery. The spinal cord itself cannot regenerate; after the effects of concussion and swelling have subsided, the spinal cord injury is permanent. The patient makes the greatest gains in recovery in the first 6 months after injury, with a plateauing of recovery after that. At 18 months, little additional neurologic return can be expected (Zigler, Capen, Atkins, & Resnick, 1991).

# SURGERY AND CONSERVATIVE THERAPY

## Surgical Considerations

The patient with a spinal cord injury will have bony or ligamentous damage accompanying the neurologic lesion. This may or may not correspond to the person's neurological level of injury. Spinal cord injuries are high impact injuries and can result in multiple trauma requiring emergency care. In the early evaluation period, the patient's surgeon will decide whether the individual's spine is mechanically stable or unstable; that is, whether the bony elements of the spinal column are stable enough to permit sitting and other activities without causing further damage to the neural elements and additional loss of function. The physician will also determine the extent of injury and whether the patient has a complete or an incomplete spinal cord injury (Benson & Keenen, 1990; Pierce & Nickel, 1972).

At the same time, the surgeon decides whether the patient needs an operation (spinal fusion) to stabilize the spine and prevent further neurological damage. Alternatively, it may be decided that a body jacket or halo vest will be sufficient to permit healing. For some patients, spinal fusion with implantation of rods, hooks, screws, or wires may allow rehabilitation without the cumbersome use of a brace or halo. In certain cases, patients may require surgical decompression to relieve pressure on the neural elements of the spine and maximize neurological recovery.

## Physical and Occupational Therapy

Once the acute emergency is over and the patient has been medically stabilized, physical and occupational therapy begin the programs for maximizing the patient's function. After the effects of the acute trauma (bleeding, swelling) subside, many patients gain some function in the early months following the injury. Thereafter, the functions remain stable. Therapists usually work to help maximize function of muscles that are present. The role of the physical therapist for a person with quadriplegia includes maintenance of range of motion and strengthening of respiratory muscles. The therapist works towards improving the patient's remaining function, including wheelchair mobility. Additionally, for the person with paraplegia, leg muscle strengthening and ambulation are also included in the program. Physical therapists work closely with the spinal cord injured in most rehabilitation centers to help determine wheelchair needs. This requires the expertise of a therapist knowledgeable in spinal cord injury as the selection of an appropriate wheelchair makes a crucial difference in job capabilities and life activities.

Occupational therapists specialize in the development of maximal skills in the shoulders, arms, and hands. To accomplish this, they may fabricate orthoses or recommend equipment to compensate for motor loss. They also may work with the surgeon to determine those cases where upper extremity tendon transfers will improve a patient's hand function (McDowell, 1988). For all persons with spinal cord injury, occupational therapists provide instruction on self-care personal activities, dressing, and home and community skill acquisition.

# LEVELS OF INJURY AND FUNCTION

The following discussion applies to patients with complete severance of the spinal cord at the level noted and are only guidelines, as no two injuries are identical. All muscles are supplied with multiple levels of enervation and the table listings are according to the main nerve supply (see Table 1) (Hussey, 1982).

## Table 1
## CAPABILITIES AND CONSIDERATIONS ACCORDING TO LEVEL OF SPINAL CORD INJURY (COMPLETE LESIONS)

| Level of Injury and Corresponding Musculature | Functional Activity | Capabilities and Considerations |
|---|---|---|
| C1, 2, or 3 | | |
| Possibly limited neck muscles repirator dependent | Mobility- | Possible candidate for electric wheelchair with portable respirator and tongue switch control/breath control. |
| | All Transfers- | Dependent requiring a lift. |
| | Skin Pressure Relief- | Independent with power reclining chair. |
| | Self Care- | Dependent. |
| | Desk Skills- | May be able to type, use computer, or write with a mouthstick and proper set-up. May be able to read with electric page turner and proper set-up. May be able to use telephone with proper set-up, gooseneck or speaker phone. |
| | Transportation- | Dependent requiring van with built-in lift and respirator back-up. |
| C4 | | |
| Neck Trapezius Functional Diaphragm | Mobility- | Electric wheelchair with chin, tongue, or breath switch control. |
| | All Transfers- | Dependent requiring a lift. |
| | Skin Pressure Relief- | Independent with power recliner. |
| | Self Care- | Dependent. |
| | Home Skills- | Dependent. |

|  |  |  |
|---|---|---|
|  | Desk Skills- | Able to type, write, read, and use telephone with proper set-up and equipment - mouthsticks, electric page turner or bookrack, gooseneck or speakerphone. |
|  | Transportation- | Dependent requiring van with lift. |

**C5**

Same muscles as above and:
<u>Deltoids</u> (shoulders)
<u>Biceps</u>

|  |  |
|---|---|
| Mobility- | Electric wheelchair with hand control or possible candidates for manual wheelchair with handrim projections (pegs). |
| Bed Transfers- | Dependent requiring lift. |
| Bath and Toilet Transfer- | Dependent requiring lift. |
| Car Transfer- | Dependent with sliding board. |
| Skin Pressure Relief- | May be independent with loops, power recliner. |
| Self Care- | Assisted with light hygiene and self-feeding with proper set-up and equipment. |
| Home Skills- | Basic counter top activities with proper equipment and set-up, but mostly dependent. |
| Desk Skills- | Independent-assisted, computer, typing, writing, reading, phone with proper set-up and equipment. |
| Transportation- | Independent with van with lift and sensitized controls. |

**C6**

Above muscles and:
<u>Wrist Extensors</u>
<u>Clavicular Pectoralis</u>
<u>Serratus Anterior</u>

|  |  |
|---|---|
| Mobility- | Manual wheelchair with friction surface handrims. May need power chair for community mobility. |
| Bed Transfers- | Independent with sliding board. |
| Bath Transfers- | May be independent with sliding board and tub seat or roll in shower. |
| Toilet Transfers- | Independent in transfers to commode chair with sliding board. May be independent to raised toilet seat. |
| Car Transfers- | Assisted-independent with sliding board. |
| Skin Pressure Relief- | Independent. |
| Self Care- | With proper equipment, independent in light hygiene, grooming, bathing, upper body dressing, and self-feeding. Independent-assisted in lower body dressing, and bowel and bladder management. |
| Home Skills- | With proper equipment, independent in light meal preparation and light housekeeping |
| Desk Skills- | Independent with proper equipment. |

| | Transportation- | Independent with van with lift and hand controls. May be independent with automobile with hand controls if able to place the wheelchair into the car. |
|---|---|---|

**C7**

Same as above and:
Triceps
Wrist Flexors
Sternal Pectoralis
Latissimus
Finger Flexors

| | | |
|---|---|---|
| | Mobility- | Manual wheelchair may require friction surface handrims. |
| | Bed Transfers- | May be independent with sliding board and tub seat. |
| | Toilet Transfers- | May be independent to commode chair and/or toilet; may require equipment. |
| | Car Transfers- | Independent, may require sliding board. |
| | Skin Pressure Relief- | Independent. |
| | Self Care- | With proper equipment, independent in light hygiene, bathing, grooming, dressing, and self-feeding. May be independent in bowel and bladder management. |
| | Home Skills- | With proper equipment, independent in light meal preparation, light housekeeping, shopping, and laundry. |
| | Desk Skills- | Independent with proper equipment. May require friction surface handrims. |
| | All Transfers- | Independent, may require sliding board and tub seat. |
| | Skin Pressure Relief- | Independent. |
| | Self Care- | With proper set-up and/or equipment, independent including bowel and bladder management. |
| | Home Skills- | Independent with proper set-up and/or equipment. |
| | Desk Skills- | Independent with proper set-up and/or equipment. |
| | Transportation- | Independent with hand controls. |

**T1 to T8**

Above muscles and:
Hand Instrinsics
Chest

| | | |
|---|---|---|
| | Mobility- | Manual wheelchair with standard handrims. |
| | All Transfers- | Independent, requires tub seat for bath transfers. |
| | Skin Pressure Relief- | Independent. |
| | Self Care- | Independent, including bowel and bladder management. |
| | Home Skills- | Independent with equipment as needed. |
| | Desk Skills- | Independent with equipment as needed. |
| | Transportation- | Independent with hand controls. |

**T9 to T12**

Above muscles and:
Trunk

| | | |
|---|---|---|
| Mobility- | | Manual wheelchair with standard handrims, some T12 individuals may ambulate. |
| All Transfers- | | Independent. |
| Skin Pressure Relief- | | Independent. |
| Self Care- | | Independent. |
| Home Skills- | | Independent with equipment as needed. |
| Desk Skills- | | Independent. |
| Transportation- | | Independent with hand controls. |

**L1 to L2**

Above muscles and:
Hip Flexors

| | | |
|---|---|---|
| Mobility- | | Manual wheelchair with standard handrims, may be a household or limited community ambulator with crutches and proper long leg orthoses (braces) and training. |
| All Transfers- | | Independent. |
| Skin Pressure Relief- | | Independent. |
| Self Care- | | Independent. |
| Home Skills- | | Independent with equipment as needed. |
| Desk Skills- | | Independent. |
| Transportation- | | Independent with hand controls. |

**L3 to L5**

Above muscles and:
Knee Extensors

| | | |
|---|---|---|
| Mobility- | | If wheelchair is needed, manual wheelchair with standard handrims, may be a community ambulator with proper equipment and training. |
| All Transfers- | | Independent. |
| Skin Pressure Relief- | | Independent. |
| Self Care- | | Independent. |
| Home Skills- | | Independent with equipment as needed. |
| Desk Skills- | | Independent. |
| Transportation- | | Independent with hand controls. |

**Sacral Segments**
**S1 to S5**

Individuals with injuries at the sacral segment levels are very independent functionally. They will probably be ambulatory, but may still need hand controls for driving. Sexual, bowel and bladder function may be severely compromised. With regard to bladder function, because of the bladder management required, they may be more susceptible to chronic urinary tract problems.

---

Courtesy of Rodney Adkins, Ph.D., and the Spinal Cord Injury Model System at Rancho Los Amigos Medical Center, Downey, California.

## Upper Cervical Injuries

The first two cervical nerve roots supply the upper neck muscles and the skin on the back of the head. These muscles assist in head control. Patients with complete injuries at this level are respirator-dependent. They may benefit from an electric wheelchair with a portable respirator and tongue switch control.

The diaphragm, the major breathing muscle, is controlled at the level of C3-4. The actual amount of diaphragmatic function will determine whether a patient is respirator-dependent. These patients can use either a sip-and-puff device that a patient controls by inhaling and exhaling air, a chin control, or a mouthstick to perform functions. These functions may involve controlling an electric wheelchair, using remote-control devices, writing, or turning pages of a book.

If the patient is respirator-dependent, speech will be affected, although some patients can communicate clearly. Patients with borderline diaphragmatic function, though not respirator-dependent, may have problems coughing and clearing lung secretions. While not a significant problem on a daily basis, after the acute post-injury stage, these patients may have a more difficult time recovering from minor respiratory ailments. Patients with upper cervical injuries are completely dependent upon others for transfers, pressure relief, and self-care.

## Lower Cervical Injuries

A C5 spinal cord injury patient has deltoid and biceps muscle enervation. These patients can flex their shoulders forward and to the side (abduction) with their deltoid muscles, and can flex the elbow and turn the forearm in an outward direction (supination) with biceps muscle function. The person can manipulate a manual wheelchair with modified handrims but, because of muscle weakness and limited endurance, often uses an electric wheelchair. Assistance will be required for all transfers (e.g., bed to wheelchair).

Many patients can lift their bodies from their wheelchairs to relieve skin pressure and avoid pressure sores. This is performed by use of a loop attachment through which patients hook their arms. Light hygiene, feeding, and desk and countertop activities can be performed with proper set-up and equipment. At this functional level, some individuals can drive with the use of sophisticated adaptations.

At C6, the key muscle group is the wrist extensors. This level permits a significant improvement in function for several reasons. The action of extending the wrist results in the fingers naturally falling together (the "tenodesis" effect). This can allow a person to pick up objects, though the finger flexors are not functioning. Orthoses can be designed by the occupational therapist to harness this wrist extension to help in the tenodesis. Most personal self-care activities can be performed by a person with C6 quadriplegia. The muscles about the shoulders have normal strength; in addition, other muscles that gain enervation at this level can improve wheelchair endurance. These patients can often perform transfers to and from their wheelchairs and in and out of vehicles. They can also perform pressure relief maneuvers to avoid pressure sores. Independence with transportation is possible if a van with a lift and hand controls is appropriately fitted.

With C7 level function, additional shoulder muscles are enervated, plus the triceps muscles. This allows the patient to perform more advanced transfers independently. Increased shoulder strength allows many of these persons to roll up inclines in their wheelchairs.

The key muscles of the C8 level are the deep finger flexors, that of T1, the hand intrinsics. The former are responsible for grip strength, the latter for much of the fine motor control of the fingers.

## Thoracic Level Injuries

Thoracic level paraplegias can be divided into high thoracic (T1-T8) and low thoracic (T9-T12). This categorization is due to the differences in trunk control in the two groups. The thoracic nerve roots each supply sequential segments of the trunk musculature so that a person with a high thoracic spinal cord injury has significantly reduced trunk control. A person may not be able to perform advanced wheelchair skills. Someone with a low thoracic spinal cord injury can transfer to the floor or bathtub and generally do wheelies (leaning back on the back wheels to elevate the front end of the chair), permitting them to handle curbs.

## Lumbosacral Injuries

Persons with paraplegia secondary to lumbar level injuries may be able to walk. Those with L1-L2 level function can flex their hips and learn to walk with braces that include the knee, ankle, and foot (called knee-ankle-foot orthoses [KAFOs]) or long-leg braces. This requires a great deal of energy and most patients with complete upper lumbar lesions choose to use wheelchairs for ambulation involving any significant distances.

L3-L4 is responsible for the quadriceps muscle function. This muscle straightens the knee and allows the patient to stabilize the knee and ambulate with only an ankle-foot orthosis (AFO). The tibialis anterior muscle, which lifts the foot at the ankle, receives its main enervation from L4. The extensor hallucis longus muscle, which lifts the great toe against gravity, and additional hip stabilizing muscles, receives enervation from L5. These patients also walk with AFOs.

The S1 nerve root level enervates the gastrocnemius and soleus muscles, calf muscles that are responsible for pushing-off from the floor. Those patients with adequate gastrocnemius strength can walk without the use of braces. Patients with sacral level injuries are very independent from a functional standpoint. However, they may have significant compromise of sexual, bowel, and bladder function, and may require a program to manage these. Again, it should be cautioned that the above descriptions apply to complete spinal cord injuries and that each spinal cord injury patient must be evaluated individually.

## Anatomic Spinal Cord Lesions

Sometimes, clinical pictures correspond to classic anatomic lesions, such as central cord syndrome, Brown-Sequard syndrome, and anterior cord syndrome (Figure 2). Central cord lesions are due to damage being greater in the central portion of the spinal cord. Since the nerve tracts controlling upper extremity muscles are more centrally located in the cord, injuries in this area result in the lower extremities being stronger than the upper extremities (e.g., a patient with quadriplegia who can ambulate). This may occur in somewhat older patients with underlying cervical arthritis who suffer a hyperextension neck injury.

Brown-Sequard syndrome or cord hemisection results in muscle paralysis on the side of the injury and sensory loss on the opposite side. This is because of the crossover of fibers within the spinal cord. Anterior cord syndrome results in paralysis with sparing of the sensory function.

The conus medullaris and cauda equina can be injured as well. The former is the region where the spinal cord itself ends and all the lumbar and sacral roots exit within the short segment of the conus medullaris, within the T12-L1 region. An injury in this area can result in paraplegia and an areflexic (without reflex) bowel and bladder. Injury to the cauda equina, where only nerve roots exist, can result in varying levels of paraplegia, including an areflexic bowel and bladder.

# Figure 2
## ANATOMIC CLASSIFICATION OF INCOMPLETE SPINAL CORD INJURIES

**Brown-Sequard Syndrome:** A lesion involving primarily one side of the cord which produces ipsilateral paralysis and loss of proprioception and contralateral loss of pain and temperature sensations.

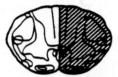

**Neuroanatomic Description of Incompleteness**
Incomplete injuries can be further classified on the basis of recognizable clinical syndromes produced by abnormal or absent function in some major tracts and cells yet normal function in others.

**Anterior Cord Syndrome:** A lesion involving the anterior two-thirds of the cord which produces paralysis and loss of pain and temperature sensations, while preserving proprioception.

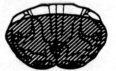

**Central Cord Syndrome:** A lesion. occurring almost exclusively in the cervical region, involving the central grey matter and the more medial white matter producing greater weakness in the upper limbs than in the lower limbs and sacral sensory sparing.

**Posterior Cord Syndrome:** A lesion involving the dorsal columns which produces loss of proprioception while preserving other sensory and motor function (very rare).

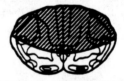

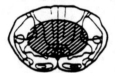

This information was obtained from the "Publication Standards for Neurologic Classification of Spinal Injury Patients," American Spinal Injury Association, pp. 16-17. Reprinted with permission.

## *Significance of Reflexes*

Presence of reflexes exists when a stimulus, often a noxious one, initiates an impulse from a peripheral nerve to the spinal cord. A neurologically intact patient conducts this impulse up the cord to the brain where the appropriate processing occurs. This results in the transmission of an impulse response down the spinal cord for the subsequent occurrence of a purposeful action. If the impulse cannot be transmitted up to the brain because of a severed cord, yet the nerve leaving the spinal cord is intact, a reflex arc is set up. This results in a non-purposeful action, ranging from a small twitch to simultaneous activity of many muscle groups, called spasticity. This action can be quite violent in some patients. If severe enough, the individual may require medication, nerve blocks, or even nerve resection (neurectomy).

The presence of reflexic contractions can be utilized to help patients perform certain functions. A patient with a reflexic bladder can learn to elicit a reflex, and "kick off" to empty the bladder when desired. Patients who are areflexic have flaccid extremities. An areflexic bladder is flaccid and requires external manual compression or catheterization to empty. The presence of reflexes in the extremities also can be utilized: patients have been known to use quadriceps spasms to help in pushing off and thus transferring from floor to chair. One can apply the law of the spinal cord: reflexes are intact above the level of injury, absent at the level of injury, and present below, usually (A.E. Comarr, Personal Communication, 1989). Exceptions may occur with a vascular injury so that even below the level of injury the cord is affected.

## Sexual Function

Sexual functioning is also affected in persons with spinal cord injury. In males, five areas are subject to potential dysfunction: erection, coitus, ejaculation, orgasm, and fertility. Most can have erections and intercourse. Completeness of the injury will determine whether there is sensation during sexual activity. In many males, the erection is due to a reflex and is not dependent on sensation. The possibilities for ejaculation, orgasm, and fertility are individual and vary from patient to patient. Still, for some males, new techniques and research are making parenthood possible.

Most women with spinal cord injury retain their ability to bear children. This underscores the importance of appropriate birth control counseling. The degree of sensation and pleasure will vary with the level and completeness of the injury. This also impacts positioning and other physical aspects of functioning. For both sexes, orgasm should be regarded as a cerebral event; many persons with spinal cord injury report a less physical, yet satisfying sensation, during lovemaking.

A broader definition of sexuality must be conceptualized wherein not only physical intercourse, but also communication, experimentation, and imagination will enhance sexual well-being. It is important that physicians and therapists give persons with spinal cord injury the knowledge of how their physical condition will affect their sexual functioning.

## Genitourinary Care

In persons with spinal cord injury, the genitourinary system is prone to frequent infection. This occurs when the bladder remains excessively full and urinary stagnation promotes bacterial growth. In addition, in the acute months after spinal cord injury, there are increased levels of calcium in the urine; this can lead to kidney stone formation. In previous times, these problems were responsible for premature mortality in these patients because of urosepsis (systemic poisoning due to urine retention) or renal failure. Today, with better understanding of these problems, patient education, and aggressive early treatment of urinary tract infections, patients can anticipate near-normal life expectancies.

If areflexic (without reflex), a patient may need to do self-catheterization or be helped in intermittent catheterization to empty the bladder. Patients who have absent or decreased bladder sphincter tone will need external catheters (for males) or diapers (for females). Other patients may be able to use intact abdominal musculature function as an adjunct to strain out urine; others, if reflexic, may, as mentioned above, be able to "kick off" to void (urinate). A few patients, unable to self-catheterize and in social or vocational situations where a caregiver may not be available frequently enough, will choose to have an indwelling catheter (one that remains permanently in place). A urologist experienced in the care of spinal cord injured patients may suggest surgery or medications to help patients manage these problems satisfactorily.

Each patient will require a personalized bowel hygiene program, usually designed by the nursing staff, to include an appropriate combination of stool softeners and suppositories, according to a patient's individual needs. In difficult cases, manual evacuation may be necessary, either by the patient or a caregiver. Since bowel and bladder control is affected in most persons with spinal cord injury, management with the least amount of inconvenience possible is important.

## Autonomic Dysreflexia

Autonomic dysreflexia is a potential catastrophic complication in spinal cord injury patients which may occur in those who have injuries at T7 and above. It is caused by abnormal stimulation of the autonomic nervous system, which controls many body functions such as regulation of blood pressure and heart rate. Because of the spinal cord injury, the patient cannot invoke normal counter-regulatory mechanisms to stimuli. As a consequence, the person experiences increased blood pressure, severe headaches, sweating, flushing, low pulse rate, goosebumps, and nasal congestion.

If the elevated blood pressure is not controlled, a cerebrovascular accident (stroke) can occur. Dysreflexia (the abnormal increase in blood pressure) can be set off by bladder distension or infection, kidney stones, spasm, colonic distension secondary to hard stools, and other noxious stimuli. Autonomic dysreflexia is a medical emergency and must be addressed immediately by reviewing all potential sources of irritating stimuli, particularly bladder distension, which is the most common inciting cause.

## Skin Care

The care of the skin is another crucial aspect of patient education. With impaired or absent skin sensation, the person does not feel irritation and pain. As a result, pressure applied to skin regions for prolonged periods of time can result in skin breakdown involving even underlying muscle with the development of decubitus ulcers (pressure sores). Appropriate cushions can decrease such problems and help avoid breakdown of the skin.

Patients with decreased sensation should be taught to perform pressure relief at regular intervals. This is done by lifting oneself from the wheelchair or leaning forward to shift weight. While a seemingly simple measure, patients have lost jobs due to frequent periods of bedrest or hospitalization for complex reconstructive surgery for their pressure sores. Patient education is important in preventing these devastating complications from occurring. This problem has economic implications as well: one pressure sore can result in both hospitalization expenses and loss of income and employment.

## Respiration

The diaphragm is the major respiratory muscle and its function is essential for normal breathing. However, other accessory respiratory muscles also play a role. They are controlled by lower nerve root levels so that patients with cervical and high thoracic lesions still have varying amounts of compromise of pulmonary function. While this may not be a problem on a daily basis, it may affect their ability to combat respiratory infections. Patients with such impairment are instructed in the use of the spirometer (a device that measures lung capacity), as well as coughing to clear the airways and deep breathing exercises to maximize pulmonary function.

## Bone Metabolism

Osteoporosis (the relative lack of bony mass) is a known occurrence after spinal cord injury; only recently have researchers begun to quantitate and define it. Bone loss appears to affect nearly the entire skeleton and occurs rapidly after injury. This loss of mineral can predispose bones, particularly in the lower extremities (long bones), to fracture from minimal trauma. This is a serious condition since fractures in patients with spinal cord injury have a much higher complication rate than fractures in the general population.

Patients with spinal cord injury have additional problems in bone metabolism. This involves a propensity for depositing bone in the soft tissues about the joints, called heterotopic ossification (HO), most frequently occurring about the hips. While many patients with HO have minimal functional limitations in range of motion, severe HO can result in a marked decrease in range of motion that results in a nearly rigid joint. This can cause difficulty in dressing, transfers, or may even preclude sitting. Surgery to resect HO has a high incidence of complications and should only be undertaken with a clear understanding of the goals and risks of surgery.

## Chronic Pain

Many spinal cord injured patients have problems with chronic pain. The incidence is higher in patients with spinal cord injury from gunshot wounds. Many patients have an eventual diminution of their pain symptoms, either spontaneously or with the help of modalities such as transcutaneous electric nerve stimulation (TENS), biofeedback, and medications. There are some patients who must learn to live and deal with chronic pain.

## Acute Versus Chronic Complications

One can summarize the complications seen after spinal cord injury and divide them into acute (within one month of injury) and long-term, as follows:

**Acute:**
1) Respiratory: pneumonia, pulmonary embolus
2) Genitourinary: kidney infections, kidney stones, bladder distension
3) Cardiovascular: autonomic dysreflexia, postural hypotension (decreases in blood pressure upon sitting or standing due to the lack of ability for blood vessels to accommodate to such changes), thrombophlebitis (blood clots in the leg veins, which can lead to pulmonary embolus, a potentially life-threatening event)
4) Skin: pressure sores
5) Gastrointestinal: stress-induced ulcers, decreased bowel motility
6) Musculoskeletal: heterotopic ossification, joint contracture

**Chronic:**
1) Respiratory: pneumonia
2) Genitourinary: bladder and kidney infection, prostatitis, bladder reflux (backflow up toward the kidney)
3) Cardiovascular: autonomic dysreflexia, postural hypotension, thrombophlebitis
4) Skin: pressure sores
5) Gastrointestinal: decreased bowel motility
6) Musculoskeletal: osteoporosis and consequent fractures, heterotopic ossification, joint contractures (secondary to muscle imbalance).

## Complications and Rehabilitation

Patients with spinal cord injury also are affected in other ways and are educated and instructed by the rehabilitation facility to manage their bowel/bladder, skin, respiratory system, and extremities. The rehabilitation counselor must be well aware that the medical stability of a client may override all other factors relating to employment because medical problems alone can lead to failure, even if all other conditions are optimal. Pressure sores, urinary tract infections, and lack of appropriate bowel management are all problems that can adversely affect persons with spinal cord injury and their employment. While not all spinal cord injured have to be concerned about these problems, the vast majority must be extremely vigilant to insure continued good health. This is more difficult for persons with quadriplegia than for those with paraplegia because of greater physical limitations and potential respiratory problems.

With appropriate preventive medical care and the correct equipment, most individuals can avoid complications. Since many health professionals have little exposure to people with spinal cord injuries, it is important that the person has access to a specialist or to a comprehensive medical facility experienced in spinal cord injury care. Minor conditions such as the flu or an ingrown toenail, if not properly managed, can seriously impact the health of a spinal cord injured person. The spinal cord injury Model Systems, sponsored by the Rehabilitation Services Administration, has gained much expertise with the centralization of a large volume of patients. Persons referred to these centers often benefit from evaluations to ensure maximization of their functional capabilities. A readily available resource for rehabilitation facilities that are accredited is the Commission on Accreditation of Rehabilitation Facilities (CARF).

History of repeated occurrences of preventable complications should alert the counselor to be especially careful when evaluating someone for employment. For example, if a person has a history of recurrent pressure sores, all details of this problem should be investigated and resolved before the rehabilitation counselor invests any significant energy toward helping the person attain employment. Since simple pressure relief requires only a few seconds, recurrent problems often suggest the person has not yet taken sufficient responsibility for self-care and may require psychological intervention before employment is considered an option.

Physical and occupational therapy, so essential in the spinal cord injury patient's recovery for the maximization of function, are also ongoing considerations in the patient's life. Most patients will leave the rehabilitation center with exercises or skills that must be practiced daily to ensure maintenance of optimal function.

Clearly, rehabilitation of the spinal cord injury patient is one that requires a team approach beginning at the time of injury. Many rehabilitation centers have regular "team meetings" where health care providers from appropriate disciplines meet and discuss short and long-term accomplishments and goals for each patient. This multidisciplinary approach has been very successful. For a full program of rehabilitation from the time of injury, a person with paraplegia can anticipate a 3-4 month stay in a rehabilitation facility; a person with quadriplegia can expect a stay of 5-6 months.

# VOCATIONAL REHABILITATION

## Employment

Estimates of employment rates among individuals with spinal cord injury vary from 13-48%. This wide range is due to differing levels of injury, time since injury, selection of population, definition of employment, and other factors. For many individuals, employment is a vital concern, either for the pragmatic necessities of wage earning, the emotional gratification of self-worth, or both (Lonnquist, 1979; Pati, Adkins, & Morrison, 1991; Weidman & Freehafer, 1981). Marcel (1949) in his book **The Philosophy of Existence** stated, "Modern man knows himself not as a man, or as a self, but as a ticket seller in the subway, a grocer, a professor, a vice-president of A.T.& T., or by whatever his economic function may be" (p. 1). While this may not be a fair assessment of character, it is frequently used.

It is also true that one should be cautioned against assuming that success in life post-injury is measured only by employment. Rehabilitation and vocational rehabilitation need not be synonymous. A successful life involves many activities; employment is only one of these. For many, avocational pursuits, volunteer work, family responsibilities, or other activities are fulfilling. For these people, rehabilitation outcome cannot be effectively measured by employment status alone (Parker, 1987; Rubin & Roessler, 1987).

## Functional Limitations

Appropriate dress, punctuality, reliability, and other basic work habits are all prerequisites to successful employment (Crewe, Athelstan, & Bower, 1978). A person with a spinal cord injury will have to get up earlier in the morning to manage self-care. Depending on the degree of impairment, it is not unusual for a spinal cord injured person to take 2-4 hours to prepare for work. Bathing, dressing, and bowel and bladder management are time and energy consuming. The ability to manage self-care functions is crucial to sustaining employment and activities of daily life.

**Activities of daily living (ADL).** The maximizing of activities of daily living skills is very important. Eating, bathing, grooming, and dressing are a struggle for many and impossible for others. The individual's ability to complete these activities should be evaluated before seeking competitive employment. The higher the level of injury, the more complex the problems. Orthotic and assistive devices are provided to make these tasks easier, but they require practice for proficiency.

For those who require attendant care for ADL, the selection of a good, reliable attendant is essential. Hiring someone to provide very personal care is difficult; there is a high turnover rate. Locating and retaining the services of a highly reliable attendant for a low paying job is an additional burden faced by most persons with quadriplegia.

**Level of physical impairment.** Among the most important factors is the level of physical impairment. Data on the effect of level of injury relative to employment is conflicting. Some studies have shown that persons with paraplegia fare better in employment than persons with quadriplegia (DeVivo, Rutt, Stover, & Fine, 1987). Yet, Goldberg and Freed (1982) reported no correlation between vocational adjustment and level of injury. El Ghatit and Hanson (1978) found that while persons with paraplegia had a greater success rate of securing employment, persons with quadriplegia maintained employment at an equal rate. Level of injury may not be as important as the person's desire and ability to be independent, either directly or with the assistance of an attendant.

Most persons with paraplegia will not be able to do jobs requiring lifting, carrying, standing, walking, or operating controls with their feet. Occasionally, job modification may permit a person with paraplegia to accomplish these tasks. Many skilled and semiskilled jobs require hand and arm function. Likewise, many jobs that emphasize intellectual skills but still require filing, typing, or traveling may be difficult for most persons with quadriplegia, unless appropriate equipment and site modifications can be applied (Pinkerton & Griffin, 1983).

**Mobility.** The degree of mobility achieved by a person using a wheelchair depends on the level of injury and the type of wheelchair used. New ultralite wheelchairs give a person with a spinal cord injury the ability to propel the chair over greater distances with less effort and more maneuverability. For those who do not require electric wheelchairs, use significantly enhances mobility and minimizes fatigue. Most persons with paraplegia can use a manually propelled wheelchair and become proficient to the point of handling very difficult terrain.

Some persons with paraplegia may require the use of electric wheelchairs because of activities involving increased energy and time expenditure. Examples of this would be a hilly college campus, a rural residence, and large areas of uneven or rough terrain. Some individuals with paraplegia can ambulate with crutches; their ability to negotiate difficult terrain depends on their level of proficiency and the amount of energy expended. In addition, some may be able to stand and work with their hands free.

It is not unusual for some persons with quadriplegia to be able to use manual wheelchairs. Yet, many choose to use electric wheelchairs to save energy. For the person accustomed to using the manual wheelchair, there may be resistance to using an electric one. It is often beneficial to use an electric wheelchair for energy efficiency and to minimize the development of chronic strain. Studies on aging in the spinal cord injured have shown that overuse of shoulders, elbows, and wrists can result in chronic fatigue, pain, and possible injury.

A standing wheelchair or standing frame may allow a person with quadriplegia to work in the upright position, depending on the individual's balance and hand function. Irrespective of level of injury, it is important that equipment and medical support are adequate to maximize the person's vocational potential.

**Additional factors.** Many persons with quadriplegia can benefit from hand orthoses; occasionally, surgical procedures can improve hand function. A person with a high level injury may have problems with sitting tolerance. Often, a different chair, cushion, or adjustment in posture may improve sitting tolerance.

Spinal cord injury may also affect the sense of balance. Those who have little or no trunk muscle function may have difficulty bending over, performing rapid upper body movements, lifting with two hands, and other similar tasks.

Another area of potential difficulty involves problems with thermoregulation (heat regulation). Many persons with spinal cord injury cannot tolerate extremes of temperature. In these cases, an indoor job is preferable. Spinal cord injured individuals will benefit from dressing in layers of clothing to insure comfort with temperature changes.

Recurrent autonomic dysreflexia can be a problem in the workplace. For those affected, it is advisable that they carry an information sheet with them to alert staff at hospital emergency rooms who may not be aware of this life-threatening condition.

The ability to be a creative problem solver greatly enhances the employability of persons with spinal cord injury. There is often a difference between the proper medical way to do things and the pragmatic way dictated by the necessities of independent living. Those persons who can identify and solve problems related to their care and mobility have a distinct advantage over those who cannot. The rehabilitation counselor may be able to help the process by developing creative alternative solutions to resolve problems the client faces.

Among the spinal cord injured, there are some individuals that sustain a concomitant brain injury. A minimal brain injury may be overlooked during hospitalization. These individuals require appropriate neuropsychological testing to determine how any deficits relate to employability.

## Rehabilitation Potential

**Pre-injury work history.** This is an important component of vocational potential. If a person was highly motivated prior to injury and had good work habits, these characteristics should carry over into post-injury development (DeVivo & Fine, 1982). Conversely, if a person exhibited lack of responsibility, undesirable social and work habits, and poor attendance, these traits will carry over post-injury. Since spinal cord injuries typically happen to young individuals, a relevant work history may not exist.

Those spinal cord injured persons with a limited work history may benefit from a job exploration phase and an interest inventory as the first stage in counseling. In addition, the rehabilitation counselor may need to assist the individual in improving job-seeking skills (Bolton, 1981, 1982). Typically, the interview process, development of a resume, filling out the application, and other skills should be addressed and reviewed.

**Motivation.** Perhaps the most crucial component for vocational rehabilitation is the motivation of the client. If the person lacks a work history but has developed specific vocational plans, this may indicate a greater chance for success. Alfred, Fuhrer, and Rossi (1989) showed that previous vocational plans and work interests were the most reliable predictors for the attainment of post-injury employment for persons with spinal cord injury.

The motivation to work is difficult for others to generate and usually must come from within the individual. An explanation of the alternatives and a supportive position by the counselor is helpful. An adjustment period following the injury may be necessary before the person is motivated to work; in some, the motivation may never develop.

**Education.** Persons who improve their educational level after injury have a better chance of employment than those who remain at the same level. There are many reasons for this. Most spinal cord injured have been physically active at the time of injury; many held manual labor jobs that required little or no education. Additional education may help many in obtaining employment in areas where the focus is on intellectual skills. For some, technical vocational training in a realistic and practical area may be more effective than in a traditional academic setting. It should be cautioned that for those who return to or initiate academic pursuits, graduation does not guarantee employment.

**Suitability of vocational goal.** In order to have a greater chance for success, the chosen field of study should lead to employment that suits the individual and the individual's current lifestyle. The counselor needs to be careful not to automatically place spinal cord injured persons into the category of sedentary work. For many years, there was a tendency to channel spinal cord injured into watch repair or radio dispatching. These are valid occupations, but are clearly not the only alternatives.

**Psychological adjustment.** Following are some psychological considerations important to the vocational rehabilitation process. It is well established that a person's emotional well-being correlates with vocational success (Trieschmann, 1980, 1988).

The stages that a person with a spinal cord injury goes through have been well described and are similar to the stages of grieving: denial, anger, bargaining, depression, and adaptation, as defined by Kubler-Ross (1969). While these are helpful in understanding the emotional response to severe disability, they should not be interpreted literally. If someone does not become depressed, it does not mean that they are hopelessly stalled in the "adjustment process." Everyone has a unique way of adjusting to a major disability such as a spinal cord injury; professionals must be sensitive to the total needs of each individual. It will take time before the person can concentrate on residual capacities and abilities, not on the disability and loss of function. Unfortunately, some persons never adjust to the consequences of severe disability.

Another problem area related to the psychological adjustment process is the prevalence of substance abuse. This is partially due to the young age of this population, combined with the isolation that frequently accompanies a major injury. The person with a spinal cord injury has limited mobility and disrupted patterns of socialization. The counselor can encourage and facilitate involvement with family, friends, and the community. This mainstreaming process may decrease depression which frequently is the cause of substance abuse. The aim is to relieve the client of the substance abuse problem before any vocational plan is finalized.

Body image and self-esteem relate to general adjustment and to employment. It takes time for the injured person to realize that, despite a change in body image, there is still significant potential for vocational achievement.

The degree of disability does not necessarily correlate with psychological adjustment to disability (Cook, Bolton, & Taperek, 1981). Some individuals with paraplegia, with greater residual function, may be more emotionally affected than individuals with quadriplegia. The effects of the injury should be viewed functionally, not anatomically. Kemp and Vash (1971) noted that persons with spinal cord injury who viewed their post-injury goals in terms of anatomic function (i.e., "I want to walk"), were less successful vocationally than those who viewed their goals more in functional terms (i.e., "I want to learn to support myself and my family").

The adjustment to a spinal cord injury is an ongoing process. Maintaining a steady job and assimilating into the traditional role of wage earner can greatly ease this process.

## Social and Economic Considerations

Transportation, family support, and living arrangements also influence employability. A highly qualified person who cannot get to work on time because of difficulty with attendants or transportation will be unable to sustain employment.

**Transportation.** The ability to drive correlates with sustained employment (Poor, 1975). With the proper equipment, those persons with injuries at C5 and below can learn to drive. A person with quadriplegia requires a van with a lift, hand controls, and other modifications. Individuals with paraplegia usually only need hand controls on a regular vehicle; most can transfer and get the wheelchair into the car independently. Since accessible and efficient public transit is not available in many areas, owning a vehicle is an important asset in finding and maintaining employment. With the passage of the Americans with Disabilities Act in 1990, transportation is becoming more readily accessible and available.

Many persons with quadriplegia do not have the considerable financial resources needed to purchase a modified van. Some states furnish vans for persons with spinal cord injury who attend school or work. Another option for some individuals is to join a car pool. This is only feasible if the person can transfer independently and does not require an electric wheelchair to be placed in an automobile trunk. Family members also may provide transportation to school or the workplace. Any form of transportation that increases the person's dependence is less than optimal. An important goal for spinal cord injured persons who are able to drive is owning a vehicle and providing their own transportation.

**Economic considerations**. A significant problem in the area of vocational development continues to be economic disincentives (Trieschmann, 1988). For many, the prospect of returning to work and relinquishing medical benefits represents a great risk. The rules and regulations governing these benefits vary from state to state and even amoung different counties. Federal benefits, however, are consistent throughout the country.

The costs of living with a spinal cord injury are considerable. In 1987, the average annual disability-related expenses for a person with T3 paraplegia was estimated at $10,200, and for a person with C6 quadriplegia, $21,100. Medical care, hospitalization, wheelchairs, attendant help, transportation costs, home modification, and bowel and bladder supplies contribute to this high cost.

Many spinal cord injured receive their income from federal public assistance. The qualifications for Social Security Disability Insurance (SSDI) are based on work history. Supplemental Security Income (SSI) is based on financial need. Cash assets, retirement plans, spouse's wages, and almost all assets except a principle home, are included in evaluating financial need. Many persons receive Medicare (or state medical assistance) as part of their Social Security benefits; if they lose Social Security, they also may lose all or part of their medical coverage. Part-time work and most entry-level salaries are insufficient to compensate for lost benefits. Even marriage to a working spouse can have a serious negative financial impact on the benefits received. Keeping these facts in mind, it is not difficult to understand why the prospect of losing benefits has kept many persons from seeking employment.

To maintain health insurance, most people seek employment where group medical coverage is available. Yet, many policies do not cover pre-existing conditions or medical equipment and supplies. Medical coverage is now generally linked to earnings of severely disabled persons so that many of these individuals cannot afford to work if it involves giving up their medical benefits.

**Employer attitudes**. Attitudes of employers also affect opportunities for employment. Many employers are reluctant to have someone in a wheelchair interact with the public. Yet, many people with spinal cord injury are trained to do this type of work. Prospective employers may be unfamiliar with individuals who have disabilities and have unrealistic fears. Concerns about office or job-site modification, relations with other employees, and capabilities can usually be remedied by a positive experience with an employee who has a disability. There are laws that prohibit discrimination which can be invoked to protect persons with disabilities where necessary. The Americans with Disabilities Act is having a significant impact on hiring practices.

**Sexuality**. This is a subject that needs consideration. Appropriately defined, sexuality is not just the physical act of sex, but includes a person's sense of self-esteem and body image. Naturally, these feelings have an impact on relationships. The person with a spinal cord injury requires access to accurate information concerning sexual problems and how injury may affect functioning. Counselors who are uncomfortable or not knowledgeable in this area would do well to make an appropriate referral. Misinformation can be considerably worse than lack of information. Sexuality is a very important component of everyone's life and must be addressed if the rehabilitation process is to be complete. While there are no known studies relating sexual satisfaction and success in employment, sexual fulfillment improves self-image and thus fosters reintegration into society.

**Other factors**. Family and interpersonal support also relate to successful employment. The rehabilitation counselor needs to interact with the person's parents, spouse, other family members, or friends to determine the amount of support or resistance that may be encountered and to clarify expectations. Some families may be overprotective and consider employment too stressful for the spinal cord injured person. Family reactions vary, but are always relevant and must be taken into careful consideration.

The physical living arrangement of the person influences employment. Accessibility within the residence is important. If the person lives with family members who provide care, one may want to recommend a professional evaluation of the home situation or possible alternatives available.

## Vocational Intervention

**Early intervention.** There are two schools of thought on when the individual with a spinal cord injury should be approached for vocational rehabilitation services. One theory states vocational intervention should begin as soon as possible after injury. Such early intervention informs the person vocational counseling services are available. For others, the counselor may suggest non-vocational community involvement as a way to avoid isolation during the early months after hospitalization. The second theory states most persons are not ready for employment for 18-24 months after injury and vocational efforts can wait until that time. When the injured person is concerned with the restoration of physical losses during the medical rehabilitation process, it is very difficult to be realistic regarding future employment.

Providing introductory vocational information early after injury serves to help the person recognize the potential employment possibilities. A discussion of pre-injury goals and plans and how they relate to the present physical condition may help formulate a program to be initiated later. One can increase the intensity of vocational intervention when the person recognizes the need for realistic alternatives in life with the new physical condition. For most individuals, this seems to fall into the 18-24 month post-injury period. There are those individuals who may be ready for vocational intervention earlier. The appropriate time for intervention must be individually determined dependent on the progress the client has made both physically and emotionally, and the vocational services that are available. Clearly, rehabilitation is an ongoing process.

**Questions relating to intervention.** Shaw and McMahon (1985) suggested that rehabilitation specialists consider the following questions when attempting vocational intervention:

1. Are expressed and assessed vocational interests being considered and weighed in the occupational selection process?

2. Is the process of vocational choice negatively affected by preconceived notions about performance capabilities held by the counselor, the client, or both?

3. Are the income levels associated with the vocational objective sufficient to provide a meaningful wage beyond additional medical and transportation needs?

4. Would retraining or additional education substantially enhance the client's value in the job market?

5. In the process of occupational selection, is sufficient attention being given to job modification, job restructuring, and alternative schedules of work so that the field of occupational alternatives is not prematurely or routinely restricted?

These questions relate not only to employment, but whether employment best suits the spinal cord injured person. Shaw and McMahon (1985) reported that of all spinal cord injuries occurring in mid-career, only 1% of these individuals ever returned to work at the same job. Further, persons with paralysis have lower median incomes than any other disability group. The emphasis should not be on any employment, but directed toward appropriate employment. Before reaching vocational decisions, the counselor and client need to realistically view various potential employment opportunities. If there exists an incorrect idea by either the client or the counselor of the potential for returning to work, the client's best interests will not be served.

**Maximizing potential.** The utilization of personal and worksite adaptive equipment can help insure sustained employment or even allow for a return to previous employment. Provision of medical and personal equipment and training are essential to help maximize vocational or ADL skills (Felice, Muthard, & Hamilton, 1976; Lassiter et al., 1983). Such devices as a tape recorder, personal computer, or electric wheelchair can provide a significant improvement in vocational training or employment. Environmental controls that allow for the independent operation of lights, office equipment, and telephones can be used in the workplace to make tasks feasible.

Modern technology allows persons with high level quadriplegia to interface with computers. Many devices for individuals with high level quadriplegia are expensive and not covered by third-party payers. It may be necessary to look for alternative sources of funding to pay for such equipment, but it may make the difference in employability. It is crucial to provide these in a timely fashion, whenever possible.

Although mainstreaming remains the preferred option, the advent of computers with modems and fax machines makes home employment an option. This may allow some persons a high level of productivity, yet the freedom to work at their own schedule. Persons with high level quadriplegia will benefit most from this option.

Most employers are unaware of modifications needed to accommodate an employee who uses a wheelchair. Simply widening a doorway or raising a desk may be all that is required. Expensive remodeling should be avoided; the counselor and client should jointly discuss the needs and come to a mutual solution. Of course, accessible bathroom facilities are essential.

There are several other areas where vocational intervention can be enhanced. Many rehabilitation counselors have not worked with persons with spinal cord injury. A knowledgeable professional, familiar with spinal cord injury, will maximize the potential for employment.

It is good practice for counselors to keep files active for clients with severe disabilities even after the completion of several months of employment. With the severity of spinal cord inury, it is probable that the person may require further medical or vocational assistance. These services often require immediate attention to insure an individual's continuing employment. Lastly, it should be emphasized that the refinement of job-seeking and interviewing skills, job performance and social skills, the provision of medical and therapeutic support, and the use of creative problem-solving, all enhance the person's employability.

**Legislation.** It is crucial for the rehabilitation counselor to be familiar with the laws and regulations relating to employment, especially the Rehabilitation Act of 1973 and the 1990 Americans with Disabilities Act. These regulations are frequently very complex, especially when they involve return to work guidelines and how this will affect a person's benefits. Accurate information is difficult to obtain and the need for an advocate is crucial in making an informed choice about employment. It is also beneficial for the counselor to be aware of federal and state legislation related to tax credits for employers who hire workers with disabilities.


# CASE STUDY


Mike McDonald is a single, 21 year-old who finished high school with a "B" average, completed real estate school, and received a real estate sales license. While in high school, he enjoyed mathematics and social science classes and was active in the drama department.

Immediately prior to the accident, Mike worked as a real estate salesperson for 4 months. Before this job, he worked for one year as a waiter in an expensive, gourmet restaurant. Mike enjoys working with people and works well with others. He possesses the work personality needed to keep a job and has not had problems with co-workers or supervisors.

Six months ago, Mr. McDonald sustained a cervical spine injury in a motor vehicle accident. The lesion is at C6 and is incomplete. There has been a return of partial function in the lower extremities, but not enough to allow for independent ambulation. Mike's arms are affected, the left more than the right. There is spasticity and contractures of the left hand and an inability to perform any fine motor skills with that hand. His right, dominant hand has residual weakness with some impairment of fine motor skills. While Mike is continuing to show neurological recovery, there is no question he will have some permanent and irreversible paralysis of both upper and lower extremities.

Due to his concerns regarding sexuality, Mike's physician referred him to a specialist, Dr. Green at the outpatient spinal cord unit, for consultation. Although you have only seen Mike on two occasions for rehabilitation counseling, he has asked you to attend this medical consultation with him.

## Questions

1. Provide a vocational profile for this client, including age category, educational level, and work history (skill and exertional levels).

2. What kinds of adaptive equipment and devices would you recommend to increase independence?

3. Does Mr. McDonald possess transferable skills? If so, identify these skills and explore employment alternatives using transferable skills.

4. Will you attend the medical consultation with Dr. Green? Discuss.

5. If Mike requires sexual counseling, will you provide it? If not, what will you advise?

6. Outline three rehabilitation plans, one involving further education, one providing short-term training, and one offering on-the-job training or immediate job placement.

# REFERENCES

Alfred, W.G., Fuhrer, M.J., & Rossi, C.D. (1987). Vocational development following severe spinal cord injury: A longitudinal study. **Archives of Physical Medicine and Rehabilitation, 68,** 854-857.

American Spinal Injury Association Standards (1990). **Publication standards for neurologic classification of spinal injury patients.** Atlanta, GA: American Spinal Injury Association.

Benson, D.R., & Keenen, T.L. (1990). Evaluation and treatment of trauma to the vertebral column, Chapter 7. **Instructional course lectures** (Vol. 39). American Academy of Orthopaedic Surgeons, pp. 577-589. St. Louis, Mo: C.V. Mosby.

Bolton, B. (1981). Assessing employability of handicapped persons: The vocational rehabilitation perspective. **Journal of Applied Rehabilitation Counseling, 12,** 40-44.

Bolton, B. (1982). **Vocational adjustment of disabled persons.** Baltimore, MD: University Park Press.

Cook, D.W., Bolton, B., & Taperek, P. (1981). Rehabilitation of the spinal cord injured: Life status at follow-up. **Rehabilitation Counseling Bulletin, 25**(2), 110-122.

Crewe, N.M., Athelstan, G.T., & Bower, A.S. (1978). **Employment after spinal cord injury: A handbook for counselors.** Minneapolis, MN: University of Minnesota.

DeVivo, M.J., & Fine, P.R. (1982). Employment status of spinal cord injured patients 3 years after injury. **Archives of Physical Medicine and Rehabilitation, 63,** 200-203.

DeVivo, M.J., Rutt, R.D., Stover, S.L., & Fine, P.R. (1987). Employment after spinal cord injury. **Archives of Physical Medicine and Rehabilitation, 68,** 494-498.

El Ghatit, A.Z., & Hanson, R.W. (1978). Variables associated with obtaining and sustaining employment among spinal cord injured males: A follow-up of 760 veterans. **Journal of Chronic Disease, 31,** 363-369.

Felice, K.A., Muthard, J.E., & Hamilton, L.S. (1976). The rehabilitation problems and needs of the spinal-cord injured: A pilot study. **Journal of Applied Rehabilitation Counseling, 7,** 76-87.

Goldberg, R.T., & Freed, M.M. (1982). Vocational development of spinal cord injury patients: An 8-year follow-up. **Archives of Physical Medicine and Rehabilitation, 63,** 207-210.

Hussey, R.W. (1982). Spinal cord injuries. In V.L. Nickel, (Ed.), **Orthopaedic rehabilitation** (pp. 209-230). New York, NY: Churchill Livingstone.

Kemp, B.J., & Vash, C.L. (1971). Productivity after injury in a sample of spinal cord injured persons: A pilot study. **Journal of Chronic Disease, 24,** 259-275.

Kubler-Ross, E. (1969). **On death and dying.** New York, NY: Macmillan.

Lassiter, R.A., Lassiter, M.H., Hardy, R.E., Underwood, J.W., & Cull, J.G. (1983). **Vocational evaluation, work adjustment and independent living for severely disabled people.** Springfield, OH: Charles C Thomas.

Lonnquist, D.E. (1979). Employment rates among severely disabled and nondisabled college graduates and dropouts. **Journal of Applied Rehabilitation Counseling, 10,** 24-27.

Marcel, G. (1949). **The philosophy of existence.** London, England: Harvill Press.

McDowell, D.L. (1988). Tetraplegia. In D.L. Green (Ed.), **Operative Hand Surgery** (2nd ed., pp. 1597-1617). New York, NY: Churchill Livingstone.

Parker, R.M. (1987). **Rehabilitation counseling: Basics and beyond.** Austin, TX: Pro-ed.

Pati, G.C., Adkins, J.I., Jr., & Morrison, G. (1981). **Managing and employing the handicapped.** Lake Forest,IL: Brace-Park.

Pierce, D.S., & Nickel, V.H. (1977). **The total care of spinal cord injuries.** Boston, MA: Little, Brown.

Pinkerton, A.C., & Griffin, M.L. (1983). Rehabilitation outcomes in females with spinal cord injury: A follow-up study. **Paraplegia, 21**(3), 166-175.

Poor, C.R. (1975). Vocational rehabilitation of persons with spinal cord injuries. **Rehabilitation Counseling Bulletin, 18**(4), 264-271.

Rubin, S.E., & Roessler, R.T. (1987). **Foundations of the vocational rehabilitation process** (3rd ed.). Austin, TX: Pro-ed.

Shaw, L.R., & McMahon, B.T. (1985). Jobs obtained by spinal cord injured rehabilitants: Implications for job placement practices. **Journal of Applied Rehabilitation Counseling, 16**(2), 48-51.

Trieschmann, R.B. (1980). **Spinal cord injuries: Psychological, social, and vocational adjustment.** New York, NY: Pergamon.

*390*

Trieschmann, R.B. (1988). **Spinal cord injuries. Psychological, social, and vocational rehabilitation**. New York, NY: Demos.

Weidman, C.D., & Freehafer, A.A. (1981). Vocational outcome in patients with spinal cord injury. **Journal of Rehabilitation, 47**(2), 63-65.

Zigler, J.E., Capen, D.A., Atkins, M.S., & Resnick, C.D. (1991). Rehabilitation, In S. Garfin, F. Eismont, & A. Levine (Eds.), **Spine Trauma**. Orlando, FL: W.B. Saunders.

## *About the Authors*

Serena S. Hu, M.D., is an orthopaedic surgeon and an Assistant Professor at the University of California, San Francisco. She completed her fellowship in spine and scoliosis surgery at Rancho Los Amigos Medical Center in Downey, California.

Jeffrey M. Cressy is the Community Liaison for the Spinal Cord Injury Project at Rancho Los Amigos Medical Center in Downey, California. He is a former President of the Board of Directors of an independent living center in the Los Angeles, California area. Mr. Cressy has quadriplegia as a result of an automobile accident that occurred in 1976.

# Chapter 25

# EVALUATING HAND FUNCTION AND IMPAIRMENT

by
*George W. Balfour, M.D.*

## INTRODUCTION

The American Medical Association (AMA) Guidelines (Engelberg, 1988) for the Evaluation of Impairment assigns a single upper extremity a value of 60% of the function of a whole person. Ninety percent of the function of the upper extremity is defined to be in the hand and, therefore, hand function represents 54% of that of a whole person. Impairment, however, differs from disability. Impairment is the loss of function in the physical sense and disability is the inability to overcome or compensate for that impairment. Oskamp (1988) defines impairment and disability as follows. **Impairment** describes an abnormality or a loss of a physiological structure or function. **Disability** refers to the consequences of an impairment - a restriction or lack of ability to perform some activity that is considered normal function. A new term, physically challenged, suggests an ability to perform, but with increased difficulty.

Injuries occur for the most part in the home, at work, in vehicle accidents, or in sports activities. Industrial statistics, well studied because of the expenses involved when injury occurs, show that in every industrialized nation, injuries to the hand and upper extremity represent approximately one-third of all work-related injuries (Absoud & Harrop, 1984). Every year, about 100,000 industrial workers in the United States sustain injury severe enough to result in permanent impairment; more than 2 million miss more than a day of work because of occupational accidents. In 1980, about 400,000 of these 2 million work-related injuries involved the hand and fingers (Baxter, 1986). Besides being common, the recovery time for significant upper extremity injury may be prolonged. This is another reason for economic concern. The better we understand these injuries, the more we can contribute to the rehabilitation process and lessen the economic and social consequences of the impairment (Schultz-Johnson, 1987).

## FUNCTION AND ANATOMY

### Function of the Hand

The hand has a variety of functions. It is in many ways a sensory organ in that it has a high concentration of nerve endings that provide information about the environment. Watch an infant at play. The infant looks at an object, picks it up and feels it, learning its weight, hardness, surface texture, temperature, size, and shape. Lastly, the infant puts the object in the mouth, further feeling and tasting it. The somatosensory surface of the brain receives and processes the sense of touch. Almost as much brain area is devoted to the hand as the rest of the body (excluding the face and mouth). Figure 1 is a schematic picture of the somasensory area of the brain. It depicts the relative importance and proportions of brain tissue devoted to the sense of touch. Note that only the lips and face are given

---

### Figure 1
### SOMASENSORY AREA OF THE BRAIN

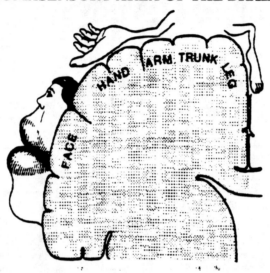

Manikin illustration of the sensory surface of the brain devoted to the sense of touch for the various parts of the body.

---

From **Human neuroanatomy** (6th ed., p. 559) by R.C. Truex & M.B. Carpenter, 1969, Baltimore, MD: Williams and Wilkins. Reprinted by permission.

---

more area than the hand. Put your hand in your pocket and feel a coin. You can recognize what kind of coin it is by its feel; you can almost read its face. In a sense, you can see it with your fingers. Rub that same coin across your face or your thigh. You cannot read the face of the coin or even tell what kind of coin it is.

The hand's sensitivity to touch is due to a high concentration of nerve endings in the skin, particularly in the palmar skin. The amount of brain surface devoted to a body part is in proportion to the part's ability to receive sensation (sensibility). A hand with significant sensory impairment can be thought of as "blind." Besides sensory functions, our hands serve as the terminal devices of the upper extremities in activities such as lifting, carrying, and grasping. Hands do fine manipulative tasks such as turning a key, holding a glass, doing fine crafts, writing, using tools, and operating office equipment. We use our hands in a social role: shaking hands, holding hands, and gesturing. The hand also has a cosmetic function. We paint finger nails, wear rings and decorative gloves. Hands function in gross strength: in lifting, carrying, pushing, pulling, and when working with large tools and equipment. The hand functions in the use of shovels, hammers, and saws in grip with the principle force and motion being at the wrist, forearm, elbow, and shoulder. The physician needs to consider each of these functions when assessing the degree of impairment and rehabilitation potential.

Another way of understanding the hand is by comprehending its component anatomical parts and the role each part has in the total function of the hand. Proximal to the hand is the rest of the upper extremity, the wrist, elbow, arm, shoulder, and neck. These areas provide muscle mass and power, and the ability to put the hand anywhere in a large global area or space surrounding the individual.

This chapter addresses the anatomy of the hand, its function, and the function of the entire upper extremity. It explains medical assessment of impairment in the upper extremity. We will look at typical injuries, including their care, treatment, prognosis, and time to final healing. Also, we will discuss residuals, sequelae, impairments, and their effects on vocational rehabilitation.

## Practical Anatomy and Physiology of the Hand and Upper Extremity

Hand function starts in the brain, the location of sensory and motor control. Afferent nerve fibers conduct impulses to the brain; efferent nerve fibers carry impulses from the brain to the rest of the body. The efferent fibers pass down the brain stem through the spinal cord and exit at the nerve roots of the fourth through seventh cervical vertebrae (C4-C7) and the first thoracic vertebrae (T1). On either side of the cervical spine, in the neck, these nerve roots combine to form the brachial plexus of nerves. From this plexus, three major nerves reach the forearm and hand: the median, ulnar, and radial nerves.

**Anatomy.** Discussion of anatomy requires some understanding of descriptive terms. In the trunk (upper body), we use the term volar (anterior) for the front or face side of the body and dorsal (posterior) for the back. Medial and lateral refer to closer to and farther away from the midline of the body. In the hand, we talk about the palmar (instead of volar) and dorsal surfaces or sides of the hand. In the forearm, we again use the terms volar and dorsal surfaces.

**The forearm.** In the forearm, there are two sets of extrinsic muscles, the volar or flexion group and the dorsal or extensor group. The term extrinsic means the muscles in the group are outside the hand itself (in the forearm), but produce function in the hand. The volar extrinsic forearm muscles are flexors. These muscles are outside of the hand, but reach the hand by tendons. They act in the hand to flex or bend the fingers and wrist. The median nerve controls most of this function. An extensor group of extrinsics function principally to extend the fingers, thumb, and wrists. This function is controlled by the radial nerve. The intrinsic muscles are located below the wrist, in the hand itself. They are innervated principally by the ulnar nerve (except those to the thumb) and balance the finger motion, add strength to grip, and abduct and adduct the fingers. Abduction and adduction of the fingers is the spreading and side to side closing motions of the fingers.

**The median nerve.** This nerve supplies sensation to the palm and palmar sides of the thumb, index, long, and radial half of the ring finger. It is the most important sensory nerve to the hand and is the motor nerve for the majority of the muscles of the volar forearm, the forearm flexors. These are the muscles that bend or flex the wrist and flex or close the fingers and thumb. These median nerve controlled flexors provide the power of grip, wrist flexion, and function in lifting and carrying. Below the wrist, the median nerves supply muscle innervation to the small or intrinsic muscles of the thumb (the thenar muscles). The median nerve innervates the intrinsic muscles of the thumb. This is important in rowing the thumb out of the palm into opposition; it contributes to the power of pinch (Truex & Carpenter, 1969).

**The ulna nerve.** This nerve passes behind the elbow, behind the medial epicondyle (the bony bump on the medial side of the elbow), and through the cubital tunnel. It runs down the ulna (little finger) side of the forearm to the hand. In the hand, it provides sensation to the little finger, the ulna half of the ring finger, and muscle innervation and control of the small intrinsic muscles of the hand. The intrinsic muscles help provide balance to the fingers and fine manipulative control of the hand.

**The radial nerve.** This is the sensory nerve for the back (dorsum) of the hand and thumb. In the forearm, it supplies muscle innervation to the extensor muscle group. These muscles allow extension of the wrist, fingers, and thumb. A radial palsy results in a wrist drop. Wrist drop means the hand droops toward the ground and the individual is unable to support the hand or fingers straight against gravity. This inability to position the hand correctly against gravity can cause a marked impairment in function. A wrist drop implies an injury to the radial nerve. A lower radial nerve injury will cause numbness only.

**Median nerve injury.** There may be high or low median nerve injuries. A high median nerve injury causes inability to flex the wrist, fingers, and thumb, makes grip impossible, and causes numbness to the thumb, index, long, and half the ring finger. A lower median nerve injury causes the numbness and weakness of the intrinsic muscles of the thumb only. Thumb intrinsic muscles function in pinch as in turning a key, and in opposition as in touching the tip of the thumb to the tip of the little finger. Substitution (finding ways to work around such an impairment or nerve deficit) is easier with a low median nerve defect than with a high one.

There are quick medical tests for muscle motor function of these three nerves. For radial nerve function, one looks for wrist extension; for median nerve function, the physician tests for thumb flexion. In the case of ulnar nerve function, one examines for isolated abduction of the index finger.

The blood supply to the upper extremity enters the arm as the large single axillary artery, and continues as the brachial artery. At the elbow, it splits into the radial and ulnar arteries, which run down their respective side of the forearm. They reconnect in the hand through deep and superficial arches. From these arches, two digital vessels supply each digit, one to each side of a finger. A single vessel is adequate to supply a hand, but the hand may then have some cold intolerance. A single digital vessel is usually adequate blood supply for a finger.

**Arterial injuries.** These include laceration, thrombosis, and aneurysm. Lacerations can be either complete or partial. Complete lacerations mean the blood supply to a part may be interrupted. If there is no collateral circulation, that part will become ischemic (deficient in blood) and die. Multi-source or collateral circulation (the alternate blood supply pathway) is where two vessels supply the same body part or area. If damage occurs to one vessel, the collateral circulation is adequate to keep the part alive.

**Vessel damage.** Completely severed vessels usually retract, rapidly clot, and quickly stop bleeding. Partially severed vessels cannot retract and may cause serious blood loss. Thrombosis involves the formation, development, or existence of a blood clot or thrombus in a blood vessel. Often caused by trauma, it can block the vessel and prevent blood from reaching a body structure. Aneurysm is a localized abnormal dilatation of a blood vessel, usually an artery. It is often due to a congenital defect or a weakness of a vessel wall. The weakened wall of the blood vessel may rupture and bleed into the surrounding area. The expansion of a vessel, like a balloon, though a weak wall, can rupture and cause significant internal bleeding.

**Upper extremity function.** The combined function of the shoulder, elbow, and wrist is to move the hand anywhere in a large globular area and position it for function. The shoulder girdle consists of the arm, the scapula, and the clavicle. The clavicle attaches at one end to the sternum and, at the other, to the scapula. It functions as a tie rod, keeping the shoulder girdle out to the side. In persons lacking a clavicle, the shoulder collapses inward toward the midline of the body, giving a narrow shoulderless appearance. The scapula (the winged bone) lays on the thorax (upper and posterior chest wall) and glides back and forth across it. The muscles located on the back, the anterior chest wall, and the upper arm all contribute to shoulder motion. Most of the muscles in the upper arm function in elbow motion, a few in shoulder motion and one, the bicep, in both (Luck & Anderson, 1990).

**The elbow.** The elbow is a complex joint (a set of three joints). The radius rolls or radiates around the ulna creating the palm up, palm down (supination, pronation) motion. The motor, muscle power to the elbow comes from muscles above the elbow for flexion and extension, and below the elbow for supination and pronation.

**The wrist.** The wrist is a complex of joints that function in supination and pronation, the turning of the hand palm up and palm down. It functions in dorsiflexion and palmarflexion movement of the hand upward and downward (as in the act of saying good-bye), and in radial and ulnar deviation (the motion of the hand from side to side). There are eight small bones that make up the carpal bones. These form the wrist joint and lie between the forearm bones (the radius and ulna) and the bones that form the palm of the hand (the metacarpal bones). The joints of the fingers are basically hinge joints that function in flexion, extension, limited abduction, and adduction (Truex & Carpenter, 1969).

**Skin function.** Skin serves as an outer covering of the body and protects if from the external environment. It is a constantly renewing wear surface and contains terminal sensory nerve endings. The palmar skin is specialized in that it is thicker than normal skin. It is more rigidly fixed to the deeper palmar fascia and moves less freely. This area is hairless, but contains many sweat glands and has a rich supply of sensory nerve endings. Scars in the palmar skin initially are very sensitive; as they mature, they become durable and non-tender. This early healing phase typically takes three months to resolve, an important characteristic for the rehabilitation counselor to know when providing vocational services.

Defects in palmar skin caused by injuries such as tears, lacerations, or burns can be covered or replaced with grafted skin or by skin flaps. Skin graft is a thin layer of skin that a surgeon removes, with a razor or a dermatome (a special machine for taking skin grafts), from one site of the body and places it in another site that needs skin coverage. Skin grafts cover defects and close wounds. Better skin can be provided by a variety of flaps. Defects in palmar skin, replaced with skin graft, skin from the dorsum, or a distal site, will retain the characteristics of its site of origin (the donor site).

Transferred skin as compared to palmar skin will be thinner, more mobile, and less adherent to the deep structures. If it is full thickness, it may have hair follicles; in dark skin persons, it often becomes hyperpigmented (increased coloration). The skin on the back of the hand (on the dorsal surface) is thinner, more pliable, and can stretch. It allows the fingers to close easily without being tight and allows the wrist to palmarflex; this area has hair follicles, in contrast to palmar skin that does not.

The nails are specialized structures that act as protective covering at the tip of each finger. An open wound can be a source of pain or route of infection. Nail injury may heal with ridges or with splits (bifid nail) (Guy, 1990).

# THE APPROACH TO TREATMENT OF INJURY

A surgeon's treatment of injury follows a consistent approach and order of priorities. The first step is to obtain as detailed a history and physical examination as possible and as emergency circumstances allow. Physical examination starts with inspection, which involves simply looking at the injury. The physician categorizes the injury including an evaluation of the skin, tendons, and bones. Palpation can demonstrate losses of tendon continuity, fractures, dislocation, and torn ligaments. The physician tests loss of sensation by touch or pinprick. Radiologic examination (x-ray) gives detail of bony injury and shows metallic and other foreign bodies that are present.

## Treatment

Once the surgeon understands the injury, a treatment plan can be formulated. If the injury involves an open wound, the first step is to clean the wound to remove bacterial contamination. A complicated fracture, such as at a joint, will require stabilization, usually with metal internal fixation. If there is injury to arteries and veins, they may need immediate repair. This is followed by the repair of injuries to tendons, nerves, and lastly, skin. The surgeon will make sure there is adequate skin coverage to avoid infection and problems due to scarring. The simplest replacement is with skin graft, usually split thickness. Split thickness skin graft is a very thin slice of skin, onion skin thin, taken from one place on the body (by use of a dermatome) and sewn over a defect or open wound. There are many other techniques used in skin grafting.

## Stabilization

A surgeon does a fracture stabilization if there is a deformity that cannot be corrected by nonoperative methods. The usual reason for instability is unopposed muscle or ligament forces creating and maintaining the deformity. Another indication for fracture fixation is when the fracture occurs within a joint surface. Joints are like machine parts. If their smooth surfaces heal unevenly, joint wear will be accelerated leading to painful arthritis. The simplest method of internal or metal fixation is with straight smooth pins drilled across a fracture to stabilize it until healing is complete. Alternative methods of stabilization include insertion of intramedullary rods, metal plates, and screws.

## Ligaments

Similarly, ligaments (the tissue holding joints together) can be torn. Many ligament injuries heal spontaneously, others require casting or surgical repair. The most common example of this, in the hand, is the large ulnar collateral ligament of the thumb. This ligament stabilizes the metacarpal phalangeal joint in pinching or in pushing buttons or twisting door knobs. Incomplete tears heal spontaneously with time, but complete tears need surgical repair. Torn ligaments that are not repaired become sources of chronic instability and impairment; if neglected long enough, they will lead to arthritis.

## Tendons

Tendons can be injured by acute laceration, rupture, avulsion from their bony sites of attachment, erosion as occurs in rheumatoid arthritis, attrition, or can become painful as in tendonitis. They can be repaired end-to-end, replaced by tendon graft, or substituted for by tendon transplant. Other conditions causing pain can be acute or chronic inflammation (tendonitis).

For purposes of prediction of outcome and planning of tendon surgery, one divides the palmar surface of the hand into five tendon zones. Zone I is from the pip joint (middle joint of the finger) to the end of the finger. In this zone, tendon repairs usually do well. Zone II is from the midpalm to the pip joints. In zone II, the results of tendon repair are far less predictable, and complications are most common. These complications involve scarring, stiffness, and adhesions. The proximal palm is zone III. In this zone, tendon repairs usually do well. The area of the carpal canal, from the wrist crease distally to the palm, is zone IV. Because of tightness, tendon repairs can be complicated by the formation of tendon adhesions. Zone V is the forearm which usually has a good response to surgical intervention.

Surgeons use tendon graft operations to avoid problems of scarring by placing tendon suture lines outside tight areas to lessen the risk of adhesion. A tendon transfer procedure involves the rerouting of a muscle tendon complex to a new site of action to replace lost motor function.

# EVALUATION OF IMPAIRMENT

Evaluation of impairment (Engelberg, 1988; Herbin, 1987) is similar to a scoring system, which assigns values to various functions and their loss. In the hand, those functions that can be evaluated include loss of parts (amputation), cosmetic defects, pain, tenderness, decreased sensation, limited range of motion, and loss of strength. An evaluation needs to describe subjective pain, including intensity and frequency. It needs to be descriptive regarding the appearance of the hand, calluses or their absence, cleanliness or the presence of dirt, and the condition of the nails. An evaluator describes sensation by a variety of testing methods. The evaluator's report measures losses of parts and scars, and measures range of motion and strength of grip, pinch, lifting, and resistance.

The first part of the evaluation is the individual's present activities and functional history. The physician asks the person about functional limitations and remaining abilities. A medical history needs to describe what activities an individual can do, how often, and for what length of time. Similarly, it needs to explain what activities cannot be done. One must find out how long the person can carry out certain activities. What can the individual do at table height? Overhead? How much can be lifted? How many repetitions? One asks the person about grip, pinch manipulation, and sensation.

## Pain and Sensory Deterioration

**Pain**. Pain is an entirely subjective experience. Nosocomia is a physically unpleasant experience; pain is the individual perception of that experience. If you take a standardized large needle and stick it an equal depth at an equal rate into a dozen individuals, each will experience an equal amount of nosocomia or unpleasant stimulation. Yet, each might describe a different degree of pain. Swanson, Goran-Hagert, and Swanson (1987) defined pain as "a disagreeable sensation that has as its basis a highly variable complex made up of afferent nerve stimuli interacting with the emotional state of the individual and modified by past experience, motivation, and state of mind." Though pain is entirely subjective, the individual's complaints have some physical coordinates. An individual complaining of severe pain will have a clean soft hand; a dirty, calloused, thickened, well used hand should raise doubts about the intensity of the subjective complaints. Similarly, some individuals will have few or no complaints, but portions of the hand will show evidence of disuse or avoidance.

Pain can be classified according to how it interferes with the individual's performance of activities. "Minimal" pain is an annoyance (0-25% factor of impairment in the American Medical Association Guidelines). "Slight" pain interferes with activity (26-50% factor of impairment), while "moderate" pain prevents activity (51-75%). "Severe" pain prevents activity and causes distress (76-100%). Besides describing pain by intensity, physicians describe pain by duration. Severe pain lasting a few seconds per week is of much less significance than moderate constant pain. Pain is described as "occasional" when it lasts up to 25% of the time; as "intermittent," if it lasts 25-50% of the time; as "frequent," lasting 50-75% of the time; and as "constant" lasting 75% or more.

**Sensory deficits**. Sensory deficits are a subjective complaint, but can be measured and, in reliable patients, can be quantified. Sensory testing includes distinguishing sharp from dull, static fixed two-point discrimination, moving two-point discrimination, Von Frey hair testing, hot versus cold discrimination, proprioception, coin discrimination, and vibration. Proprioception is that sense that tells us our body's position. It tells us if our hand is open or closed, if our hand is below our waist or over our head, and allows us to perform activities such as typing without looking at the keyboard.

Placing the hand behind a screen to hide it from visual feedback allows testing of proprioception. Stereoagnosis is the sense that allows us to read or see objects by feel; it is how we tell a dime from a quarter in our pockets without visual feedback, and is how a person reads Braille. Individuals without good sensation in the hand can be thought of as having a "blind" hand. Patients, after nerve laceration with poor recovery, or following a stroke or a spinal cord injury, may have severe sensory impairments. A severely sensory-impaired hand may be so "blind" as to be ignored by the patient; the hand may be nonfunctional on a sensory basis only. A physician usually records the results of sensory testing on a diagram of the hand.

**Nerve compression**. Individuals with nerve compression syndrome, such as herniated discs (causing pressure on nerve roots), thoracic outlet syndrome, cubital tunnel syndrome, and carpal tunnel syndrome, also experience decreased sensibility (the ability to feel or perceive). One loses vibration sense more often than two-point sensation loss. Anyone can experience the sensation of a compression syndrome by crossing the legs until one leg "falls asleep." That "pins and needles" sensation, deep aching, a loss of the sense of position, of dropping things are all associated with compression syndromes. In compression syndrome, the involved nerve is longitudinally intact but nerve impulse transmission is impaired by local pressure on a nerve at some point along its path into the hand.

**Reporting**. To report the results of inspection of the cosmetic appearance of the hand, the physician draws a diagram of both the palmar surface and the dorsal surface. The diagram illustrates amputations, nail deformities, scars, pigmentation alterations, calluses, and smooth areas. Finger amputations can be expressed by measuring the residual finger length and comparing with the same digit on the opposite hand. Another method is to describe the level of bony amputation by naming the most distal residual bone and what portion of that bone remains. One can draw nail clefts, ridges, grooves, and bumps on an illustration. Scars are drawn showing length, width, keloids (raised scar tissue), and tender spots (neuromas).

## Range of Motion

A physician measures the range of motion of each joint. The American Academy of Orthopaedic Surgeons has published standards for the measurement of joint motion. Each joint has a typical normal range of motion. The national standard defines full extension as $0^\circ$ of flexion. In some states, such as California, this is called $180^\circ$ of extension. Range of motion of the opposite hand is measured as a comparison to normal. One records results of these measurements on a standard "range of motion chart" (see Chart 1). Included with the range of motion chart should be the distance in flexion between the finger tips and the midpalmar crease as another illustration of finger flexion. Normally, a finger can touch the palm at the midpalmar crease. The distance that a digit fails to touch the palm is a measure of impaired flexion.

## Grip Loss

Forearm circumference is measured as an estimation of atrophy; one compares the uninvolved extremity to the involved side. Atrophy is precipitated by disease, disuse, and impaired function. The physician measures grip strength with a dynamometer (a calibrated instrument to measure grip), often a Jamar dynamometer. Usually, the examiner obtains and records a minimum of three good efforts on each hand. If the patient is making maximum effort, the Jamar readings are consistent; if less than maximum effort is made, the readings will be variable. The ratio between the involved and uninvolved hand is the best measure of grip loss; the absolute numbers are not important. Similarly, one measures pinch strength with a pinch meter. Individual muscles can be tested on a 1-5 grading system, but such testing is subjective and imperfectly reproducible.

## Radiological Assessment

An examination also requires radiological evaluation to define the status of the skeletal system and the degree of joint injury, disorganization, and degeneration. The physician needs to note any bone shortening or angulation. One reports shortening in millimeters and angulation in degrees. Rotational errors cannot be seen on x-rays. Density changes, for example, disuse loss of bone (osteopenia), are seen on x-rays as thinner, less dense, more radiolucent bone. Joint surface changes, narrowing, sclerosis, fractures, osteophytes (new, abnormal bony formation), lipping, arthritic changes, joint displacement (subluxations), and any other x-ray findings are mentioned.

## Work and Physical Capacity Evaluation

Work capacity evaluation measures the capacity of a person to function over time. Under the direction of a physician, occupational therapists do the actual evaluation by observing the person performing tasks over several days. By doing specific capacity testing, one is able to quantify the individual's ability to do a specific job (Herbin, 1987).

Physical capacity evaluation documents a person's objective hand function, including strength and range of motion. There are three components to physical capacity evaluation. These are (1) administration of hand function tasks; (2) standardized tests; and (3) observation of the person performing the physical demands of the job. Through observation of the person performing simulated job duties, the occupational therapist can assess functional limitations concerning job requirements. An accurate, highly descriptive, and detailed job description (job analysis), tailored to the injured worker's impairment, is of great help. The physician can then determine if the individual can return to a specific job (Baxter, 1986). An accurate and detailed job description also can assist a rehabilitation counselor to provide job modification or accommodation (Kasdan & McElwain, 1986).

# Chart 1

## MEASUREMENT OF ACTIVE MOTION

Patient Name: _____      _____ involved/ _____

Date of Exam: _____      MAJOR HAND: _____

Shoulder: F F_____ / _____      Elbow: Ext_____ / _____

  ABD _____ / _____          Flex_____ / _____

  E R _____ / _____

  I R _____ / _____      Forearm: Pronation _____

                                                    Supination _____

Wrist:  D F _____ / _____      Thumb: ABD_____ / _____

  P F_____ / _____          ADD _____ / _____

  R D_____ / _____      (tip misses distal palm at base of small finger)

  U D_____ / _____

| | | (MCP) Proximal | (PIP) Middle | (DIP) Distal | |
|---|---|---|---|---|---|
| Thumb | Ext | | | | Pulp of finger fails to touch composite transverse crease of the palm. |
| | Flex | | | | |
| Index | Ext | | | | |
| | Flex | | | | |
| Long | Ext | | | | |
| | Flex | | | | |
| Ring | Ext | | | | |
| | Flex | | | | |
| Small | Ext | | | | |
| | Flex | | | | |

# FUNCTIONAL LIMITATIONS IN COMMONLY
# OCCURRING HAND INJURIES

Hand surgery is a broad field dealing with many different problems. There will be a variety of injuries causing different functional limitations. The attitude and motivation of the patient will play a significant role in rehabilitation potential (Blumental, 1987; Kasdan & McElwain, 1989). This section discusses a few typical, common problems often seen in rehabilitation.

## *Finger Tip Injuries*

These are often seen industrial accidents and the most common reason for amputation. The variables involved include the level of amputation, the amount of soft tissue coverage on the remaining stump, the presence or absence of tender neuromas (abnormal nerve growth) or bone prominences, and nail deformities. Involvement of flexor tendons influences strength and range of motion. An example is an injury involving amputation though the middle of the nail bed. Half the nail bed has been destroyed and half the distal part of the finger is gone. Treatment includes providing adequate soft tissue padding. There is some decreased sensitivity. Since both flexor tendons are still intact at this level, there is no loss of grip strength. The finger may fail to touch the midpalmar crease by 0.5 centimeter (cm); tenderness is variable. Most laborers with this injury take about 12 weeks to return to work. Even at 12 weeks, the majority of individuals have some tenderness for several months longer. Few at this level of injury have much functional impairment, nor do they require rehabilitation (Guy, 1990).

An amputation proximal to the distal joint means the loss of the nail. With this type of injury, the profundus tendon (the stronger of the two tendons to the finger) is lost and with it some decrease in grip strength. Most individuals regain sufficient strength in 12 weeks or so to return to hard labor; some cannot or will not do so, and require different work, involving less dexterity and strength. For each digit involved, the impairment is different. As a guide, the entire thumb contributes 40% of hand function; the long and ring finger 20% each, and the border digits, the index and little finger, 10%. The loss of several digits increases the impairment even more than the sum of the parts lost. Multiple digit injuries take longer to heal, require more hand therapy to regain motion and strength, have greater residual impairment, and are more likely to require job change.

## *Hand Fractures*

Fractures are another common hand problem. Each kind of fracture has a different treatment and prognosis. A physician can splint simple non-displaced, non-angulated, and non-articular fractures and they usually heal in three weeks. Most of the stiffness will resolve in 3-4 weeks; minor residuals take much longer. Even laborers can usually return to work in 6-8 weeks. If the fracture was displaced, angulated, intra-articular, and required reduction or surgery, the patient will take significantly longer to heal.

Some of these residual impairments can be permanent, while others may prevent a return to customary work. The most common problem following a finger or hand fracture is stiffness. Most stiffness resolves with time and exercise; if the cause is tendon adherence (scar between tendon and bone), the only way to regain motion may be through surgical intervention. The most common site for tendon adhesions is the extensor tendons over the middle and proximal phalanges. Following surgery, patients rarely regain full range of motion. Some decreased residual dexterity from such complications causes little difficulty in jobs requiring gross lifting and carrying, but impairs manipulative tasks.

## Wrist Fractures

The most common significant wrist fracture is that of the waist of the scaphoid. The scaphoid is 1 of the 8 small bones of the wrist or carpus. This fracture is most often found in otherwise healthy young men. The median time to union (healing) in non-displaced fractures is 14.5 weeks, and the non-union (non-healing) rate is high (in some reports as high as 40%). Following such injury, stiffness and weakness are common.

## Carpal Tunnel Syndrome

This is another problem and is the most common nerve compression syndrome. It occurs in the wrist. Thyroid disease, masses, extra muscles, rheumatoid arthritis, amyloidosis, vibration disease syndrome, synovial hypertrophy, and prior wrist fractures are a few of the causes. Many conditions are idiopathic, that is the causes are unknown. Repetitive use of the hand, as in cashiers using optical scanners, typists, clerical file clerks, or factory assemblers are often the cause of industrial injury insurance claims.

Young men may develop the syndrome as the result of vibratory tools such as pneumatic tools, jackhammers, and power wrenches. Risk factors include age near or in the 40s, generalized mild synovitis (inflammation of the synovial membrane covering bones), and emotional problems. Women develop carpal tunnel syndrome more frequently than men. Initial conservative treatment consists of decreased use of the affected wrist, splints, non-steroid anti-inflammatory medication, and diuretics.

A physician makes the diagnosis of carpal tunnel syndrome based on appropriate history, complaints, and physical findings. Testing may include abnormal nerve conduction time and abnormal vibratory sense testing. If the diagnosis is confirmed, the next treatment step will be steroid injections into the area of pain and inflammation. If that fails and if symptoms are severe enough and prolonged, the person may need surgical decompression. Following the operation, the surgeon splints the patient in dorsiflexion for about a month. The scar can be tender for as long as 6 months. Return to work will take 2-12 weeks, depending on the physical demands of the job. Individuals with clerical and professional occupations take less time for recovery than those with more physically demanding jobs. Persons with carpal tunnel syndrome, aggravated by vibration, such as mechanics and pneumatic tool operators (jack hammer operators), may need occupational change if they cannot tolerate return to tasks requiring use of vibratory equipment (Blair & McCormick, 1985; King, 1988; Steinberg, 1989).

Carpal tunnel syndrome is one example of a cumulative trauma disorder. Practitioners believe these disorders are caused by the sum of multiple microtraumas. While this undoubtedly does occur, it probably occurs less frequently than diagnosed.

Other conditions that may occur as the result of cumulative trauma include tendonitis, tennis elbow, and trigger finger. Arthritis is rarely caused by cumulative trauma but can be aggravated by repetitive activity. In many of these conditions, the precipiting event is a nonspecific synovitis or thickening. This irritation or thickening contributes to the carpal tunnel syndrome, the tendonitis, or the trigger finger.

# REHABILITATION POTENTIAL

Potential for rehabilitation will vary depending on many factors. One of the most important of these is whether the dominant or non-dominant hand is involved. Injuries resulting in severe impairment of the dominant hand will be more disabling than injuries to the non-dominant hand. When a person has a severe injury to the dominant hand, training to improve use of the opposite hand is appropriate. Such a program may include:

1.  strengthening exercises

2.  development of skills in activities of daily living

3.  improvement in writing abilities

4.  enhancement of manual dexterity

Motivation and attitude are crucial aspects in the assessment of rehabilitation potential. For serious injuries resulting in major impairment, the motivation and attitude of an individual may make the difference between successful medical and vocational rehabilitation and failure. Highly motivated individuals with severe impairment seem to do better in rehabilitation than poorly motivated persons with significantly less impairment.

Other factors to be considered are age, educational level, and work history. Younger, more educated persons with skilled or professional work backgrounds can adjust more readily to impairment. Older workers seem more tolerant of residual discomfort and pain.

Many people who have serious hand injuries are unable to return to previous work activity because of residual impairment. Some employers will offer lighter duty work or other types of accommodation. A few companies will provide an entirely different job. The rehabilitation counselor can offer suggestions on alteration of the work environment to accommodate the impairment. With passage of the Americans with Disabilities Act in 1990, more employers are investigating the provisions of reasonable accommodation to workers with disabilities. This applies to both currently employed workers and to perspective employees.

There is a variety of orthotic and prosthetic devices for the hand and fingers that can provide improvement in function. Orthotists and prosthetists custom make many of these devices to accommodate specific jobs. One example of this involves a car wash attendant who lost two fingers of his dominant hand in an industrially-related accident. He was unable to operate the gasoline pump, a primary part of the job. A metal device worn on the injured hand, which enabled him to pump gasoline, was made that allowed him to do this function and remain employed at this job. He wore the device only for this job function.

Emotionally, every individual reacts differently to injury and impairment. Psychological counseling may be an important and necessary aspect of rehabilitation for particular individuals. There are some persons that view appearance as more important than function (Horovitz & Casler, 1986). The counselor must evaluate the impairment considering the needs of the individual. Many persons with disfigured hands can do a variety of activities and are not self-conscious in public. Others with even minor injuries, attempt to keep their hand out of sight.

The ability to use the hand involves sensibility, dexterity, and mobility. Rehabilitation of hand injuries may often require time and effort - maximum return of function is the goal of the hand surgeon teamed with hand therapists and rehabilitation counselors. The counselor needs to work closely with the other professionals in returning the person to maximum gainful employment.

# CASE STUDY

Mr. Jose Montoya is a 27 year-old married printer who sustained an injury to his right non-dominant hand while working in his profession. Born and educated (completed the 9th grade) in Mexico, his primary language is Spanish; he speaks and understands only minimal English. His wife is not currently employed as she spends her time taking care of their two children, ages 3 and 5. In the past, she worked as a child care attendant, a job she thoroughly enjoyed. Born and raised in Los Angeles, California, Mrs. Montoya became proficient in both the English and Spanish languages.

During the previous 7 years, Mr. Montoya worked for a printing and publishing company that specialized in printing material in the Spanish language. He began work with this company as a helper, learned to operate the various printing and publishing machines (printing press operator), and later became a printer, also supervising the helpers and press operators at the company.

As a printer, he set and assembled type, composed type by operating various typecasting machines, and printed the material. The work involved publishing a daily newspaper, several magazines, and books, all in the Spanish language.

While at work, a book binding machine closed on his right, non-dominant hand, severely crushing all four of his fingers, sparing only the thumb. Mr. Montoya had emergency surgery. The surgeon found the ring and little finger and portions of their metacarpals beyond salvage and surgically amputated these two fingers. There were multiple fractures of the index and long fingers, which the surgeon stabilized with pins. By the third month following injury, the wounds and fractures healed. After several months of physical therapy, the two digits were still very stiff and functioned as static posts against which the thumb could pinch. Mr. Montoya could hold objects between the thumb and index finger, but his grasp was weak. In an attempt to improve his limited grip, the surgeon detached the abductor pollicis longus from the base of the thumb and transferred it, through a tendon graft extension, to the radial side of the index finger. Four months later, the transfer was working reasonable well and the physician recommended vocational rehabilitation services.

## Questions

1. Since the injury occurred on the job, the workers' compensation system provided coverage. The workers' compensation system in California, where the injury occurred, provides both medical treatment and vocational rehabilitation. If you were the workers' compensation insurance claims adjuster, at what point would you recommend vocational rehabilitation intervention? Support your response.

2. Assign Mr. Montoya a vocational profile, including age level, educational category, and work history (including skill and exertional levels). Comment on the significance of this client's inability to communicate in the English language.

3. What are the occupationally significant characteristics of the worker's employment, and which ones are relevant in terms of the injury?

4. Can Mr. Montoya return to any of his prior jobs? Discuss.

5. Does Mr. Montoya have transferable skills? If so, identify these skills. Suggest several vocational rehabilitation plans for this injured worker.

# REFERENCES

Absoud, E.M., & Harrop, S.N. (1984). Hand injuries at work. **Journal of Hand Surgery, 9,** 211-215.

Baxter, P.L. (1986). Physical capacity evaluation and work therapy for industrial hand injuries. In C.A. Moran (Ed.), **Hand rehabilitation** (pp. 137-146). New York: Churchill Livingstone.

Blair, S.J. & McCormick, E. (1985). Prevention of trauma: Cooperation toward a better working environment. **Journal of Hand Surgery, 10**(6), 953-957.

Blumental, S.M. (1987). Vocational rehabilitation with the industrially injured worker. **Journal of Hand Surgery, 12**(2), 926-930.

Engelberg, A.L. (Ed.). (1988). **Guides to the evaluation of permanent impairment** (3rd ed.). Chicago, IL: American Medical Association.

Guy, R.J. (1990). Etiologies and mechanisms of nail bed injuries. **Hand Clinics, 4**, 9-19.

Herbin, M.L. (1987). Work capacity evaluation for occupational hand injuries. **Journal of Hand Surgery, 12a**(5), 958-960.

Horovitz, E.R., & Casler, P.T. (1986). Replantation: Current clinical treatment. In C.A. Moran (Ed.), **Hand rehabilitation** (pp. 91-116). New York: Churchill Livingstone.

Kasdan, A.S., & McElwain, N.P. (1989). Return to work programs following occupational hand injuries. **Occupational Medicine State of the Art Reviews, 4**(3), 539-546.

King, N.N. (1988). Practical considerations for the physician concerning workers' compensation law. **Hand Clinics, 2**(3), 503-610.

Luck, J.V., Jr., & Anderson, G.B.J. (1990). Occupational shoulder disorders. In C.A. Rockwood, Jr. & F.A. Matsen, III (Eds.), **The shoulder** (pp. 1088-1103). Philadelphia, PA: W.B. Saunders.

Oskamp, S. (1988). The editor's page. **Journal of Social Issues, 44**.

Schultz-Johnson, K. (1987). Assessment of upper extremity-injured persons' return to work potential. **Journal of Hand Surgery, 12a**(5), 950-957.

Steinberg, F. (1989). The law of workers' compensation as it applies to hand injuries. **Occupational Medicine State of the Art Reviews, 4**(3), 559-571.

Swanson, A.B., Goran-Hagert, C., & Swanson, G.D. (1987). Evaluation of impairment in the upper extremity. **Journal of Hand Surgery, 12**(5), 896-925.

Truex, R.C., & Carpenter, M.B. (1969). **Human neuroanatomy** (6th ed.). Baltimore, MD: Williams and Wilkins.

## *About the Author*

George W. Balfour, M.D., is an orthopaedic surgeon specializing in surgery of the hand and is in private practice in Van Nuys, California. He is an Assistant Professor of Surgery and Director of the Hand Clinic at the Charles R. Drew School of Medicine, Martin Luther King, Jr. Medical Center in Los Angeles, California.

# Chapter 26

# ORTHOTICS AND PROSTHETICS

by
*Darrell R. Clark, C.O.*

## INTRODUCTION

It is estimated about 3% of the civilian, non-institutionalized population in the United States use some type of orthopedic aid. Today, this means about 7.5 million people. These aids range from simple ambulatory devices, such as canes and walkers, to more complex systems, which include computerized controls to manipulate a client's environment.

Orthopedic aids include artificial braces and limbs, or orthoses and prostheses. An orthosis is an external device applied to the body to restrict or enhance motion to or support a body segment. A prosthesis is a replacement of a missing part by an artificial substitute, as in an artificial extremity. Orthotists and prosthetists are the practitioners in each specialty area who provide services to clients (Shurr, 1990).

Orthotists and prosthetists typically have 4 or more years of college education and specialized training in the field. The American Board for Certification in Orthotics and Prosthetics is the national certifying organization, in existence since 1948, which certifies these professionals. This permits orthotists and prosthetists to add the title of Certified Orthotist (CO), Certified Prosthetist (CP), or Certified Prosthetist-Orthotist (CPO) after their names.

The patient's physicians, and possibly a physical therapist or an occupational therapist, evaluate needs. The orthotist or prosthetist is often consulted in the process of defining the best treatment approach. The physician orders orthoses and prostheses by prescription.

Orthoses typically fall into 1 of 3 categories: lower limb, upper limb, and spinal. One classifies prostheses by the amputation level: below-knee (BK), above-knee (AK), below-elbow (BE), above-elbow (AE). This chapter presents an overview of some individual systems and their components to provide a better understanding of their use.

The status of orthotic and prosthetic design is constantly changing as new techniques and materials come into use (American Academy of Orthopedic Surgeons, 1985, 1992; Shurr, 1990; Veterans Administration, 1982; Wilson, 1989). The orthotic and prosthetic practitioner is the best source of information regarding these changes. Rehabilitation counselors can stay current with major advances by referring to publications in the field. These include the **Atlas of Orthotics** (American Academy of Orthopedic Surgeons, 1985) and the **Atlas of Limb Prosthetics** (American Academy of Orthopedic Surgeons, 1992), both published by the American Academy of Orthopedic Surgeons. Also useful are **Prosthetics and Orthotics** (Shurr, 1990) and **Limb Prosthetics** (Wilson, 1989). With some basic understanding of orthotic and prosthetic systems, counselors can better assist their clients during the rehabilitation process and help their transition to productivity.

# ORTHOSES

Orthoses are used for a variety of reasons. These include relief of pain (by limiting motion or weight bearing); immobilization and protection of weak, painful, or healing musculoskeletal segments; reduction of axial load; prevention and correction of deformity; and improvement of function (American Academy of Orthopedic Surgeons, 1985; Redford, 1986).

## Systems of Identification

In the past, professionals identified orthoses by a vague nomenclature based on the inventor's name or on some component of the system. This created some obvious difficulty in communicating exactly what the physician desired. The current system of identification is by the joint(s) that the orthosis usually supports and crosses. For example, the traditional "short leg brace" is an ankle-foot orthosis (AFO); the "long leg brace" is a knee-ankle-foot orthosis (KAFO). The upper limb and spine follow a similar approach (see Table 1). There are several design variations within these generic categories; close communication between the orthotist and the treatment team members is crucial to ensure maximum benefit for the client.

## Table 1
## CATEGORIES OF ORTHOSES

| | |
|---|---|
| Ankle-Foot Orthosis | AFO |
| Knee-Ankle-Foot Orthosis | KAFO |
| Hip-Knee-Ankle-Foot Orthosis | HKAFO |
| Wrist-Hand Orthosis | WHO |
| Wrist-Driven Wrist-Hand Orthosis | WDWHO |
| Shoulder-Elbow Orthosis | SEO |
| Lumbosacral Orthosis | LSO |
| Thoraco-Lumbo-Sacral Orthosis | TLSO |
| Cervico-Thoraco-Lumbo-Sacral Orthosis | CTLSO |

## Lower Limb

Clients who, through disease or accident, have weakness or paralysis in one or both legs must often use orthoses to walk. Ambulation is one of the most frequent goals of orthotic treatment. Depending on the extent of the paralysis, the client will generally need an AFO or a KAFO.

AFOs. The AFO is typically used to substitute for muscle weakness around the ankle. The muscles across the ankle provide two significant benefits during ambulation: (1) the muscles in front of the ankle lift the foot during the "swing phase" of gait (the time when the foot is off the floor and moving forward); and (2) the muscles in back of the ankle provide stability during the "stance phase" of gait (the time when the foot is on the floor and weight-bearing) to prevent uncontrolled forward motion at the ankle joint (Redford, 1986; Shurr, 1990).

In paralysis, two gait-related problems exist: (1) the foot may drag on the floor during the swing phase of gait; and (2) the person may experience excessive forward motion at the ankle during the stance phase of gait. This will result in a loss of stability and balance. By modifying the amount of motion allowed at the ankle joint, the orthosis can hold the foot up in a normal position to prevent tripping or falling during swing and prevent uncontrolled forward motion during stance. Typical AFOs are either metal or plastic and may have ankle joints that allow varying amounts of motion (Figure 1a & 1b).

---

## Figure 1

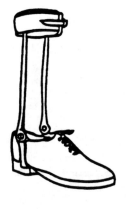

1a - Conventional metal AFO

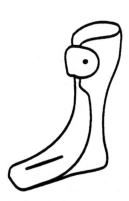

1b-Plastic AFO

---

**KAFOs.** If the client also has weakness at the knee joint, there will be danger of falling because of knee collapse during the stance phase. One may use a KAFO (Figure 2) to prevent this possible collapse. By holding the knee securely in its fully extended position, the knee will not bend and cause the person to fall. Various types of locking mechanisms are available to keep the knee extended in a secure manner. A common type is the "drop lock" (Figure 3) where the locking component drops into place and locks the knee joint. In order to sit, the client raises the drop lock, which allows the knee to bend.

Like the AFO, KAFOs are often plastic to decrease weight and reduce the energy demand when the individual is walking. Structural plastics allow the orthotist to produce a system that is as strong as the traditional metal systems, while being lighter in weight and more cosmetically acceptable. A potential problem with plastic components is that they do not allow for easy evaporation of perspiration and some clients may feel the orthosis is too hot to wear.

A more common disability requiring KAFOs is paraplegia due to spinal cord injury. The level of injury is crucial in determining whether a client can use KAFOs effectively. Clients most likely to be able to use orthoses for effective ambulation are those whose injuries are below the 12th thoracic vertebra (T12), since the hip muscles are still intact below that level. Hip control is crucial for functional ambulation and injuries above T12 will result in varying degrees of weakness in the hip muscles and in the lower abdominal muscles (which contribute to pelvic stability). Below T12, energy demands of walking are greatly increased and functional ambulation may be impossible. A wheelchair will then be required for mobility. A client with paraplegia ambulating with KAFOs has significantly decreased energy and speed.

While wheelchair use is the most practical means of mobility for most clients with paraplegia, limited ambulation as a form of exercise can be beneficial because it maintains upper limb strength, prevents contractures,

---

## Figure 2

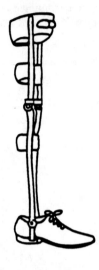

Metal KAFO

---

## Figure 3

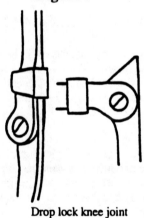

Drop lock knee joint

---

and may reduce the possibility of osteoporosis in the lower extremities. An individual also may use KAFOs when working, even if they are not used to get to and from the job.

## Spine

**Back immobilization**. Orthoses are often used to support and immobilize the spine during healing, to control pain, or to control or correct a deformity. The physician will prescribe limitations on lifting and movement; it is very important that clients follow physicians' instructions.

There are many types of orthoses used to immobilize the spine, ranging from a simple corset to more complex systems. The basic idea is to provide stability to the spine by encompassing the controlling motion of the affected segment. Orthoses with rigid components against the client's back for support are often utilized (Figure 4). The front also may be rigid or may be a softer material to provide more comfort. Much of the spinal support is accomplished through pressure in the abdominal area. This creates a "column effect" against the spine from the internal organs, which helps support and immobilize the spine.

## Figure 4

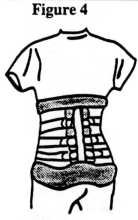

Rigid spinal orthosis

**Neck immobilization.** Injuries in the neck and upper chest area of the spine are hard to immobilize because of the difficulty in obtaining a secure position to prevent motion. The system of choice to achieve the desired immobilization is frequently the "HALO" (Figure 5). This consists of a horizontal ring which the operating surgeon attaches directly to the skull with pins. A plastic vest is fit to the client's chest and vertical bars go from the vest to the skull ring to prevent the head and neck from moving. The HALO is often used after surgery to maintain position during healing of the vertebrae. After the client discontinues use of the orthosis, the physician may prescribe an exercise program to gradually restrengthen the muscles of the head and neck.

## Upper Limb

Upper limb orthoses can substitute for absent muscle power, assist or support weak segments, or be used for the attachment of specialized devices. They typically help position the hand for some useful activities of daily living, such as eating, dressing, grooming, and writing. The complexity of the orthosis depends on the severity of the disability.

**Arm and hand function.** Disease or accident can often result in limitations in arm and hand function. These limitations are often more functionally disabling than leg injuries because of the importance of the upper extremities in activities of daily living. Orthotic management of the arm and hand is difficult due to the intricate fit and function that is necessary and the potential for skin problems. There is also a problem in the limited number of orthotists trained to provide complex hand orthoses.

Many factors affect a client's willingness to accept an orthosis. The most important is whether the orthosis allows the client to perform activities that are not otherwise possible. Others are the appearance, ease of application, and function of the opposite arm. If a client still has one good hand, it will be used and the disabled hand neglected. This phenomenon also applies to persons with upper limb amputations. These factors contribute to a high rejection rate on the part of the client of upper limb orthotic devices.

## Figure 5

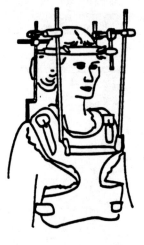

Halo

There are three major nerves supplying the hand and arm, each with a different pattern of functional distribution. Depending on how much the disease or injury affects that distribution, the client may need only a simple system to support the hand or wrist for function. Otherwise, the client may need a system which not only holds the hand in the correct position, but helps initiate hand and finger motion to pick up and hold objects.

**Static and dynamic upper limb orthoses.** There are two broad categories for upper limb orthoses, static and dynamic. Static orthoses do not allow motion but simply provide support to maintain proper position. An example is an orthosis that holds the wrist immobilized during healing following surgery (Figure 6). Dynamic orthoses allow some motion and their effectiveness relies on that motion. For example, a wrist-driven wrist-hand orthosis provides

## Figure 6

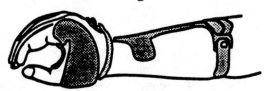

Wrist-hand orthosis, static

finger pinch by the motion of wrist extension (Figure 7). This motion utilizes a natural action of the tendons of the fingers and wrist and harnesses the energy for functional use.

**Mobile arm supports.** Other systems attach to the wheelchair and support the arms when the muscle power required to do so is absent. These systems, called Mobile Arm Supports (MAS), may have separate joints at the wrist and elbow. A more recent design, called the Linear Mobile Arm Support, eliminates the need for an elbow joint, allowing for easier access to doorways (Figure 8). Clients using the MAS also typically use some type of wrist-hand orthosis to allow hand function once the hand is properly placed through use of the MAS.

**Figure 7**

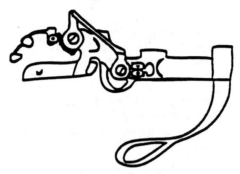

Wrist-driven wrist-hand orthosis

**Figure 8**

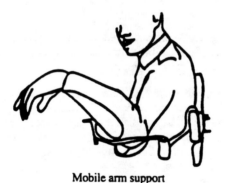

Mobile arm support

## Adaptive Equipment

Besides the above standard categories of orthotic management, two others deserve mention: self-help aids and automobile modifications. For the client who is paralyzed, the simplest tasks often require Herculean effort, if the person can do them at all.

**Self-help aids.** Specialized adaptive equipment designed to assist in specific tasks can make activities of daily living easier. Tasks such as eating, writing, grooming, and dressing are all candidates for equipment that can make life easier for the individual with a physical disability (U.S. Department of Health & Human Services, 1977).

A thorough evaluation by members of the health care team is essential to identify factors influencing the selection and acceptance of self-help aids. These factors include physical condition, mental abilities, emotional concerns, and economic and vocational situations.

Designs vary widely and are only limited by the ingenuity of the client and the health-care providers. Many items are also available commercially that will aid in accomplishing the above tasks. Often, a simple modification to an existing implement is enough. For example, a larger handle or cuff on a fork or knife makes it easier for a client with arthritis to grasp a utensil. A long-handled brush or shoehorn or a foodplate guard to help keep food on the plate are examples of effective modifications. Even clients with high-level spinal cord injury may be able to use special mouth-sticks to do some tabletop activities such writing, typing, or turning pages. Designs need to be simple and easily maintained to be effective. Client acceptance is improved if the item is as inconspicuous as possible. Factors such as cognition, age, and the likelihood of return of function affect psychological acceptance.

**Automobile modifications**. Driving a car with a manual transmission requires continuous coordination of all four extremities. People do most of the operations routinely. A disability, however, may greatly affect driving skills. Automatic functions, such as an automatic transmission, make operating the vehicle easier; and modifying or relocating controls for such items as the brakes also may help.

In recent years, the advent of the minivan has been beneficial to people with disabilities who have been unable to drive. Entry and exit for clients in wheelchairs are relatively easy and the smaller size makes it more practical and provides more space than a car; it is easier to handle and park than a full-size van. Many modifications and conversion packages are available to meet personalized needs. There are many driving aids available to persons with disabilities today, but a thorough evaluation of the capacity to drive is crucial before assistive devices can be matched to abilities.

## Functional Limitations and Rehabilitation Potential

Psychosocial problems may relate to several issues. Any significant anger, anxiety, and depression will relate to the loss rather than use of orthotic devices. The rehabilitation counselor will need to deal with these issues if the client is to make maximum use of the prescribed orthotic devices.

The physician may prescribe orthotic devices for low back injuries to increase function by providing support during the healing process through immobilization of the spine. This also may decrease pain thereby allowing the individual greater functioning. The client needs to be cognizant of the physical limitations imposed by the physician so as not to exceed these limitations and cause increased pain and possible physical damage to the area that is healing. One of the reasons for temporarily limiting use is the long-range goal of improved function and greater mobility, and hence, increased rehabilitation potential.

Orthoses for the upper extremities can decrease functional limitations and increase use, thereby increasing the client's rehabilitation potential. Weak and dysfunctional muscles can become more functional with proper use of orthoses to support the weak muscles. Adaptive equipment can help the client conduct activities of daily living that were previously impossible. They can also help some individuals perform work tasks and increase vocational opportunities. A modified van may enable a client to drive. This increases independence and allows for greater opportunities for gainful employment, where previously the client had to rely on others for transportation.

Applied to a partial hand, orthotics may enable increased manual dexterity and eye-hand coordination. The orthotist may be able to increase functional ability in a hand by providing a device that allows a client to continue essential work functions. A rehabilitation counselor can be instrumental in coordinating these efforts and intervening with the present or prospective employer.

Orthoses applied to the lower extremities may allow an individual greater and more reliable ambulation. By supporting weak lower extremity muscles, the client may be able to ambulate independently and with confidence. With appropriate application, the client may decrease functional limitations, increase independence, and improve vocational outlook. Improved function is the uppermost goal of the orthotist.

# PROSTHESES

Over 60% of amputees are candidates for vocational rehabilitation. The ratio of lower limb amputations compared to upper limb is 9:1. Ambulation is an important goal for lower extremity amputees. Incidence of limb amputation is difficult to determine precisely, but national health statistics estimate there are approximately 43,000 new amputees per year.

Amputations may be surgical or traumatic. The need for surgical amputation is usually associated with cancer or peripheral vascular disease, often a result of diabetes. A third category, congenital limb deficiency, results from problems that occur to a fetus during pregnancy (Friedmann, 1981).

Phantom limb is a sensation, following amputation of a limb, that the limb still exists. This is a normal phenomenon and usually decreases over time. Phantom-limb pain, as differentiated from phantom limb, is a sensation of pain in the missing extremity. Depending on the intensity of the pain, it can be a disabling condition. Phantom pain also may diminish over time. There are surgical procedures that alleviate some types of phantom pain.

The vocational implications of amputation are generally the same despite the cause. Many factors must be considered in meeting the client's needs, from psychological to functional limitations and prosthetic design (American Academy of Orthopedic Surgeons, 1992; Wilson, 1989).

## Lower Limb

**Levels of amputation.** Lower limb amputations are classified according to level of limb lost (see Illustration 1). Hip disarticulation (HD) is the highest level of lower extremity amputation and occurs through the hip. The next levels down are the above-knee (AK), knee disarticulation (KD), and below-knee (BK) amputations. The "Syme" amputation occurs through the ankle joint. The lowest level of amputation is called the partial foot, where only a portion of the foot is removed. A partial foot amputation may occur at various levels. This amputation permits easy fit of a prosthesis. The higher the level of amputation of the lower extremity, the greater functional limitations will occur and the more difficulty there will be in fitting and wearing of a prosthetic device.

**Functional restoration.** This is strongly·related to amputation level. The more involvement there is of the anatomical joints, the more difficult it is to regain maximum function. Another major factor affecting residual function is whether one or both legs are involved. Bilateral lower limb amputation makes independent ambulation extremely difficult. Torres and Esquenazi (1991) found that many clients with bilateral lower extremity amputation achieved limited household ambulation and a few achieved limited community ambulation. Those with below knee amputations were significantly more ambulatory than those with amputations above the knee.

The more severe the involvement, the more likely the client will need a cane or crutch to aid in balance. After prosthetic fitting and training, the unilateral amputee typically achieves independence in most activities. The higher the amputation level, the more difficult will be the training. Bilateral amputation presents a far greater challenge for the client to again achieve an acceptable level of functioning, since it is more difficult to regain ambulation and transfer abilities. While the unilateral amputee can at least stand on one leg to transfer in and out of the wheelchair, the bilateral amputee cannot start training until some type of prosthesis is provided.

A temporary prosthesis may be fitted immediately after surgery to allow early standing, weight-bearing, and walking with crutches. This is both physiologically and psychologically beneficial. One may also prescribe an exercise program to strengthen the body generally and to work on the specific muscle groups used in ambulation, balance, and the use of crutches. In some situations, clients choose to abandon their prostheses part of the time in favor of crutches or a wheelchair to permit quicker and less energy-consuming mobility. They may continue to use their prostheses in social settings, mainly for cosmetic reasons.

## Illustration 1

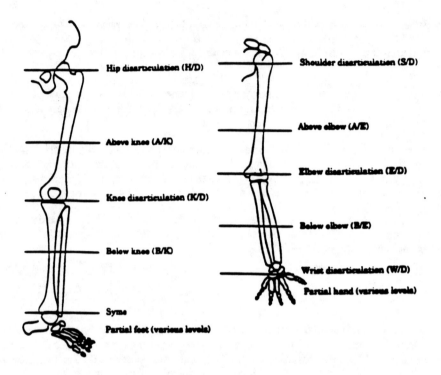

| | |
|---|---|
| Hip disarticulation (H/D) | Shoulder disarticulation (S/D) |
| Above knee (A/K) | Above elbow (A/E) |
| Knee disarticulation (K/D) | Elbow disarticulation (E/D) |
| Below knee (B/K) | Below elbow (B/E) |
| | Wrist disarticulation (W/D) |
| Syme | Partial hand (various levels) |
| Partial foot (various levels) | |

Levels Of Typical Amputation Sites

**Components of lower limb prostheses.** These include the socket, mechanical joints, and foot assembly. Above the knee (AK) sockets are typically plastic, although some long-time wearers may have wood sockets. The plastic socket is fabricated from a plaster model taken of the client's residual limb; if the limb is long enough, it is frequently held in place by suction. This design uses a one-way valve to evacuate air as the prosthesis is applied but prevents air from re-entering. This creates a negative pressure on the thigh tissues to hold the socket in place. In other cases, the client uses a special belt. The socket of a new amputee must be adjusted periodically to accommodate changes in limb volume due to swelling, or weight gain or loss during the post-amputation period.

**Above the knee prostheses.** The traditional AK socket design is the quadrilateral socket. This four-sided design is an improvement over the earlier round design and provides specific anterior-posterior pressure to position the ischial tuberosity of the pelvis on the posterior wall of the socket so the patient can sit comfortably. A recent development in AK socket design is the CAT-CAM socket, which provides for more natural shape and alignment of the leg and attains a bony lock to afford better control of the residual limb.

A variety of knee and ankle joint designs are available and the prosthetist will determine which is most suitable. A recent advance in foot design is the "energy-storing" foot, formulated to provide improved shock absorption, smoother gait, and increased responsiveness while walking and running. This prosthetic foot typically has a flexible component in the mid-section of the foot which deflects during walking. It provides a smoother, more natural gait pattern, especially in the swing phase, and reduces stress on the knee joint.

**Below the knee prostheses.** BK prostheses (Figure 9) utilize either supracondylar or suprapatellar suspension, both of which rely on contact with bony prominences in the knee area to keep the prosthesis in place. A third method utilizes a strap above the patella.

**Figure 9**

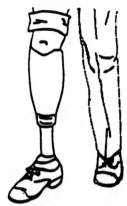

Below-knee prosthesis (no cosmetic cover)

## *Upper Limb*

**Levels of amputation.** Like lower limb, designation of amputation level varies with the length of the residual limb (Illustration 1). The highest amputation level is through the shoulder, called a shoulder disarticulation (SD). An above-elbow (AE) amputation occurs between the shoulder and elbow, an elbow disarticulation (ED) through the elbow, and a below-elbow (BE) amputation occurs between the elbow and wrist. An amputation through the wrist is called a wrist disarticulation (WD). A partial hand amputation involves removal of a portion of the hand or one or more fingers.

**Functional restoration.** The higher the amputation level on the arm, the more difficult it is for the client to adapt to the limb loss, the greater functional limitation will be present, and the more difficulty there will be in fitting a prosthetic device. Clients with unilateral amputation of the nondominant arm will tend to adapt well because they still have their dominant arm and hand, and can learn to modify their usage patterns and better accommodate the loss. This improved adaptation often means that a prosthesis will be rejected as unnecessary, even when its use could improve function. Conversely, a high level bilateral amputee will have the most difficulty in adapting, and may never achieve real functional independence in all activities.

Normal arm function is very complex and presents formidable challenges to replace prosthetically. This is especially true of the intricate movements of the hand, which are not yet available in a prosthetic "terminal device" (the component that replaces the hand). The standard components of the upper limb prosthesis include the socket, mechanical joints, terminal device, and suspension system (Figure 10).

**Components of upper limb prostheses.** Like the lower limb socket, the upper limb socket is typically plastic or metal, fabricated from a plaster cast taken of the residual limb. Joints historically are of simple design and move in only one plane. They frequently have a friction component to maintain stability and position. Although electric power has been available for prosthetic joints for some time, it is only in recent years that systems have become sophisticated and reliable enough to begin to provide more complex motion and function.

**Figure 10**

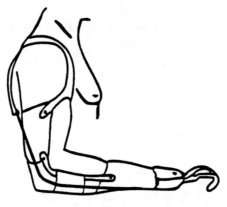

Below-elbow prosthesis

The terminal device gives the client an ability to grasp and hold objects and may resemble either a hook or a hand in appearance. Hooks are more functional and various designs are available for specific types of tasks. The prosthetic hand resembles a normal hand in appearance, but does not have the same dexterity. Passive, cosmetic hands have no real function and are simply used for appearance. A functional hand allows the thumb and at least the second and third fingers to move and provide a three-finger pinch or grasp. Prosthetic hands can be covered with a cosmetic glove to enhance their appearance. Clients sometimes use a hook for work and a cosmetic hand for social engagements.

Power for the upper limb prosthesis is typically provided by a harnessing system operated by the client's normal muscles; it also can be supplied through myoelectric amplification of the client's muscle activity or by batteries built into the prosthesis. The myoelectric arm, a recent innovation, functions through electrical potentials produced by remaining muscles in the arm. There are electrodes placed within the prosthesis and over the skin of the muscles in the arm that will pick up the electrical impulses and close or open the prosthetic hand. The myoelectric arm is very expensive and suitable for BE amputations only. It allows some dexterity and power, but only on a very limited basis (Falvo, 1991).

**Coping.** The client needs to realize that no prosthesis will match the appearance and ability of a natural limb. There is always a trade-off between function and appearance. Many adjustments must be made to begin coping with an amputation. It takes several weeks to become accustomed to wearing and using a prosthesis. The prosthesis does not provide any sensory feedback and will seem heavy at first. With practice and patience, the client will develop skill with the prosthesis and can resume many activities he or she was formerly able to accomplish before the amputation.

## Functional Limitations and Rehabilitation Potential

There are psychosocial implications involved in individuals using prostheses. In the case of a recent amputation, the client may have hostility, anger, fear, anxiety, and depression (Friedmann, 1981). These and other emotions may help contribute to nonuse of a prescribed prosthetic device. Acute and chronic pain may complicate adjustment to disability and the use of a prosthesis. Acute pain occurs immediately after the traumatic event; chronic benign pain, such as phantom-limb pain, is a more complicated and difficult issue. It may prevent the individual from wearing the prosthesis and, therefore, disrupt a potential plan to decrease functional limitations and thereby, increase vocational rehabilitation potential. Phantom-limb pain itself may be disabling. The rehabilitation counselor may need to refer the client to a specialist skilled in the area of chronic pain management if the pain does not subside. Inability to tolerate a prosthesis will increase functional limitations.

A lower extremity prosthesis is designed to make independent ambulation possible. This functional capacity will increase vocational potential by increasing independence and mobility. Use of crutches at a worksite decreases the ability to ambulate quickly and diminishes the client's use of both hands while walking or standing. Most clients will be limited to sedentary work, but may occasionally stand and walk. A client with a bilateral lower extremity amputation will typically use a wheelchair for ambulation, especially at the worksite. These clients are limited to sedentary work activity.

Complications at the site of the amputation, such as edema (swelling), ulceration, and infection may temporarily interfere with the ability to wear the prosthesis. Significant weight gain or loss is a factor that interferes with proper fit and leads to complications at the amputation site.

The use of upper extremity prostheses increases manual dexterity, bilateral dexterity, and eye-hand coordination. Some upper extremity prostheses are quite functional and useful on the job. The client may choose to use a functional prostheses while working and a cosmetic one for social events. Although an upper extremity prosthesis can be functional, the client will have significant limitations in dexterity and complex functions of the hand, especially with AE amputations. A hook device will allow for lifting, carrying, and grasping of objects. A client may be able to learn to write and use small hand tools with this device. The myoelectric arm will have less function but has the appearance of a natural arm and hand.

# CASE STUDY

Amy is a 22 year-old who has a Bachelor of Arts degree from a local state university. She is living with her parents in a large metropolitan city. Several months ago, she was in a car versus bicycle accident. A serious right leg injury resulted in an AK amputation. She has had great difficulty accepting the loss of the leg, although she has now begun to work with the prosthetist for fitting of a prosthesis. At present, she experiences "phantom pain," a well documented, but poorly understood phenomenon of the sensation of pain in the missing limb.

Having recently graduated from college with a degree in liberal arts, Amy would like to become an elementary school teacher. She needs to attend one more year of college that will include student teaching, and pass a certification examination. The only work Amy has done has been on a temporary or part-time basis. She has worked as a salesperson during several Christmas seasons, a cashier and hostess in several restaurants, and a part-time cashier/ticket taker for a movie theater during summer vacations and occasionally on a part-time basis during the school year.

## Questions

1. Assign Amy a vocational profile including an analysis of age, education, and work history.

2. Discuss the occupationally significant characteristics of her past work and how these may relate to the disability.

3. Describe the functional limitations of a person with an AK amputation. Will Amy be able to drive an automobile?

4. Amy is having great difficulty with adjustment to her disability. She is also experiencing "phantom pain." As her counselor, offer recommendations in regard to these two conditions.

5. Discuss Amy's vocational objective and, if you recommend pursuing it, how you would help her implement this rehabilitation goal. Suggest other possibilities.

# REFERENCES

American Academy of Orthopedic Surgeons (Ed.). (1985). **Atlas of orthotics** (2nd ed.). St. Louis, MO: C.V. Mosby.

American Academy of Orthopedic Surgeons (Ed.). (1992). **Atlas of limb prosthetics: Surgical and prosthetic principles** (2nd ed.). St. Louis, MO: C.V. Mosby.

Falvo, D.R. (1991). **Medical and psychosocial aspects of chronic illness and disability.** Gaithersburg, MD: Aspen.

Friedmann, L.W. (1981). Amputation. In W.C. Stolov & M.R. Clowers (Eds.), **Handbook of severe disability** (pp. 169-188). Washington, DC: U.S. Department of Education, Rehabilitation Services Administration.

Redford, J.B. (Ed.). (1986). **Orthotics, etcetera** (3rd ed.). Baltimore, MD: Williams and Wilkins.

Shurr, D. (1990). **Prosthetics and orthotics.** Norwalk, CT: Appleton and Lange.

Torres, M.M. & Esquenazi, A. (1991). Bilateral lower limb amputee rehabilitation - A retrospective review. **The Western Journal of Medicine, 154**(5), 583-586.

U.S. Department of Health and Human Services (1977). **Use of special aids** (Publication No. PHS 81-1563). Washington, DC: Author.

Veterans Administration, Department of Medicine and Surgery (Ed.). (1982). **Bulletin of prosthetic research.** Washington, DC: Rehabilitative Engineering Research & Development Service.

Wilson, A.B. (1989). **Limb prosthetics** (6th ed.). New York, NY: Demos.

## *About the Author*

Darrell Clark, C.O., is the Director of Orthotics at Rancho Los Amigos Medical Center in Downey, California. He also directs the Orthotic Certificate Course at Rancho Los Amigos Medical Center and serves as an adjunct faculty member for the Orthotics-Prosthetics Program at California State University, Dominguez Hills.

# *Chapter 27*

# NEUROLOGICAL CONDITIONS

by
*Joshua Goldman, M.D.*

## INTRODUCTION

Neurology is the specialty of medicine that deals with the study and treatment of the nervous system and its disorders. The practice of neurology requires specialized knowledge of the anatomy and physiology of the nervous system and familiarity with many diseases rarely encountered in general medicine. It is a challenge for future scientific research to explain the brain's miraculous processes of thought, memory, judgment, and motor function. The complexities of the neurological system challenge the expertise of the most experienced clinicians.

The purpose of this chapter is to familiarize the rehabilitation counselor with aspects of the neurological examination, neuroanatomy, and some frequently diagnosed neurological illnesses and conditions. It is not an all inclusive discussion of neurology. References to standard neurological textbooks can be reviewed (Adams & Victor, 1989; Joint, 1990; Rowland, 1989) for a more extensive and comprehensive understanding of the diseases affecting the neurological system.

## NEUROLOGICAL EXAMINATION

In the usual situation, an individual with complaints suggesting disease of a neurological origin sees a general practitioner. These complaints vary widely but commonly include headaches, motor weakness, pain, sensory disturbance, vertigo, and difficulties in cognition and speech. The general practitioner may refer the patient to a neurologist for further evaluation.

The neurologist first attempts to determine the specific anatomical location of the abnormality within the nervous system. Secondly, the neurologist will assess the possible etiology (cause) of the lesion. The cause or origin of the problem may be trauma, tumor, immunological, infection, hereditary predisposition, or other diseases and disorders. The neurologist proceeds with the evaluation in the following manner:

1. Obtains a neurologically-oriented history.

2. Performs a neurological evaluation.

3. Decides on and orders laboratory tests, imaging procedures, and other needed testing.

4. Coordinates all clinical and laboratory findings.

Based on the evaluation, course of the illness, and special testing, the neurologist can often establish a specific diagnosis (Andreoli, Carpenter, Plum & Smith, 1990; Schroeder, Krupp, Tierney, & McPhee, 1990; Wyngaarden & Smith, 1988). The neurological examination undertakes a systematic evaluation of the following areas:

1. mental status

2. cranial nerves

3. gait and station

4. cerebellum

5. motor and sensory function

The following discussion provides important aspects of neurological evaluation for rehabilitation counselors to consider in reviewing medical records.

## Mental Status

The mental status examination evaluates mental function, such as the ability to follow commands, speak, and do arithmetic. It will reveal gross abnormalities of mental function and difficulties in speech. When dysfunction of cognition and judgement exists, return of function is dependent on the cause. Depending on the illness, function may worsen, improve, or remain unchanged over time. Once the condition has become stable, neuropsychological testing may help in assessing mental status in a more thorough manner to establish the person's remaining functional capacity.

The speech centers of the brain are located in the left hemisphere and are named after the scientists that originally described them. Broca's area, in the left frontal lobe, is connected by means of nerve pathways to Wernicke's area in the left temporal lobe.

**Wernicke's aphasia.** A lesion in Wernicke's area will produce a specific speech defect called Wernicke's aphasia (receptive aphasia). Wernicke's aphasia involves a disturbance of comprehension in terms of spoken and written language. The individual is unable to produce understandable speech or write.

There is fluent but paraphasic speech (the misuse of words or phrases). As it becomes worse, this pattern involves the patient speaking fluidly with normal inflection and sentence patterns but in an incoherent manner. Over time, with appropriate treatment, Wernicke's aphasia may improve but some residual speech deficit remains. In these cases, word substitution is typical in that the person is unable to produce a given word and substitutes another word for the appropriate one. Difficulty following verbal commands due to misinterpretation of words may occur.

Individuals with this speech problem may have functional limitations in the area of communication with others, depending on the extent of the speech and comprehension difficulty. For persons with minor residual deficits, the problem may go unnoticed. Rehabilitation counselors can suggest to the individual alternative ways to express ideas. If the problem is moderate to severe and the person relies on verbal communication for employment, simple modifications may not be sufficient and a change in occupation is advisable. Through analysis of job functions, the counselor can recommend jobs that do not require extensive verbal discourse.

**Broca's aphasia.** In Broca's aphasia (expressive aphasia), the abilities to comprehend and conceptualize speech are relatively intact. There is a problem in the capability to form language and express oneself. Over time, the ability to speak major words may return; often, minor words disappear from speech. Adjectives and adverbs are the words that typically disappear. An individual might say "weather hot" instead of "the weather is hot." A person with Broca's or expressive aphasia can return to employment without job modification, providing writing or speaking with other individuals is not required to any significant degree. For example, the person would have difficulty over the telephone or working with customers, but should be able to follow verbal orders.

**Conduction aphasia.** A third form of speech disturbance is conduction aphasia. The cause of conduction aphasia is an interruption of the conducting fibers between Wernicke's area and Broca's area. This causes a speech disturbance in which an individual receives the information but has difficulty reacting to it. Frequently, the person is able to copy and mimic sounds but cannot comprehend the information. Clearly, this is a severe, disabling speech impairment.

**Global aphasia.** Large frontal-temporal lesions cause global aphasia. Serious deficits will be seen in both expression and comprehension of language. This is also a severe disability that creates major functional limitations. The individual may need a rehabilitation counselor to recommend possible accommodations for this disability.

## Cranial Nerves

This involves evaluation of the nerves that serve the areas of the face including the sense of smell, vision, eye movement, face movement, and sensation on the face. Of particular importance are (a) visual disturbances and (b) disturbances in speech formation (dysarthria).

A frequently encountered neurological finding in the examination of the eyes is homonymous hemianopsia. In this condition, there exists a state of blindness in one-half of the vision of both eyes. There is an inability to see to the right in the right eye and to the right in the left eye or vice versa. The ability to read and see with the other half of the visual field of each eye remains intact.

With abnormalities of the facial nerve, there are disturbances of facial movements which may result in difficulty in pronunciation or in slurred speech. There is a functional limitation in the ability to produce understandable speech (dysarthria).

## Gait and Station

Disorders of gait and station include various disturbances of walking, such as ataxic (defective coordination), spasticity, and steppage gait (high-stepping gait). Clearly, gait disturbance may cause limitations in the ability to walk, particulary long distances. If a significant gait disturbance is present, vocational rehabilitation to work involving limited ambulation, such as sedentary work activity, is appropriate.

## Cerebellum

Evaluation of cerebellar function is included in this category in the neurological examination. The cerebellum controls movement and coordination; a person with cerebellar disease may have an unsteady gait, lack coordination, and have difficulty with fine movements. This may affect one side of the body (upper and lower extremity) or both sides. With involvement of the dominant hand, the degree of disability and resulting limitations will be significantly more severe. The individual may need to transfer hand dominance to the previously nondominant hand.

## Motor and Sensory Function

In the motor/sensory function evaluation, the medical examiner tests for disturbances of the motor system and sensory system. The examiner systematically tests each group of muscles (e.g., about the elbow, wrist). Also tested are reflexes and muscle tone. The sensory examination tests pin sensation, touch, proprioception (the ability to tell where a finger or toe is in relation to the rest of the body), and vibration. The motor system consists of upper motor neurons (nerve connections to the central nervous system from the spinal cord) and lower motor neurons (nerve connections to the spinal cord and periphery). Upper motor neuron dysfunction occurs in illnesses involving the spinal cord, brain stem, and brain. This often produces abnormalities involving at least one limb or one-half of the body. There is a characteristic loss of strength, increase in reflexes (hyperflexia), and spasticity associated with these disorders.

Lower motor neuron diseases typically include the nerve roots, peripheral nerves, or both. This produces a smaller area of deficit which affects a specific group of muscles, resulting in abnormal muscle functioning. Characteristically, there will be muscle weakness, a lack of muscular tone (hypotonicity), and no reflexes (areflexia). The sensory system also has central nervous system and peripheral nervous system components. In a central sensory nervous system disorder, sensory loss is present and affects one limb or one-half of the body. In peripheral nervous system disease, a small area of the skin may show decreased sensation corresponding with an abnormality of the specific nerve or nerve root that supplies that given skin area (Berkow, 1987; Wilson et al., 1991).

# NEUROLOGICAL DISORDER CLASSIFICATION

Neurological illnesses can be classified as acute, subacute, and chronic conditions. **Acute** neurological disorders involve symptoms of illness that occur with a sudden and severe onset, over minutes or several hours. There is a rapid and dramatic deterioration of the person's neurological function. Examples include stroke, seizure disorders, and severe headaches.

**Subacute** illnesses evolve over days to months. Various forms of infection (e.g., meningitis), brain tumor, and peripheral nerve pain may occur in this manner.

**Chronic** neurological conditions most often have a progressive course that may extend over many years. They typically are of long duration and have a slow progression. Degenerative conditions of the nervous system such as muscular dystrophy, myasthenia gravis, Alzheimer's disease, Huntington chorea, amyotrophic lateral sclerosis, and Parkinson's disease are typically chronic in nature.

Knowledge of the history, onset, and course of the disease process is important in rehabilitation. In order to maintain employment or to return a person to work, the neurological disorder must be stabilized or very slowly progressive. If a patient has had an acute episode that has run its course and reached maximum improvement, the counselor can formulate a rehabilitation plan based on the knowledge that the deficit will not worsen. If an individual is under the best medical control possible, but continues to have debilitating neurological symptoms, the frequency and intensity of these events is important in determining the feasibility of providing vocational rehabilitation services.

# NEUROLOGICAL TESTING

The following will familiarize the rehabilitation counselor with the commonly encountered neurological tests used in clinical practice. Various types of electrodiagnostic tests, the electroencephalogram, magnetic resonance imaging (MRI) scans, and computerized axial tomography (CAT) scans of the brain and spine are tests physicians frequently request and are seen in clients' medical records (Conn and Conn, 1985).

## Description

**Electromyography.** Electrodiagnostic testing includes electromyography. This procedure involves inserting needles into various muscles to amplify the electrical activity of the muscles. Electromyographic examination will reveal abnormalities suggestive of muscle or nerve disease. This procedure aids in the diagnosis and pinpointing of a disturbance of a particular nerve, nerve root (radiculopathy), or muscle. It is most useful in myopathy and radiculopathy.

**Nerve conduction study.** Nerve conduction study, on the other hand, is a test which delivers small electric shocks via electrodes placed on the skin. The electrical stimulation can then be followed as it travels along the nerve. Motor and sensory nerve fibers are tested. This test is most useful for mononeuropathy (e.g., carpal tunnel syndrome) or peripheral neuropathy.

**Electroencephalogram (EEG).** This involves the use of scalp electrodes. It provides an amplification and summation of the activity of the brain as measured at the scalp level. There are several patterns in the electroencephalogram that are normal. Other patterns correlate with either diffuse or local pathology of the brain. Electroencephalogram patterns divide into normal, abnormal, and a pattern of uncertain clinical significance. Physicians frequently use electroencephalograms to aid in the diagnoses of focal brain disturbances and seizures.

**MRI and CAT scans.** Both MRI and CAT scans provide pictures of the brain. They are useful in detecting large focal anatomic lesions of the brain or spinal cord. Brain tumors, intracerebral hemorrhage, and spinal disc disease are detectable using this means. The MRI and CAT scan procedures are replacing the less frequently performed myelography (injection of a radiopaque substance into the spinal column, followed by x-ray).

# ANATOMY AND PHYSIOLOGY

Anatomically, the nervous system is composed of the central nervous system (CNS), peripheral nervous system (PNS), and autonomic nervous system (ANS).

Before describing the signs and symptoms of diseases and injuries of the nervous system, two basic principles of neurophysiology should be emphasized (Felton, Perkins, & Lewin, 1966, p. 60):

1. The brain must receive a constant supply of oxygen and glucose in order to meet its incessant metabolic needs. If, because of a vascular or metabolic disorder, this supply is interrupted, the brain will metabolize its own proteins and fats, and rapidly destroy itself. Without oxygen, the brain dies in 6 minutes.

2. Unlike most tissues of the body, the cells of the brain are not capable of regenerating themselves. Nerve cell death is irreversible. To some extent, the functions of an injured or dead area can be assumed by other uninjured areas.

## The Central Nervous System (CNS)

The brain and the spinal cord compose the CNS. There are three parts to the brain: the cerebrum, the cerebellum, and the brain stem. The cerebrum is the largest section of the brain and consists of two hemispheres. Each hemisphere further divides into four lobes: frontal, parietal, temporal, and occipital. Each of these lobes has specific functions (Williams, Warwick, Dyson, and Bannister, 1989). A discussion of the effects of damage to the specific lobes will follow under the section "Abnormalities of the Brain Hemispheres."

The brain contains deep and superficial gray matter as well as white matter. Gray matter receives and processes messages from the nerves of the body. White matter conducts the nerve messages. Gray matter consists of nerve cells, while white matter is composed of myelinated fibers (axons). The cerebellum is part of the brain stem and helps control coordination and movement. The brain stem and deep gray matter interact with the spinal cord and gray matter of the brain.

## The Peripheral Nervous System (PNS)

The peripheral nervous system begins in the spinal cord at which point a spinal nerve forms from anterior and posterior roots. There are 8 cervical roots, 12 thoracic roots, 5 lumbar roots, and 6 sacral roots. Anterior roots involve motor function and posterior roots involve sensory function. The roots form a spinal nerve as they exit through the spinal column. Spinal nerves then converge in the brachial and lumbosacral plexus. The spinal nerves are integrated at this point and leave the plexus as peripheral nerves. Each nerve and nerve root serves a specific cutaneous area of the skin and a specific set of muscles (Williams et al., 1989).

The neurologist becomes familiar with each pattern of abnormality seen for each nerve and nerve root. For instance, root involvement at the fifth lumbar level (L5) causes weakness in the ability to lift the ankle and toe from the floor. The forearm involvement of the ulnar nerve (neuropathy) produces weakness in the intrinsic muscles of the hand and an inability to move the hand outward.

Twelve pairs of cranial nerves, 31 pairs of spinal nerves, and the nerves of the autonomic nervous system compose the peripheral nervous system. The 12 cranial nerves are designated either numerically or by descriptive names. These nerves and their related functions are illustrated in Table 1 (Felton, Perkins, & Lewin, 1966, p. 60). Each of the 31 pairs of spinal peripheral nerves connect to their roots within the spinal cord and are made up of a posterior root (sensory) and an anterior root (motor).

## Table 1

### THE CRANIAL NERVES AND THEIR RELATED FUNCTION

| Nerve and Number | Related functionally to— |
|---|---|
| I. Olfactory | sense of smell. |
| II. Optic | vision. |
| III. Oculomotor | movement of eye muscles. |
| IV. Trochlear | movement of one eye muscle. |
| V. Trigeminal | sensation over skin of face, lining of mouth and nose, tongue, and muscles used in chewing. |
| VI. Abducens | movement of one eye muscle. |
| VII. Facial | muscles of the face, salivary glands, and sense of taste in anterior part of tongue. |
| VIII. Auditory (with a vestibular branch) | hearing, sense of balance, and sense of rotation. |
| IX. Glossopharyngeal | salivary glands, muscles of the pharynx, swallowing, and sense of taste in pharynx. |
| X. Vagus | heart action, peristalsis of small intestine, speech, swallowing, secretion of gastric glands, and respiratory rhythm of lungs. |
| XI. Spinal Accessory | muscles of the shoulder and neck. |
| XII. Hypoglossal | musculature of the tongue. |

## The Autonomic Nervous System (ANS)

The nerves of the autonomic nervous system supply internal organs of the body and control vital involuntary or autonomic body functions such as respiration, heart rate, digestion, defecation, urination, sweating, and other autonomic functions. The system is made up of the sympathetic and the parasympathetic components. In body functions, one acts to control or antagonize the other, e.g., one nerve (sympathetic) increases heart rate, while another nerve (parasympathetic) decreases heart rate (Williams et al., 1989).

## Abnormalities of the Brain Hemispheres

Abnormalities involving all hemispheres will produce a decrease in mental or cognitive function. The brain hemispheres discussed below include the frontal, parietal, temporal, and occipital lobes.

**Frontal lobe.** Clinical syndromes resulting from disorders affecting the precentral gyrus portion of the frontal lobe of the brain include motor abnormalities of the opposite side of the body or hemiparesis (paralysis affecting only one side of the body). Lesions of the dominant frontal lobe may cause Broca's aphasia. In more extensive lesions of one or both frontal lobes, there may be impairment of cognitive and behavioral functions with a specific dull affect, resulting in symptoms including lack of initiative and spontaneity. Poor attention to personal hygiene is also a frequent residual. Individuals often display socially unacceptable behavior such as improper remarks, coarse jokes, and impulsive conduct, without being aware of it.

**Parietal lobe.** Abnormalities of the parietal lobe typically affect sensation on the opposite side of the body (hemianesthesia). There also may be a homonymous hemianopsia present. Disease of the dominant parietal lobe, most commonly in the left hemisphere, produces problems in recognizing reading and in writing (alexia). It also may result in a peculiar symptom in which the individual has difficulty recognizing objects through the sense of touch (agraphia). Disease of the nondominant parietal lobe (typically, the right side) often produces a lack of recognition of the non-dominant side of the body (apraxia). This condition causes an inability to perform purposive movements, such as involved in the act of dressing.

**Temporal lobe.** Abnormality of the temporal lobe of the dominant hemisphere produces Wernicke's aphasia, as discussed earlier, and an inability to produce or appreciate musical sounds (amusia). Lesions in the nondominant temporal lobe produce difficulty with spatial relationships. Dysfunction of either temporal lobe can produce auditory hallucinations and psychosis or depression. Bilateral disease of the temporal lobe may produce difficulty with retaining new information (Korsakoff's amnesia).

**Occipital lobe.** Abnormalities of the occipital lobe result in homonymous hemianopsia and may produce other visual illusions or hallucinations. Disease of both occipital lobes may cause cortical blindness where the pupils remain reactive, but the individual cannot see or react to visual stimuli (Anton's syndrome).

# DISORDERS OF THE CENTRAL NERVOUS SYSTEM

The neurologist must first determine whether the central nervous system (CNS) disease is a **stable** or **progressive** illness. These are discussed below.

**Nonprogressive** disease of the CNS causes neurological deficit that is not anticipated to change over time. Individuals with this kind of CNS condition, depending on the extent of the impairment, can benefit from rehabilitation efforts. Alternatively, **progressive** illness of the central nervous system, having a steady downhill course, will make rehabilitation efforts more difficult and may require short-term goals at best. One must consider whether the disease is a generalized brain disease in which there is some degree of impairment, or a focal involvement of the brain which affects one specific area of the brain. Stroke (cerebral vascular accident) is an example of a fixed nonprogressive neurological disease resulting from a focal abnormality. Brain tumor is an example of a slowly progressive focal neurological disease, worsening, in many cases, over years.

## Infection

Various types of infection can affect the central nervous system. Usually, bacteria and viruses are involved. Patterns of infection include a focal inflammation site (cerebritis) or abscess, most frequently bacterial in origin. An inflammation of the meninges (the membranes enveloping the brain and spinal cord) may be bacterial or viral (meningitis). Finally, a meningoencephalitis is usually viral in origin and affects the brain and meninges. Most central nervous system infections result in residual deficits. These may be subtle with personality change and sleep disturbance being prominant. Viral meningitis never causes residual deficit. One must keep in mind there is no specific treatment for viral diseases. When complications occur, damage to cranial nerves and the brain may result in permanent deficit.

A most common residual deficit is a permanent hearing loss. Other serious deficits may occur. In addition to personality change and sleep disturbance, one may also see behavioral changes, particularly decreased cognitive capability, and seizures. Neuropsychological testing is helpful to ascertain the remaining functional capacities and limitations.

## Focal Brain Disease

Traumatic brain injury is the most common disorder of the nervous system in younger individuals. Stroke and brain tumors also may be considered under focal neurological brain disease.

Brain trauma includes closed and open head trauma. Closed head trauma implies that the skull remains intact; open head trauma involves a breech of the integrity of the scalp and skull.

Both closed and open head trauma may be severe and result in significant deficit and possible death. Clinicians are aware of potential life threatening conditions in cases of traumatic brain injury. Closed head trauma can produce focal brain abnormalities, particularly when the trauma involves contusion, intracerebral hemorrhage, or edema (swelling).

Speech deficit, difficulty with spatial relationships, incoordination, personality change, sleep disturbance, and irritability are common residual symptoms from this type of injury. Closed head trauma has a spectrum of symptoms that may range from very mild impairment to extremely severe deficits. Those individuals who may benefit from rehabilitation services will range from mild to moderate in impairment. Neuropsychological evaluation may be very helpful in determining their rehabilitation capabilities and potentials.

## Post Concussion Syndrome

Persons with head trauma have a constellation of symptoms called post concussion syndrome or post traumatic brain injury syndrome. After even minor head trauma (trauma with no apparent neurological deficit at the onset), the patient may develop headaches, nausea, vomiting, dizziness, sleep disturbance, and irritability. There can be forgetfulness and decreased eye-hand-foot coordination. This symptomatology persists for several weeks, generally resolving with only minor symptoms remaining or a complete lack of complaints. In about 5% of individuals, post concussion syndrome symptomatology is chronic and persists beyond 6 months. These individuals may continue to have headaches and related behavioral problems that negatively affect the personality. They may experience forgetfulness, irritability, and decreased stamina. Sometimes, they require medication to maintain daily activities.

A major factor in post concussion syndrome is a loss of stamina. There may be significant vocational implications in that an individual may not be able to work for a complete 8-hour day.

**Stroke.** The aging process results in many medical complications in the elderly person. Hardening of the arteries (arteriosclerosis) and hypertension (high blood pressure) are common disorders found in the elderly. These conditions predispose an individual to arterial vessel abnormalities that may result in a rupture, causing a stroke. Occasionally, a younger person has a stroke. This may produce focal brain damage and, depending on the severity, result in loss or diminished use of one side of the body due to paralysis (hemiplegia). Speech disturbance often occurs with damage to the dominant hemisphere. Even in mild cases, one may observe a loss of stamina and incoordination on the affected side. Improvement after stroke may occur for 3-6 months.

Once stabilized, these patients may benefit from rehabilitation evaluation. Many stroke patients are elderly and may not need or request vocational rehabilitation, although stroke does occur in individuals of working age. The direction of rehabilitation will depend on the functional limitations, both physical and psychological.

**Brain tumor.** Brain tumor, because of its usually pervasive features, particularly into the deeper structures of the brain, often denotes a poor prognosis with progressive deterioration. Brain tumors include primary tumors which are those arising directly from brain cells and metastatic tumors (spread from a tumor elsewhere in the body). Metastatic disease by far comprises the largest percentage of brain tumors. The brain is affected in approximately 20% of individuals with cancer. In most cases, once the brain is affected, the prognosis is extremely poor and death will follow rapidly, often times within several months of diagnosis.

Alternatively, primary brain tumors are less common, with an incidence of 15 per 100,000 people. Generally, brain tumors grow and cause local destruction within the brain. The rate of growth is variable, at times very rapid with death ensuing after several months or sometimes more slowly with death occurring after several years. In individuals with brain tumors, attempts at continuing their current employment may be appropriate, depending on the symptoms and the rate of growth of the tumor. Retraining is probably not appropriate. Occasionally, very slowly growing tumors are found in younger people. In this situation, the counselor should obtain information regarding prognosis from the treating physician.

## Spinal Cord Disorders

In younger individuals, especially males, spinal cord injury is frequently the result of acute trauma. Multiple sclerosis is another common cause of spinal cord dysfunction in younger individuals, both male and female. The residual muscular and sensory defects are dependent on the level of injury to the spinal cord and on the number of nerve fibers injured within the cord. The physician describes the injury by the vertebral level of the lesion. For example, a cervical (neck) injury in the area of the fifth cervical vertebra is expressed as a C5 myelopathy. A thoracic injury in the area of the fifth thoracic vertebra is expressed as a T5 myelopathy.

Trauma to the spinal cord may result in paralysis of the lower extremities (paraplegia) or both upper and lower extremities (quadriplegia), depending on the location of the injury. Injury to the thoracic spine and spinal cord may produce abnormalities involving the legs and cause incontinence. Trauma to the cervical spine typically produces abnormalities involving at least some function of the arms and hands, as well as incontinence. These individuals will often require light or sedentary types of work and may have fatigue, loss of stamina, and incoordination. All of these are factors for the rehabilitation counselor to consider.

## Multiple Sclerosis (MS)

Multiple sclerosis is an inflammatory disease of the central nervous system that destroys the lining covering the axons, the myelin sheath. This occurs in localized areas of the brain and spinal cord. MS is a disease characterized by remissions and exacerbations. After each exacerbation, new neurological deficit occurs which remains stable until the next exacerbation. Frequency of exacerbation is unpredictable. The cause of MS is unknown and there is no specific treatment. After each exacerbation, loss of function of the affected part of the brain or spinal cord occurs. Frequently seen symptoms include spasticity, weakness, incoordination, incontinence, and speech and visual disturbances. Fatigability is a frequently overlooked complication of this disease.

## Inherited and Degenerative Diseases of the Central Nervous System

A number of diseases of the central nervous system are inherited. They show progressive deterioration that may occur rapidly or slowly over many years. Huntington's chorea is a slowly progressive inherited neurological disorder. A second type of disorder described in this category are the degenerative disorders. Medical researchers have not identified a true cause for most of the diseases within this area. As with the inherited type, these diseases also are slowly progressive. Classic examples of diseases in this group are Parkinson's and Alzheimer's disease.

## Parkinson's Disease

Parkinson's disease is a condition in which there is a degeneration of unknown etiology involving the substantia nigra, a small area in the upper brain stem. The substantia nigra produces a neurotransmitter called dopamine, necessary for normal functioning. The typical features of Parkinson's disease include bradykinesia (extreme slowness of movement), rigidity, and a resting tremor. Onset typically occurs between the ages of 40-70, most often in the 50s and 60s. It is a slowly progressive disease, becoming severe over several years. Treatment with medications will temporarily improve the physical manifestations. There is no treatment for the underlying disease and progressive degeneration of the substantia nigra is relentless in this disease.

## Dementia

Dementia is a loss of global intellect. All aspects of intellectual function are diminished, although the absolute decrease varies with the different aspects of intellectual functioning and the particular individual. There are several different diseases associated with dementia. Approximately 10% are specifically treatable and relate to illnesses such as vitamin $B_{12}$ deficiency and hypothyroidism.

The remainder of dementias are not specifically treatable. There are illnesses, such as subcortical dementia or multi-infarct dementia, caused by either small lacunar strokes in the deep gray matter of the brain or by multiple small strokes in various other areas of the brain. In these diseases, progression may be decreased by medication or possibly carotid endarterectomy (surgical removal of the carotid plaque to improve circulation). Those illnesses, not specifically treatable, are described as nontreatable dementia (e.g., Alzheimer's disease). Alzheimer's disease is a slowly progressive degenerative condition in which nerve cells within the brain die. There is no treatment available. Presenile dementia (beginning in middle age) and senile dementia (occurring in people over 60) are arbitrary divisions of this disease. Presenile dementia is not a commonly encountered disease.

## Motor Neuron Disease

There are three specific forms of motor neuron disease. In the bulbar form, abnormalities begin in the brain stem and affect the face, tongue, and the ability to swallow. The onset of amyotrophic lateral sclerosis is typically on one side of the body and involves one arm and leg. Progressive muscular atrophy begins in both hands and progresses. No specific treatment is available for any form of this disease.

Lou Gehrig (a famous New York Yankees' baseball player) brought attention to a motor neuron disease, which became identified with his name. Lou Gehrig disease is amyotrophic lateral sclerosis (ALS). It is a disease of the alpha motor neurons involving specific cells in the brain stem and spinal cord. This disease is degenerative, of unknown etiology, and is rapidly progressive. There is loss of strength with hyperreflexia and fasciculations (involuntary small movement of muscles) present. The disease is progressive and individuals frequently use wheelchairs for mobility. Sometimes the downhill progression can be such that the person cannot eat or swallow within 12 months of onset.

## Developmental Diseases

Developmental diseases may be genetic in origin or may include maternal or fetal events occurring prenatally, perinatally, or immediately postnatally. Genetic disease is typically progressive over time. If the causative factor is a specific event, such as intrauterine hypoxia or viral infection, the disease usually results in a finite deficit.

**Cerebral palsy.** Cerebral palsy results from injury to the brain occurring during the period of development. The usual cause is hypoxia (deficiency of oxygen). Usually, weakness and spasticity are present with the arms affected more than the legs (spastic diplegia-congenital spastic stiffness of the limbs).

**Mental retardation.** Mental retardation implies below average intellectual ability. It is usually detected in infancy and causes abnormal development, difficulty in learning, and problems with social competency. Mild retardation is usually related to a combination of causes. Severe retardation is often caused by a specific severe disease.

## Epilepsy

Epilepsy is caused by damage to the brain. It involves transient electrical disturbances in the brain resulting in various types of seizures. This condition occurs at all ages. Seizures may range from mild to severe, may occur often or rarely, and may be partial (in a given area) or generalized (affecting the total body). Seizures may be caused by trauma, tumors, high fevers, or drugs. The most common form of seizure, partial complex seizure disorder with secondary generalization, occurs in the teenage years. It is usually ideopathic (cause undeterminable). The counselor must be aware of the sedative effects of the medications that are prescribed to control this condition. Medication can control most seizures, although some individuals have seizures that are difficult to control. Persons with seizures should avoid situations where they would injure themselves or others should a seizure occur.

## Headaches

Headaches usually do not indicate there is significant intracranial or brain pathology. Less than 1% of individuals with headaches have serious central nervous system abnormalities. The neurologist must deal with persons experiencing an acute or chronic headache on an individual basis and be alert for clues that point to the possibility of serious pathology. One also must realize that although headaches may not be the basis for eligibility in vocational rehabilitation systems, they do play a role in aggravating the impairment of any disability. Stress may precipitate or aggravate headaches.

There are two classifications of the common headache: migraine and tension headaches. Migraine headaches are predominantly frontal and may be unilateral. Frequently, an aura or a focal neurological deficit precedes these headaches. Just before onset, the individual may experience a visual disturbance such as flashing lights. Some patients complain of blind spots (scotomata), while others experience nausea and vomiting. Although it occurs rarely, patients may experience generalized weakness or sensory changes involving one side of the body, primarily an arm and leg. Following these early symptoms, the person may develop a severe, throbbing headache. Most often, finding a quiet environment and resting is helpful. Most migraine headaches resolve spontaneously with sleep.

Tension headaches frequently occur in the back of the head. Also, generally affected are the muscles of the neck and upper back. The person complains of neck stiffness. These headaches are not generally alleviated by sleep and may last for several days.

Headaches may be associated with a major disability or complaint but generally are not the primary disorder. This condition, coupled with the side effects of medication taken to control symptoms, can contribute to and aggravate the primary disability. Factors that are important in evaluating functional limitations are the type, dosage, and frequency of medications required to maintain the person free of symptoms. Also important is the individual's attitude and ability to tolerate the pain.

## Vertigo

Vertigo is a sensation of spinning and a feeling that oneself or the environment is unstable. The individual may experience a loss of balance. Causes of vertigo include disturbances of the vestibular apparatus within the inner ear and a variety of central nervous system conditions involving the brain stem. Vertigo is divided into peripheral and central nervous system causes. Generally, peripheral nervous system vertigo will be intermittent and experienced as the result of rapid head movement. Vertigo from central nervous system causes is generally persistent irrespective of head movement or head position. It may be a persistent symptom of a disease process with some individuals having mild, intermittent symptoms and others having persistent ongoing complaints.

Clients requesting rehabilitation will usually have at least moderate symptomatology. They should avoid working at heights and around dangerous equipment where injury may occur should they become dizzy or disoriented. Driving commercial vehicles is contraindicated. If head movement brings on symptoms, employment in which a person must move the head frequently and rapidly needs to be avoided.

## Nervous System Disease Related to Drugs

A variety of chemicals and drugs affect the central nervous system. These substances can cause a multiplicity of side effects and reactions. Typical abnormalities include cognitive and behavioral deficits, seizures, and peripheral neuropathies.

Predictable side effects related to drug intoxication and idiosyncratic reactions to medication are the two areas relating to drug and chemical effects on the nervous system. Predictable side effects are related to the amount of drug ingested (dose). Idiosyncratic reactions are peculiar to an individual and are unpredictable and unrelated to the amount of drug taken.

Cocaine, for instance, will cause a central nervous system vasculitis (inflammation of the vessels) in a few individuals that may lead to small strokes. This is not a predictable side effect of the drug. These individuals will generally have diffuse brain involvement and may have decreased cognition and deteriorated intellectual functioning as the principle finding.

Chronic alcohol abuse may cause several specific neurological problems, such as peripheral neuropathy, cerebellar degeneration, and alcohol-related dementia. These are predictable side effects of alcohol. They are related to amount and duration of alcohol intake. With abstinence, improved nutrition, and rehabilitation, these are usually partially reversible.

# DISEASES OF THE PERIPHERAL NERVOUS SYSTEM

Peripheral nervous system (PNS) disease involves the nerves, nerve roots, and associated muscles. These diseases may be progressive or nonprogressive.

## Disease of Muscle

**Muscular dystrophies.** Muscular dystrophies are inherited or genetically determined illnesses involving a progressive weakening of muscles. The etiology is unknown. These diseases usually begin in childhood or in the teens and are slowly progressive. Individuals with muscular dystrophy usually require sedentary work. As the condition progresses, short-term goals need to be established; periodic reevaluation, and modification of these goals will be necessary. The more sedentary the work activity, the longer the individual may be able to maintain the particular employment situation. Prescribed exercise is important as prolonged inactivity leads to worsening of the disease state. Maintaining activities and possible physical therapy during non-work hours will be very beneficial for most persons.

**Primary myopathies.** Primary myopathies are a rare group of diseases in which there are histological abnormalities involving the muscle fiber or muscle cell mitochondria. These produce mild diffuse weakness and mild diffuse decrease in stamina. The abnormalities are slowly progressive, although typically life expectancy is not significantly affected. No specific treatment is available. Individuals with primary myopathies do best in light and sedentary types of employment.

**Myasthenia gravis.** This is a disease of the myoneural (muscle-nerve) junction. It can occur at any age. Initial normal strength with rapid loss of strength with use of affected muscles is characteristic of individuals with myasthenia gravis. There is restoration of strength with rest. Periods of exacerbation and remission may occur. Medication may help prevent loss of strength. Individuals who seek rehabilitation usually will have a more severe form of the disease and will require sedentary types of work. They may need pauses and rest periods while at work as the muscles weaken with use and become restored with rest. For some persons, the counselor should consider employment that can be done at home to accommodate the rest periods that may be needed.

## Cranial Neuropathies

Each of the 12 cranial nerves may manifest its own specific symptomatology when involved in a disease process. In rehabilitation, abnormalities involving eye and face movement may present significant handicaps for employment. Cranial nerves three, four, and six control eye movements. Abnormalities of these cranial nerves will cause a variation of eye movement, including diplopia (double vision). Often, the physician prescribes an eye patch for an individual with this condition, leaving the person monocular as long as the patch is worn. Eighth nerve or auditory nerve abnormalities may be associated with hearing deficits and vertigo.

Seventh nerve (the facial nerve) abnormalities cause difficulty in moving the face muscles and closing the eyes. Individuals with this problem will need protective glasses and must avoid environments where particles of dust can irritate the eyes. Additionally, they may have some degree of dysarthria (difficult and defective speech).

## Radiculopathy

There are various causes for radiculopathy (an abnormality of a nerve root). Degenerative changes in the spine with the formation of bony osteophytes (outgrowths) may cause radiculopathy. A ruptured or bulging disc is also a frequent cause of radiculopathy. Radiculopathy will cause pain in the affected region of the spine. This will be accompanied by limited motion of the spine, muscle spasm, and nerve root pain radiating down an extremity. Sensory and motor loss may occur in the affected area. Pain generally will be experienced below the knee in lumbar radiculopathy, and below the elbow in cervical radiculopathy.

Individuals with radiculopathies may require surgery to help alleviate symptoms. This depends on the pathology and severity of the condition. Work limitations for individuals with radiculopathies frequently involve limitation to light or sedentary work. Since many jobs in these categories involve extensive sitting, the person may need to alternate positioning between sitting and standing. The frequency of change in position is dependent on the individual's tolerance to discomfort. Generally, it will be beneficial to avoid prolonged sitting or standing.

Back and neck pain is a major employment problem in most industrialized countries. Workers frequently have chronic back and neck pain complaints without having objective findings of disc disease or radiculopathy. Often, there will be an initial injury, possibly a strain, with ongoing complaints of severe pain. For rehabilitation purposes, one must distinguish between the actual physical limitations and pain complaints. A thorough medication history should be obtained with particular attention to addicting or sedating drugs.

## Peripheral Neuropathy

Peripheral neuropathy is a disease that can affect any nerve in the body. Frequently, peripheral neuropathy affects lower extremity nerves more than the nerves of the upper extremities. Weakness, sensory loss, and incoordination will be noted. There are multiple causes of peripheral neuropathy. Approximately one-third are due to systemic disease, such as diabetes. Another one-third are due to autoimmune inflammation, such as Guillain-Barré syndrome. The last one-third are due to multiple causes, often inherited and/or degenerative.

It is important for the physician to understand the underlying cause of the illness, since peripheral neuropathy due to a systemic disease or autoimmune abnormalities may be ameliorated by treatment of the underlying disease process. Despite medical treatment, some mild residual symptoms may persist and the person may have symptoms such as mild incoordination, weakness, decreased stamina, and decreased sensation in the extremities. These persons require lighter types of employment that do not involve frequent use of fine coordination and manual dexterity. At the time of referral for rehabilitation, the level of dysfunction is stable and not anticipated to change. Therefore, the counselor can usually provide vocational rehabilitation services based on the current limitations.

## Mononeuropathy

Mononeuropathy involves injury or disease of a single nerve. These usually involve compression of a nerve in a specific area of the body (segmental mononeuropathy). The most frequently seen mononeuropathies involve the medial nerve of the wrist (carpal tunnel syndrome), ulnar nerve at the elbow (cubital tunnel syndrome), and peroneal nerve at the head of the fibula.

**Carpal tunnel syndrome.** This condition involves compression of the median nerve in the carpal tunnel of the wrist. It causes numbness and pain in the thumb, palm, and second through fourth fingers. The person may experience night pain and radiating pain. Carpal tunnel syndrome may be caused by repetitive wrist motion, sustained grip and pinch activities, continuous wrist angulation, poor posturing, repetitive vibration, physical injury, or muscle weakness. There will be weakness in the affected hand and a loss of grip strength. Individuals with carpal tunnel syndrome need to avoid frequent pronation, supination, and extension of the wrist. Repetitive activities such as using a screwdriver for long periods of time, operating a typewriter or a computer terminal, may need to be avoided or modified.

**Ulnar neuropathy.** Individuals with ulnar neuropathy typically have decreased strength in the muscles of the hand. There will be weakness of grasp and frequently a decreased coordination of the hand. Sensory disturbance occurs in the fourth and fifth fingers. Usually, the nerve is injured at the elbow level; the individual should avoid activities where the elbow rests on a firm surface or in which minor trauma to the elbow occurs repetitively.

**Peroneal neuropathy.** In the lower extremity, peroneal neuropathy causes a foot drop. Thus, the individual will not be able to lift the foot against gravity and will walk with a peculiar gait termed a steppage gait. Often a brace is used to maintain a 90° angle of the foot with the ankle. Individuals with peroneal neuropathies will have difficulty with ambulation and stair climbing; they should have jobs that primarily require sedentary work. Sensory disturbance is usually not significant.

Rehabilitation potential for persons with mononeuropathies is generally good. Functional disability is limited to one specific area of the body. These conditions are often stable and may improve with treatment. The condition typically does worsen over time; yet, temporary exacerbation may be experienced. Rehabilitation counselors working with individuals who have these conditions need to consider job modification with the current employer, whenever possible.

# CASE STUDY

Ms. Nancy Smith is a 48-year old married woman with three children. Two of the children are living at home and dependent on their parents for financial support. Mrs. Smith's husband is working full-time as a machine operator. She has an Associate of Arts degree. Ms. Smith has been a grocery checker for 12 years. The **Dictionary of Occupational Titles** (1977, 1981) classifies the work as GROCERY CHECKER (retail trade), **D.O.T. #** 211.462-014. It is light, semiskilled work. The **D.O.T.** provides the following description:

**211.462-014 CASHIER-CHECKER** (ret. tr.)

Operates cash register to itemize and total customers' purchases in self-service grocery or department store. Reviews price sheets to note price changes and sale items. Records prices and departments, subtotals taxable items, and totals purchases on cash register. Collects money from customers and makes change. Stocks shelves and marks prices on containers. May weigh items, bag merchandise, issue trading stamps, and redeem food stamps and promotional coupons. May cash checks. May be designated according to items checked as GROCERY CHECKER (ret. tr.) (U.S. Department of Labor, 1977, p. 167).

Before this job, Ms. Smith worked as a nursing assistant in a convalescent home for 3 years and as a pharmacy technician in a retail drugstore for 5 years. For the past year, Ms. Smith has had complaints of pain and numbness in her left nondominant hand, primarily in the second through fourth fingers. She also has night pain and pain radiating into the right shoulder. Recently, Nancy has had low back pain and states she is unable to lift and carry more than 25 pounds.

Currently, Ms. Smith receives physical therapy three times a week at 5:00 p.m. on Monday, Wednesday, and Friday. Her work hours are 8:00 a.m. to 5:00 p.m. She leaves work early, at 4:30 p.m., to attend physical therapy. The employer has concerns about her missing 1 1/2 hours of work each week.

The physical therapist suggested to Ms. Smith she see a rehabilitation counselor for advice. Ms. Smith has followed through with this suggestion.

## Questions

1.  Assign Ms. Nancy Smith a vocational profile, including age category, educational level, and work history (skill and exertional levels).

2.  What medical condition(s) do Ms. Smith's symptoms indicate she may have?

3.  Describe Ms. Smith's functional limitations in regard to her job.

4.  Should she attempt to continue working as a grocery checker for the current employer?

5.  If you recommend she continue her employment, what advice would you give her and her employer regarding reasonable accommodation?

6.  Describe the occupationally significant characteristics (worker traits) and possible transferable skills of Ms. Smith.

7.  Suggest rehabilitation possibilities if she does not continue working for this employer.

# REFERENCES

Adams, R.D., & Victor, M. (1989). **Principles of neurology** (4th ed.). New York, NY: McGraw-Hill Information Services.

Andreoli, T.E., Carpenter, C.C.J., Plum, F., & Smith, L.H., Jr. (1990). **Cecil essential of medicine** (2nd ed.). Philadelphia, PA: Harcourt Brace Jovanovich.

Berkow, R. (Ed.). (1987). **The Merck manual of diagnosis and therapy** (15th ed.). Rathway, NJ.: Merck Sharp & Dohme Research Laboratories.

Conn, H.F. & Conn, R.B., Jr. (Ed.). (1985). **Current diagnosis-7**. Philadelphia, PA: W.B. Saunders.

Felton, J.S., Perkins, D.C., & Lewin, M. (1966). **A survey of medicine and medical practice for the rehabilitation counselor**. Washington, DC: U.S. Department of Health, Education, and Welfare.

Joint, R.J. (1990). **Clinical neurology**. Philadelphia, PA: J.B. Lippincott.

Rowland, L.P. (Ed.). (1989). **Merritt's textbook of neurology** (8th ed.). Philadelphia, PA: Lea & Febiger.

Schroeder, S.A., Krupp, M.A., Tierney, L.M., Jr., & McPhee, S.J. (1990). **Current medical diagnosis and treatment**. Norwalk, CT: Appleton and Lange.

U.S.Department of Labor (1977). **Dictionary of occupational titles** (4th ed.). Washington, DC: Author.

U.S.Department of Labor (1981). **Selected characteristics of occupations defined in the dictionary of occupational titles**. Washington, DC: Author.

Williams, P.L., Warwick, R., Dyson, M., & Bannister, L.H. (Eds.). (1989). **Gray's anatomy** (37th ed.). New York: C. Livingstone.

Wilson, J.D., Isselbacker, K.J., Petersdorf, R.G., Martin, J.B., Sauci, A.S., & Root, R.K. (Eds.). (1991). **Harrison's principles of internal medicine** (12th ed.). New York: McGraw Hill.

Wyngaarden, J.B., & Smith, L.H., Jr. (Eds.). (1988). **Cecil textbook of medicine** (18th ed.). Philadelphia, PA: W.B. Saunders.

## *About the Author*

Joshua Goldman, M.D., is a neurologist in private practice in Las Cruces, New Mexico. He is on the medical staff at the Memorial Medical Center in Las Cruces and is on the Panel of Medical Experts of the Social Security Administration.

# Chapter 28

# EPILEPSY

by
*Robert T. Fraser, Ph.D., C.R.C.,*
*Elaine Glazer, M.S.W., L.C.S.W.*
*and*
*Barbara J. Simcoe, B.S.*

## INTRODUCTION

The word "epilepsy" derives from the Greek word meaning "to be seized" and is a generic term that refers to a wide variety of seizure conditions. As early as 150 A.D., Galen recognized seizures may originate in the brain and result from some underlying disease (Wannamaker, Booker, Dreifuss, & Willmore, 1984). Several well known individuals in history such as Socrates, Leonardo de Vinci, Charles Dickens, Thomas Edison, and Julius Caesar had active seizure conditions. A seizure involves a disruption of the normal activity of the brain through neuronal instability. Neurons become unstable and fire in an abnormally rapid manner. This excessive electrical discharge results in a seizure. A seizure may be confined to one area of the brain (partial seizure) or may take place throughout the entire brain (generalized seizure).

The extent to which seizures affect brain functioning relates to both duration and location within the brain. Consequently, some seizures impair brain functioning slightly, while others result in a complete cessation of normal activities.

Causes of epilepsy include traumatic brain injury, birth trauma, anoxia (insufficient oxygen), brain tumors, infectious diseases in the pregnant mother, parasitic infections, vascular diseases affecting the brain's blood vessels, and substance abuse. Only a small portion of patients with epilepsy (1-2%) will have a diagnosable genetic etiology for their seizure occurrences (Anderson, 1988).

A seizure is a discrete event and is a symptom of brain dysfunction; it takes many seizures to establish a diagnosis of epilepsy. Epilepsy is a chronic disorder that involves recurrent, unprovoked seizures (Pedley & Hauser, 1988). The incidence of recurring seizures or epilepsy in the general population is between 1-3% and tends to vary with age groupings (Hauser & Hesdorffer, 1990).

## SYMPTOMATOLOGY

Seizures are generally classified by review of clinical symptoms and supplemented by electroencephalogram (EEG) and sometimes videotape monitoring. There are two types of seizures:

1. Generalized seizures that affect both cerebral hemispheres.

2. Partial (focal) seizures that affect a specific part of one cerebral hemisphere.
   a. simple partial seizures with elementary symptomatology, in which consciousness is not impaired
   b. complex partial seizures, which involve more than one symptom (complex symptomatology) and in which consciousness is impaired
   c. partial seizures which evolve into secondarily generalized seizures

It is important to note many partial seizures may secondarily evolve into generalized seizures. The most recent classification proposed by the International League Against Epilepsy (ILAE) Commission on Classification and

---

## Table 1
## AN ABBREVIATED CLASSIFICATION OF EPILEPTIC SEIZURES

**I.  Generalized Seizures of Non-Focal Origin**
   1.  Tonic-clonic
   2.  Tonic
   3.  Clonic
   4.  Absence
   5.  Atonic/akinetic
   6.  Myoclonic

**II.  Partial (Focal) Seizures**
   1.  Simple partial seizures with elementary symptomatology (consciousness is not impaired)
      a.  With motor symptoms (including Jacksonian, versive, and postural)
      b.  With sensory symptoms (including visual, somatosensory, auditory, olfactory, gustatory, and vertiginous)
      c.  With autonomic symptoms
      d.  With psychic symptoms (including dysphasia, dysmnesia, hallucinatory, and affective changes)
      e.  Compound (i.e., mixed) forms

   2.  Complex partial seizures with complex symptomatology (consciousness is impaired)
      a.  Simple partial seizures followed by loss of consciousness
      b.  With impairment of consciousness at the outset
      c.  With automatisms

   3.  Partial seizures evolving into secondarily generalized seizures

**III.  Unclassified Seizures**

*Reprinted with permission of the Epilepsy Foundation of America as found in Pedley & Hauser (1988, p. 3).*

Terminology, published in 1981, is provided in Table 1. This table gives a basic overview of the different types of seizure conditions.

## Generalized Seizure Conditions

These types of conditions tend to involve both cerebral hemispheres and several areas of the brain (cerebral cortex, thalamus, and brain stem structures), and are sub-categorized into several specific types.

**Tonic-clonic seizures.** The most common form of generalized seizure is the tonic-clonic convulsion (formerly known as grand mal seizure), which occurs in 10% or less of epilepsy cases (Penry, 1986). Although this type of seizure is not always the most difficult to treat, it is the stereotypic seizure with which most people are familiar. This type of seizure involves two stages. The tonic stage, in which the body becomes rigid, lasts for a few seconds. A clonic stage follows in which the person endures a series of convulsive and jerky movements. The entire seizure generally lasts about 2-3 minutes.

From a rehabilitation perspective, the severity of the seizure may leave some individuals disoriented or fatigued following cessation. Some clients can return to work immediately while others may require a full day of rest to return to work activity. Approximately 50% of those with tonic-clonic seizures have them early in the morning when first awakening. Usually, this does not interfere with their ability to arrive on time at the job site. Although most tonic-clonic seizures last for just a few minutes, it is important to note some individuals enter an emergency state called "status epilepticus." This involves a continuing, prolonged seizure or recurring seizures within a brief period. This is an emergency situation and requires immediate hospital care.

**Absence seizures.** The other commonly known type of generalized seizure is the simple absence seizure (traditionally known as petit mal). These seizures take only a few seconds and involve a brief disruption of consciousness (10-20 seconds). There are mild rhythmic movements of the eyelids and autonomic symptoms such as pupil dilation. These seizures show three-per-second spikes on wave tracings on the electroencephalogram (EEG). Most patients with this type of epilepsy begin having these seizures before age 12. This category involves less than 5% of epilepsy cases (Penry, 1986). They are often not identified for years and eventually may transition into generalized tonic-clonic seizure conditions. From a functional perspective, absence seizures may not be very vocationally limiting, especially if there is no memory loss experienced. Exceptions occur when an individual is experiencing many seizures of this type throughout the day or has a physically high risk occupation, where even brief losses of consciousness affect job performance.

**Other types.** Other types of seizures include tonic or clonic seizures, which are limited tonic-clonic or grand mal seizures. In a tonic seizure, the person may fall to the ground and experience rigidity without the convulsive movements. Conversely, in a clonic seizure, they may experience convulsive activity without the earlier period of rigidity.

Other types of generalized seizures include atonic seizures or brief drop attacks. These tend to affect children under 5 years of age. Adults can experience generalized myoclonic jerks that are brief shock-like contractions and may affect the entire body or only a part of the body.

## Partial Seizures

As represented in Table 1, partial seizures can be divided into three categories: (a) simple partial seizures with elementary symptoms; (b) complex partial seizures; and (c) partial seizures evolving into generalized seizures. Each of these categories is discussed below.

**Simple partial seizures.** These seizures may be motor, sensory, autonomic, or involve some combination of symptoms without impaired consciousness. They are linked specifically to an affected area of the brain. Most partial seizures last less than 30 seconds and, due to unimpaired consciousness, are often not a significant problem in regard to job performance. Some individuals who may experience partial seizures may have time to pull over to the side of the road while driving a vehicle, and then proceed when the seizure ends.

**Complex partial seizures.** Impairment of consciousness accompanies complex partial seizures; they are usually associated with temporal or frontal lobe foci. These seizures have an associated aura or warning that can involve a strange odor, aphasia, dizziness, nausea, headaches, unusual stomach sensations, or deja vu experience. Common events include the patient having repetitive motor movements, fumbling with one's hands or clothing, lip-smacking, or aimless wandering. Partial complex seizures without motor components are less common. When they do occur, they can involve impaired consciousness and complex symptoms such as rapid sensory or emotional changes.

From a functional perspective, complex partial seizures can be impairing due to both loss of consciousness and the odd symptoms expressed by the person. It is fortunate many people have a brief aura or warning that enables them to take safety precautions or alert others of their oncoming seizure status. It should be noted approximately 60% of those with epilepsy have seizures classified in the partial seizure category (Pedley & Hauser, 1988).

**Partial seizures evolving into generalized seizures.** Several of these individuals have partial seizures, which if not controlled, spread into generalized seizures. These individuals are often not appropriately treated for their partial seizures, but only for the later observed generalized seizure activity (e.g., a tonic-clonic or grand mal seizure).

# DIAGNOSIS AND TREATMENT

When individuals first experience a seizure, they usually consult their personal or primary care physician. This can involve hospitalization; if the seizure occurred several days previous, an outpatient evaluation may be adequate. The physician may begin a medical treatment program or refer the individual to a general neurologist. If the person does not achieve seizure control within 3 months, the personal or primary care physician should recommend a general neurological referral (National Association of Epilepsy Centers, 1990).

Neurological consultation includes a physical examination and patient history taking, metabolic studies, and other evaluations including EEG testing. The EEG provides the physician a clearer definition of the nature of the abnormal neuronal discharging, often confirming a seizure diagnosis. The physician uses more specialized and noninvasive techniques, such as computerized tomography (CT) scans or magnetic resonance imaging (MRI) of the head when the diagnosis remains unclear. The former is a noninvasive, neuroradiological technique and the latter is non-neuroradiological; both are helpful in identifying small focal lesions or tumors that may be the cause of the partial seizures.

MRI is a technique helpful in identifying lesions in different areas of the brain not clearly seen on CT scans. MRI scans provide better information in cases where bone interference hinders CT scans; they also appear to be more sensitive to certain tissue. Conversely, CT scans are superior in detecting calcified lesions in the brain (Penry, 1986). When seizure control cannot be achieved and more information is needed, the physician may use other types of testing (e.g., positron emission tomography - PET).

As recommended by the National Association of Epilepsy Centers (1990), when the general neurologist does not achieve seizure control within 9 months, a referral to a tertiary or fourth-level epilepsy center should be made. These centers have neurologists who specialize in epilepsy treatment within an allied health center that has specialized teams devoted to the medical and psychosocial needs of persons with epilepsy. The National Association of Epilepsy Centers indicates referral to a center should be made based upon continuing areas of difficulty. These include pharmacological problems; possible psychogenic or pseudoseizures; the potential for epilepsy surgery; the need for invasive, intracranial video/EEG recording; and the need for complementing psychological or psychiatric expertise.

## Treatment Principles

As indicated by the Epilepsy Foundation of America (Wannamaker et al., 1984), it is important to acknowledge that anti-epileptic medications are selectively effective for one or more different types of seizures. It is necessary the neurologist match the appropriate drug to the specific seizure type. Table 2 reviews the primary and secondary drugs that are most useful for different seizure categories.

It is desirable that individuals use one medication (monotherapy) whenever possible to control symptoms. This is because one drug can often be most effective, it is easier to manage, and it has less toxicity. To achieve optimal daily life functioning for a person, the normal course of treatment is to prescribe the maximum effective tolerable dosage of one medication. A dosage should be established that maintains clinically effective concentration within the blood throughout the day. The major recommended drugs have therapeutic ranges and toxicity levels. Table 3 overviews pharmacological data on the major antiepileptic drugs.

### Table 2
### SEIZURE TYPES AND INDICATED ANTIEPILEPTIC DRUGS

| Seizure Type | Effective Antiepileptic Drugs (listed alphabetically) |
|---|---|
| Simple partial or complex partial | **Primary Drugs** |
| | Carbamazepine (Tegretol) |
| | Phenobarbital (Luminal) |
| | Phenytoin (Dilantin) |
| | Primidone (Mysoline) |
| | **Secondary Drugs** |
| | Clonazepam (Clonopin) |
| | Methsuximide (Celontin) |
| | Valproic acid (Depakene) |
| Generalized tonic-clonic (Primary or secondary generalized) | **Primary Drugs** |
| | Carbamazepine |
| | Phenobarbital |
| | Phenytoin |
| | Valproic acid |
| | **Secondary Drugs** |
| | Primidone (Mysoline) |
| Generalized absence | **Primary Drugs** |
| | Ethosuximide (Zarontin) |
| | Valproic acid |
| | **Secondary Drugs** |
| | Acetazolamide (Diamox) |
| | Trimethadione (Tridione) |
| Myoclonic | Clonazepam |
| | Valproic acid |

*Reprinted with the permission of the Epilepsy Foundation of America as found in Leppik (1988, p. 13).*

It is important to note that the time to reach steady-state, the appropriate drug blood serum level, varies across medications relative to number of days. The physician needs to take periodic blood levels of the antiepileptic medication to ensure the person is maintaining an adequate dosage for seizure control and yet has not reached a toxic range concentration. Toxic ranges of medication (excessive drug concentrations) can result in double vision, lethargy, cognitive impairment, coordination difficulties, weight gain, and other medical complications. Medication levels require periodic laboratory monitoring for assessment of appropriate ranges. Even within appropriate ranges, drug side effects may require intervention.

## Surgery

Surgical treatment for epilepsy has been experimental; however, is now becoming better established. There is a growing number of epilepsy centers and neurosurgical groups around the country that perform this operation. The Epilepsy Foundation of America maintains a directory of centers that perform the surgery. Surgery may be considered only when thorough trials on the best available anticonvulsant medications are not successful in controlling seizures. When seizures are cognitively or physically markedly impairing independent living, school performance, work capacities, and social activities, the physician may recommend a surgical consult.

## Table 3
## COMMON ANTICONVULSANT PROPERTIES

| Drug | Therapeutic range (ug/ml.) | Time to reach Steady therapeutic range (in days) |
|---|---|---|
| Ca~ | 6 - 12 | 3 - 4 |
| Clon. | 25 - 0.075 | - - - |
| Ethos. | 0 - 100 | 7 - 10 |
| Phenob. | 15 - 30 | 14 - 21 |
| Phenytoin. | 10 - 20 | 7 - 28 |
| Valproic A. | 50 - 100 | 1 - 2 |

*Note: This information is current at the time of publication (1992). Guidelines for optimal therapeutic ranges can fluctuate based on medical advances. The reader is encouraged to contact the Epilepsy Foundation of America, Landover, Maryland for the most current information. Reprinted with permission.*

In order for surgery to be performed, there must be a clear lesion on the surface of the brain cortex, which can be surgically removed without producing substantial negative consequences. For some persons, although surgery could be helpful in reducing seizures, they may be left with significant language, memory, or other functional deficits. A series of diagnostic tests that include neuropsychological and continuous EEG/video monitoring are conducted so the medical staff and the person have a clear understanding of the absolute need and prognosis of surgical intervention. Some individuals and families will choose to have minor memory deficits as a trade-off for possible seizure-free status achieved by surgery. As physicians choose patients more selectively for the surgical procedure, cognitive deficit problems after the operation may be avoided or diminished. As a result, patients may perform better following surgery.

There are two different approaches to surgery. As described by Schaul (1987), these include (1) a standard temporal lobectomy and (2) the Penfield technique, in which the surgical procedure is tailored to the individual's seizure focus. Results of surgery throughout the country suggest more than 70% of patients achieve a seizure-free or almost seizure-free outcome, with the remaining group having a moderate or less beneficial reduction (Schaul, 1987). Schaul estimates there may be up to 120,000 people within the United States who could benefit from this type of surgery.

## Medical Prognosis for Patients with Epilepsy

It appears 60-70% of those with epilepsy can achieve complete seizure control. Annegers (1988) indicated that 10 years after epilepsy diagnosis, 65% of patients seen are in seizure remission; at 20 years, 76% (of the 65%) are still in remission. The most important prognostic indicator for the eventual control of seizures is the duration of seizure occurrences. Other factors include seizure causality, seizure type, and age at onset of seizures (Annegers, 1988).

# FUNCTIONAL, ENVIRONMENTAL, AND PSYCHOSOCIAL ISSUES

## Functional Issues

Clients with epilepsy generally have no physical limitations, unless their seizures are due to stroke or cerebral trauma. They are fully independent in eating, dressing, walking, personal hygiene, and communication abilities. While the person usually has unimpaired mechanical driving skills, the laws of each state dictate the seizure free status required for issuance or maintenance of a driver's license. This varies from the physician's discretion to a maximum of 3 years of seizure free status, depending on state law.

At times, excessive blood levels of anticonvulsant medication may impair the individual's physical and intellectual functioning. Even low grade toxicity can produce some awkwardness of gait, coordination problems, and eye-focusing difficulties. Higher levels of toxicity can create problems in physical functioning, memory, and attention span. These usually can be resolved with medical treatment and an alteration in drug regimen, if necessary.

## Emotional and Social Issues

Although epilepsy is a hidden disability, clients with this disorder will have many of the same insecurities and fears that other individuals might have. They may be dealing with one or more of the specific emotional problems that occur from having a seizure disorder.

There are three prominent special adjustment problems persons with epilepsy face:

1. The epileptic seizures are episodic; consequently, a person may be functioning normally one minute and be totally nonfunctional the next. This is not true for persons with orthopedic or audiovisual/speech disabilities. Although these disabilities may be more limiting, individuals with these disabilities have opportunities to develop adaptive reactions to their disorders. For the person with an active seizure condition, there is always the possibility of an occurrence. Because the time, place, and circumstances are often unknown, the individual lives with a great degree of ambiguity and anxiety.

2. The epileptic seizure itself is often an alien, unusual, and frightening spectacle. This is one main reason epilepsy carries the stigma it does. A convulsion is a traumatic and unknown event, which can terrify the observer.

3. The person experiencing the convulsion is not in control. Not only does the individual lose control during the seizure, but there is a lack of control of the actual initiation of the seizure. All societies desire and respect predictability and regularity, particularly in one such as ours which stresses self-control and responsibility.

## Family Response to Epilepsy

Family response to the child or adolescent with epilepsy has great impact on the young person's future. As part of the assessment process, it is helpful to evaluate a client's developmental history. The following illustrates some common family response styles:

1. **Overprotective:** The family is unwilling to risk any physical or emotional damage and is reluctant to set reasonable expectations for the child, expectations that might encourage a youngster to reach the limits of social, educational, and vocational potential.

2. **Reality-Oriented Action:** This group is composed of families and others in the child's world who accurately assess the young person's abilities and potential, while not letting their fears and anxieties hamper growth.

3. **Spartan Orientation:** This type of family believes the child with epilepsy can progress further if strongly pressed to achieve.

4. **Rejecting:** The family believes itself to be defective because it produced a "deviant" child. The depression the family feels can become internalized by the child.

If seizures begin in adulthood, the situation is different. The individual may have developed a solid self-concept and benefitted from a supportive home and work environment. Some individuals may still practice disability denial or experience stages of adjustment.

# VOCATIONAL LIMITATIONS AND REHABILITATION POTENTIAL

## Seizure Status

A careful review of the functional seizure-related considerations is very helpful in establishing a client's employment potential. For those who do not achieve seizure control, it is a combination of seizure type, duration, frequency, pattern of occurrence, and job goal context that most effect employability. For example, an individual can have generalized tonic-clonic seizures weekly, but have them nocturnally (at night) in a fashion that does not affect employment. The treating physician, on a regular interval basis, must evaluate the therapeutic blood levels of the medications and also assess compliance.

## Neuropsychological and Psychosocial Assessment

As discussed earlier in this chapter, seizures are not always the primary issue. Concerns about brain functioning and psychosocial adjustment can be prevalent among those referred to specialized epilepsy medical and vocational rehabilitation programs. Clients with prior head injury should be routinely referred for neuropsychological assessment. Psychosocial adjustment difficulties can be identified through use of the Washington Psychosocial Seizure Inventory (Dodrill et al., 1980) as an initial screening device. This inventory is a Minnesota Multiphasic Personality Inventory-like questionnaire that is used with other tests to assess different areas of psychosocial maladjustment. It was developed specifically on an epilepsy population and has been translated into more than 20 languages.

Many clients will benefit from individual counseling. Group sessions can be beneficial for some people, although cognitive level and emotional integration are factors in considering the appropriateness of group counseling. Sometimes epilepsy is a symptom but not the primary disability. For example, cerebral palsy or mental retardation may be the major disabling condition (Fraser, Clemmons, Trejo, & Temkin, 1983).

## Work History and Prior Training

It is important to carefully review the person's employment history and determine reasons for any job changes or job terminations. Sometimes the individual had adequate abilities, but lost employment due to discrimination because of occasional seizures while at work. Conversely, some clients indicate the seizures were the reason for termination, when difficulties related more to abilities or to interpersonal issues. Information from family members, prior employers, and other third parties can be helpful in clarifying job performance issues. For many clients with epilepsy and associated brain impairment, on-the-job training and supported employment are more effective avenues to placement than formal academic or technical training. Also, the person's education may have ended early due to memory retention or other related problems. On-the-job-training can be effective for people who have had negative experiences in school.

## Environmental Considerations

When beginning vocational rehabilitation services, the counselor carefully evaluates the client's financial needs. Those on a federal subsidy such as Social Security Disability Income (SSDI), if facing significant seizure associated impairments, may want to seek part-time work in order not to jeopardize their funding. Those on Supplemental Security Income (SSI) may need to use the Work Incentives Program in order to establish their capacity for self-support and not jeopardize their living subsidy prematurely. In relation to families, it is helpful to determine how much financial support the family provides. Some of these clients can be financially supported by the family to such an extent it may curtail the incentive for job seeking activity.

For people with epilepsy, the ability to drive is often affected. In some states, this is at the discretion of the physician, based on review of seizure information. In other states, an individual must achieve several years of fully controlled seizures before a driver's license can be secured. If driving is not possible, access to public transportation can be critical. In some instances, employers may be requested to make shift changes as a reasonable accommodation for employees with epilepsy.

## Considerations for the Rehabilitation Counselor

Each client must be evaluated individually with job skills and experience carefully appraised. The assets and liabilities of clients will vary widely. For the individual with epilepsy, it is not so much the type of seizure that influences the person's functioning level as it is the frequency of seizures. Frequently occurring absence or petit mal epilepsy can pose more problems than a well-controlled case of tonic-clonic (grand mal) epilepsy. When working with an individual with epilepsy, the following are critical questions to ask concerning the person's seizure status:

1. What type of seizure(s) does the client have? It is helpful to have a clear description of the seizure activity. If there is a loss of consciousness, how much time is involved?

2. How well controlled are the seizures? If the client does have active seizures, at what time(s) of day do they occur?

3. Does the client have a warning or aura before the seizure? How consistent is the warning and how much time does it provide the client?

4. Are there certain precipitants (e.g., flickering lights, stress, fatigue) to seizure events?

5. What types of medication is the client taking? Is there consistent medication compliance and are there any prominent side-effects? Does the client complain of side effects of medication; if so, what are they? How specialized was the medical evaluation? Did a general practitioner, neurologist, or an epileptologist (a neurologist specializing in epilepsy) perform the evaluation?

6. When was the last evaluation by the client's physician?

7. What is involved in the recovery period? What is a reasonable time in which a client can return to work?

8. Does the client have any other physical or mental disabilities?

Information in the above areas can be very helpful in establishing an individual's daily functional capacities despite the existence of a seizure condition. Motor performance can sometimes be slowed, primarily in cases involving repeated severe seizure activity over time, but also due to side-effects or toxicity of medication.

# JOB DEVELOPMENT AND PLACEMENT

## *Service Methodology*

As discussed earlier, interpretation of data and individual counseling can be very helpful to clients with epilepsy. Sometimes, simply establishing a reasonable job goal is a major step for an individual. The philosophy of the Epilepsy Foundation of America's vocational programs is generally that of shared responsibility between employment services staff and client. There is a philosophical emphasis on personal empowerment.

Most clients with epilepsy benefit from job finding and job seeking skills provided within the job club format. Job clubs are typically modifications of the highly successful program developed by Azrin, Flores, and Kaplan (1977) used nationally with hard-core unemployed and rehabilitation populations. This type of group activity reinforces diverse job seeking activity such as "cold calling" and scheduling of interviews. The job club setting provides emotional support and encouragement in addition to basic skills teaching and ongoing organization of job search activities.

Since a segment of epilepsy clients will have brain impairment affecting memory and other cognitive functions, reinforcing information from individual counseling sessions within the group setting helps to assure information is retained. Handouts and attractive visual aids also can be very helpful, as well as weekly reminders about job club meetings and appointment schedules with vocational staff.

The issue of disclosure of epilepsy to a potential employer is a very important area for discussion within the job club setting. Although an individual may have a seizure condition that does not affect job performance, existing data suggest more than two-thirds of those with epilepsy would prefer to disclose the condition to the perspective employer. Job seekers with seizure conditions have a responsibility to consider various work-related factors. These include the type of seizure they have, the frequency of occurrence, and the risk associated with specific job duties. Also important is whether the person experiences an aura or warning before a seizure occurs. For some individuals with no significant safety issues in the workplace, disclosure may not be an important issue either on the application or in the interview.

Recently, at one epilepsy center, a patient who was a medical assistant was terminated from two different medical clinics because she had not disclosed her epilepsy at the time of hire. Since her job involved frequent taking of blood samples, the disclosure issue was an important one. If she had discussed her epilepsy at the time of hire, reasonable accommodation may have been possible with another staff member taking responsibility for taking the blood samples. Job restructuring or modification may have helped her retain the job.

People with frequent seizures occurring during the work day need to discuss their epilepsy with perspective employers. Some individuals have decided not to disclose their seizure condition on the job application but discuss it and have the information added to their application form during the actual interview process. This enables them to discuss their skills and aptitudes in relation to the job before mentioning their seizure status. Other individuals decide to disclose their epilepsy after they have been hired. There is no one strategy that is appropriate for most people with epilepsy. The Americans with Disabilities Act of 1990 states that employers cannot discriminate because of a person's disability. If the seizure disorder does not affect performance of the job, the job seeker may chose to reveal the disability immediately after the employer has made a decision to hire the person.

Applicants should be able to discuss their seizure condition clearly, positively, and succinctly, in terms that can be understood by the lay person, keeping the information job-related. For example, people who have absence or petit mal seizures may describe periods lasting a few seconds in which they may look distracted. Following the seizure, they are able to resume work quickly. A job seeker with a seizure condition needs to practice disclosure to present the information comfortably and clearly to a perspective employer.

A successful placement program will include active job development and a job bank with integration of employers on an advisory board. Private sector firms and public agencies have become accustomed to hiring from specialized vocational rehabilitation programs.

## Interacting with Employers

Although employer attitudes are improving in certain areas of the United States (Hicks & Hicks, 1991), a study by John and McLellan (1988) in England indicated only 58% of employers surveyed felt they had jobs that could be handled by a person with a seizure condition. In approaching the employment market, it is important to stress the individual nature of a client's seizure condition and emphasize pre-screening the counselor has done to present a qualified applicant. Information that can be presented to the employer to affect positive hiring behaviors includes the following:

1. **Working around machinery** - In consideration of today's safety standards, it is rare that machinery will require special modifications. Plastic guards on hazardous machinery or rubber matting on a concrete floor area are examples of inexpensive job-site modifications. In other cases, assigning driving tasks to a different worker produces a simple job restructuring. Both job-site modifications and job restructuring are examples of reasonable accommodation.

2. **Attendance and job performance** - Most studies suggest attendance and performance records for those with epilepsy are equal to or better than the general working population (McLellan, 1987).

3. **Accident rates** - Risch (1968) demonstrated the actual time lost due to seizures was approximately 1 hour for every 1,000 hours worked for individuals with active seizure conditions. Sands (1961), in comparing

workers' compensation cases over a 13-year period in New York, indicated accidents caused by sneezing or coughing on the job were twice as frequent as those related to seizure occurrences.

4. **Insurance rates** - Hiring a person with epilepsy within the United States does not increase industrial insurance rates. These rates are linked to hazards of specific occupational classes. Health insurance providers generally link rates to age and sex in larger companies, while among smaller companies, the providers usually pool claim experiences and no one employer is penalized. Epi-Hab, a United States sheltered work system for those with seizure disorders, reports receiving significant insurance premium reductions due to outstanding safety records. It is important to note that people with epilepsy generally refrain from drinking alcohol or using illegal drugs since these aggravate their condition. Thus, they are often safer on the job than the average employee.

## *Predictors of Successful Placement*

Factors that influence successful vocational rehabilitation can be considered across different categories: demographic, neuropsychological, and psychosocial. The Epilepsy Foundation of America has found that individuals with less than one seizure per month, 12 years of education, no additional disability, and the ability to drive are more successful. Other factors associated with employment outcome include the recency of employment before program entry, previous salary earned, and compliance with an anticonvulsant medicine regimen. The Training and Placement Services (TAPS) program of the Epilepsy Foundation of America provides placement services for persons with epilepsy.

A University of Washington program compared early program dropouts to those people successfully securing jobs. This program found that psychosocial variables were the best discriminators of successful outcome. The Washington Psychosocial Seizure Inventory identified these psychosocial variables, which included increased depression, anxiety, financial distress, and lack of adjustment to a seizure condition (Fraser, Clemmons, Dodrill, Trejo, & Freelove, 1986). Although seizure variables have not consistently shown discriminatory capability between successful and unsuccessful program participants, they deserve more attention.

## *Existing Programs*

In 1976, the Epilepsy Foundation of America (EFA) established a national network of employment programs for individuals with epilepsy. This Department of Labor funded program has grown from five original sites to a network of 14 EFA-administered programs in local EFA affiliates. There are also 25 locally funded programs based on the same employment preparation model. The Training and Placement Services (TAPS) program funded by the grant is highly successful. The program has an overall successful placement rate of 65-75%, including those enrolled either securing employment or entering a training program.

Other program model types include a job center, offering clients information on local service and training programs or job leads; teen centers focusing on the needs of young job seekers transitioning from school to work; and a STEPS (Skills Training and Employment Preparation Service) program, designed to meet the needs of clients with brain impairment or associated retardation who cannot work effectively under the other models. (This STEPS program has a supported employment emphasis).

The Rehabilitation Services Administration (RSA) has always advocated for and supported vocational rehabilitation on a national level for clients with epilepsy. Many state-funded vocational rehabilitation programs assign specialized counselors with particular expertise to clients with epilepsy. New directions include the development of a national employer advisory board and refinement of a cooperative agreement between the Epilepsy Foundation of America and the Council of State Administrators of Vocational Rehabilitation Services (CSAVR). Rehabilitation counselors seeking additional information can contact the Epilepsy Foundation of America to identify the nearest specialized epilepsy vocational rehabilitation program and for information on new models or services offered.

# CASE STUDY

Ronnie is a 35 year-old single male, who lived with his parents until they recently passed away. After their deaths, he inherited their home and now lives there by himself. Because of epilepsy and current seizures, Ronnie does not drive. Ronnie's social skills are under-developed as a result of living in such a protected environment for so many years and his reaction to the death of his parents was aggravated by the fact that he had developed no independent living skills.

Despite adherence to a medical regimen, Ronnie has complex partial seizures several times a month. He takes several doses of his tegretol anticonvulsant medication daily. Occasionally, he requires hospital visits in order for his physician to monitor medication level and make adjustments. Seizures consist of his wandering around, looking dazed and confused. During a seizure, he does respond to gentle coaxing without exhibiting any anger or aggression. The recovery after each seizure is rapid and he is able to return to his activities quickly.

Ronnie is somewhat paranoid, expecting problems before they occur, taking offense easily, and tending to blow negative interpersonal encounters out of proportion. These characteristics and his lack of response to social cues, make him somewhat difficult to deal with on a personal level.

Ronnie recently began work in the nursery of a large retail home and garden store (this store has five other locations throughout the city) as a Horticultural Worker II (D.O.T. # 405.687-014), where he is responsible for planting, spraying, weeding, and watering plants, shrubs, and trees; planting shrubs and plants in containers; tieing, bunching, wrapping, and packing flowers, plants, shrubs, and trees to fill orders; assisting customers in choosing purchases and transporting the purchases to vehicles; arranging and positioning plants and plant care products in order to artistically display them; and occasionally, acting as a runner, going for change from the front cash registers to fill the plant department registers. He has no problem with the physical aspects of the job which involves hauling large bags of soil and plants (weighing up to 60 pounds). Working in the nursery requires little customer contact; there is no driving on the job.

Certain simple accommodations are required. You are a rehabilitation counselor working at a Department of Rehabilitation office. The employer has contacted you requesting information on epilepsy and advice about how to proceed with Ronnie if problems occur.

## Questions

1. Give a vocational profile for this rehabilitation client, including age category, educational level, work history (exertion and skill levels), occupationally siginificant characteristics, and transferable skills, if any.

2. Describe Ronnie's functional limitations as they relate to the job.

3. What advice would you give to Ronnie's employer regarding reasonable accommodations as they relate to:
   a. medication schedule on a daily basis and occasional need for physician visits.
   b. social skill level and interaction with customers.

4. Describe the type of follow-up services, if any, you would suggest.

5.  After responding to the above questions, answer the following. Because of financial problems, the facility will permanently close in the near future. Discuss possible vocational rehabilitation services you will now provide this client.

# REFERENCES

Anderson, V.E. (1988). Genetics of the epilepsies. In W.A. Hauser (Ed.), **Current trends in epilepsy: A self-study course for physicians, unit III** (pp. 1-12). Landover, MD: Epilepsy Foundation of America.

Annegers, J.F. (1988). The natural history and prognosis of patients with seizures and epilepsy. In W.A. Hauser (Ed.), **Current trends in epilepsy: A self-study course for physicians, unit I** (pp. 16-28). Landover, MD: Epilepsy Foundation of America.

Azrin, N.H., Flores, T., & Kaplan, S.J. (1977). Job finding club: A group-assisted program for obtaining employment. **Rehabilitation Counseling Bulletin, 21**, 130-140.

Dodrill, C.B., Batzel, L.W., Queisser, H.R., & Temkin, N.R. (1980). An objective method for the assessment of psychological and social problems among epileptics. **Epilepsia, 21**, 123-135.

Fraser, R.T., Clemmons, D.C., Dodrill, C.B., Trejo, W., & Freelove, C. (1986). The difficult to employ in epilepsy rehabilitation: Predictors of response to an intensive intervention. **Epilepsia, 27**, 220-224.

Fraser, R.T., Clemmons, D.C., Trejo, W., & Temkin, N.R. (1983). Program evaluation in epilepsy rehabilitation. **Epilepsia, 24**, 734-736.

Hauser, W.A., & Hesdorffer, D.C. (1990). **Epilepsy: Frequency, causes, and consequences.** New York: Demos.

Hicks, R.A., & Hicks, M.J. (1991). Attitudes of major employers toward the employment of people with epilepsy: A 30-year study. **Epilepsia, 32**, 86-88.

John, C., & McLellan, D.L. (1988). Employers' attitudes to people with epilepsy in the Southampton district. **British Journal of Industrial Medicine, 45**, 713-715.

Leppik, I.E. (1988). Drug treatment of epilepsy. In W.A. Hauser (Ed.), **Current trends in epilepsy: A self-study course for physicians, unit II** (pp. 12-22). Landover, MD: Epilepsy Foundation of America.

McLellan, D.L. (1987). Epilepsy and employment. **Journal of Social and Occupational Medicine, 3**, 94-99.

National Association of Epilepsy Centers (1990). Recommended guidelines for diagnosis and treatment in specialized epilepsy centers. **Epilepsia, 31**(suppl. 1), S1-S12.

Pedley, T.A., & Hauser, W.A. (1988). Classification and differential diagnosis of seizures and of epilepsy. In W.A. Hauser (Ed.), **Current trends in epilepsy: A self-study course for physicians, unit I** (pp. 1-15). Landover, MD: Epilepsy Foundation of America.

Penry, J.K. (Ed.). (1986). **Epilepsy: Diagnosis, management, and quality of life.** New York: Raven.

Risch, F. (1968). We lost every game . . .but. **Rehabilitation Record, 9**, 16-18.

Sands, H. (1961). Report of a study undertaken for the committee on neurological disorders in industry. **Epilepsy News, 7**(abstr.), 1.

Schaul, N. (1987). Epilepsy surgery. **The New York Journal of Epilepsy**, 5, 14-15.

Wannamaker, B.B., Booker, H.E., Dreifuss, F.E., & Willmore, L.J. (1984). **The comprehensive clinical management of the epilepsies**. Landover, MD: Epilepsy Foundation of America.

## *About the Authors*

Robert T. Fraser, Ph.D., C.R.C., is an Associate Professor within the University of Washington Department of Neurological Surgery and Rehabilitation Medicine in Seattle, Washington. Dr. Fraser began the Vocational Services Unit of the University of Washington Regional Epilepsy Center in 1976, which has expanded to provide vocational services for the Department of Neurological Surgery.

Elaine Glazer, M.S.W., L.C.S.W., is the Director of Social Services at The Epilepsy Society serving Los Angeles and Orange counties in southern California. Her principle areas of activity within the society include counseling individuals, facilitating support groups, and conducting educational seminars.

Barbara J. Simcoe, B.S., is the Employment and Training Coordinator for the Training and Placement Services (TAPS) Program of the Epilepsy Foundation of America, located at the Los Angeles affiliate, The Epilepsy Society serving Los Angeles and Orange counties in southern California.

# Chapter 29

# MULTIPLE SCLEROSIS

by
*Harry L. Hall,*
*Shirley M. Rohaly, M.S.W.*
*and*
*Myra A. Shneider, M.S.W., L.S.W.*

## INTRODUCTION

Multiple sclerosis (MS) is a variable and unpredictable disease, often with both visible and invisible symptoms. Onset usually occurs in early adulthood; exacerbations and remissions are the usual pattern and generally symptoms increase over time. Most persons with MS have lost jobs due to the direct and indirect affects of multiple sclerosis, and many others are having difficulty retaining employment.

While traditional vocational rehabilitation approaches have experienced some success in helping people with MS obtain employment, the authors belive that most persons with MS will benefit from an approach concentrating on enhancing self-assessment, self-management, and self-advocacy. This chapter discusses this and other issues pertinent to MS.

## HISTORY AND EPIDEMIOLOGY

### Description and Overview

The French neurologist Charcot first identified multiple sclerosis in 1868. It is an adult-onset, chronic, sometimes progressive disease of the central nervous system (brain and spinal cord) that interferes with nerve function, distorting or blocking nerve signals to and from the brain. Symptoms can come and go unpredictably and may vary widely both in intensity and location in the body. They may include: fatigue, weakness, numbness, impaired vision, difficulty with coordination, loss of balance, gait problems, bladder and bowel dysfunction, impaired sexual function, and cognitive dysfunction. Combinations and intensity of symptoms vary from imperceptible to catastrophic.

The cause of multiple sclerosis remains unknown. Yet, there have been recent developments in the understanding of multiple sclerosis as a result of advances in fundamental science, particularly in the fields of immunology, virology, and genetics. MS may involve a combination of a slow-acting virus (or similar environmental factor) encountered before or during adolescence, abnormal immune response, and genetic predisposition. There is no known treatment that will prevent or reverse the course of the disease. However, over the last 10-15 years, there has a been dramatic expansion in knowledge and skill in treating and managing symptoms and their complications. People with multiple sclerosis can now anticipate a near normal life span.

## Who Gets Multiple Sclerosis?

This disease affects an estimated 250,000 to 350,000 persons in the United States today. Symptoms generally appear between the ages of 15-55. The average age of onset in women is just before 30 years of age; in men, age of onset is slightly later. The average age at diagnosis is 33. More women than men have MS (1.8:1) (Rosner & Ross, 1987).

Multiple sclerosis becomes more prevalent (the proportion of a total population who have MS at a given time) the further one lives from the equator. Therefore, it is more prevalent in the northern United States, Canada, northern Europe, southern New Zealand, and Australia (colder climates) than in southern regions (warmer climates). Within the United States, the likelihood of having MS is four times greater in Minnesota than in Louisiana (National Institute of Health, 1984).

Whites have a much higher prevalence rate than Blacks in the United States. MS is minimal among Asian groups (Japanese and Chinese) and unmixed Indians of North and South America. It is unheard of in Eskimos and Yakuts of Siberia, Bantus in Africa, and Gypsies (Rosner & Ross, 1987).

Since multiple sclerosis is usually diagnosed in the late 20s and early 30s, many individuals have completed their education or vocational training and begun their careers. Thus, persons with MS tend to have higher educational levels and more work experience than most persons with disabilities, and the majority have not experienced difficulties before adulthood.

Because life expectancy is nearly at the national average, persons with MS experience impact of the disease for many years. This produces a comparatively high socio-economic impact. A national survey (National Institute of Health, 1984) undertaken in 1976, found 93% of persons with multiple sclerosis have work experience and approximately 60% are working at the time of diagnosis. Yet, at any time, only 25% of these people are working and, of those, at least 2 in 5 report being in trouble on the job because of MS symptoms (Rosner & Ross, 1987).

No one knows what causes MS, but we do know that it is an acquired disease. A person is not born with it; one contracts MS from the outside. However, this disease is not contagious.

## Physiology Altered by Disease: How Does Multiple Sclerosis Affect The Body?

Multiple sclerosis is a disease of the central nervous system (brain, brain stem, and spinal cord), which controls the movements and functions of the entire body. As the brain sends and receives signals, the spinal cord transmits them in and out, to and from different parts of the body through a network of nerves. The peripheral nervous system is not directly affected by multiple sclerosis.

Myelin is a soft, white, fatty substance that surrounds the nerves. The myelin sheath, which develops in the first 10 years of life, insulates the nerve fibers and helps conduct signals through the body. In multiple sclerosis, the myelin breaks down and is replaced by scar tissue (often called a lesion or plaque). How this happens is still imperfectly understood. This demyelination can slow down or even block the flow of signals to and from the central nervous system to the rest of the body, impairing such functions as vision, strength, and coordination (Scheinberg & Holland, 1987).

One important characteristic of myelin is that it can partially repair itself. Remyelination is one reason MS is usually characterized by many attacks or exacerbations and remissions.

# DIAGNOSIS

A neurologist usually diagnoses multiple sclerosis, although other medical practitioners are often involved in the process. The person with multiple sclerosis may have seemingly unrelated symptoms, and may see various specialists in the effort to find out the cause of the symptoms.

To diagnose multiple sclerosis, the physician must establish: (1) a history of attacks and remissions (at least two events, separate in time); and (2) symptoms that suggest the existence of lesions in two different sites of the central nervous system. To document these clinical criteria, the neurologist examines the medical history in detail and conducts a neurological examination. The physician also may administer a variety of tests to further document the presence of multiple sclerosis (Calvano & Gresser, 1991).

Before the early 1980s, MS was diagnosed by "exclusion". Besides the history and neurological examination, the physician administered a variety of tests to "exclude" other possible diagnoses. There was no single test that could confirm a diagnosis of multiple sclerosis. With the use of magnetic resonance imaging (MRI) in the late 1980s, the process of diagnosis has become more exact. This procedure can detect lesions in the brain and spinal cord. MRI scans are confirmatory in 70-95% of persons with suspected MS. Due to the expense of administering an MRI scan, some physicians defer the use of it and conduct less expensive procedures (e.g., spinal tap, myelogram, and evoked response tests) to collaborate clinical findings (Waksman, Reingold, & Reynolds, 1987).

Practitioners classify multiple sclerosis in one of three categories: definite, probable, or possible. This has been a cause of confusion for the person with MS. In receiving a diagnosis of **possible** MS, it is commonly perceived as, "the doctor said I **possibly** have MS." This change in emphasis inaccurately represents the diagnosis.

MRI testing has shortened the length of time needed to make a definitive diagnosis. A process that in the past took years may now take only months. This has major implications for the rehabilitation counselor in that people with multiple sclerosis are now being diagnosed at a younger age and at an earlier stage in the disease process. This often occurs before the individual has many functional limitations.

## *Patterns*

After a period of time (5-10 years in most persons), one can identify an individual pattern; continuation of that pattern is only a probability, not a certainty. It is medically impossible to project a specific prognosis for any individual.

Statistically, researchers have found patterns commonly listed as follows (Scheinberg, & Holland, 1987; Schapiro, 1987, 1991):

1. **Benign:** sudden onset, 1-2 mild attacks, near complete remission, no long-term disability. Approximately 20% of people with MS have this pattern.

2. **Exacerbating-Remitting:** most common, sudden onset, relapses and remissions, usually no permanent damage, no restrictions in daily activities, remissions are often over long periods. Affects 20-30% of people with MS.

3. **Remitting-Progressive:** begins as exacerbating-remitting, after 5 or more years, turns chronic (with some permanent damage) or slowly progressive. Affects 40% of people with MS.

4. **Chronic Progressive:** slow worsening without remission, onset slower. Affects 10-20% of people with MS.

*Symptoms*

Symptoms of MS correspond with four specific areas of the central nervous system. Fatigue, a fifth symptom, is generalized and not attributable to a specific area of the CNS. The symptoms associated with each are as follows:

I. **Spinal Cord Involvement.** This produces sensory and motor symptoms, bowel and bladder difficulties, and sexual dysfunction.

    A. **Sensory symptoms** are disturbances in feeling (sensation) in the limbs or trunk. They include numbness or loss of feeling, unpleasant sensations, and Lhermitte's sign. **Numbness** may include the inability to feel a light touch, sensations of hot and cold temperatures, or movement of a toe or finger up or down (position sense). **Paresthesias** (or unpleasant feelings) include "pins and needles" or tingling sensations, hot and burning feelings, feelings of wetness, girdle sensations, or feelings of swelling. **Lhermitte's sign** feels like a brief electric current or buzzing that travels down the spinal cord when a person bends the head forward.

    B. **Motor symptoms** are disturbances in moving one or more limbs. These may include weakness or spasticity. **Weakness** may vary from the limb feeling tired or heavy to it being very difficult to lift. Weakness can affect legs or the upper extremities. Spasticity is rigidity or stiffness, most commonly found in the legs.

    C. **Bowel and bladder** symptoms may occur. **Bladder** problems include hesitancy (slowness in starting urination), increased frequency of urination, urgency, retention, or episodic incontinence. **Bowel** symptoms involve constipation, urgency, and incontinence. **Sexual** dysfunction may be a lack of feeling in the genitals, difficulty getting or maintaining an erection, or difficulty achieving orgasm.

II. **Brain Stem and Cerebellar Involvement.** The cerebellum is the center of muscle coordination. Demyelination in this area produces defects in the range, rate, and force of movement of certain body parts.

    A. **Eye movement abnormalities** include **double vision** (diplopia) or **nystagmus** (jerking of the eye muscle).

    B. **Imbalance and incoordination** symptoms are called **ataxia.** Balance problems occur both with and without **vertigo.** Incoordination may be reported as clumsiness, shakiness, or slowness in movement. **Intention tremor** is a tremor reported when attempting to touch a target.

    C. **Speech disorders** consist of a disturbance of pronunciation (slurring) or speech rhythm (scanning) called **dysarthria.**

    D. **Facial nerve abnormalities** include facial weakness, numbness, spasms, or pain. **Trigeminal neuralgia** is characterized by sharp jabs of pain that follow a nerve root down the side of the face.

    E. **Emotional disturbances** may include depression, emotional lability, (including inappropriate or excessive laughing or crying) and infrequently, euphoria. These symptoms represent organic changes caused by the disease process. Emotional responses to MS that include similar symptoms will be discussed later.

    F. **Other brain stem cerebellar symptoms** include **tinnitus** (loss of hearing and ringing in the ears) and **dysphagia** (difficulty swallowing).

III. **Optic Nerve Involvement.** Typical symptoms in this area include vision described as blurry, foggy, cloudy, fuzzy, or distorted. Clinicians report the presence of visual loss in one central spot, loss of peripheral vision, and impairment in depth perception for some individuals. Symptoms can occur in one or both eyes, simultaneously or successively. Some persons with MS meet the legal definition of blindness.

IV. **Cerebral Involvement.** Cerebral symptoms, which are less frequent in MS, include mental disturbance, seizures, loss of speech expression or comprehension (aphasia), one-sided visual field loss, and sensory loss or weakness in the face, arm, and leg on one side. These symptoms tend to occur like those of a stroke (Rosner & Ross, 1987).

A. **Cognitive difficulties** may involve short-term memory loss, disruption in verbal fluency, and difficulty in abstract reasoning and problem-solving. For many years, the dissemination of information on MS downplayed the existence of **cognitive symptoms**. One reason for this was that we knew very little about how MS affected intellectual functioning. The only cognitive problem identified was short-term memory loss; we now know this is only one symptom. Today, there is much research that clearly shows that MS lesions in the brain and fluctuating inflammations affect certain intellectual functions.

Estimates of the frequency of intellectual dysfunction in MS have ranged from 0-100%. Most recently, Dr. Stephen Rao of the Medical College of Wisconsin, concluded that about 45% of people with MS show no evidence of intellectual dysfunction. Of those with detectable evidence, most have only mild dysfunction, some of which may vary with the location and amount of inflammation corresponding to a lesion. Less than 10% have moderate to severe dysfunction (LaRocca, 1990). Further discussion follows later in this chapter.

V. **Fatigue.** The most prevalent symptom in MS is **fatigue**. It is untraceable to any one location in the nervous system. Because it is invisible to others, it is particularly troublesome for the person with MS. The person with MS and those people close to the individual frequently misunderstand and discount this problem.

Besides the fatigue of normal, everyday activity and the fatigue which is symptomatic of depression, two other types of fatigue may affect persons with multiple sclerosis.

A. **Fatigue of handicap.** To overcome weakened muscles or muscles that no longer work, the person with MS uses more energy to perform everyday activities. To walk across a room using a cane or crutches takes a great deal more energy than typical ambulation.
B. **Nerve fiber fatigue.** This type of fatigue is almost exclusive to MS. Nerve fibers damaged by multiple sclerosis tend to conduct nerve impulses poorly or not at all. When they do conduct, they tend to fatigue rapidly; this results in weakness. Nerve fibers are also very temperature sensitive. Any increase in body temperature (including a fever, sitting in the sun, a hot shower or bath, or the normal fluctuation in body temperature) will reduce the conductivity of nerve impulses. It is common for people with MS to "run out of gas" late in the afternoon and get a "second wind" in the evening. This parallels the typical increase and decrease in body temperature throughout the day.

Unless fatigue is severe, it usually can be relieved by cooling the body and resting. In the late 1980s, practitioners found that two medications were useful in alleviating fatigue in some persons with MS. When fatigue occurs throughout the day, is unrelenting or completely debilitating, it can be the primary factor that keeps an individual from working (Herndon, 1991).

## External Factors Impact Symptoms

It is important to note that there are some environmental conditions that tend to intensify the symptoms of multiple sclerosis. Extreme heat and extreme cold, an infection in the body, and intense and prolonged exercise may cause body temperature to rise. When this occurs, symptoms may worsen. This is usually transient.

Many people with multiple sclerosis report that symptoms also may worsen if they are experiencing unusual stress. Yet, there is no scientific information proving a direct link between stress and the symptoms of multiple sclerosis.

# TREATMENTS

In any discussion of treatments for multiple sclerosis, it must be noted that there is no known cure. While a person with MS is in exacerbation (having a flare-up of symptoms), corticosteroids (ACTH, prednisone) are often routinely administered and may shorten the duration and lessen the intensity of symptoms. There is no evidence that corticosteroids alter the long-term course of the disease. Although research is ongoing, no medication is now known that will stop the onset or the progression of the disease.

## Knowledge Base

During the past 10 years, there has been an explosion in knowledge about MS and in the development of medications to treat symptoms. This new information has vastly increased the individual's ability to manage symptoms more effectively, to forestall complications of the disease, and ultimately, to minimize the affects caused by the advancement of functional disabilities. Drug therapy has been effective in treating bladder problems, spasticity, tremors, fatigue, and some emotional symptoms. Medications affect individuals differently; what is effective for one person may not be for another. Medications also will generally have some side effects, which may prove to be problematic. For these reasons, drug therapy must be administered and carefully monitored by a physician (Rosner & Ross, 1987; Shapiro, 1987).

## Physical Therapy

Physical therapy that has as a goal to increase strength and endurance can be useful both during acute exacerbations and during periods of remission. It is also valuable in treating weakness, spasticity, balance problems, and other walking difficulties. Physical therapists employ a variety of techniques including range of motion exercises, stretching, hydrotherapy, gait training, and recommendation of and training in the use of mobility aids (canes and walkers). In working with an individual with MS, the physical therapist helps the person achieve the objectives, while avoiding fatigue.

## Occupational Therapy

The occupational therapist focuses on helping the individual continue to do as many activities of daily living as possible. Occupational therapy is helpful in managing hand tremors, incoordination, sensory symptoms in the upper extremities, fatigue, and some cognitive problems. The techniques include strengthening exercises and assisting the individual in reorganizing living and work areas to maximize function. Occupational therapists also recommend assistive devices to aid in ambulation.

If complicating cognitive problems are suspected, persons with MS with employment goals should be advised to obtain professional neuropsychological testing and evaluation, preferably by someone with specific knowledge of MS cognitive difficulties (LaRocca, 1990; Shapiro, 1987). There is no broadly based knowledge of effective therapeutic remediation, but current research holds promise both for strategies of intervention and specific drug therapy (Waksman, Reingold, & Reynolds, 1987). There are techniques to compensate for the limitation if the individual is aware of the specific nature of the problem.

## Self-management

Self-management strategies are equally important as the interventions just described to manage MS symptoms effectively. These can include getting adequate rest, controlling one's environment, using stress and time management techniques, exercising appropriately, and maintaining a healthy diet. Learning what works and what is ineffective is a continual process. Community resources such as the local multiple sclerosis society can give help. Programs providing interaction with others with MS in self-help groups are beneficial. To help in the management of the emotional problems, many persons have also found benefit in psychological counseling (Scheinberg & Holland, 1987).

Most symptoms of multiple sclerosis can be less problematic using combinations of these self-management techniques. Persons with MS find that working as a team with medical professionals is the most effective way to manage their condition.

# THE SPECIAL IMPACT ON EMPLOYMENT OF MS SYMPTOMS

The functional limitations of fatigue and cognitive dysfunction have the most complicating impact on employment because of the direct effects and because they make dealing with all the other symptoms more difficult. In the workplace, problems faced by an individual with fatigue symptoms may include (but are not limited to): decrease in ability to perform tasks (including fine and gross motor skills and cognitive tasks), miscommunication with supervisors and co-workers, resentment of co-workers, inability to sustain work effort for an entire work period without rest breaks, and an inability to maintain a regular work schedule. Fatigue is not typically visible. Supervisors and co-workers may not realize there is anything wrong and expect the individual to perform on the normal schedule. Communicating to co-workers and supervisors one's ability to maintain general productivity despite variations from the normal schedule is often difficult (Herndon, 1991).

For many people with multiple sclerosis, managing fatigue becomes the single most important adaptation they must make to remain employed. The individual needs to become aware of the affects of fatigue and what actions can be taken to accommodate it. Often the accommodations needed can be made in private (e.g., relaxation exercises); sometimes, they are more apparent (e.g., lying down to rest). Individuals who can manage fatigue on the job remain productive employees.

People also misunderstand and misinterpret cognitive dysfunctioning. What may appear to be a personality problem (stubbornness, hostility, inability to follow through, or indifference) may be indications that there are problems in memory or reasoning. These symptoms can be incorrectly labeled as "personality" problems and may cause the most difficulty while returning to or retaining employment (LaRocca, 1990).

The intellectual dysfunctions that are most problematic for people with multiple sclerosis include the following:

1. **Memory problems.** This symptom is the most frequently reported. The problem is not in the storage of the information but in the ability to retrieve it from the brain. It is more often a problem related to information that an individual has learned in the recent past. Retrieving information stored in the distant past is not usually affected.

2. **Abstract reasoning and problem-solving abilities.** Some people with multiple sclerosis report that they have begun to exercise poor judgment; others report confusion when given complex tasks. Difficulties can occur in the ability to analyze situations, identify important points, or plan and carry out a course of action.

3. **Verbal fluency.** Persons with MS report knowing the word is "on the tip of my tongue" but not being able to retrieve it.

4. **Speed of information processing.** The recall of information and word finding require rapid processing of verbal information. People with MS report that they are unable to think through and respond to events as quickly as they once did.

# WHY MULTIPLE SCLEROSIS IS SO PROBLEMATIC

An appreciation of psycho-emotional reactions to receiving a diagnosis of multiple sclerosis is vital to understanding the person with MS. The unpredictable nature and course of MS coupled with the fact that no cure currently exists makes the diagnosis a particularly devastating one. Additionally, two non-physical characteristics of the disease pose a unique challenge. These two characteristics are variability and uncertainty (unpredictability) (Shuman & Schwartz, 1988).

## *Variability*

On a daily basis, the newly diagnosed person with MS does not know what to expect. While some experience the same symptoms as others, there is always variation that makes each person different. Besides, the individual symptoms may fluctuate, sometimes as frequently as daily. People with MS generally do not get sick and then get well and stay that way. To live with MS requires continual adaptation. If the adaptation is effective, MS becomes a chronic condition; if the adaptation is ineffective, MS becomes a long-term crisis.

## *Uncertainty*

No one ever knows what life will bring. This engenders some discomfort. Yet, we usually adapt by learning to live with that "edge" in our lives. We adapt so well that we are no longer aware that this is even a problem. With the diagnosis of MS, fears and insecurities that we once dealt with come flooding back, and now have new components. Some persons adapt to this new situation by choosing to incorporate the uncertainty factor in their redeveloping psyche; others choose to deny the disability and refuse to incorporate it in any reevaluation of self.

These two characteristics, variability and uncertainty, force the person with multiple sclerosis to attempt to make new sense out of life and struggle to find new meaning. The diagnosis of MS usually occurs between the ages of 15-55, a range of years during which most adults are accomplishing significant life tasks. Sometimes the MS diagnosis interrupts the completing of education, getting married, creating a family, and starting a career. More often, it begins after an individual has recently accomplished these tasks.

## *The Reasons Why MS is Problematic for Rehabilitation Professionals*

The historic record documents that MS has been problematic for rehabilitation professionals and provides some clues about why. Recent experience in developing successful programs provides additional answers.

The delay in diagnosis, which had been characteristic of multiple sclerosis, made vocational rehabilitation intervention unlikely before diagnosis and more complicated after diagnosis (Calvano & Gresser, 1991). The multifaceted impact of MS on individuals created many difficulties for the general rehabilitation services approach. Many people with MS do not seek rehabilitation services until late in the course of the disease. By this time, disability is more severe, and the person may have lost employment, have diminished self-esteem, and have a significantly decreased potential for successful reemployment.

Multiple sclerosis is different from most other disabling conditions for the following reasons:

* Multiple sclerosis is a permanent disability, but not a static condition.

* There are some long-term needs, many that change over time.

* Changing cognitive and fatigue problems complicate physical symptoms and functional limitations.

* Good medical care is important, but medical interventions are often disconnected with vocational potentials.

* People who have multiple sclerosis are, on the average, better educated and have good vocational histories; many have useable transferable skills.

* Neither entry-level employment nor traditional placement approaches fit the skills and needs of most persons with MS.

There are many persons with multiple sclerosis who have unmet employment needs. These are people who have stopped working or are in serious danger of losing their current jobs and want to work. Yet, they need to develop personal skills, self-management skills, job readiness skills, and often, job seeking skills. There are other persons with MS who have the same levels of motivation, but need additional and more extensive support. Finally, there are others, who do not want to work, do not need to work, or have no interest in any type of employment.

# EMPOWERMENT: A KEY FOCUS

## An Empowerment Model

Earlier in this chapter, we examined factors that affect employment for people with multiple sclerosis. The variation of those factors strongly suggest maximum investment in the capacity of individuals to self-assess, self-manage, and self-advocate (i.e., an "empowerment model").

The core of an employment-related "empowerment model" is developing and strengthening the array of skills and capabilities that enable individuals to compete effectively for jobs they want to do and can perform. It also helps individuals deal with disability-related aspects so that disability is minimized. Self-assessment, self-management, and self-advocacy are essential to the model and group process is the primary means to achieve success. Also, an empowerment model permits a full range of disclosure options.

* **Self-assessment.** There is no one who can better assess how all the factors affecting employment interrelate than the person with MS. Issues in self-assessment include: interest in working, financial considerations, physical ability, job qualifications, realistic employment goals, readiness to work, job seeking skills, willingness to use job search contacts, and commitment to participate in an empowerment program.

* **Self-management.** This includes management of schedule, time, fluctuations of the impact of the disease, fatigue, stress, symptomatic treatments, and independent living support systems. Self-management can be developed to a more competent level in nearly all individuals. Self-management includes full participation in rehabilitation planning through and including job search activities. Decisions about whether, when, and to whom to disclose information about MS are important reasons to develop self-management skills.

* **Self-advocacy.** It is important the job seeker and the job retainer develop the capacity to intervene with employers and discuss reasonable accommodation in a practical way.

* **Group process as a "means" to achieving self-empowerment.** A most significant value of group process for persons with multiple sclerosis is that the group process facilitates self-empowerment. The interrelationships involved in participating in a group enhance motivation, discipline, and follow through. The group process helps promote the acceptance of responsibility and provides for reality testing by one's peers. It requires and generates a commitment to each others' success. Developing a belief that one can successfully acquire job seeking skills and secure employment enables individuals to feel confident when initially seeking new employment. The need to reconsider and seek employment may recur related to changes in MS symptoms.

Besides the above empowerment model, there are other aspects for a rehabilitation counselor to consider that deal with special employment-related impacts of MS. These are described below.

1. **Outreach to persons with MS should include staged levels of response.** A formal outreach effort for persons with MS is necessary; the process for initial expressions of interest should be very simple. Such persons may be inhibited from seeking help or pursuing eligibility because of uncertainty and ambivalence. They may have problems with assertiveness, self-image, communication ability, and awareness of social stigma toward people with MS. Explaining a special MS program in written form and requiring a very simple expression of interest (checking a box on a self-addressed postcard) has been an effective broad outreach technique in the programs managed by the authors. The screening process follow-up should be a personal contact (telephone call). A telephone interview gives the individual a one-to-one opportunity to explore the issues and determine whether to undertake a more extensive in-person screening session. The process should include increasing levels of commitment and avoid long intervals between stages. As MS fluctuates, so do times of readiness. When readiness is evident, long delays before action begins often leads to failure. The outreach and screening process should culminate in a formal contract.

2. **Group process - neither totally didactic nor therapeutic.** Group process is a key technique of the empowerment model, but it also responds to the substantial need for both detailed knowledge and genuine understanding. The best approach is midway between didactic and therapeutic with strong group session objectives providing for both improvements in knowledge and in personal skills leading to employment goals.

3. **Thoroughly prepared group session materials.** Projects with Industry (PWI) is a national program managed by The Development Team of Baltimore, Maryland. The program produced a JOB RAISING Participant Manual, covering 10-12 sessions of approximately 3 hours each - spaced weekly. In the manual are session outlines, reading materials, exercises, and various programmatic and background materials. These resources provide a long-term support where participants can come back periodically to review information.

   Although very different subjects are the primary focus of each session, there is an ongoing need for participants to see where each session fits into the whole and identify when other issues about which they have concerns will be covered. The materials are extensively, but not entirely, focused on multiple sclerosis. Many materials have been adapted from non-MS sources.

4. **Reality testing.** The spaced repetition of self-management techniques within the group setting and the constant attention to reconsideration of decisions provide a setting in which group members, more than facilitators, can help each other approach reality more effectively.

5. **Gradual and recurrent self-evaluation.** A one-time vocational evaluation process is often unreliable due to the rapid variability in the effects of the disease in the brain. Also because of the complexity of the interrelationships among the factors and use of the empowerment model, the primary person who must understand the assessment is the participant. The group training program focuses on the factors that must be integrated in a coherent assessment and plan.

6. **Confrontation of demoralizing attitudes.** The combined on-going affects of MS often result in major demoralization (which is different from organically-based or emotionally-related depression). Identifying the factors involved in demoralization and confronting these with knowledge and well developed personal skills are important elements.

7. **Program scheduling factors.** Scheduling a group training program for unemployed persons with MS desiring to return to work involves the balancing of many factors, including fatigue. The Projects With Industry experience has shown that one group training session of 3 hours once a week for 10-12 weeks is the most appropriate schedule; a consistent weekday morning has had the most success. Evening sessions present many problems. The time needed between sessions for "processing" and work at home is important; experience suggests that twice a week is usually too frequent, although eventually individuals will usually involve themselves in daily work activities. Thus, the program should be regular, but not overscheduled.

8. **Medically-related considerations.** Most functional limitations have not proven to be a primary or dependable predictor in explaining employment outcomes. Certain limited medical situations rule out participants as good candidates.

   These include:
   a. medical crisis presently occurring.
   b. time-limited heavy medication which seriously changes the temporary potential.
   c. functional/medical realities that are in serious conflict with the only employment options a participant will consider.

   Various practices of good health, including appropriate diet and exercise, may give an additional needed edge in competing for jobs. It is also important for the program to urge individuals to obtain specialized medical care, rehabilitation aids, and technologies as available, and to understand the assessments that their physicians are presenting.

9. **Improving personal skills and self-marketing approach.** Partly because most people do not understand multiple sclerosis, persons with this disease often find it necessary to modify existing interpersonal skills and adapt new ones to increase their capacity to market themselves effectively.

10. **Focus on a plan for change and uncertainty.** In many respects, it is possible for individuals with MS to plan for uncertainty and to position themselves for more flexibility. This is true with respect to employment options, emotional responses, financial and insurance possibilities, and adaptations at home and at work. Similarly, incorporating uncertainties in establishing employment plans of persons with MS gives a stronger sense of security and minimizes necessity for future adaptations. Incentives and disincentives in income maintenance, medical insurance programs, and pension plans take on a different light when viewed from the perspective of uncertainty.

11. **Develop special skills to manage stress, fatigue, and possible cognition changes.** Developing specific insights and special skills to manage stress, fatigue, and cognition changes are an important aspect. Keeping a diary of the impacts of various factors and attempted resolutions has proven to be an important technique, as has advanced planning to limit potential crises.

12. **A long-term connection and a regularized follow-up program.** Local chapters of the National Multiple Sclerosis Society or similar organizations that have ongoing programs of contact are an important assurance and long-term resource. The Projects with Industry program's formalized system of tracking participants regularly for two years has shown the need for long-term follow-up.

## Some General Reccommendations to Vocational Rehabilitation System Professionals

* Support (a) special recruitment of groups of persons with MS, (b) group programs, and (c) "packaged services" defined as core vocational rehabilitation services that are not "means" tested.

* Develop PWI verification and vocational rehabilitation eligibility procedures and purchase of service strategies which accommodate group programming schedules.

* Concentrate on employment needs rather than degree or type of current symptoms; symptoms will change.

* Early intervention is usually more strategic and less costly; treat MS as a "severe" disability in terms of priority for service despite current symptoms.

* Wherever JOB RAISING type programs exist, consider collaboration. If they do not exist, find ways to help develop them.

* Develop programs with probabilities of success for those persons with MS who have more extensive needs. The general approach we believe will be most successful is to incorporate the "services" of the PWI Job Raising Program into an empowerment-type model, being careful to maintain the acceptance of self-management responsibility by the participants.

# FUNCTIONAL LIMITATIONS

Multiple sclerosis symptoms, in combination, can result in a wide variety of functional limitations. Yet, functional limitations, with the exception of cognitive and neurological fatigue, have not proven to be a primary or dependable predictor in explaining employment outcomes. Many people with multiple sclerosis develop self-management and coping techniques that enable them to carry out employment and other activities effectively in the face of changing and fluctuating limitations.

In addition to the intellectual dysfunctions previously discussed, specific functional limitations that may exist singly or in combination include:

1. **Fatigue and lack of energy**. Fatigue from multiple sclerosis can be severely debilitating. It can cause severe limitation in a person's ability to work and carry out activities of daily living. Other symptoms may temporarily worsen when fatigue is severe (i.e., visual impairments, incoordination, among other symptoms). Heat can intensify fatigue. The earlier discussion of fatigue explained why it occurs and some self-management and medical strategies that can impact it. Ultimately, only the person with MS can determine how limiting it is in terms of employment.

2. **Weakness, especially of the extremities**. Weakness may be mild so the person's limbs just tire easily or feel heavy. It may be severe and make the legs feel too heavy to lift, and make walking difficult. When it affects the arms, it may cause small motor movements to become more difficult (e.g., handwriting, lifting, and carrying).

3. **Hand tremors and lack of coordination**. Clumsiness, shakiness, slowness, and disturbance in the rhythm of movement when using a limb will affect fine actions such as writing, fastening buttons, picking up objects, and eating.

4. **Problems of balance**. Disturbance of balance and coordination may cause the person to sway, tilt, weave, or stagger when walking. Problems with balance associated with vertigo may occur primarily with changes of position, such as when first standing up to walk.

5. **Spasticity (rigidity or stiffness).** The leg is most commonly affected especially in walking speed or ease and climbing stairs. It also may cause a "drawing up" involuntarily ("charley horse") resulting in falling without warning.

6. **Problems with standing or walking.** Problems with standing or walking usually result from a combination of MS symptoms which may include weakness, vertigo, ataxia, and spasticity. The patterns are different. They frequently cause an inability to stand for an extended period or to balance without holding on to something. Problems with walking are varied, depending upon the combination and degree of symptoms. The ability to walk only short distances and the inability to use stairs is quite common.

7. **Visual Impairments.** Double vision (diplopia) or eye muscle jerking (nystagmus) are visual symptoms caused by brain stem and cerebellar involvement. They may cause only mild functional problems, such as blurred vision or overlapping images, or may be more marked and cause the perception of objects jumping. Depending on the severity, these symptoms can be very limiting.

Visual symptoms caused by involvement of the optic nerve may include: blurry, foggy, or cloudy vision; visual loss in one central spot or in the entire eye; impairment in depth perception; and pain and tenderness in the eye. These symptoms usually improve after a short period. There may be some permanent loss of vision. Some individuals with MS have visual impairments so limiting they are legally blind and require large type or magnification aids. There is seldom a total loss of vision.

8. **Emotional lability and depression.** Emotional disturbances associated with MS may be caused by organic changes in the brain. Some psychological manifestations are related to trying to cope with an unpredictable and variable chronic disease. Less common problems associated with organic brain stem and/or cerebellar involvement are emotional lability or euphoria.

9. **Exacerbations and remissions.** The course of multiple sclerosis may have a sudden onset (an "attack") followed by remissions, often with no residual functional limitations. There are often long periods of remission. Sometimes remissions are not total and mild permanent disability remains (e.g., weakness in one leg). Most gainfully employed people with MS can handle their periods of exacerbation within the framework of sick leave and vacation time, and will not have prolonged absences from work.

# REHABILITATION POTENTIAL PREDICTABILITY

There is very little that can be predicted on an individual basis. While it is often true that the pattern of disease demonstrated over the first 5-10 years is a strong indicator of future probabilities, it is not certain. A reasonable and appropriate approach to providing services for persons with multiple sclerosis is to take chances, and not expect each person to achieve employment objectives. The degree, combination, and nature of symptoms at one time may be quite different from another time.

## *Motivation*

The combination of various demoralizing factors of multiple sclerosis undermines motivation, but for those who want to work, it is possible to confront and deal effectively with many of these factors. There are opportunities inherent in SSDI and SSI work incentive programs to deal partially with some financial disincentives of these systems. This is problematic in the sense that the so-called incentives require a type of risk-taking, which is more difficult for those already living an uncertain life related to an unpredictable disease.

A successful rehabilitation approach will include the genuine potential of individuals achieving or reachieving employment opportunities of which they are capable, usually substantially above entry-level employment. Also, because of the general lack of understanding of multiple sclerosis and the wide range of symptoms, enhancing motivation is usually best achieved in a group process in which individuals interact with each other (Wolf, 1991).

## *Symptoms and Physical Limitations*

For the majority of persons with MS who believe they could work, the exact nature of present symptoms, with the exceptions of severe fatigue and extensive cognition problems, does not have major relevance in terms of successfully obtaining employment. Career planning should anticipate changes in symptoms and provide maximum flexibility. Career shifts from heavier types of work or from the types of work where undependability of physical traits would endanger the public are obvious. Most persons with MS can develop techniques and accommodations to perform work similar to their former occupations in which they have experience or expertise.

## *Special Impact of Fatigue*

The most difficult part of fatigue and MS is the type of fatigue (sometimes called neurological fatigue) that is not related to exertion or psychological factors such as depression. An individual maximizes employment potential in several ways. One is by understanding the pattern of fatigue through a diary and other processes. Another is by developing techniques and schedules that limit and deal with fatigue. Other ways include receiving medical therapy to assist with neurological fatigue and selecting types of employment opportunities where there is an opportunity to rest briefly, usually in the early to mid-afternoon.

# CASE STUDY

Ms. Estelle Watson is 35 years old and has an M.S.W. degree (Master of Social Work). Her treating neurologist diagnosed multiple sclerosis when she was 29 years of age. She is single, lives alone, and is employed as a social worker with a small community agency. Ms. Watson has lived in the community for many years and is involved in community life (church, YWCA, and other philanthropic organizations).

The counselor she saw for rehabilitation stated she appeared somewhat distraught and confused. Estelle describes her experiences with MS as follows:

* Once or twice a year, I had some brief episodes of numbness and tingling in either leg or a hip. These would last 2-3 weeks and then disappear. They didn't affect my ability to walk; they were just uncomfortable. The doctor I saw thought I might have done something to bruise a nerve in my back. Since these episodes sometimes occurred when I was moving to a new apartment, this made sense.

* Five years after the numbness began, it recurred in both legs, from my waist down. After 1 week, I began to stumble and catch my right leg on carpeting or cracks in the sidewalk. My legs got very wobbly and collapsed under me a couple of times. The treating neurologist hospitalized me and ordered a spinal tap and myelogram. By this time, I could barely walk, even with the use of crutches. Needless to say, I was really frightened.

* The testing confirmed my doctor's suspicions. He shared the diagnosis and discussed the treatment with me immediately. Following a long course of steroids and physical therapy, I regained my ability to walk independently.

* I felt very relieved now to have a name for what was wrong with me. I read everything I could on multiple sclerosis and was determined that I was going to do all that was suggested to avoid getting sick again (reduce stress, simplify my life, avoid exposure to heat). I had been unable to work for 6 weeks, but my employer was very supportive.

* Six months later, the vision in my right eye became blurred. I was again given steroids and my vision returned to normal. For the first time, I began to believe that there was something wrong with me and that it was not going away. I found myself getting very frustrated, angry, and depressed. It must have presented some problems with my work but my employer said nothing.

* Two years later, symptoms of numbness and tingling began in my right arm and hand. Within one week, I was unable to write my name or hold an object. I again began to stumble as I walked. My physician hospitalized me a second time, for 3 weeks, during which I received both physical therapy and occupational therapy. I regained the use of my hand and arm but had constant numbness, weakness, and inability to sense temperature in the affected arm and hand. In addition, fatigue had become a major problem. I could not function for about an hour during the afternoon; a nap became necessary. At the time, I was working with children and adolescents. It became very difficult for me to be functional in the afternoon when they were present. My agency was able to find another social worker on staff to assume some of my responsibilities during the afternoon. It was no longer possible for them to pay me for full-time work; I went to 3/4 time shortly after that.

* Two years later, I had another attack. I am now having difficulty walking any distance and my handwriting has deteriorated. Even more problematic is that I am having trouble remembering things. It may be impossible to continue to work with clients. I cannot always remember what clients said from week to week. So far, no one at work has said anything but I can tell that it is only a matter of time. My performance is slipping and that makes me anxious, which makes everything worse.

* I really thought I had multiple sclerosis beaten. There would be an attack for which I would receive treatment with steroids, and I got well. It just is not working out that way. It is impossible to know daily or weekly what is going to happen next. I find I have to make continuous changes in how I do things. Just when I think I have something mastered and am ready to get on with life, something new occurs and I have to readjust and readapt. It gets to be very tiresome.

* By this time in my life, I had planned to be in a serious relationship, maybe even married, and well on my way to a successful career in social services. None of that is happening. It is very hard to maintain an active life when my energy is so limited. Now my professional skills are being affected and I am concerned about being able to support myself.

* All this make me very angry, although I know I am not alone. I have been to MS support groups and have listened to other people so I know that these are not just my "demons." It is my belief I can still work and probably full-time, given the right situation. I want to continue being productive and do not want to give that up just because of MS."

## Questions

1. Assign Ms. Watson a vocational profile, including age category, educational level, and skill and exertional levels of her work.

2. What are Estelle's current functional limitations? Do the symptoms of multiple sclerosis prevent her from continuing employment? Discuss any possibilities of reasonable accommodation.

3. Identify the occupationally significant characteristics of Ms. Watson's work, noting which characteristics relate to her present and possible future functional limitations.

4. Did this client acquire skills that are transferable to other jobs? If so, identify these skills and suggest possible occupations.

5. As her rehabilitation counselor, recommend several possible rehabilitation programs. These programs may involve use of transferable skills, additional training, or further education.

6. What additional information would be useful to your analysis of this case?

# REFERENCES

Calvano, M., & Gresser, B. (1991). Diagnosis...the whole story. **Inside MS, 9**(3), 16-17.

Frankel, D, (Ed.) (1982). **Maximizing your health.** Waltham, MA: National Multiple Sclerosis Society, Massachusetts Chapter.

Herndon, R.M. (1991). Fatigue in MS (revised). **JOB RAISING Participant Manual.** Baltimore, MD: The Development Team, Inc.

LaRocca, N.G. (1990). The mind and MS. **Inside MS, 8**(1), 24-28.

National Institute of Health, NINCDS, (1984) **Multiple Sclerosis: A national survey** (Highlights of the 1976 Survey). NIH Pub. 84-2479. Prepared by Biometry and Field Studies Branch, International Research Program, NINCDS.

Rosner, L.J., & Ross, S. (1987). **Multiple sclerosis.** New York: Prentice Hall.

Schapiro, R.T., (1991). **Multiple sclerosis: A rehabilitation approach to management.** New York: Demos.

Schapiro, R.T., (1987). **Symptom management in multiple sclerosis.** New York: Demos.

Scheinberg, L.C., & Holland, N.J. (Eds.). (1987). **Multiple sclerosis: A guide for patients and their families** (2nd ed.). New York: Raven.

Shuman, R. & Schwartz, J. (1988). **Understanding multiple sclerosis.** New York: Macmillan.

Waksman, B.H., Reingold, S.C., & Reynolds, W.E. (1987). **Research on multiple sclerosis** (3rd ed.). New York: Demos.

Wolf, J.K., (Ed.), (1988). **Mastering multiple sclerosis.** (2nd ed.). Rutland, VT: Academy Books.

Wolf, J.K., (1991). **Fall down seven times, get up eight: Living well with multiple sclerosis.** Rutland, VT: Academy Books.

## *About The Authors*

Harry L. Hall, a former Assistant Commissioner of the Rehabilitation Services Administration, served as Washington Representative for the National Multiple Sclerosis Society for 6 years. Since 1983, he has been President of The Development Team, Inc. (TDTI), a non-profit corporation located in Baltimore, Maryland, which developed an employment services program, JOB RAISING, for people with multiple sclerosis and closely related disabilities. The Development Team implements the program in collaboration with local chapters of the National Multiple Sclerosis Society, the Arthritis Foundation, and survivors related to the National Head Injury Foundation.

Shirley M. Rohaly, M.S.W., a former Director of Services for the Delaware Chapter of the National Multiple Sclerosis Society and National Staff Consultant to Chapters for the National Multiple Sclerosis Society, facilitated the collaborative working party for the 1983 Cooperative Agreement among the National Multiple Sclerosis Society, the Rehabilitation Services Administration, NIDRR, and CSA-VR. She joined The Development Team, Inc. in 1987 as JOB RAISING Project Manager.

Myra A. Shneider, M.S.W., L.S.W., formerly Director of Professional Training for The Development Team, Inc. directed the vocational rehabilitation group program model known as JOB RAISING in the Chicago-Northern Illinois Chapter of the National Multiple Sclerosis Society for several years. She is a member of the Consumer Task Force of the Illinois Attorney General's Disabled Persons Advocacy Division.

# Chapter 30

# ACQUIRED TRAUMATIC BRAIN INJURY

by
*Susan Vanost Wulz, Ph.D.*

## INTRODUCTION

Injury to the brain causes some of the most pervasive and significant disabilities that a rehabilitation counselor is likely to encounter. "In one sense, vocational rehabilitation represents the 'final frontier' in the rehabilitation of the head injured adult; it is the ultimate goal of comprehensive rehabilitation, but the one that may be the hardest to achieve" (Rosenthal, 1987, p. 57).

Even mild brain damage may interfere with the behaviors that are necessary for successful employment (O'Shaughnessy, Fowler, & Reid, 1984). Rimel, Giordani, Barth, Boll, and Jane (1982) studied the outcome of a mild head injury 3 months after injury. All the individuals were unconscious less than 20 minutes. However, 3 months after injury, 78% of them continued to have headaches, 59% complained of memory problems, and 15% had trouble with activities of daily living or transportation. A full 34% had not returned to work within the first 3 months after their mild injury. Although neuropsychological testing identified a variety of mild deficits in problem-solving, attention, and concentration, only 2% of these individuals showed positive neurological signs.

Fraser, Dikmen, McLean, and Miller (1988) examined the employment status of 102 head-injured adults to identify factors that correlated with successful return to work. They found that neurological functioning one month post-injury was the best predictor of subsequent return to work. Seventy-three percent of the individuals studied returned to work within the first year, but nearly half of them reported some residual difficulties at work because of their injury.

Strub and Black (1988) reported that even someone with a mild concussion may experience difficulty concentrating for several weeks after injury. They warned: "If such a person returns to work prematurely, the difficulty he experiences in carrying out his work can easily be very frustrating to him and will often be misinterpreted by his employer as being a deliberate attempt to receive additional compensation or time off from work" (p. 314).

Yarnell and Rossie (1988) studied 16 patients with whiplash injuries and found that none of them had returned to their prior level of occupational functioning. Although neurological tests showed minimal deficits, they had impairments in attention, memory, cognitive flexibility, and stamina.

The most common causes of traumatic brain injuries are automobile accidents and falls. Although the death rate from accidents has dropped 21% since 1980, accidents are the leading cause of permanent total disability for individuals under the age of 35. Estimates of the number of individuals with significant brain damage each year vary from 350,000 (Rosenthal, 1987) to 8.8 million people (Shordone, 1987). Durgin, Rath, and Dales (1991) estimated that the costs of health care related to head injury now exceed $500 billion per year, or 12% of the Gross National Product (GNP). Most of the people who suffer brain damage each year are children and young adults under the age of 35. There are twice as many men as women who suffer head trauma.

A vocational rehabilitation referral following an automobile accident or fall may not identify the individual as brain injured. Except when the brain damage is severe, there may be multiple diagnoses and frequent references in medical reports to secondary gain factors. Physicians often attribute fatigue and behavioral changes to non-organic psychological problems. Furthermore, it is not uncommon for intelligence and aptitude test results to be within normal limits, even where there is significant brain damage (Parker, 1990). Lezak (1983) adds:

> Yet many of these patients continue to suffer frontal apathy, memory deficits, severely slowed thinking processes, or a mental tracking disability that makes them unable to resume working or, in some instances, to assume social responsibility at all. Insufficient or inappropriate behavioral examinations of head trauma can lead to unjust social and legal decisions concerning employability and competency, can invalidate rehabilitation planning efforts, and can confuse patient and family, not infrequently adding financial distress to their already considerable stress and despair. (p. 174)

Caplan and Schechter (1991) warn: "The lesson from recent research about the consequences of minor head injury is that clinicians must be quite cautious about invoking malingering as an explanation of deficient performance" (p. 164).

The multiple and confusing diagnoses may complicate the counselor's efforts in many ways. First, the party with monetary responsibility for the claim may have unreasonable expectations. From their perspective and based on their forensic medical reports, vocational rehabilitation should be a relatively easy task because it is simply a matter of controlling someone who is seeking secondary gain from the symptoms.

On the other hand, injured workers are confused and uncertain about changes in their personality and behavioral functioning. Their stress, fear, and anxiety are further exacerbated by the skepticism of the people around them. Often they become insecure and afraid to try anything at all because they cannot understand what is happening to them and why. The counselor is similarly unable to predict what types of problems will be encountered in developing and implementing a vocational rehabilitation plan. Unaware of the deficits caused by the head injury, the counselor cannot assist the injured worker in adapting to the injury. A counselor may even exacerbate the situation by placing the injured worker into situations where success is not possible.

# MECHANISMS OF INJURY

Traumatic brain injuries are usually divided into two types: closed head injury and penetrating injury to the skull. These are discussed below.

## Closed Head Injury

The most common type of head injury may show no external evidence of damage and does not involve penetration of the skull. It occurs in a situation of rapid acceleration and deceleration, where movement in one direction is stopped or started suddenly. This is the typical mechanism of head injury in an automobile accident. The person is in a car that is moving forward at a consistent speed. The car stops suddenly, and the person's head continues to move forward until it encounters a force that stops it (either a dashboard or steering wheel). In whiplash, the head is stopped because it is restrained by the neck. Because the upper portions of the brain are surrounded by fluid, the brain does not move with the skull. Instead, when the skull stops suddenly, the brain crashes against it and then rebounds against the other side of the skull.

The possible sites of injury are extensive, including where the brain initially hit the skull, where it rebounded against the other side of the skull, and the base of the brain where it attaches to the spinal cord. Most frequently, the sites of injury include the frontal and occipital regions of the brain, which may cause the most pervasive and subtle behavioral changes (Walsh, 1990). A similar type of injury occurs when the person slips, and falls against a solid object.

The damage in a closed head injury is generally diffuse. In some cases, the immediate damage may seem to be minimal, with very brief or no loss of consciousness. Yet, there is usually bleeding (hemorrhage), tearing (laceration), bruising (contusion), and swelling (edema). The bleeding creates a pocket of blood called a hematoma which pushes against the skull and the brain. Increased pressure also occurs when the injured cells of the brain swell. Because the skull does not yield, the pressure of the bleeding and swelling squeezes nerve cells and blood vessels in the brain, interfering with the circulation of uninjured parts of the brain. As a result, the damage continues beyond the point of immediate injury. In addition, there may be significant scarring or dead brain tissue, which interferes with the circulation, chemical functioning, and metabolism of the surrounding tissue (Brodal, 1981).

Diagnosis following a mild closed head injury is difficult. Strub and Black (1988) pointed out:

> Findings on the neurologic examination and CT scan are usually normal, as are the EEG and other neurodiagnostic tests. For this reason, some physicians consider any patient who has symptoms lasting longer than a few weeks or a month after injury to have emotional or other reasons (e.g., a desire for compensation) for the perpetuation of symptoms (p. 322).

The issue of secondary or monetary gain is encountered in nearly all forensic evaluations regarding head injury, but appears to be a less frequent occurrence than was previously believed (Parker, 1990).

## Penetrating Injury

Penetrating injuries may appear more dramatic than closed head injuries because the skull is fractured and there is visible bleeding. There is usually little dispute about the diagnosis when there is an obvious penetrating injury. However, the damage to the brain may be less serious than in a closed head injury because the damage may be confined to a particular area of the brain.

Even though it appears that the injury impacted only one area of the brain, one may observe a widespread range of dysfunctions. This is because the functions of the brain interrelate. Clear independent functioning is the exception, not the rule. Penetrating injuries also may be complicated by infection, scarring, and hemorrhage. Infections in the spinal fluid can lead to swelling that impacts the entire surface of the brain. As with closed head injuries, hemorrhage may increase the damage by decreasing circulation to the areas of the brain not otherwise impacted. The presence of dead or diseased brain tissue affects the biochemical balance of the brain and is associated with increased impairment (Brodal, 1981; Lezak, 1983).

The prognosis for recovery from a penetrating injury to the head depends on the location of the injury, the extent of damage, and the type of lesion. The likelihood of seizures is much higher with a penetrating injury than one in which the skull was uninjured (Wasco, 1991).

# PREDICTION OF IMPAIRMENT

"The usual criterion of good outcome for younger adults, and therefore for most head trauma patients, is the return to gainful employment" (Lezak, 1983, p. 213). Caplan and Schechter (1991) stated: "Among the factors that seemed to predict successful resumption of work were younger age, superior intelligence, greater education, professional training, absence of premorbid psychopathology, and shorter duration of post-traumatic amnesia" (p.

153). Other factors that appear to affect the outcome of brain injury are the severity of the lesion, location of the injury, duration of symptoms, and the environment to which the injured person will return.

## *Severity of the Lesion*

The prognosis for recovery is closely related to the severity of the injury (Strub & Black, 1988). The best measurements for this are the duration of unconsciousness and post-traumatic amnesia.

The duration of the coma or period of unconsciousness is the most common measurement of severity (Walsh, 1990). These are reliable measures in a severe injury where the individual is unconscious when hospitalized and recovers in the hospital. It is rarely accurate in mild injuries when there was no observation of the individual's condition immediately after the injury. Parker (1990) stated: "Significant brain damage may occur without loss of consciousness, e.g., penetrating head injuries or when there is no transmission of injury to the brainstem" (p. 100). False reports of no residual brain damage are often made because of the observation that there has been no loss of consciousness. In contrast, the coma may be of long duration with no associated cognitive problems, if the injury is limited to the brainstem, which directly affects the level of alertness.

Brooks, Aughton, Bond, Jones, and Rizvi (1980) found that duration of post-traumatic amnesia was more closely related to cognitive status 2 years later than length of coma. "The amnesiac period is measured from the last memory before the trauma (retrograde amnesia) to the point of complete return to continuous memory (anterograde amnesia); the term post-traumatic amnesia includes retrograde and anterograde amnesia" (Strub & Black, 1988, p. 316). Again, this measure is only reliable if one makes a thorough and accurate assessment of the period of post-traumatic amnesia.

## *Areas of Damage*

The breadth of the damage and the areas involved may be predictive of the nature of deficits caused by the injury. In an intact human brain, the effects of lateralization and specialization of function are insignificant; the different parts of the brain interact with one another smoothly to produce integrated behavior. It is only when there is an injury to the brain that the specialized functioning of the different parts of the brain is observed and becomes important.

The cerebrum is divided into right and left hemispheres joined by the corpus colosseum. In an uninjured person, the two hemispheres work together and the separation of functions is not relevant. Motor and sensory parts of the brain are organized in a point-to-point representation of the opposite side of the body. Thus, when there is an injury to the left side of the brain, it may affect the motor control of the right side of the body and vice versa. Similarly, sensory data from the right side of each eye enters the left side of the brain (Brodal, 1981).

Even though specialization is well-established, it does not have a direct one-to-one relationship with deficits. For example, the primary motor area of the cerebral cortex includes sensory cells, while the sensory area contains some motor cells. The actual integrated functions of a primary location for motor behavior are also dependent upon secondary zones which provide perceptual feedback and tertiary zones which integrate the information (Walsh, 1990). Therefore, it would be inaccurate to assume that there would be no motor problems if the injury was in the sensory part of the brain, or vice versa.

The left side of the brain is dominant for speech and all verbal activities, even with the majority of left-handed people, while the right hemisphere appears to be dominant in non-verbal activities. However, even this is not a clear distinction, as the right side of the brain appears to be involved in comprehending complex sentences, humorous material, and speech intonation. Individuals with left hemisphere damage may show clear impairments in speech and language-related activities, while people with right hemisphere damage may be verbose but unable to understand humor or generalized concepts (Lezak, 1983).

The vast majority of left-handed people still have left brain lateralization of speech and language functions. Damage to the left side of the brain will affect speech and language usage. Left-brain injured people are more likely to be depressed shortly after the injury, aware of their disabilities. Some people with right-brain injuries are unaware of their disabilities and are insensitive to other people's reactions to their behavior. After a long period of disability, individuals with right-brain injury may show more depression and poorer outcome than those with left-brain injury (Lezak, 1983).

"In cases of diffuse impairment, there will usually be deficits in many functional areas with relatively few areas of cognitive/behavioral functioning remaining intact" (Jarvis & Barth, 1984, p. 53). In these cases, the counselor is likely to receive detailed neuropsychological reports to identify the types of deficits that the injured person is likely to exhibit.

Many head injuries involve damage to the frontal and temporal lobes. The frontal lobe is the primary area of the brain that integrates the "higher" intellectual functions, such as abstract thinking, planning, and problem-solving. "Changes in personality after brain injury are most often noted after damage to the frontal lobes" (Walsh, 1990, p. 126). In addition to the visual and auditory perception, the temporal lobes integrate sensory stimuli, motivational, and emotional aspects of experience. Temporal lobes also have a direct impact on memory functions. Walsh (1990) warned: "Because of this anatomical and functional complexity, one must be cautious of over-simplified conceptions based on examination of lesions in specific parts of the temporal lobes" (p. 169).

## Stabilization of Deficits

Rapid improvements may be observed on a daily basis once the traumatically brain injured person has emerged from a coma. The rapidity of the return of functioning is a positive prognostic indicator. The sooner the individual recovers functioning, the more functioning is likely to be recovered. Conversely, the longer the problems persist, the less functioning is likely to be recovered (Anderson, 1981).

If the injury was mild, many of the more diffuse symptoms will have gone within the first 3-6 months. However, Strub, and Black (1988, p. 333) warn: "Estimates of overall functional recovery can be given accurately at six months, whereas a prognosis after three months or less is unnecessarily pessimistic." Similarly, Lezak (1983) stated:

> Intellectual functions, particularly those involving immediate memory, attention and concentration and specific disabilities associated with the site of the lesion generally continue to improve markedly during the first six months or year, and improvement at an increasingly slow rate may go on for a decade or more following a stroke or other single-event injury to the brain... However, improvement probably never amounts to full recovery, even when the insult may appear to be slight (p. 211).

Lezak concluded: "Unless the patient's handicaps are so severe as to be permanently and totally disabling, it is unwise for binding decisions or judgments to be made concerning his legal, financial, or vocational status until several years have passed" (p. 214). Some behaviors may actually deteriorate over time. Parker (1990) suggested that this could be due to a pathological process or to continuing frustration secondary to impaired neuropsychological deficits. The abilities most at risk are social behaviors, learning and recall, reasoning, mental flexibility, and judgment.

## Pre-Injury Functioning

In general, the more skilled the individual prior to injury, the better the outcome. Fowler (1987) stated: "The brighter, better educated, productive person with excellent family support will tend to perform at a higher functional level, given the same injuries, than his duller, less well-educated, less productive, more lonely counterpart" (p. 127).

Similarly, Anderson (1981) indicated that those persons with higher socioeconomic and educational background usually show greater use of their potential.

Highly skilled and intelligent individuals may be less likely to be identified as significantly impaired in the initial evaluations. Their superior fund of knowledge may allow them to demonstrate normal or near normal test results following injury. In these cases, many significant impairments will not be identified until the individual returns to home or work and attempts to resume pre-injury tasks and responsibilities.

In addition, sometimes the higher achievers experience more frustration and anger with their deficits, leading to greater emotional problems in adapting to the deficits (Michael, 1985). As stated in the **DSM-III-R** (American Psychiatric Association, 1987):

> Severe emotional disturbances may accompany cognitive impairment in a person who views it as a loss, a serious threat to self-esteem, or both. Anxiety, depression, irritability, and shame of varying degrees of intensity may be present. Compulsive individuals tend to be particularly intolerant of and disturbed by their reduced cognitive capacity or by perceptual abnormalities . . . There may also be severe depression leading to suicidal attempts . . (p. 99).

On the other hand, because basic personality patterns may remain intact, the overall prognosis is better for someone with a high level of motivation and skills prior to the injury (Caplan & Schechter, 1991). Frontal lobe damage, which is the most common in closed head injuries, directly impacts motivational factors and may reduce the predictive factors related to pre-morbid functioning. The very characteristics that led to high achievement in the past are affected by the injury and personality change may be marked.

## Age

A general rule with brain traumas of all types is the younger the person at the time of injury, the better the prognosis for recovery. Strub and Black (1988) explained that "Symptoms are definitely increased in older patients, a finding that may be of multifactorial cause but certainly suggests that the older, less plastic brain cannot adjust to trauma as well as the younger one can" (p. 322).

On the other hand, Parker (1990) pointed out that young individuals have less stored information and experience to rely on after the injury. Older individuals may be able to function with the stored information (experience) that they have developed over the years. Often, well-established skills, such as speech and self-care routines, are less affected than more recently developed skills. To that extent, a younger individual may suffer more problems than the older individual. Nonetheless, among adults there appears to be a clear advantage for the under-40 adults versus over-40 adults sustaining injuries to the brain (Strub & Black, 1988).

# FUNCTIONAL LIMITATIONS

There is extreme variability of symptoms and deficits following brain injury that make it nearly impossible to predict the impact on any particular individual. Lezak (1983) stated: "Few symptoms distinguish the behavior of persons suffering chronic brain damage of adult onset with sufficient regularity to be considered characteristic." An evaluation of a brain-injured individual must include an assessment of physical restrictions, stamina, work adjustment, and cognitive abilities.

## Physical Problems

Someone who has suffered a head injury also may have all of the physical problems seen in the non-injured population. As stated by Anderson (1981): "Patients who have suffered an injury severe enough to result in cerebral trauma have often sustained injuries to other parts of the body as well and these injuries may cause symptoms unrelated to the area of the brain damaged" (p. 119). Often, these physical problems are not given the necessary attention when there has been a severe head injury. This may occur because of the individual's impaired ability to communicate clearly and meaningfully. Often, people suffering from traumatic brain injury are perceived as exaggerating symptoms, and physical complaints are basically ignored (Lezak, 1983).

Some physical problems are frequently the direct result of the injury to the brain. The most common problems are apraxia (defined below) and paralysis, which may affect any part of the body. Generally in a localized injury, the impact will be greatest on the side of the body opposite the injury to the brain.

**Apraxia.** This is an inability to perform movements independent of physical deficits or disabilities. A person who has apraxia may be able to perform the movement, but not when making a conscious effort to do so. This is frequently observed when attempting to speak or write or to use an object in a familiar manner. Imitation is also limited, which reduces the value of this technique in teaching new behaviors.

**Dysarthria.** Speech also may be affected by dysarthria. Dysarthria is weakness and slowing in the muscles related to speech. The person appears to slur words and have significant articulation problems.

**Paralysis.** There may be paralysis on the side opposite of where the brain injury occurred (hemiplegia). For example, an individual with an injury to the right side of the brain may experience motor dysfunction on the left side of the body. Even where there is no paralysis, there still may be a weakness limiting strength and endurance (paresis). In most cases, there are no specific medical restrictions requiring the avoidance of jobs using body parts affected by apraxia, dysarthria, or paralysis. Injured workers are encouraged to use their limbs to the extent that they are able. A functional evaluation is necessary to determine the types of activities in which they will be able to engage.

**Balance and coordination.** These are frequent problems, even following relatively mild injuries. These symptoms usually occur within 24 hours, but may begin several days or weeks after the injury. Headaches are experienced by 60-95% of patients suffering closed head injury. Headaches may be aggravated by activities requiring concentration or attention to multiple stimuli. Over half of the people seen after injury report experiencing dizziness. Approximately half of the individuals will be symptom-free in 6 weeks. Others continue to have problems for over a year (Strub & Black, 1988).

**Motor speed.** Physicians commonly observe a decrease in speed of motor behaviors and cognitive processing following an injury to the brain (Lezak, 1983; Parker, 1990). This greatly restricts the injured worker's vocational alternatives. Most individuals with brain injury will experience decreases in speed of performance, affecting all tasks. Verbal responses and motor performances are both slower and appear difficult. This will reduce the likelihood of success in occupations requiring production work (e.g., assembly) or social responses (e.g., receptionist). Fowler (1981) stated:

> The majority of these clients do not function as rapidly as they did prior to their stroke or brain injury. Some of them work so slowly that it is preferable for them to be employed in a sheltered setting. Others can produce high quality work as long as they did not feel they need to hurry. The pressure of trying to hurry may itself decrease quality (p. 134).

## Stamina/Fatigue

Fatigue is a common characteristic of the majority of people who have suffered cerebral trauma. Their best efforts and strongest results are likely to be achieved in the morning. Many of these individuals do not appear to be directly aware of the fatigue. Instead, they may indicate that they have a headache after extended activity, have increased frustration or irritability, show decreased motor ability, or their performance illustrates a marked deterioration over time. The counselor needs to keep cognizant of the fact that verbal expression is one of the areas usually affected by head injury. Therefore, they may not be able to reliably report their own condition.

Fatigue will become more pronounced with complex tasks requiring concentration and memory. It can be assumed that, as the task becomes easier and more automatic, the worker will be able to perform it for a longer time. This is a strong argument for gradually increasing work activity when people are participating in vocational rehabilitation following brain injury.

## Sensory Limitations

Where sensory and perceptual functioning is affected, the damage may be dissimilar to most of the types of problems vocational rehabilitation counselors encounter. Anderson (1981) pointed out that the most disabling residuals from stroke and cerebral trauma may be sensory problems, such as touch, pain, temperature, pressure, vibration, vision, hearing and position.

**Vision.** A lateralized injury may show lateralized visual field defects in both eyes. For example, an injury to the right side of the brain can lead to blindness in the left side of each eye. Even without a lateralized injury, there may be inattention to the missing visual field, such that the person appears unaware that there is part of the visual picture missing. In an assembly task, stimuli placed to the left might be completely ignored by someone suffering right-side neglect. Visual scanning (search) and tracking may also be affected by the injury (Lezak, 1983).

Individuals with predominant right brain injury will show more difficulty working with non-verbal visual materials. They may have difficulty recognizing, copying, matching, or discriminating patterns or faces. Injuries to the left brain may cause problems with reading, interpreting signs, drawing angles, and itemizing characteristics of a visual stimulus. A thorough neuropsychological test battery by a qualified professional is the best resource for the rehabilitation counselor.

**Hearing.** The most obvious auditory problems occur when speech is disrupted. A lesion in the left hemisphere will affect both expression and comprehension of speech. In contrast, someone with a right hemisphere lesion may speak a great deal, but much of what is said is not meaningful or logical. An experienced speech and language pathologist is an essential resource for the counselor to understand and deal with these problems.

Another frequent complication of head injury, regardless of the location of the lesion, is an inability to tolerate a noisy environment (Caplan & Schechter, 1991). The intolerance for noise may be due to an overall increased irritability, fatigue due to the increased effort required to concentrate, or an inability to screen out distractions.

**Pain.** Pain is a neurological function that involves multiple parts of the brain but requires left parietal lobe response (Strub & Black, 1988). Some individuals may lose the ability to recognize painful stimulation completely, or there may often be a predominance of pain sensation. Any kind of stimulus to the patient's involved side may be recognized as pain.

Chronic pain is a common problem with individuals who have suffered traumatic brain injury and are referred to vocational rehabilitation. This may be a function of the mechanism of injury (e.g., car accident or fall) in which multiple parts of the body are injured. The person's difficulty with verbal expression may interfere with medical attention or treatment to other involved areas of the body. Depression, which is a common aftermath of head injury, sometimes aggravates the perception of pain.

## Emotional Factors

While cognitive functioning may improve over time, psychological and behavioral problems may worsen. Brooks et al. (1980) interviewed close relatives of adult patients 5 years after injury. Some relatives noted more problems 5 years after the injury than at one year post-injury.

Emotional characteristics and social behaviors may interfere with employability more than any other disability resulting from the brain damage. The vast majority of employment involves some interaction with people.

**Depression.** The most common mood disorder observed after injury is depression. Varney, Martzke, and Roberts (1987) interviewed 120 patients with closed head injuries two or more years after the date of injury. Of these, 76% met the **DSM-III-R** (American Psychiatric Association, 1987) criteria for major depressive disorder. Over half of the patients suffering depression did not demonstrate these symptoms until 6 months or more after injury. Generally, people with injury to the left side of the brain exhibit depression sooner because they are more aware of their problems. However, people with injury to the right side of the brain may show more chronic depression.

**Indifference reaction.** People with injury to the right brain may experience euphoria or an unawareness of their problems, rather than depression or anxiety. While depression interferes with the individual's progress, the lack of depression may be a poor prognostic sign:

> Patients whose permanent disabilities are considerable and who have experienced no depression have either lost some capacity for self-appreciation and reality testing, or are denying their problems. In both cases, rehabilitation prospects are significantly reduced, for the patient must have a fairly realistic understanding of his strengths and limitations to cooperate with and benefit from any rehabilitation program. (Lezak, 1983, p. 212).

These individuals tend to be unaware of other people's reactions to them. They are not able to identify emotional tones in speech, do not observe subtle reactions of people around them, and remain oblivious about their impact on people. As a result, social behavior rarely improves through the natural consequences of their actions.

Because people with right hemisphere damage are not able to assess the extent of their disability, they frequently set unrealistic goals for themselves. Some people may be completely unaware of their physical problems, to the extent that they do not recognize even paralysis or visual loss (Lezak, 1983).

**Hesitancy.** There is a certain level of insecurity or hesitancy that impacts nearly everyone who has sustained serious injury. This is evident following head trauma where the individual may feel strange or confused because of the unfamiliarity of an environment that was once familiar. There may be a hyper-sensitivity to every memory problem or disruption in concentration, even those that had been experienced before the injury.

**Flat affect.** The most common characteristic after brain injury is a flattening of emotional response. Emotions are expressed in less intense form. The person appears bland and without substantial personality.

**Emotional lability.** Brain injured persons frequently show partial loss of emotional control. They may begin crying or laughing without any clear change in stimuli or situation. Behaviors such as laughing, crying, or moaning, may usually be interrupted through diversion. When asked, the brain injured individual will often be unable to explain the sudden emotional outburst.

**Frustration/anger.** Emotional outbursts are not uncommon, especially when the brain injured person is faced with frustration. There may be a very low frustration tolerance, reduced further by fatigue. The individual may be agitated and combative when unable to perform tasks or confused by multiple stimuli. Task-oriented frustration is an indication that an activity is too difficult for the brain-damaged person at that time. This reaction is more common with people who have suffered left-hemisphere injury. Left-hemisphere damage causes a much higher incidence of both catastrophic anxiety reaction and depression. Sometimes the person will cry because of the deficits that are being observed in a task.

**Irritability.** General irritability is a common outcome of brain injury. It will frequently be observed when the injured individual faces frustrating situations.

## Social Behaviors

Very few jobs lack contact with people. Even jobs on assembly lines, where the primary activity is well-defined and routine, requires working in proximity with people, taking breaks with others, and following verbal instructions. Brain injury may impact all areas of working with and around people.

To return someone to a job involving a high level of social interaction, an assessment must be made of the individual's verbal flexibility and fluency, ability to change tasks rapidly, facial recognition, memory for prior conversations, and ability to concentrate. In general, jobs with social interaction involve multiple interruptions or changes in direction. An evaluation by a speech pathologist is beneficial to the rehabilitation counselor.

Inappropriate social behaviors may pose a major barrier in returning to work, even in jobs involving minimal interpersonal interactions. Socially inappropriate statements, sexually suggestive remarks, and emotional outbursts may require job coaching to provide on-site social training. The person may appear very child-like, coarse, or rude in interactions with others. The brain injured individual may be socially isolated, which further reduces the opportunity to acquire appropriate social behaviors.

## Motivation

Strub and Black (1988) stated, "The ultimate impediment to successful rehabilitation is often the presence of frontal lobe damage. Thus afflicted, the patient loses his basic drive, and the resultant apathy makes a productive career impossible even when the cognitive and physical problems have been overcome" (p. 341).

People with frontal lobe damage are likely to be referred to rehabilitation counseling with no work restrictions because they do not appear to have any loss of specific skills, information, reasoning, or problem-solving ability. They may perform intelligence and aptitude tests within normal limits. "Cognitive defects associated with frontal lobe damage tend to show up most clearly in the course of daily living and are more often observed by relatives and co-workers than by a medical or psychological examiner in a standard interview" (Lezak, 1983, p. 82).

Misdiagnosis is particularly pervasive with patients exhibiting these behaviors, even though this syndrome has been recognized for nearly a century. These individuals are frequently diagnosed as having a psychiatric reaction, rather than an organic problem. Strub and Black (1988) stated:

> The symptom complex may vary from patient to patient, but most commonly the patients demonstrate some degree of apathy, irritability, poor judgment, uninhibited social behavior, lack of motivation and goal direction and euphoria. The patients generally display very shallow affect and, although easily angered, do not sustain their irritation for more than a few minutes. (p. 285)

These patients show an inability to plan ahead, lack motivation, and have poor judgment.

## Flexibility

Many jobs require that the individual be able to shift responses to new problems, identify the effectiveness of the new behavior, and shift again if needed. Perseveration occurs when a person repeats or prolongs a response that was once effective but is no longer appropriate. This can lead to problems in social interactions, where repetition becomes inappropriate. It can eliminate jobs that require changes in activities or alternating activities.

Similar behaviors may be observed when the individual is unable to stop an ongoing behavior or control a response to a particular stimulus. This may interfere with teaching someone a new task in a setting or situation in which a prior task or sequence of behaviors was learned. Following a head injury, the individual will have more difficulty adapting to change.

The injured worker may have problems dissociating from the environment to deal with abstract concepts, though testing has indicated that conceptualization is intact. Thus, it is difficult to direct attention away from the immediate setting to the future, past, or another setting.

## Attention/Concentration

Impaired attention and concentration are among the most common problems associated with brain damage. Attention is the ability to focus on an activity. Concentration is intense attention, requiring the ability to selectively exclude irrelevant stimuli. The results of attentional deficits are easy distractibility and inability to follow a thought pattern or perform multiple step instructions. The environment may need to be modified to reduce the distractions. Multiple-step procedures may need to be supported by separate cues that assist the injured worker in maintaining attention.

## Memory

Caplan and Shechter (1991) stated: "Impaired memory is certainly the most disabling intellectual consequence of brain dysfunction and much of the rehabilitation process for head injured patients revolves around new learning or relearning" (p. 160). The most common complaint following brain injury is memory problems. In its most extreme form, the person with amnesia may be able to carry on a completely normal conversation but cannot learn any new material. Some people suffering this problem will confabulate (make up answers) without hesitation. Unless the counselor is able to compare the answers with fact, the extent of the problem may not be recognized.

Memory can be divided into 3 types: (a) registration which holds incoming information for 1-2 seconds in sensory storage; (b) immediate memory, short-term storage lasting from about 30 seconds to 2-3 minutes, especially if sustained by rehearsal and repetition (which lengthens the duration of the memory trace); and (c) long-term memory which stores, consolidates, and organizes information (Lezak, 1983). Remote memory is frequently less impacted by brain injury than short-term memory.

Many of the injured individuals who complain about memory dysfunction are actually experiencing difficulties with attention or concentration. The inability to maintain attention or concentration prevents appropriate responding or retrieving needed information. Another factor in memory function relates to the type of task involved. Recognition occurs when choices are available for selection, such as in a multiple-choice task. Recall is memory without any supportive stimuli, such as seen on essay tests or short-answer tasks. Some deficits are observed only when the task is unstructured.

Other deficits are specific to a particular type of information or modality. For example, individuals may have retained a fund of knowledge, such as involved in speech and reading, but not personal information related to their own lives. They may be able to spell words without recognizing their meaning. Although learning and memory problems can be distinguished in testing and structured tasks, the functional limitations are very similar. Memory problems affect the individual's ability to perform complex problem-solving or thinking (requiring chaining ideas), goal formulation, and planning.

*Seizures*

Approximately 5% of closed head injuries result in seizure disorder. In contrast, 30-45% of people suffering a penetrating injury develop seizures (Muller-Rothman, 1987). Seizures may occur very shortly after injury or as late as many years later. Over half the people who will have seizures will experience them in the first year.

The more serious the injury, the greater the risk of seizures. Seizures are a greater risk when injury is due to bullets or high velocity missiles, wounds that tear the dura mater, depressed skull fractures or foreign bodies penetrating brain tissue, intracranial hematoma and bleeding, infections or hemiplegia, aphasia, or focal effects. Forty percent of all patients who later develop seizures do not show epileptiform activity on an EEG prior to their first seizure (Newcombe, 1969).

The individual profile, types of seizures, and frequency of seizures should be evaluated when assessing vocational options for an injured worker. In general, seizures will prevent the individual from retaining a driver's license. This means that transportation will need to be provided through other means (e.g., public transit, friends or relatives, coworkers, or taxi). A person with seizures should not operate dangerous machinery or work at heights. Because seizures may render the individual unconscious or unable to function for a period of time, jobs involving working alone should be avoided (e.g., security guard, night nurse in a chronic care facility, home daycare provider). The probability of seizures are frequently increased by physical exercise, fatigue, or emotional stress. One needs to consider these factors based on the individual characteristics of the seizure profile.

# LIKELIHOOD OF FURTHER INJURY

Parker (1990) observed that the effects of brain damage are cumulative. An individual with a prior brain injury is more likely to suffer greater deficits following minor head trauma than someone with no prior history. Strub and Black (1988) similarly observed that "the effect of each succeeding injury becomes more significant, recovery is slower, and eventually permanent brain damage can result" (p. 324).

Therefore, after an injury, there should be an avoidance of occupations that have a higher likelihood of repeated injury. The counselor should evaluate carefully any jobs that involve climbing, balancing, driving, contact with aggressive people, or similar activities that increase the likelihood of head injury. Professional athletes are at a high risk of repeated injury.

# RETURN TO WORK

Injured employees frequently attempt to return to work too soon. As described by Strub and Black (1988):

> The patient feels well enough to return to work but finds that he cannot keep his mind on the job and forgets details that were easily retained previously. Because the medical release mentions no neurological abnormalities, employers often interpret the patient's complaints as a deliberate attempt to avoid work or to get a greater amount of compensation (p. 320).

As a result, the relationship between the employee and employer is damaged, perhaps irreparably. Strub and Black (1988) recommended that people be put on a gradually increasing work schedule and that both employee and employer be warned of the possible sequelae of brain injury.

Caplan and Shechter (1991) reported that many people found problems when they returned to work, such as headaches, irritability, sensitivity to noise, and impaired memory or concentration. They were initially unable to work in their former capacity. However, those who remained off work for a longer period, had fewer problems. Clinicians working with individuals who have sustained minor head trauma should use caution and a phased resumption of work, if possible. The client should not be returned to competitive work or an academic program until maximum recovery has been reached. Vocational rehabilitation counselors working with brain injured individuals are careful to pace the return to work to ensure maximum success.

# REHABILITATION POTENTIAL

A rehabilitation counselor should be involved as soon as possible with a head injured individual to work as part of the initial rehabilitation team. In the early stages, before the client's condition has stabilized, the counselor can provide a job analysis of the client's current employment for review by all the medical professionals. Using this job analysis, a clear evaluation of the client's functional skills and work restrictions can be established before attempting a trial period at work.

## *Job Analysis*

Success is most likely when the injured worker returns to a job and setting that is already familiar. Skills that have already been learned are less often affected by the head injury than the ability to learn new skills. Transferable skills are more important with clients with brain injury than with any other caseload. It is crucial that the counselor use retained information and well-learned behaviors in seeking to return the injured worker to suitable, gainful employment.

A job analysis should include a full **task analysis** of the activities that the injured worker performed on the job with consideration of the cognitive, social, and physical components of the task. In many positions, there are requirements that the employee is able to (a) interpret and analyze data, (b) make decisions based on factual data, (c) plan and schedule projects, (d) respond and adapt quickly to new information or procedures, (e) change activities rapidly, and (f) perform any or all of these activities under stress.

Social interactions are very important to include in a job analysis. Among the social factors evaluated are (a) people with whom the injured worker will interact (e.g., coworkers, customers, supervisors), (b) types of interactions (e.g., providing information, resolving problems, following instructions), (c) complexity of the verbal behaviors required, and (d) the number and speed of interactions. Some jobs require a large number of social interactions in a relatively fixed format, while other jobs may involve fewer social interactions but more complex language comprehension.

In evaluating tasks, the counselor makes certain that speed of performance is carefully evaluated. Even when this function appears otherwise normal, slowness in responding can interfere with employment.

In addition, fatigue can limit the types of jobs that the injured worker can do. Fatigue is highly detrimental to recovery. Tasks requiring high levels of concentration are likely to increase fatigue, as are tasks involving physical exertion. Even after a minor head injury, individuals are told to avoid physical or mental effort if they experience an exacerbation of symptoms. Fatigue may also affect balance and coordination, increasing the likelihood of other types of injuries in jobs that involve working with dangerous machinery or driving. As a general rule, workers who have suffered head injury should avoid jobs that involve working at heights or climbing, at least until all of the symptoms have resolved.

The type of employment setting is also important. The counselor needs to note the presence of potentially dangerous materials (e.g., moving machinery, hazardous equipment). Parker (1990) noted that the likelihood of further injury increases after brain damage because the person's judgment and coordination may be somewhat more deficient. While some people with head injury have good tolerance for outside work, the majority should seek protection from the weather and more sedentary work with less physical activities.

The employee's performance in a noisy and confusing setting is likely to be diminished following brain injury. The effort to screen out distractions while concentrating will increase fatigue and reduce frustration tolerance.

## Evaluation Techniques

During the medical recovery period, the injured worker may be seeing a cognitive psychologist, occupational therapist, physical therapist, and speech pathologist. These professionals provide the rehabilitation counselor with extensive test results and information regarding functioning. The most valuable information will be given if they use a detailed job analysis to assess the injured worker's skills and abilities.

## Work Hardening

The best method of work hardening is a part-time, trial period at work or school. After obtaining a job analysis and reviewing it with the treatment team, the counselor and the employer can design a return to work plan which will maximize the injured worker's success. For maximum effectiveness, the specific tasks and daily hours of employment will be controlled in the beginning and the counselor will observe the injured worker's performance on-site. Additional tasks and time can be added as the injured worker demonstrates the ability to assume these tasks. The counselor's role is gradually decreased as the injured worker becomes more proficient at the job.

## Retraining

Where retraining is necessary, it should follow the same principles of utilizing the injured worker's transferable skills, and careful introduction of tasks as the worker demonstrates an ability to perform them. The counselor is instrumental in selecting appropriate and realistic training programs.

# CASE STUDY

Ms. Sylvia Blanco is a 28 year-old loan officer who worked for a bank at the time of injury. Raised in Mexico, she immigrated to the United States with her family when she was 16 years of age. While in the United States, she learned English and received an Associate of Arts (A.A.) degree at the age of 20. She began working for the bank as a teller when she was 20 and had been promoted consistently during her 8 years of employment.

Bank teller, **D.O.T.#** 211.362-018 (U.S. Department of Labor, 1991), involves lifting and carrying a maximum of 15 pounds, with repetitive lifting and carrying of 5-10 pounds. Ms. Blanco performed the job standing or sitting, as the bank provided a stool for the tellers that wanted or needed to sit. Most of the tellers alternated sitting and standing throughout the work shift. It typically takes 6-12 months to learn this job. The bank promoted Sylvia consistently during her 8 years of employment. Her most recent position at the bank was loan officer.

Sylvia was injured in a car accident when delivering some loan documents to a bank customer. Following the injury, she was unconscious for 4 days.

When referred for vocational assessment approximately 8 months after the injury, Sylvia reported that she was not able to return to work. She suffered headaches on a daily basis and spent most of the day lying down, rarely watching television or reading, because both activities increased her headaches. Ms. Blanco could not walk for long periods because of dizziness, fatigue, and back pain. Noise and large groups of people gave her headaches, so she avoided people. Her speech was slow but appeared fluent; physical movements were slow and she frequently touched walls or furniture for balance when walking. A housekeeper was paid by the workers' compensation carrier to clean her house, but Sylvia had resumed responsibility for shopping and cooking.

Medical reports indicated that she had a light work restriction due to a back injury that was diagnosed 6 months after the original injury. The cognitive assessment conducted 6 months after the accident showed problems with concentration, memory, attention, and word retrieval. Physical therapy, speech pathology, and other ancillary services had ended before the referral for vocational rehabilitation. Ms. Blanco had participated in biofeedback to reduce her headaches and provide pain control; she refused to take medications for pain.

On untimed multiple-choice academic tests, Sylvia had above average skills in vocabulary, reading, spelling, grammar, arithmetic operations, and problem-solving. Especially strong in mathematics, she reported liking work with numbers. However, she took approximately three times the average amount of time to complete these tests. After an hour of concentration, she would have a headache and terminate the testing. She had typing skills but could not tolerate the noise of a typewriter.

The rehabilitation counselor conducted a thorough job analysis of her job as a loan officer, (DOT #186.267-018), shortly after the vocational referral. As a loan officer, Sylvia examined, evaluated, authorized, or recommended approval of customer applications for lines or extension of lines of credit, commercial loans, and real estate loans. This involved reviewing the loan application for completeness, analyzing the applicant's financial status, credit, and property to determine the feasibility of granting the loan request. She interviewed applicants applying for loans to elicit information, prepared the loan request papers, and obtained related documents from applicants, such as blueprints and construction reports. The loan officer corresponded with the applicant or creditors to resolve questions regarding applications and investigated the applicant's background to verify credit and bank references. The applicants were then informed whether the loan requests had been approved or rejected. If the loan was accepted, the loan office completed the loan agreement. Ms. Blanco prepared forms for forwarding to insuring agencies. The job involved supervising a loan assistant and a secretary.

The work of a loan officer at the bank involves lifting and carrying a maximum of 20 pounds with frequent lifting of paperwork. It is primarily a seated job and takes over 2 years to learn.

Data analysis was a major part of the job and there were continual interruptions, multiple ongoing projects, and complex interactions with applicants and loan agencies. The job involves decision-making and analysis with no clear-cut guidelines or standards. There were stringent deadlines that had to be met in funding or approving loans. Sylvia's secretary reported that the telephone rang 3-4 times per hour and each call involved a new problem or task. Prior to her injury, Ms. Blanco frequently worked 10 hours per day. A general survey showed that most banks were as fast-paced and stressful as where Sylvia worked.

Ms. Blanco frequently drove to people's homes and to lenders' offices. Although she was able to drive, she reported that she was frightened when driving because it was difficult to pay attention to the cars, the road, the lights, and where she was going. The counselor observed that she drove slower than the speed limit and tended to stop too far behind stop signs and traffic lights.

When specific documents were brought to Sylvia, she demonstrated an understanding of the purpose for the document and the standards to be met in completing the forms. She was unable to take messages over the telephone or to follow rapid speech. Her total span for continuous activity was approximately one hour with rest periods up to 30 minutes.

Contact was made with the employer. The employer was unwilling to offer modified work even for 1-2 hours per day. A slow course of rehabilitation was begun through classes at the local college. The coursework included basic skill development courses in mathematics, spelling, and vocabulary to increase her speed and fluency. At the same time, Ms. Blanco was adapting to the group setting and learning to concentrate in a relatively distracting environment. Initially, she experienced an increase in headaches and fatigue, which stabilized after about two months. At the end of one semester, she was able to maintain her attention and concentration levels for 4 hours on a consistent basis.

## Questions

1. Provide a vocational profile for Ms. Sylvia Blanco, including age category, educational level, and work history (skill and exertional levels).

2. What are the occupationally significant characteristics of her jobs? Which characteristics may impact employment considering her disability and limitations?

3. What are the skills that Sylvia has acquired in her prior occupations that might be transferred to other employment?

4. What are the barriers this client faces in returning to suitable, gainful employment?

5. What other methods could be used to increase Sylvia's stamina and improve her ability to work consistently?

6. What types of jobs might be appropriate for Ms. Blanco when her stamina improves if she still has difficulty concentrating in the presence of multiple stimuli and continues to process information slowly?

# REFERENCES

American Psychiatric Association (1987). **Diagnostic and statistical manual of mental disorders (DSM-III-R)** (3rd ed). Washington, DC: Author.

Anderson, T.P. (1981). Stroke and cerebral trauma: Medical aspects. In W.G. Stolov & M.R. Clowers (Eds.), **Handbook of severe disability**. Washington, DC: U.S. Department of Education, Rehabilitation Services Administration.

Brodal, A. (1981). **Neurological anatomy in relation to clinical medicine**. New York: Oxford University Press.

Brooks, D.N., Aughton, M.E., Bond, M.R., Jones, P., & Rizvi, S. (1980). Cognitive sequaleae in relationship to early indices of severity of brain damage after severe blunt head injury. **Journal of Neurology, Neurosurgery, and Psychiatry, 43**, 529-534.

Caplan, B., & Schechter, J.A. (1991). Vocational capacity with cognitive impairment. In S.J. Scheer (Ed.), **Medical perspectives in vocational assessment of impaired workers.** Gaithersburg, MD: Aspen.

Durgin, C.J., Rath, B., & Dales, E. (1991). The cost of caring. **Continuing Care, 10**, 20-29.

Fowler, R.S. (1981). Stroke and cerebral trauma: Psychosocial and vocational aspects. In W.G. Stolov & M.R. Clowers (Eds.), **Handbook of severe disability**. Washington, DC: U.S. Department of Education, Rehabilitation Services Administration.

Fraser, R., Dikmen, S., McLean, A., & Miller, B. (1988). Employability of head injury survivors: First year post-injury. **Rehabilitation Counseling Bulletin, 31,** 276-288.

Jarvis, P.E., & Barth, J.T. (1984). **Halstead-Reitan Test Battery: An interpretive guide.** Odessa, FL: Psychological Assessment Resources.

Lezak, M.D. (1983). **Neuropsychological assessment.** New York: Oxford University Press.

Maloney, M.P. (1985). **A clinician's guide to forensic psychological assessment.** New York: The Free Press.

Muller-Rothman, J. (1987). The medical aspects of disabling conditions. In B. Caplan (Ed.), **Rehabilitation psychology desk reference.** Rockville, MD: Aspen Publications.

Newcombe, F. (1969). **Missile wounds of the brain.** London: Oxford University Press.

O'Shaughnessy, E.J., Fowler, R.S., & Reid, V. (1984). Sequelae of mild closed head injuries. **Journal of Family Practice, 18,** 391-394.

Parker, R.S. (1990). **Traumatic brain injury and neuropsychological impairment.** New York: Springer-Verlag.

Rimel, R.W., Giordani, B., Barth J.T., Boll, T.J., & Jane, M.A. (1982). Disability caused by minor head injury. **Neurosurgery, 11,** 221-228.

Rosenthal, M. (1987). Traumatic head injury: Neurobehavioral consequences. In B. Caplan (Ed.), **Rehabilitation psychology desk reference.** Rockville, MD: Aspen.

Shordone, R.J. (1987). A neuropsychological approach to cognitive rehabilitation within a private practice setting. In B. Caplan (Ed.), **Rehabilitation psychology desk reference.** Rockville, MD: Aspen.

Strub, R.L., & Black, F.W. (1988). **Neurobehavioral disorders: A clinical approach.** Philadelphia, PA: F.A. Davis.

U.S. Department of Labor (1991). **Dictionary of occupational titles** (4th ed., revised). Washington, DC: Author.

Varney, N.R., Martzke, J.S., & Roberts, R.J. (1987). Major depression in patients with closed head injury. **Neuropsychology, 1,** 7-9.

Walsh, K. (1990). **Neuropsychology: A clinical approach.** New York: Churchill Livingstone.

Yarnell P.R., & Rossie,, G.V. (1988). Minor whiplash head injury with major debilitation. **Brain Injury, 2,** 255-258.

## *About the Author*

Susan Vanost Wulz, Ph.D., is in private practice in rehabilitation counseling in Santa Ana, California. She is an independent vocational evaluator for the Rehabilitation Unit, Division of Industrial Accidents, State of California. Her book, **Rehabilitation: The California System,** co-authored with Leonard Silberman and published in 1988, is widely used by workers' compensation professionals throughout California.

# Chapter 31

# LEARNING DISABILITIES

by
*Jack Little, Ph.D.*

## INTRODUCTION

Learning disabilities are not a new phenomenon. It has long been recognized that some individuals fail to master basic academic skills, although provided with adequate instruction. It was noted more than 300 years ago that some individuals lose reading abilities due to head injury. In 1676, Schidt described this, while in 1877 Kussmaul referred to such a reading loss as **alexia** or word blindness. Berlin, in 1877, suggested the use of the term **dyslexia** for the partial loss of reading ability (Critchley, 1970).

The British physician James Hinshelwood (1917) supported the earlier findings when he described the loss of the ability to read in a group of brain-damaged adults. Hinshelwood coined the term "word blindness" which he defined as the inability to interpret written or printed language, while possessing normal vision.

Kurt Goldstein (1936, 1939) working with brain-damaged World War I soldiers, noted a set of behaviors which included preservation, distractibility, inability to deal with abstractions, figure-ground problems, and catastrophic reactions. Alfred A. Strauss and Heinz Werner, a neuropsychiatrist and developmental psychologist who had worked with Goldstein, fled Germany after the start of World War II. Influenced by Goldstein's work, Strauss and Werner began working with brain-injured, mentally retarded children at the Wayne County Training School in Northville, Michigan. They noted that many of these children demonstrated behaviors similar to those noted by Goldstein in brain-damaged soldiers and, from their findings, inferred underlying brain damage (Strauss & Werner, 1942; Werner & Strauss, 1940, 1941). Their findings led to the development of new concepts regarding the treatment and educational needs of children with nongenetic retardation and set the foundation for what was to become the field of "Learning Disabilities."

Strauss went on to establish the Cove School in Racine, Wisconsin. There, with the educational director Laura Lehtinen, he developed further refinements to the definition and treatment of the brain-injured child. The work of Strauss, his associates, and students at the Wayne County Training School and Cove School, was summarized in the classic **Psychopathology and Education of the Brain-Injured Child** (Strauss and Lehtinen, 1947).

While much of what Strauss and Lehtinen reported was based upon work with post-natally, brain-damaged, mentally retarded children, they recognized that some nonretarded children exhibited similar patterns of behavior. They attributed this to unidentified or undiagnosed brain injury.

William Cruickshank, a scholar at the Wayne County Training School, was the first to apply the findings of Werner and Strauss to individuals who were not retarded. Cruickshank, Bentzen, Ratzeburg, and Tannhauser (1961) designed the Montgomery County Project to study the educational innovations suggested by Strauss and Lehtinen. The children who were the subjects of the study were of normal or near normal intelligence. While the children were not retarded, they exhibited the behavioral characteristics associated with brain injury although this could not be demonstrated in all cases. Their work, along with that of Norris Haring, E. Lakin Phillips, Marianne Frostig, Samuel Kirk, and Helmer Myklebust brought still further attention to this group of individuals.

Prior to 1950, those children who appeared to lack the ability to master specific academic skills, while demonstrating normal behavior in other aspects of their lives, were often placed in educational programs for the mentally retarded. During the decade between 1950 and 1960, parents, educators, and other professionals demonstrated an increasing awareness of the inappropriateness of such placements. The increased awareness of the differences between the population of individuals with mental retardation and those of average or near average intelligence who failed to learn, resulted in the establishment of numerous special programs. These programs were designed to meet the unique learning needs of this group.

Causative factors were (and are) poorly understood although it is assumed by many that the basis of the learning problems is in some way neurological or the result of some type of brain injury. Labels such as Strauss Syndrome, Minimal Brain Dysfunction, Brain Injured, Brain Damaged, Neurologically Handicapped, and Psychoneurological Dysfunction were frequently used to describe this population. In some instances, labels which described behavioral characteristics seen in some of these individuals were used (e.g., the Hyperactive Child Syndrome or the Clumsy Child Syndrome). The debate as to what these children should be called to differentiate them from other groups of special needs children continued until the latter part of the 1960s.

## *Definitions*

Dr. Samuel Kirk of the University of Illinois first suggested the term "learning disabilities." His suggestion was in response to a meeting of concerned parents and professionals who were attempting to find a term to describe that group of children who experience school failure but do not demonstrate primary mental retardation, brain damage, sensory deficit, physical disability, or emotional disturbance (Kirk, 1963). The term was readily accepted but lead to an on-going controversy regarding the most appropriate definition.

In 1968, the National Advisory Committee on Handicapped Children (NACHC) was formed, under the leadership of Kirk, to develop a definition of "Learning Disabilities" which would be generally acceptable. The NACHC definition was included in the **First Annual Report of the National Advisory Committee on Handicapped Children:**

> Children with special learning disabilities exhibit a disorder in one or more of the basic psychological processes involved in understanding or in using spoken or written language. These may be manifested in disorders of listening, thinking, talking, reading, writing, spelling, or arithmetic. They include conditions which have been referred to as perceptual handicaps, brain injury, minimal brain dysfunction, dyslexia, developmental aphasia, etc. They do not include learning problems which are due primarily to visual, hearing, or motor handicaps to mental retardation, emotional disturbance, or to environmental disadvantage. (p. 34)

The NACHC definition was incorporated into Public Law 91- 230, **The Learning Disability Act of 1969.** There has been considerable dissatisfaction with the NACHC definition.

The primary issues of debate surrounding the NACHC's 1968 definition are the following:

1. The limit imposed by the use of the term **children**. Learning disabilities occur at all age levels.

2. The term **basic psychological processes** has resulted in ongoing controversy due to its association with the neurological orientation and **abilities model** related to learning disabilities.

3. The parallels drawn between learning disabilities and other conditions is misleading and inexact.

4. The fact that learning disabilities may be present with other handicapping conditions, but do not result from such conditions as mental retardation or sensory impairment, has been obscured.

After numerous unsatisfactory attempts to improve the NACHC definition, it was incorporated into Public Law 94-142, the **Education for All Handicapped Children Act** (1975) with only minor changes. Public Law 94-142 became effective in 1977. The definition was not changed in the **Reauthorization of the Education of the Handicapped Act** (1986). However, there is an on-going debate as to the accuracy and appropriateness of this definition of **learning disabilities**. Alternatives have been suggested, but at the present time the NACHC definition, as modified, is still the most accepted definition.

## *Increased Understanding*

During the 1960s and through the 1970s it was generally assumed that learning disabilities could be "cured." The assumption was that basic psycholinguist and perceptual-motor dysfunctions resulted in the failure of the child to develop skills prerequisite to academic success. It was believed that early identification and intervention through the perceptual-motor skill and psycholinguistic training programs (ability training) would result in remediation of the dysfunctions. The development of a greater knowledge base, through research and application of various remedial practices, has forced a reconsideration of this position.

Efforts to remediate learning disabilities through ability training, have been demonstrated to be less effective than originally thought. Consequently, attention has shifted to behaviorally and cognitively oriented instruction. There has been considerably more interest in strategies for learning, and the recognition and regulation of how individuals learn (Reid, 1988). Additional emphasis is also being placed upon teaching individuals to circumvent their deficits by learning alternative approaches to problem solving through the application of technology (Mercer, 1987).

The 1980s was a period in which both professionals and the public became increasingly aware that learning disabilities are not confined to early or middle childhood, but persist into adolescence and adulthood. It also became obvious that learning disabilities not only involve academic areas, but extend into all aspects of the affected individual's life.

The psychosocial implications of learning disabilities are becoming better understood. Individuals with learning disabilities have deficits in their ability to activate and utilize the processes of attention, perception, and memory in an interactive manner. Consequently, they are limited in their ability to process information as do the majority of the population. Individuals who perceive the world, or process information, differently from the general population behave differently. Therefore, individuals with learning disabilities must frequently be taught specifically what the majority of the population learn incidentally.

# ETIOLOGY OF LEARNING DISABILITIES

The causes of learning disabilities are at best unclear. There is evidence that some learning disabilities appear to be the result of acquired trauma. Drug and alcohol consumption during pregnancy, as well as exposure to other toxic substances may cause harm to a fetus. Gold and Sherry reviewed the literature and found a direct relationship between maternal consumption of alcohol during pregnancy and later learning disabilities (Mercer, 1987).

Birth complications have frequently been associated with later problems in learning. The reduction in oxygen supply (hypoxia) or total loss of oxygen (anoxia), prematurity, extended labor, induced birth, forceps deliver, and other birth complications are more frequent in individuals who are identified as having learning disabilities than in the population.

Postnatal traumas resulting in head injuries, or diseases resulting in high fevers, have frequently been assumed to cause learning disabilities. It appears that while this may be so in some cases, not all such experiences result in learning disabilities. The diseases or accidents that result in learning disabilities appear to have to be specific to a certain area of the brain or occur at a particular age. It is not questioned that such damage may result in learning disabilities, but at the present time, just when and under what circumstances is unknown.

There are on-going investigations designed to explore support for the hypothesis that heredity plays a part in learning disabilities. Hermann's (1959) twin studies indicated that all the identical twins he studied (12 pairs) appeared to have similar problems with learning, while fraternal twins (33 pairs) yielded only a 33% chance of having similar problems. While there have not been sufficient studies to substantiate that heritability factors are related to learning disabilities, evidence does support such a relationship.

There has been a great deal of speculation about the possible relationship of learning disabilities to biochemical imbalance. However, there is little support in the literature for this position. Feingold (1976) postulated a theory of allergic response to certain foods and food additives. Allergic reactions to foods, milk, wheat, and other substances have been noted and linked to learning problems, but the evidence of such a relationship is inconclusive.

# SYMPTOMATOLOGY

Learning disabilities may occur in isolation from, or in the presence of, other handicapping conditions. Such disabilities may be identified in the intellectually gifted or in the mentally retarded. However, such disabilities are discrete. That is, they are separate from other disabilities and are not caused by, nor do they cause, other disabilities. Learning disabilities are frequently not obvious to the casual observer. They are demonstrated through inefficient and ineffective learning strategies which frequently result in school failure. Further, productivity is a frequent problem. Many individuals with learning disabilities do not use the knowledge or strategies they have.

## Characteristic Behaviors

Behaviors characteristic of individuals with learning disabilities can be discerned in several areas:

1. Pre-academic or Academic Performance

2. Social Competence

3. Self-control

4. Self-concept

5. Motivation

**Identification.** Individuals with learning disabilities are usually first identified as a result of their failure to master those skills which are age or grade-appropriate. In more severe cases, parents report delays in the development of independent eating skills, toilet training, and both language acquisition and competence. It is reported that these children often demonstrate frustration and respond impulsively, appearing to lack the ability to concentrate on any one thing for more than a short period. They are frequently demanding, obsessive, and dependent, yet inquisitive and eager to please.

The less severe cases are usually not recognized until the child enters school. The early signs of learning disabilities are often dismissed as developmental lags, or due to inexperience. Recently, there has been an increased emphasis on early identification and intervention with children who appear to be at risk of developing learning disabilities.The majority of children are identified due to their repeated failures to achieve in the areas of reading or mathematics. However, on closer observation, other deficiencies are usually noted. Deficits are observed in the ability of the child to strategize, organize, and execute tasks in an efficient, effective, age-appropriate manner. This frequently results in both academic and social failure.

**Social skills.** Social competence is built upon the ability of the individual to perceive that which is occurring within a social environment, determine an appropriate response, and take action accordingly. Individuals with learning disabilities frequently demonstrate deficient or distorted social perception. Without intervention, both academic failure and social incompetence become more acute, hence more observable, with age.

Social skills and social competence in adolescents and young adults with learning disabilities has been the focus of considerable recent research. White, Schumaker, Warner, Alley, and Deshler (1980) reported that young adults with learning disabilities are less likely to participate in social activities and more likely to be underemployed than their nonhandicapped peers. Deshler and Schumaker (1983) reported that learning disabled adolescents participated less in school activities than any other group. Schumaker and Hazel (1984) found that individuals with learning disabilities tended to exhibit deficits in both social skills and social competence.

**Self-control.** With increasing age, many individuals with learning disabilities display an increase in the lack of self-control. They frequently do not take the time to assess a situation and develop an appropriate response strategy. Gresham (1986) proposed four causes for four types of social deficits. Among those proposed were **self-control skill deficit** and **self-control performance deficit**. A self-control skill deficit is the result of inadequate learning of a social skill due to emotional interference. Self-control performance deficits occur when the person is incapable of performing a social skill which has been learned due to behavior occurring just prior to the demand for a specific social skill, or what is perceived as the consequence of performing the social skill.

Many adolescents with learning disabilities tend to act on impulse. This is demonstrated by the number of errors, or social "blunders" made in attempting to accomplish an assignment or social goal without attending to the response requirements of the task prior to attempting it. Inappropriate social and nonsocial responses may be the result of the same type of behavior. The result of such behaviors is a predictably high rate of failure, both socially and academically.

**Learned helplessness.** Repeated failure often results in learned helplessness, behavior problems, or both. Learned helplessness is a strategy used by students who have not developed more appropriate problem-solving. It is typified by the individual who requires or demands constant supervision and direction to accomplish a task. They assume a roll of helplessness, hence dependency. The dependency upon external sources for direction reduces the individual's need to develop efficient organizational skills and problem-solving strategies. Further, it reduces the necessity of being responsible for one's own behavior. Such behavior is consistent with locus of control factors typical of many children and adults with learning disabilities. That is, they tend to perceive their successes and failures as resulting from **external** rather than **internal** forces - they are controlled by fate rather than controlling their own fate. The outcome of abdicating responsibility for one's own behavior and assuming a role of helplessness, is usually reduced self-esteem and the development of a poor self-concept.

**Behavior problems.** Many individuals with learning disabilities present significant behavior problems. Repeated failure experiences resulting from both affective and learning problems, may produce a high level of anxiety. Anxiety can interfere with the attention and concentration to task, producing more failure and increased anxiety. This destructive cycle may produce still greater fear of failure and feelings of hopelessness as well as helplessness and depression. Anxiety also can result in what appears as hyperactive, defiant, or aggressive behavior. Increased irritability, distractibility, and resistance to structure are common. The introduction of a new task or new routine may produce increased or renewed anxiety. Repeated failure experiences tend to reduce the willingness of individuals with learning disabilities to take risks. Noncompliance, disruptive behavior, or withdrawal may be used as a strategy to escape new tasks, or tasks where failure has been previously experienced.

## Self-Concept

How one perceives oneself, or self-concept, is primarily a cognitive function (Bandura, 1977). Self-concept is developed over time, based upon life experience. Adolescents and adults with learning disabilities often recognize their own strengths and weaknesses. They recognize that they have problems related to organization and the execution of specific tasks. Also, they may be aware that they have difficulty in the direct application of many of the strategies they have developed, or the knowledge they have acquired, when confronted with problems to solve. This leads to frustration and threatens self-esteem. Many adolescents and adults with learning disabilities will refuse to perform a task or pretend ignorance rather than attempt tasks which they believe may result in failure. While this behavior may be observed as a lack of motivation, it is more probably a way of coping with self-perceived deficits (Pullis, 1983).

## *Motivation*

This comes from within. That is, when an individual is confronted with a moderate level of the unfamiliar, within a familiar setting, there is a drive to seek a balance. When a task or situation is very familiar, or very unfamiliar, this drive is weakened. Individuals who have not developed adequate organizational skills, or efficient and effective problem-solving strategies, tend to look upon each new encounter as highly unfamiliar. They do not have the prerequisite skills necessary to plan and execute the actions required to adequately respond to the situation. Consequently, motivation to seek a resolution is diminished and the encounter may elicit no response or an impulsive, non-strategized response.

## *Feelings of Inadequacy*

Individuals with learning disabilities are used to failure. They have experienced the embarrassment, guilt, ridicule, and frequent rejection from their peers, associated with both academic and social incompetence, from their earliest school experiences. This, naturally, leads to feelings of failure, depression, and helplessness. Such feelings, in turn, tends to substantiate their feelings of inadequacy and negatively affect their motivational set.

# DIAGNOSIS, EVALUATION, AND ASSESSMENT

The identification and assessment of individuals with learning disabilities is an area of on-going debate for which there is no easy answer. The debate centers on several issues:

1. Professionals in the field of learning disabilities have not been able to agree on a definition. This has resulted in different interpretations from state to state and considerable variation in the criteria used to determine the existence of a learning disability.

2. The within group differences found among individuals with learning disabilities has made the task of developing consistent identification criteria extremely difficult. Criteria which identify all individuals with learning disabilities, but do not include individuals who do not have learning disabilities, have not been developed.

3. The identification and determination of a significant discrepancy between achievement and ability has not been adequately defined or operationalized.

4. The adequacy of the procedures and instruments used for the determination of the existence of a learning disability is still to be determined. The lack of valid, reliable procedures and instruments to be used to identify individuals with learning disabilities may have resulted in frequent misdiagnoses.

Regardless of the debates over definition and criteria to be used to determine eligibility to receive special education services, Mercer (1987) reported that if mildly disabled learners are included, the prevalence figure would probably be between 4-5%. This figure appears to be growing. Reynolds (1985) indicated that the number of individuals with learning disabilities is growing so rapidly as to jeopardize the existence of learning disability programs.

# THE PURPOSE OF ASSESSMENT

Assessment is accomplished for a purpose. Salvia and Ysseldyke (1988) specify the purposes:

1. Screening - a review of student performance characteristics used to detect those students who require more in-depth study due to possible learning problems.

2. Referral - a request for assistance from other professional personnel. This includes observation, and review of classroom performance leading to a request for evaluation.

3. Classification - assessment leading to determination of eligibility to receive special education services and determination of classification under which those services are authorized.

4. Instructional Planning - assessment information used to assist in the development of the Individual Education Plan (IEP), including goals and objectives.

5. Monitoring Student Progress - to maintain an on-going evaluation of student achievement and progress.

Public Law 94-142 insures that all handicapped children receive a free, appropriate public education. This includes the right to a thorough nondiscriminatory assessment, an individualized educational program designed to meet the student's specific needs, placement within the least restrictive educational environment, and designated services as required to insure the success of the educational program.

The identification and assessment of individuals with learning disabilities is a complex task. The focus of the criteria for identifying learning disabled students as stated in the **Federal Register**, December 29, 1977, is on academic achievement in relation to ability and the exclusionary provisions. However, many individuals lack social skills which may be just as debilitating as their academic problems (Schumaker & Hazel, 1984).

If assessment is to meet the purposes identified by Salvia and Ysseldyke (1988), it must be designed to identify and describe both deficits and strengths. The identification of deficits may serve as the basis for the determination of eligibility, but the identification and specification of what skills and content have been mastered provides the starting point for the development of an appropriate educational plan. Additionally, the assessment of affective and motivational factors as well as the learning strategies used, may be as significant to the development of an appropriate educational plan as is knowledge of academic achievement.

The heterogeneity of individuals with learning disabilities requires that we make generalizations regarding their learning and behavior with great caution. There is a growing body of evidence that while, by definition, poor academic achievement is characteristic of individuals with learning disabilities, deficiencies in social skills, learning strategies, study skills, and motivation, as well as cognitive deficits, must be taken into consideration when designing educational programs. Assessment in these areas is frequently neglected.

The growing emphasis on early identification and intervention with young children with learning disabilities may result in a reduction in some of the deficits observed in adolescents and young adults. The reduced self-esteem, learned helplessness, depression, and lack of motivation to learn, so often associated with older students with learning disabilities, may be prevented with early intervention.

Assessment of adolescents and young adults with learning disabilities is even more complex than with children. Adolescents and young adults with learning disabilities may already demonstrate the debilitating effects of repeated failure experiences and, as a consequence, lack the willingness or motivation, to fully participate in assessment procedures.

# ASSESSMENT FOR REHABILITATION SERVICES

The vast majority of individuals seeking rehabilitation services due to learning disabilities already will have been identified as having learning disabilities. The terms, **disability** and **handicap**, are frequently used interchangeably. However, as Westman (1990) pointed out, **disability** refers to a person's condition, while a **handicap** exists when a disability significantly interferes with a person's functional ability to perform in a social, personal, or work environment and requires special consideration or accommodation. Assessment for the development of a rehabilitation plan must be focused on the specification of functional handicaps, determining the severity of the handicaps, and the identification of strengths.

An outline for such an assessment includes:

I. Assessment of the client:
  A. Physical factors:
    1. General health
      a. Sight
      b. Hearing
      c. Weight\nutrition
      d. Strength\stamina
    2. Motor functions
      a. Gross motor skills
      b. Fine motor skills
      c. Perceptual motor skills
    3. Neuropsychological functions
      a. Attention
      b. Perception
      c. Memory
  B. Social\Emotional
    1. Social skills
      a. Mastery of daily living skills
      b. Self-perception
      c. Sensitivity to others
      d. Social judgment
      e. Social competence
    2. Emotional status
      a. Self-concept
      b. Self-regard\esteem
      c. Self-control
      d. Level of independence
      e. Stability
      f. Motivation
  C. Cognitive\metacognitive
    1. Level
    2. Metacognitive strategies

a. Preplanning
b. Planning
c. Implementation
d. Self-monitoring
e. Evaluation
D. Academic
    1. Reading
        a. Functional level
        b. Application for problem-solving
    2. Mathematics
        a. Functional level
        b. Application for problem-solving
    3. Writing
        a. Functional level
        b. Effectiveness for communication
    4. Language
        a. Functional receptive oral language level
        b. Functional oral expressive language level
E. Vocational interests\skills
    a. Vocational awareness
    b. Vocational interests
    c. Pre-vocational skills
    d. Vocational skills
F. Avocational interests\pursuits
    1. Avocational interests
    2. Recreational activities
    3. Hobbies

II. **Assessment of work demands of specific vocational\avocational activities**
A. Identification of specific vocations\avocational activities
    1. Physical demands
    2. Social demands
    3. Academic skill requirements
    4. Specific skill requirements
B. Identification of required strategies

III. **Matching specific vocational\activity requirements to client skills\competencies**
A. Interests
B. Physical requirements and capabilities
C. Social\emotional demands and characteristics
D. Academic skill requirements and functional levels
E. Specific activity skill requirements and client skills\competencies

IV. **Determination of the "fitness" of the match**
A. Determination of compatibility of client and specific job\activity
    1. Identification of areas of "match"
    2. Identification of areas of "mismatch"
    3. Identification of specific training needs
    4. Development of an individualized training\educational plan

The assessment of the strengths and weaknesses of individuals with learning disabilities must not focus on skills alone. The functional capabilities of many individuals with learning disabilities may be as dependent upon the use of the skills and strategies they have mastered as on whether they have mastered such skills or strategies.

# TREATMENT

Historically, the instructional model which has been advocated for individuals with learning disabilities has frequently centered upon remediation of what were assumed to be underlying psychological process deficits. This approach provided the basis for the more sophisticated "cognitive processing" model.

Direct instruction is advocated by many of those who have developed cognitive approaches to instruction of individuals with learning disabilities (Lloyd & deBettencourt, 1982; Deshler, Schumaker, Lenz, & Ellis, 1984). The Institute for Research in Learning Disabilities at the University of Kansas (Lawrence, Kansas) has developed a Learning Strategies Curriculum (LSC). This curriculum was designed for direct instruction and attempted to eliminate many of the problems which had been associated with cognitive skills training (Deshler et al., 1984).

Rehabilitation activities designed to ensure individuals with learning disabilities the opportunity to compete socially, or in the job market, must take the following into consideration:

1. Learning disabilities is constituted of many different disabilities. The assessment plan must be designed to be broad-based, yet focus upon those disabilities which are demonstrated through inadequate application of strategies within the context of specific activities. That is, if the individual fails in an attempt to perform a task based upon written instructions, is the problem a reading problem or inadequate, or incomplete, knowledge of the strategies necessary to carry out instructions.

2. Generic strategy instruction frequently fails to generalize. Teaching generic strategies within the context of specific activities or work assignments may be more effective.

3. Rehabilitation programs for individuals with learning disabilities must include knowledge about cognition and the regulation of cognition (metacognition). Individuals must learn to think about how they learn and develop strategies, designed not only to ensure task completion, but which are age-appropriate and efficient. This may require that the individual select, evaluate, and even discard strategies which may have been appropriate earlier, under different circumstances, at a different age.

   The regulation of cognition requires that the individual plan, monitor, and evaluate the outcomes of the application of the strategies used to solve a problem to determine their effectiveness and efficiency. Such a procedure puts the individual in charge; the individual becomes internally regulated, rather than dependent for regulation from an external source.

4. Knowledge of the tasks to be performed and the reason behind such tasks is critical. Prior knowledge about the anticipated outcomes provides a basis for planning, monitoring, and evaluation. It also increases the probability that adjustments or modifications in work approaches or habits to meet the job requirements will be made.

5. Assumptions are frequently made that individuals with learning disabilities have a limited "capacity." However, such assumptions are often wrong. The individual with learning disabilities may demonstrate a functional capacity deficit, but have no structural capacity deficit. Such individuals can be taught to demonstrate greater capacity by directing their attention to the critical elements of a task, and through the identification and instruction in those strategies essential to effective and efficient completion of the assigned task.

6.  Perhaps the single most critical consideration in the development of a rehabilitation program for an individual with learning disabilities is establishment of a "match" between the individual and the objectives of the program. The analysis of the demands or requirements of the tasks for which the individual is being trained and the assessment of the individual provides the framework for the program. The individual with dysgraphia (difficulty with handwriting) will probably not develop the strategies necessary to become an outstanding calligrapher. However, such an individual may become adept at the selection of specific type faces and print sizes necessary to produce an attractive document.

Treatment plans for individuals with learning disabilities must be designed on an individual basis. Motivation, interest, and social competence may be the primary determiners of success. The development of a treatment program for an individual with learning disabilities should follow the same design as the treatment: (1) preplanning; (2) planning; (3) implementation; (4) monitoring; and (5) evaluation.

# FUNCTIONAL LIMITATIONS

The functional limitations of individuals with learning disabilities is dependent upon the unique characteristics of each individual. Physically, the vast majority have no limitations. Minor motor dysfunctions, "soft" neurological signs, impulsivity, distractibility, and hyperactivity are all frequently observed in such individuals. Whether or not such conditions constitute a functional limitation is dependent upon what they are asked to do. Albert Einstein, Woodrow Wilson, Thomas Edison, and Auguste Roden are all said to have had learning disabilities (Lerner, 1989). Some individuals with learning disabilities may be gifted (Waldron, Saphire, & Rosenblum, 1987).

# VOCATIONAL LIMITATIONS

The vocational limitations of individuals with learning disabilities is, of course, dependent upon the type of learning disability. However, Warner, Schumaker, Alley, and Deshler (1980), reported that individuals with learning disabilities plateau at the 4th to 5th grade level in academic achievement. Schumaker, Hazel, Sherman, and Sheldon (1982) found that adolescents with learning disabilities demonstrate deficits in social skills, when compared to adolescents who do not have learning disabilities.

The limitations experienced by individuals with learning disabilities, other than those of relatively low academic performance and a general lack of social competence, are individual, not specific. Problems related to self-concept, self-regard, and self-esteem are generally acknowledged, but are frequently viewed as components of social competence or motivation. Vocational limitations must be determined on an individual basis. Some individuals will be found to be excellent readers, yet have marginal skills in mathematics, while others will be non-readers and have excellent computation skills. Similar differences in social situations will also be found. Some will exhibit no lack of social competence, while others will be highly incompetent in specific social situations, and some lack minimal social skills. Perhaps the most effective way to determine an individual's vocational limitations is to observe that individual in the work setting.

Many individuals with learning disabilities have learned, or learn, to compensate for their disabilities. Consequently, the disability may not create a limitation and, therefore, will cease to be a handicap. That is one of the objectives of rehabilitation.

# REHABILITATION POTENTIAL

The rehabilitation potential of individuals with learning disabilities is dependent upon many variables. The type, severity, and age at when intervention is initiated are especially significant to rehabilitation potential. "Learning disabilities" must be viewed as a generic term encompassing learning problems which are either inherent to the individual or induced through environmental encounters. The primary types of learning disabilities can be grouped under the headings of "Social Competence Deficits," "Language Related Learning Disabilities," and "Learning Disabilities Related to Mathematics."

## *Social Competence Deficits*

The rehabilitation potential for social incompetence is high in many individuals with learning disabilities. Social skills, from which social competence is developed, can be taught. The development of strategies which allow for the appropriate application of such skills, hence demonstration of social competence, requires practice. The social potential of the individual can be realized only when classroom instruction is augmented by "real-life" experiences (i.e., experiences within the social structures where one is expected to become an independent, contributing member).

## *Language Related Learning Disabilities*

Language related learning disabilities affect all areas of human communication. Receptive and expressive language problems, as well as reading and writing problems, constitute the basis for identification of the majority of individuals with learning disabilities. Deficits in communication result in inadequate development of personal relationships, social skills, and vocational competencies. The assumption that such disabilities result from psychological processing dysfunctions has not been dismissed. However, attempts to accurately identify and remediate such dysfunctions has met with limited success. The "direct instruction" approach, whereby communication skills are taught and strategies to use those skills developed, appears to be the most promising approach.

The rehabilitation potential of individuals with language related learning disabilities are frequently situational specific. The potential success of the individual is dependent upon the demands of the tasks which will be required. Consequently, carefully reasoned consideration of both the learning characteristics of the individual and the demands to be made of that individual, must be made prior to the initiation of the rehabilitation program.

## *Learning Disabilities Related to Mathematics*

Learning disabilities related to mathematical reasoning and function are not as frequently encountered as disabilities related to reading and writing. However, such disabilities permeate all aspects of the life of the individual with this disability. Quantitative factors including time, space, mass, volume, and number play a critical role in human communication and understanding. Virtually every word in the English language carries a quantitative, qualitative, or dimensional connotation (e.g., "the" indicates one specific thing, while "a" or "an" indicates any one of a group of things). Even when an individual has mastered the basic operations of addition, subtraction, multiplication, and division, without a recognition and understanding of mathematical-logical constructs, that individual will demonstrate critical deficits in both the social and vocational arenas.

The rehabilitation potential of the individual with learning disabilities related to mathematics is dependent upon ability to first master the concepts, and secondly to formulate and apply the operations associated with those concepts. Examples include telling time, measuring, weighing, counting, and calculating. In this area, rehabilitation depends upon severity of deficit. In the most severe cases, rehabilitation must start with concept development. Less severe cases may only require specific skill development or the development of strategies for the determination and application of those skills which are required in specific social or vocational situations.

## Early Intervention

The majority of rehabilitation programs for individuals with learning disabilities are initiated at the secondary or post-secondary level. There is a growing awareness on the part of the professional community that the earlier the initiation of such a program, the higher the probability of success. Those individuals with learning disabilities who do not receive rehabilitation services are frequently incapable of becoming productive participants within society. Initiation of services at the point of identification and diagnosis, may result in a significant decrease in the cost to the public of supporting that individual in the future. Further, such a program appears justifiable as a "quality of life" issue, if for no other reason.

# CASE STUDY

Mary, a 22 year-old woman, has just graduated from a high school special education program. It had been determined that she was eligible to receive special education services, when she was 8 years old, due to a specific learning disability. She demonstrated a significant discrepancy between ability and performance in the areas of reading and writing. This individual also had a very short attention span, had difficulty with organization and planning, and was hyperactive. However, Mary is well within the normal range of ability.

For the majority of her elementary school years, Mary was in a special day class, but was placed in a program which stressed community-based instruction when she was in the 9th grade. Mary spent 3 hours per day in the special day class program and 2 hours per day in mainstream classes. The public school allowed her to continue attending public school beyond 18 years of age because she had not met all the goals and objectives as specified on her individual educational plan.

Mary enjoys talking and will initiate conversations with anyone who will attend to her. When people "won't listen" to her, she becomes frustrated. However, she tends to jump from one subject to another. Group living has not worked out well. The others in the house objected to her erratic behaviors (getting up at all times of night and cooking, forgetting to do her chores, among other things). Mary is currently living with her parents, but is seeking a different living arrangement.

The post-secondary part of Mary's education program stressed helping to prepare her for competitive employment. Her reading abilities are currently at the 2.4 grade level on standardized tests; her math scores are considerably higher (6.5 in computation and 7.2 in mathematical reasoning). The real challenge to employment is more closely related to social competence than academic performance. Mary is seeking employment in the produce department of a supermarket. At a supermarket, she will be required to have minimal contact with the public, but will have to work in an organized, systematic fashion with others. Organization of time, the development of appropriate strategies for getting to work on time, and effective interpersonal relations are the potential problems which have been identified by her counselor.

## Questions

1.  What types of services are available to Mary?

2. What services can be provided to accommodate her needs related to living arrangements?

3. Is the type of employment Mary is seeking realistic? Why?

4. What would you predict will be Mary's future? Explain?

# REFERENCES

Bandura, A. (1977). Self-efficacy: Toward a unifying theory of behavioral change. **Psychological Review, 84,** 191-215.

Critchley, M. (1970). **Aphasiology.** London, England: Edward Arnold.

Cruickshank, W.M., Bentzen, F.A., Ratzeburg, R.H., & Tannausher, M.T. (1961). **A teaching method for brain-injured and hyperactive children.** Syracuse, NY: Syracuse University Press.

Deshler, D.D., & Schumaker, J.B. (1983). Social skills of learning disabled adolescents: A review of characteristics and intervention. **Topics in Learning and Learning Disabilities, 3,** 15-23.

Deshler, D.D., Schumaker, J.B., Lenz, B.K., & Ellis, E. (1984). Academic and cognitive interventions for LD adolescents: Part I. **Journal of Learning Disabilities, 17**(3), 108-117.

Feingold, B.F. (1976). Hyperkineses and learning disabilities linked to the ingestion of artificial food colors and flavors. **Journal of Learning Disabilities, 32,** 48-55.

Goldstein, K. (1936). The modifications of behavior consequent to cerebral lesions. **Psychiatric Quarterly, 10,** 586-610.

Goldstein, K. (1939). **The organism.** New York, NY: American Book.

Gresham, F.M. (1986). Conceptual issues in the assessment of social competence in children. In P. Strain, M. Guralnick, M., & H. Walker (Eds.), **Children's social behavior: Development, assessment, and modification** (pp. 143-186). New York, NY: Academic Press.

Hermann, K. (1959). **Reading disability: A medical study of word blindness and related handicaps.** Springfield, IL: Charles C Thomas.

Hinshelwood, J. (1917). **Congenital word blindness.** London, England: H.K. Lewis.

Kirk, S. (1963). **Proceedings of the annual meeting of the conference on exploration into the problems of the perceptually handicapped child** (Vol. 1). Chicago, Ilinois

Learner, J.W. (1989). **Learning disabilities: Theories, diagnosis, and teaching strategies** (5th ed.). Boston, MA: Houghton Mifflin.

Lloyd, J.W, & deBettencourt, L.J.U. (1982). **Academic strategy training: A manual for teachers.** Charlottesville, VA: University of Virginia Learning Disabilities Research Institute.

Mercer, C.D. (1987). **Students with learning disabilities** (3rd ed.). Columbus, OH: Merril.

Pullis, M. (1983). Stress as a way of life: Special challenges for the LD resource teacher. **Topics in Learning and Learning Disabilities, 3,** 14-36.

Reid, D.K. (1988). **Teaching the learning disabled: A cognitive developmental approach.** Boston, MA: Allyn & Bacon.

Reynolds, C.R. (1985). Measuring the aptitude-achievement discrepancy in learning disability diagnosis. **Remedial and Special Education, 5**(3), 19-23.

Salvia, J., & Ysseldyke, J. (1988). **Assessment in special and remedial education.** Boston, MA: Houghton Mifflin.

Schumaker, J.B., & Hazel, J.S. (1984). Social skills assessment and training for the learning disabled: Who's on first and what's on second? Part 1. **Journal of Learning Disabilities, 17,** 422-431.

Schumaker, J.B., Hazel, J.S., Sherman, J.A., & Sheldon, J. (1982). Social skill performance of learning disabled, non-learning disabled, and delinquent adolescents. **Learning Disability Quarterly, 5,** 388-397.

Strauss, A.A., & Lehtinen, L.E. (1947). **Psychopathology and education of the brain-injured child.** New York, NY: Grune & Stratton.

Strauss, A.A., & Warner, H. (1942). Disorders of conceptual thinking in the brain-injured child. **Journal of Nervous and Mental Disease, 96,** 153-172.

U.S. Congress, Federal Public Law 94-142, **Congressional Record,** 94th Congress, November 29, 1975, **12,** 173-196.

U.S. Office of Education (1968). **First annual report of National Advisory Committee on Handicapped Children.** Washington, DC: U.S. Department of Health, Education, & Welfare.

Waldron, K.A., Saphire, D.G., & Rosenblum, S.A. (1987). Learning disabilities and giftedness: Identification based on self-concept, behavior, and academic patterns. **Journal of Learning Disabilities, 20**(7), 422-432.

Warner, M.M., Schumaker, J.B., Alley, G.R., & Deshler, D.D. (1980). Learning disabled adolescents in the public schools: Are they different from other low achievers? **Exceptional Education Quarterly, 1,** 27-36.

Werner, H., & Strauss, A.A. (1940). Causal factors in low performance. **American Journal of Mental Deficiency, 44,** 163-168.

Werner, H., & Strauss, A.A. (1941). Pathology of figure-background relation in the child. **Journal of Abnormal and Social Psychology, 36,** 236-248.

Westman, J.C. (1990). **Handbook of learning disabilities.** Boston, MA: Allyn & Bacon.

White, W.J., Schumaker, J.B., Warner, M.M, Alley, G.R., & Deshler, D.D. (1980). **The current status of young adults identified as learning disabled during their school career** (Research Report No. 21). Lawrence, KS: University of Kansas Institute for Research in Learning Disabilities.

## About the Author

Jack Little, Ph.D., is a Professor of Education, Division of Special Education, California State University, Los Angeles, California. He coordinates the Special Education Teacher Training Program in the areas of learning handicaps and serious emotional disturbance. Dr. Little is also known for his extensive work in the area of AIDS research and case management of persons with HIV infection.

# Chapter 32

# CEREBROVASCULAR ACCIDENTS

by
*Joshua Goldman, M.D.*

## INTRODUCTION

Cerebrovascular disease is one of the major forms of neurological disorder. It includes all abnormalities of blood vessel disease within the brain and spinal cord. Commonly encountered forms of cerebrovascular disease include ischemic and hemorrhage stroke, hypertensive stroke, vascular malformations, and aneurysm with intracranial hemorrhage. There are a multitude of other diseases that affect blood vessels in the central nervous system that occur less commonly. These include various forms of vasculitis (inflammation of small blood vessels) as well as fibromuscular hyperplasia, Moya-Moya disease, lupus erythematosus, and polyarteritis nodosa (Barnett, Moler, Stein, & Yatsu, 1986; Millikan, McDowell, & Easton, 1987).

## ANATOMY

The arterial circulation of the brain is most frequently involved in cerebrovascular accidents. Occasionally, venous abnormalities occur as well. Four major arteries supply the brain: the two common carotid arteries and the two vertebral arteries. The common carotid artery in the neck divides into the internal and external carotid artery. The external carotid artery supplies blood to the extra brain structures, such as the meninges (the membrane covering the brain). The internal carotid artery passes into the skull and then branches into the ophthalmic artery, the posterior communicating artery, the anterior choroidal arteries, and then terminally branches into the anterior and middle cerebral arteries. The vertebral arteries join to form the anterior spinal artery and the basilar artery. The basilar artery supplies branches to the brainstem and cerebellum and terminates as the two posterior cerebral arteries.

Knowledge of the anatomy of the vasculature supplying the brain is important in that each artery supplies a specific area of the brain. When the artery is occluded, lack of oxygen will lead to abnormalities of brain function (ischemia) and, if persistent, death of the brain cells supplied by the specific artery. Collateral circulation is generally not a major significant factor in the central nervous system blood supply. Collateral circulation occurs in most other areas of the body except the central nervous system. Arterial and venous interconnections occur between major arterial systems so that if one artery is blocked, the area needing oxygen obtains blood via another major artery. This is termed collateral circulation.

Vertebral and basilar arteries generally supply the brainstem. Small perforating arteries, the anterior and posterior choroidal arteries, typically supply the deep brain matter such as the thalamus and basal ganglia. Anterior choroidal arteries are supplied by the carotid and the posterior communicating artery. The posterior cerebral artery supplies the posterior portion of the brain, including the posterior portions of the temporal lobe and the occipital lobe.

The middle cerebral artery supplies the middle brain regions including the parietal and portions of the frontal lobe, as well as the anterior portion of the temporal lobe. The anterior cerebral artery typically supplies the anterior frontal lobe (Adams, 1989; Joint, 1990; Rowland, 1989).

# CEREBROVASCULAR ACCIDENT (CVA) (STROKE)

## Causes of Stroke

Ischemic vascular disease of the brain (lack of oxygen) results from transient ischemic attacks or stroke. The latter is also called a cerebrovascular accident (CVA). There are two major causes of stroke, cerebral embolus and thrombus.

**Cerebral embolus.** Embolic stroke implies a particle or substance travelled from a large artery and lodged in a smaller artery, thereby obstructing it. Sources of embolus are typically the heart, aorta, or carotid vessels. Characteristically, blockage of arterial circulation results in decreased or absent blood flow. This leads to a deficit, which is greatest at the time of onset and is proportional to the length of time of the obstruction. If the obstruction lasts for just a brief period with a full recovery following, the condition is called a transient ischemic attack (TIA). Transient ischemic attacks also may be caused by transient muscle spasm of the artery without an embolus or a thrombus. If the obstruction persists beyond 6-10 minutes, brain cell death occurs leading to a stroke (CVA) and a fixed neurological deficit.

**Thrombus.** The second major form of obstructing arteries in stroke is by a thrombus. This essentially is a blood clot developing within the brain vasculature leading to obstruction of an artery. Typically, neurological symptoms are progressive over several minutes to an hour or so and become maximal as time progresses. If the obstruction lasts for a brief period, transient ischemic attack will result, with recovery of neurological function. If the obstruction is persistent, stroke with fixed neurological deficit occurs (Halperin & Hart, 1988).

Most frequently, embolic disease is caused by atherosclerotic vascular disease (hardening of the arteries) in which a small portion of atherosclerotic plaque breaks off and travels to blood vessels within the brain. Less commonly, bacterial endocarditis (an acute infection of the inner lining of the heart) can lead to clumps of bacteria breaking off and acting as emboli. In people over the age of 60, atherosclerotic vascular disease and cardiac disease are the most common causes of stroke. In the younger population, other diseases become more significant, such as fibromuscular hyperplasia, vasculitis, coagulation abnormalities, and valvular heart disease.

## Neurological Deficits

Transient ischemic attack (TIA) by definition is a cerebrovascular event with full recovery of neurological function occurring within 24 hours of onset (Meyer & Shaw, 1982). A stroke is a neurological deficit persisting beyond 24 hours. Generally, stroke occurs in people over 60 years of age. Less frequently, stroke can occur in younger individuals.

Typical clinical residual findings of the middle cerebral artery after a stroke include abnormalities of the motor and sensory cortex leading to a spastic hemiparesis (inability to move the affected arm and leg on one side of the body). In addition, there will be decreased sensation of the body on the affected side of the brain. Stroke in the right middle cerebral artery distribution is frequently associated with asomatagnosia, which is a state in which the individual does not recognize the affected side of the body as belonging to oneself. Right middle cerebral artery lesions will affect the left side of the body. Left middle cerebral artery lesions will affect the right side of the body.

Lesions of the left middle cerebral artery may affect the speech centers and typically will cause speech abnormalities as well (Adams, 1989; Joint, 1990).

Abnormalities of the posterior circulation, including the vertebral artery and the basilar artery, will cause brainstem strokes. These typically result in crossed neurological findings. There will be abnormalities ipsilateral (affecting the same side) to the side of the stroke involving the face, and contralateral (affecting the opposite side) to the side of the stroke involving the body, including the arm and leg on one side of the body.

## Complications

A major stoke is a devastating occurrence. Approximately one-third of individuals die within 7-14 days of a major stroke and the mortality rate increases with age. Approximately one-third will experience devastating neurological deficit and approximately one-third will have minor or no deficit. The extent of damage depends on the person's age, general health, and size and location of the lesion. Recurrence of stroke is common and each new one is likely to increase the neurological deficits (Berkow, 1987).

Complications of a stroke may include physical paralysis, intellectual deficits, communication or perceptual problems, emotional lability, and behavioral changes. Any or all these may occur; yet, an individual may recover fully and have no noticeable deficits or difficulties. Other problems that may be observed include contractures, seizures, bowel and bladder problems, and spasticity of the muscles. Statistically of interest in rehabilitation is that of those who survive, approximately 50% will have myocardial infarction (heart attack) within the following year. In the group that survive for one year, marked neurological deficit often occurs. All strokes, however, are not necessarily major and devastating. Frequently, small strokes occur that may result in mild or no residual deficits. Clinically, small silent (lacunar) strokes are the most often seen in the aged individual.

## Treatment

There are three phases in the treatment of stroke. These include: (1) the acute state or onset; (2) the stage of recovery and convalescence; and (3) the special problems stage (Krupp & Chatton, 1975).

**Acute state or onset** (Krupp & Chatton, 1975; Rowland, 1989). This state occurs immediately after the stroke and requires acute medical management. Various medical emergency measures are taken. These may include general life support measures (bed rest, medication, feeding tubes, and possible catheterization). Additional measures may involve lumbar puncture, anticoagulant therapy, and surgery. This stage generally lasts 7-14 days.

**Stage of recovery and convalescence** (Krupp & Chatton, 1975; Schroeder et al., 1990). Early medical rehabilitation is important for long-term recovery. This intensive program has four primary goals. One (1) is achievement of mobility and ambulation. A second (2) is achievement of self-care. The third goal (3) is to help the patient with psychosocial adjustment to disability. Lastly (4), the rehabilitation team aims to prevent secondary, permanent disability and return the individual to the mainstream of life. During this stage, the patient goes through a four-phase progressive program consisting of:

1. bed phase (exercise, self-care)

2. standing phase (exercise, self-care)

3. stair-climbing phase (exercise, self-care, bracing)

4. cane-walking phase (slow gait, fast gait)

Depending on the severity of the stroke, initial rehabilitative efforts may begin within 1-2 days of the stroke. Typically, most of the recovery after a stroke will occur within 3-6 months of the stroke.

**Special problems (stage) in patients with hemiplegia.** (Adams & Victor, 1989; Krupp & Chatton, 1975; Schroeder et al., 1990). Special problems of patients with hemiplegia may include care of the paralyzed upper extremity, treatment for aphasia, organic brain syndrome, and medications.

In most cases involving a paralyzed upper extremity, return of complete function does not occur, as opposed to lower extremity paralysis in which function returns about 90% of the time. As partial function returns, physical therapy may help improve function related to possible return to work. This is particularly significant when the dominant upper extremity is the one affected.

Aphasia, when present, can benefit from appropriate speech therapy. This should be started as quickly as possible. In these cases, when the aphasia is sensory or receptive, the person finds it most difficult to comprehend verbal communication; treatment is difficult and progress limited.

Organic brain syndrome may occur in stroke. It is unlikely these individuals will return to work activity. Yet, an active medical rehabilitation program sometimes can improve an individual's impaired mentation.

The vocational rehabilitation counselor must keep in mind that the person who has had a stroke may be taking various types of prescribed medication. Familiarity with the medications and their side effects, especially when considering return to work, is crucial.

## Evaluation

**Heart involvement.** Evaluation of a stroke may include studies of other important vascular components, including the heart. The cardiac function study includes an electrocardiogram and echocardiogram. The physician also undertakes evaluation of the carotid vessels (the major entry arteries to the head and neck). This may include a noninvasive carotid vascular study or, sometimes, an invasive carotid and cerebral angiogram (MRI angiogram is replacing these studies). If a significant cardiac abnormality is found, such as a cardiac arrhythmia or valvular disease, the physician may prescribe anticoagulation medication, such as coumadin. The individual will remain on this medication for life. If the physician finds carotid vascular disease, medical treatment with acetysalicylic acid (aspirin) is the prevalent mainstay of medical treatment. Studies suggest that aspirin will decrease the risk of major stroke by approximately one-third (Smith et al., 1990).

**Other vascular components.** Alternative treatment is to consider carotid endarterectomy (surgical removal of atherosclerotic plaque from the lining of the carotid artery). Current studies have evaluated the effectiveness of carotid endarterectomy versus medical management. If a significant stenosis is present (greater than 70%), carotid endarterctomy will decrease the risk of stroke. Although commonly performed, data does not support significant improvement considering the surgical risk. After an acute stroke, some improvement in neurological function does occur. This will range from slight improvement to substantial improvement, with minor neurological deficits persisting. Typically, after an acute stroke, optimal recovery in neurological function will take place in 3-6 months. Yet, some slight ongoing improvement is seen for a longer period after that (Johnstone, 1985; Kaplan & Cerullo, 1986; Mulley, 1985; Rowland, 1989).

Hemiplegia (hemi-half, plegia-paralysis) is a major consequence of stroke. It involves paralysis of one-half side of the body. A person is said to have right hemiplegia if the right side of the body has paralysis. The lesion in the brain will typically be on the opposite side. The upper extremity is usually more limited functionally, by paralysis, than the lower extremity (Sharpless, 1982).

When the stroke occurs on the right side of the brain, paralysis may occur to the left arm and leg. The extent of paralysis depends on the site and extent of the lesion. Visual-spatial deficits also can occur when the stroke affects the right side of the brain. The individual with visual-spatial problems may incorrectly interpret visual information and have difficulty with environmental orientation.

A stroke occurring on the left side of the brain may result in paralysis to the right upper and lower extremities. These individuals also may have deficits in the ability to solve problems. If the speech centers are affected, problems in communication also may occur. This deficit is called aphasia. It can involve either the absence or an impairment in the ability to communicate through speech, writing, or signs; this complication seriously affects vocational rehabilitation.

**Emotional problems.** Emotional instability also often occurs in persons who have sustained strokes. One may see a rapid shift and change in emotions for no apparent reason. Partial loss of emotional control may be experienced and expressed clinically as various emotional states, such as crying, sudden laughter, depression, and hostility (Cox, 1972; Mulley, 1985). Besides the clinical neurological deficit seen after a stroke due to brain damage, depression and occasionally psychosis may occur. Depression is not unusual and may interfere with rehabilitation; it responds well to antidepressant medication.

Any area of the brain may be affected by a stroke. The most common arteries involved are the middle cerebral, choroidal, and basilar system arteries. Deficit depends on size and location of the stroke. The size of stroke, as seen on CT (computerized tomography) or MRI (magnetic resonance imaging) brain scans, frequently does not correlate well with the degree of deficit seen clinically.

# INTRACRANIAL HEMORRHAGE

The three major causes of intracranial hemorrhage are ruptured aneurysm (a congenital weakness and ballooning of the vessel wall), rupture of a vascular malformation, and rupture of an artery in the brain due to high blood pressure (hypertensive hemorrhage). These three are described below.

## Aneurysm

An aneurysm commonly develops at branch points of cerebral blood vessels and represents a thinning of the arterial wall leading to an outpouching of the blood vessel. Any weakened arterial wall is at risk for rupture. Intracranial aneurysms typically rupture during the fifth decade of life, or after. Approximately 85% of cerebral aneurysms develop in the anterior circle of Willis that includes the middle cerebral artery and the anterior and posterior communicating arteries. There are multiple aneurysms in approximately one-fifth of individuals. In the basilar artery, a specific form of aneurysm develops; it is a fusiform (elliptical) aneurysm, causing an enlargement of the entire basilar artery. Basilar artery aneurysms may enlarge sufficiently to cause pressure and compress cranial nerves or portions of the brainstem. In addition, a thrombus may occur leading to a stroke involving most or all of the brainstem. This event is invariably fatal. Less common causes of aneurysms include mycotic (fungal infections) aneurysms and aneurysms associated with vasculitis (inflammation of the arteries) (Adams, 1989; Rowland, 1989; Smith et al., 1990).

When an aneurysm ruptures, it gives rise to bleeding into the subarachnoid or brain space. Blood in the subarachnoid space and spinal fluid causes an inflammatory response. All areas of the brain in contact with bloody spinal fluid become inflamed. This is a potentially reversible cause of neurological deficit. Clinically, this bleeding episode will cause the person to complain of severe headaches, eventually leading to loss of consciousness and coma. The aneurysm also may rupture into the brain substance itself in which case the nerve tissue surrounding the hemorrhage will be disrupted and become nonfunctional. This leads to local neurological deficit similar to that seen in stroke. This deficit is irreversible.

Following the rupture of an aneurysm, a blood clot forms. There are two major complications following the rupture of an aneurysm. One is the dissolution or breaking up of the clot with rehemorrhage from the ruptured site, and the second is vascular muscle spasm of intracranial blood vessels leading to ischemia and stroke. Surgical intervention does not affect survival for the first 7 days. Typically, physicians observe individuals with aneurysms for at least 7 days before attempting surgical correction of the aneurysm. A ruptured aneurysm is a catastrophic event with approximately only half the individuals surviving for 30 days. Approximately 40% of paitents survive for 6 months; of that population, approximately 25% will be totally disabled. Without corrective surgery, recurrence of bleeding is approximately 4% per year.

## Vascular Malformation

Vascular malformations are congenital abnormal collections of blood vessels. They are typically a tangled interconnected network of blood vessels in which arteries pass directly into veins without intervening capillaries and supporting brain tissue. There are several different forms of cerebrovascular malformations; the most significant are the artery and vein malformations. Approximately 50% of vascular malformations will bleed eventually, and these may occur in any portion of the brain. Vascular malformations typically bleed into brain tissue. The neurological deficit that will result depends upon the site and areas of brain where the bleeding occurs and on the extent of the hemorrhage.

## Hypertensive Hemorrhage

Individuals who have had significant hypertension over several years may develop abnormalities in small blood vessels in the brain. Physicians call this condition amyloid angiopathy. This degenerative pathological process affects and weakens small blood vessels of the brain, usually choroidal arteries. In a person with a severe sudden increase in blood pressure, a rupture may occur that leads to a hemorrhage within the brain.

The most common sites of cerebral hypertensive hemorrhage involve the deep gray matter, secondly various areas of the brain including temporoparietal or frontal lobes, and finally portions of the brainstem and cerebellum. Approximately one-third of individuals die within the first month after a hypertensive hemorrhage. In persons with minor hemorrhages, often neurological recovery occurs with minimal residual deficit. The thrust of long-term prevention is adequate control of blood pressure. Individuals experiencing difficulty in controlling high blood pressure should avoid stressful situations and heavy work, which often elevate blood pressure (Barnett et al., 1986; Millikan et al., 1987).

# FUNCTIONAL LIMITATIONS

The patient who survives the initial phase of a major stroke may improve significantly over the next 3-6 months. There may be a significant return of physical functioning, particularly when paralysis is due to edema (brain swelling), rather than permanently damaged nerve tissue. Manual dexterity and coordination also may return (Cox, 1972). During this early phase, supportive medical treatment and physical and occupational therapy are useful. Vocational rehabilitation services are best provided after 6 months, when most of the physical improvement has occurred. Early intervention by a rehabilitation counselor shortly after the stroke is beneficial, since a counselor can let the individual know that there is a possibility for a return of gainful employment. The rehabilitationist also can provide information on how to obtain vocational guidance when the client is ready.

Other residuals of stroke include problems with speech (aphasia), visual impairment, motor impairment, and generalized weakness. Each of these possible deficits needs careful assessment when considering vocational rehabilitation alternatives. Through the provision of reasonable accommodation, job modification, and job restructuring, many of the functional limitations of these deficits can be minimized.

Depending on the extent of brain damage, individuals with aphasia may benefit from speech therapy and later occupational therapy. Interaction between the rehabilitation counselor and the therapist can help direct rehabilitation efforts toward important occupational characteristics of future employment. This is one reason early intervention by the counselor can be so crucial in the overall rehabilitation effort. Aphasia deficits can involve auditory comprehension, speaking, reading, and writing. Jobs vary in the degree to which they use these four aspects of communication. A detailed job analysis will enable the counselor to determine which job functions are essential and which are secondary. This information will simplify rehabilitation planning for individuals with multiple aphasia deficits.

Hemiplegia is a common result of stroke (Carr & Shepherd, 1983; Veith, 1988). The physical therapist provides strengthening exercises for both upper and lower extremities. Interaction with the counselor helps direct the exercise program toward occupational characteristics of future employment goals. There are many orthotic devices such as leg braces that may help the person ambulate and return to work. Splints and other orthotic devices improve use of the affected arm and hand. Once the counselor and client have decided on a return to work objective, special orthotic devices may be developed to help the person with specific job functions.

Emotional lability is a difficult area since it is often unpredictable and frequently occurs for no identifiable reason. Open discussion with the client, counselor, and employer is essential in many cases. Employer understanding of the problem can help alleviate some of the client's concerns and lead to earlier successful return to gainful employment.

Stroke also may cause intellectual impairment. There can be problems with memory and with the ability to concentrate. Work evaluation provides an opportunity to observe an individual over time and may assist the rehabilitation counselor in evaluating deficits of intellectual functioning. Once one identifies and analyzes intellectual impairments, the counselor will be better equipped to assess future employment options.

Some intellectual deficits can be minimized and others circumvented. For example, the person with memory difficulties can learn to use a small notepad and write down information that may be forgotten. Certain intellectual tasks crucial to the job may be reassigned to other employees. If job modification is not possible or the extent of intellectual impairment too great, use of transferable skills or retraining may be necessary. Considering the age of many persons with stroke, extensive retraining is not feasible; use of transferable skills is usually a more realistic procedure to follow.

Stroke most often occurs in older individuals. Many will be beyond working age and others, due to advancing age, may not choose to return to work. Older workers often have many years of work experience and have developed a significant number of work skills. The counselor can use this work experience and potential array of transferable skills to help in return to work.

Early intervention by a rehabilitation counselor may be crucial, especially when considering return to work with the previous employer. Since recovery time may be prolonged, it is important for the counselor to have early contact with the employer to maintain the potential of the individual returning to previous employment.

Many patients who have had one or more strokes may be on anticoagulant medication. This may cause excessive bleeding with serious cuts and injuries. The individual may need to avoid jobs where there is a likelihood of injury, such as sheet metal work, automotive mechanics, and construction jobs.

If the individual has residual paralysis involving a lower extremity, there will be limits on standing and walking. A sedentary occupation with limited ambulation is advisable. There also may be restrictions on lifting and carrying; most individuals are restricted to a maximum of light work activity.

Upper extremity paralysis involving the dominant hand involves significantly more problems than paralysis of the nondominant hand. Although there are programs for dominance retraining, these have met with limited success. The age and intellectual capacities and deficits of the client will be considerations in evaluation this dimension.

Persons with high blood pressure may need to avoid excessively stressful work environments and heavy exertion work activity that tend to elevate blood pressure. Compliance with medication can be a problem with some patients.

As previously noted, the person may have depression or other psychological problems. Psychological counseling will help the individual develop insight to understand the condition and at least partially control emotional lability.

# REHABILITATION POTENTIAL

Only a small number of persons who have sustained stroke will be candidates for vocational rehabilitation. Many will be retired and some, because of advanced age, may choose not to return to gainful employment. For individuals with severe impairment, the provision of independent living skills and counseling may be necessary.

The variety of functional limitations that occur makes generalization difficult. Persons who have little or no deficit will not require rehabilitation counseling services. On the opposite end of the continuum, individuals with a variety of physical, emotional, and intellectual deficits may be difficult to evaluate. For some, an extensive work evaluation program will help the counselor determine the limitations and potentials of the person with multiple deficits.

For individuals who have had major strokes, the counselor must wait at least 6 months to determine rehabilitation potential, as maximum return of function takes up to 6 months. Yet, early intervention is advisable to maintain and encourage the person's desire to return to work. Prompt intervention with the previous employer may facilitate an eventual return to work.

Since many individuals with stroke are older, skills and work experience may increase rehabilitation potential. The counselor should carefully consider use of transferable skills for individuals that have a skilled or semiskilled work history.

Socioeconomic factors have a bearing on return to gainful employment. Sharpless (1982) reported that individuals with at least a high school education and a professional, managerial, or technical job returned to work significantly more often than those with only a grammar school education and manual job experience.

Vocational programs that offer a multidisciplinary approach to stroke rehabilitation have had the greatest success. The key to success is in coordination of services and team work.

The ability to drive is a determinant in successful vocational rehabilitation. The ability to travel independently to and from the work or training site is a factor in maximizing rehabilitation potential. Various comprehensive rehabilitation centers provide driver training for persons with disabilities. There are also adaptations to the vehicle to accommodate the disability.

Sharpless (1982) noted that studies have not identified specific psychological factors related to vocational success. Many studies cite motivation as a prime component of successful return to work. As with other disabling conditions, some individuals are highly motivated, despite a variety of complications and symptoms. Unfortunately, there are also clients who appear impossible to motivate and may have little potential for rehabilitation. These cases are the greatest challenge for the vocational rehabilitation counselor.

# CASE STUDY

Ms. Mary Whitworth is a secretary for a large aerospace company. Her job is described below.

SECRETARY (clerical) **D.O.T.** # 201.362-030 (U.S. Department of Labor, 1991). Schedules appointments, gives information to callers, takes dictation, and otherwise relieves officials of clerical work and minor administrative and business detail. Reads and routes incoming mail. Locates and attaches appropriate file to correspondence to be answered by employer. Takes dictation in shorthand and transcribes notes on typewriter or word processor. Composes and types routine correspondence. Files correspondence and other records. Answers telephone and gives information to callers or routes call to appropriate official and places outgoing calls. Records minutes of staff meetings. Makes copies of correspondence or other printed material, using copying or duplicating machine. May prepare outgoing mail, using postage-metering machine. Delivers mail to various departments located in different buildings.

Although the job is classified as sedentary work, Ms. Whitworth is required to deliver mail to various departments, in different buildings. This activity requires walking around the large aerospace facilities for about 1 hour per day.

This job took about 1-2 years to fully learn. The company has employed Ms. Whitworth in this position for 15 years. After finishing high school and receiving her diploma, she worked for several years in a restaurant as a short-order cook. Also, she worked in various manufacturing plants as an electronics assembler, tester, and packer. She is right-handed.

This case was referred to you by the employer. The medical file indicates that the day before Ms. Whitworth's 61st birthday, she had a stroke. Two weeks after the stroke, the company called you and requested vocational rehabilitation services. They authorized you to provide any and all services you felt would benefit this valued employee.

The stroke occurred on the right side of the brain. It was a moderate stroke that would cause some permanent functional limitations. Although unknown at the time of referral, Ms. Whitworth will recover about 80% functioning. The functional limitations would involve all the typical areas that could be affected by a stroke on the right side of the brain and would be considered mild to moderate. In reviewing the medical information of record, you note that Ms. Whitworth was hypertensive before her stroke; at this time, her physician is able to control her blood pressure with medication.

The company would like Ms. Whitworth to return to work as quickly as possible. They feel she has been an outstanding employee and is very loyal to the company. The company president understands the importance of early intervention and reasonable accommodation and is willing to consider all possibilities for rehabilitation.

## Questions

1. Give a vocational profile for this client including age category, education level, work history (exertional level & skill level), occupationally significant characteristics, and job skills. Which of the occupational characteristics and skills may be affected by the residuals of the stroke?

2. How will Ms. Whitworth's age affect your provision of rehabilitation services? Explain your response.

3. Speculate on Ms. Whitworth's probable medical problems and prognosis.

4. Indicate possible functional limitations from a physical and psychosocial standpoint?

5. Outline the vocational rehabilitation services you will provide including when they will begin and the time frames for each step in the process.

6. Discuss how and at what times you will involve the employer in the rehabilitation process.

# REFERENCES

Adams, R.D., & Victor, M. (1989). **Principles of neurology** (4th ed.). New York: NcGraw-Hill Information Services.

Barnett, H.J.M., Moler, J.P., Stein, B.M., & Yatsu, F.M. (Eds.). (1986). **Stroke pathophysiology, diagnosis and management.** New York, NY: Churchill Livingstone.

Berkow, R. (1987). **The Merck manual** (15th ed.). Rahway, NJ: Merck.

Carr, J.H., & Shepherd, R.B. (1983). **A motor relearning program for stroke.** Rockville, MD: Aspen.

Cox, B.G. (1972). **Care and rehabilitation of the stroke patient.** Springfield, IL: Charles C Thomas.

Halperin, J.L., & Hart, R.G. (1988). Atrial fibrillation and stroke: New ideas, persisting dilemmas. **Stroke, 19,** 947.

Johnstone, M. (1985). **Restoration of motor function in the stroke patient** (2nd ed.). New York, NY: Churchill Livingstone.

Joint, R.J. (1990). **Clinical neurology.** Philadelphia, PA: J.B. Lippincott.

Kaplan, P.E., & Cerullo, L.J. (Eds.). (1986). **Stroke rehabilitation.** Boston, MA: Butterworths.

Krupp, M.A., & Chatton, M.J. (1975). **Current medical diagnosis and treatment.** Los Altos, CA: Lange Medical Publications.

Meyer, J.S., & Shaw, T. (Eds.). (1982). **Diagnosis and management of stroke and TIAs.** Menlo Park, CA: Addison-Wesley.

Millikan, C.H., McDowell, F.H., & Easton, J.D. (1987). **Stroke.** Philadelphia, PA: Lea and Febiger.

Mulley, G.P. (1985). **Practical management of stroke.** Oradell, NJ: Medical Economics Books.

Rowland, L.P. (Ed.). (1989). **Merritt's textbook of neurology** (8th ed.). Philadelphia, PA: Lea and Febiger.

Schroeder, S.A., Krupp, M.A., Tierney, L.M., Jr., & McPhee, S.J. (1990). **Current medical diagnosis and treatment.** Norwalk, CT: Appleton & Lange.

Sharpless, J.W. (1982). **Mossman's a problem-oriented approach to stroke rehabilitation** (2nd ed.). Springfield, IL: Charles C Thomas.

Smith, L.H., Jr., Plum, F., Carpenter, C.C.J., Andredi, T.E. (Eds.). (1990). **Cecil essential of medicine** (2nd ed.), Philadelphia, PA: W.B. Saunders.

U.S. Department of Labor (1991). **Dictionary of occupational titles** (4th ed., revised). Washington, D.C.: Author.

Veith, I. (1988). **Can you hear the clapping of one hand? -** Learning to live with a stroke. Berkeley, CA: University of California Press.

## *About the Author*

Joshua Goldman, M.D., is a neurologist in private practice in Las Cruces, New Mexico. He is on the medical staff at the Memorial Medical Center in Las Cruces and is on the Panel of Medical Experts of the Social Security Administration.

# *Chapter 33*

# CEREBRAL PALSY

by
*Peter Kopriva, Ed.D.*
*and*
*Joseph R. Taylor, Ed.D.*

"Remember that persons with disabilities are persons first and disabled individuals secondly. These persons have the same right to self-actualization as any others - at their own rate, in their own way, and by means of their own tools. Only they can suffer their nonbeing or find their 'selves.' " (Buscaglia, 1983, p. 18).

## INTRODUCTION

This chapter is dedicated to individuals who have cerebral palsy in the hope the information provided will help in the knowledge and training of skilled and sensitive professionals providing services to persons with cerebral palsy. We believe the physical difficulties faced by persons with cerebral palsy are secondary in magnitude to how they may feel about themselves and their adjustment or maladjustment as seen through the eyes of family, peers, service providers, and society. Perhaps our society could offer no greater gift than to support the development of dignity, self-worth, and self-respect in all people. We must guard against patronizing and making assumptions in our various professional roles that we know what is "best" for a given individual. With proper interaction among service providers, agencies, families, and individuals with cerebral palsy, the likelihood of self-actualization may become a reality.

Historically, individuals in many fields have struggled to find a definition that adequately describes individuals who have cerebral palsy. We are indebted to those pioneering individuals whose interests lay in the treatment of persons with cerebral palsy. Their willingness and ability to share the knowledge gained through the treatment process led to our present level of professional understanding of cerebral palsy.

### *Definition*

An earlier contributor to the knowledge base concerning cerebral palsy was Dr. William John Little (1810-1894), an English surgeon. His was the first description of the conditions which were later to be known as cerebral palsy. However, at that time, Little's professional interest in diagnosing and treating individuals with the disorders led to their being known as "Little's Disease" (Green, 1975).

The term "cerebral palsy" was introduced by Dr. Winthrop Phelps in 1937. Phelps dedicated most of his professional career as an orthopedic surgeon to the treatment and study of cerebral palsy. He established the Children's Rehabilitation Institution of Baltimore to provide specialized treatment and training for individuals with cerebral palsy. Phelps helped provide guidance to clinics, hospitals, and special schools established to serve those with cerebral palsy throughout the United States (Bleck, 1982; Green, 1975).

Current professional literature provides numerous definitions and examples of cerebral palsy. These definitions, while having many similarities, reflect the diverse professional orientation of their authors. One definition of cerebral palsy which appears to be functional and understandable to those from a variety of working disciplines is that of Bleck (1982): "Cerebral palsy is a non-progressive disorder of movement and is caused by a malfunctioning of, or damage to, the brain (cerebral dysfunction). "(p. 59)

As this (and other) definitions imply, the disorders known as cerebral palsy have the following features in common: (a) aberrant control of movement or posture; (b) early onset; and (c) no recognized underlying progressive pathology. These disorders affect movement and posture due to damage to areas of the brain that control motor function. Cerebral palsy manifests itself in a variety of conditions that affect numerous anatomical locations throughout the human body, different levels of severity, various expressions of manifestation, and through variable associated disorders. Disorders of speech, such as dysarthria (slurred speech due to muscle tightness, weakness, or incoordination), and aphasia (impairment in ability to communicate through speech or writing) are frequently associated impairments. These manifestations of cerebral palsy are used to determine the medical classification of the condition in specific individuals (see Table 1).

## Table 1
## CLASSIFICATION OF TYPES

Classification of cerebral palsy is determined by its manifestations which depend upon the location, cause of the damage, and development of the brain at which time the damage occured. A system of classifying or describing cerebral palsy was developed by Dr. Winthrop Phelps and adopted by the American Academy for Cerebral Palsy in 1956 (Minear, 1956).

### Classification of Cerebral Palsy
   I. Physiological (motor)
        A. Spastic
        B. Athetotic
            1. Tension
            2. Non-tension
            3. Dystonic
            4. Tremor
        C. Rigidity
        D. Ataxic
        E. Tremor
        F. Atonic (rare)
        G. Mixed
        H. Unclassified

II. Topographical
        A. Monoplegia - involves one limb
        B. Paraplegia - involves the legs only and practically always of the spastic or rigidity type
        C. Hemiplegia - the lateralized one-half of the body is affected and it is usually spastic, although pure athetoid hemiplegias are occassionally seen, as are pure rigidity hemiplegias
        D. Triplegia - involves three extremities, usually both legs and one arm, usually spastic
        E. Quadriplegia - (tetraplegia) involvement of all four extremities
        F. Diplegia - affecting like parts on either side of the body
        G. Double Hemiplegia - arms are more involved than the legs

**III. Etiological** (See discussion text of chapter)
A. Prenatal
B. Natal (perinatal)
C. Postnatal

**IV. Supplemental**
A. Psychological evaluation
1. Degree of mental deficiency, if any
B. Physical status
1. Physical growth evaluation (Wetzel Grid or other)
2. Developmental level
3. Bone age
4. Contractures
C. Convulsive seizures
D. Posture and locomotive behavior patterns
E. Eye-hand behavior patterns
1. Eye dominance
2. Eye movements
3. Eye postures
4. Fixation
5. Convergence
6. Prehensory approach
7. Grasp
8. Manipulation
9. Hand dominance
F. Visual status
1. Sensory
2. Motor
G. Auditory status
H. Speech disturbance

**V. Neuroanatomical** (See figure 1 in text of chapter)
The following two headings are added for completeness, and for the use of the clinician studying the patient with cerebral palsy.

**VI. Functional Capacity** (degree of severity)
Class I.      Patients with cerebral palsy with no practical limitation of activity
Class II.     Patients with cerebral palsy with slight to moderate limitation of activity
Class III.    Patients with cerebral palsy with moderate to great limitation of activity
Class IV.    Patients with cerebral palsy unable to carry on any useful activity

**VII. Therapeutic**
Class A.     Patients with cerebral palsy not requiring treatment
Class B.     Patients with cerebral palsy who need minimal bracing and minimal therapy
Class C.     Patients with cerebral palsy who need bracing and apparatus, and the services of a cerebral palsy treatment team
Class D.     Patients with cerebral palsy limited to such a degree that they require long-term institutionalization and treatment

## Classification

In most cases, children and adults who have cerebral palsy can be divided into two major physiological categories. In one category, the structural change involves the "pyramidal" tract (pathway) of the nervous system; spasticity is a key sign. This system derives its name from the arrangement of nerve fibers (pyramid arrangement) that descend from the brain surface motor cells of the cerebral cortex through the spinal cord to the muscles they enervate (see Figure 1). These cells and nerve fibers have a primary function of the voluntary control of muscles in the limbs. Consequent damage to either the cells or nerve fibers results in spastic paralysis.

In the other category, the "extra pyramidal" tract of the nervous system is involved, with athetosis (slow, irregular, twisting movements) exhibited as the principle sign. Damage that occurs in the extra pyramidal area of the brain means the damage has taken place in the parts of the brain that exclude the pyramidal area (see Figure 1). This damage is assumed to occur in the large cell collection in the central portion of the brain (basal ganglia). A commonly used term for these disorders of movement is dyskinetic (difficulty of movement) cerebral palsy. Within this group are the athetoses (deranged physical motions) (Keats, 1965). While mixtures of these two categories can be confusing to the practitioner, they do not invalidate the distinctness of the two identifiable categories.

## Figure 1
## NEUROANATOMICAL CLASSIFICATION

Representation of the major portion of the brain involved in each of the three major types of cerebral palsy.

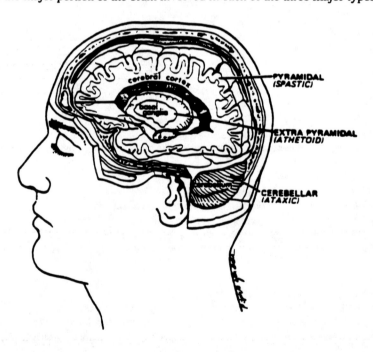

From **Physically Handicapped Children: A Medical Atlas for Teachers** (2nd ed., p. 67) by E.E. Bleck and D.A. Nagel, 1982, New York: Gruen & Stratton. Copyright 1982 by Allyn & Bacon. Reprinted by permission.

# ETIOLOGY

One may acquire cerebral palsy during the prenatal period (before birth), perinatal period (around the time of birth), or postnatal period (following birth through the early developmental years). In each of these periods, there are numerous factors which may contribute to the condition. Of growing concern is the type of damage sustained by the brain because of infections, toxins, or trauma.

Three distinct groups delineate the causes of cerebral palsy: PRENATAL FACTORS (before birth), PERINATAL FACTORS (around the time of birth), and POSTNATAL FACTORS (following birth) (Bleck, 1982).

## Prenatal Causes

1.  **Hereditary.** This rare cause of cerebral palsy is genetically transmitted, often sex-linked, with symptoms present at birth or soon after. It does not progress. The common inherited form is familial spastic paraplegia.

2.  **Infections.** Infections can cause cerebral palsy when acquired in utero (during the mother's pregnancy), such as rubella (German measles) in the first 3 months (first trimester) of pregnancy, syphilis, herpes, HIV, AIDS, toxoplasmosis (parasitic infection), and cytomegalic inclusion disease (a presumed virus).

3.  **Prenatal anoxia.** This condition involves a lack of oxygen from premature separation of the placenta, malformation of the placenta, shock due to loss of blood (injury to mother, e.g., auto accident), and kinking or knotting of the umbilical cord.

4.  **Rh incompatibility.** If the Rh factor is present in the fetus (Rh+) but not in the mother (Rh-), the mother's immune defenses manufacture destructive agents (antibodies) that destroy the infant's red blood corpuscles. This state results in an anemia (hemolytic anemia) in the infant. The blood cell disintegration products (bilirubin), when combined with a lack of oxygen, cause damage to the brain. Today, most cases of cerebral palsy due to Rh incompatibility are preventable with immunization of the mother and early exchange transfusion of the infant.

5.  **Prematurity.** This may cause cerebral palsy if the child is born before developing in the womb less than 40 weeks (gestation) and having a birth weight of less than 5 pounds. Within the United States, prematurity accounts for 33-60% of all cases of cerebral palsy.

6.  **Metabolic disorders.** These disorders are predominantly maternal diabetes or toxemia of pregnancy, occurring during the last trimester.

7.  **Unknown origin.** It is estimated that up to 30% of all prenatal cerebral palsy is in this category. Most cases exhibit abnormal development of the brain originating during the first 12 weeks of pregnancy, when the brain is completing most of its development.

## Perinatal Causes

1.  **Trauma (birth injury).** The infant skull can be injured during the delivery process. Rupture of blood vessels in the brain or compression of the brain results in sustained damage. Injury during birth is more likely when the baby's head is large in relationship to the mother's pelvis (cephalopelvic disproportion), in difficult deliveries, in breech birth, and in prolonged labor.

2.  **Lack of oxygen (fetal asphyxia, anoxia, or hypoxia).** The brain cells can survive only a few minutes without oxygen. Possible reasons for anoxia are lung collapse or pneumonia. Also, excessive sedation at the time of birth in an attempt to relieve the distress of labor can be a cause.

## *Postnatal Causes*

1. **Traumatic head injuries.** These include skull fractures and brain lacerations. There is a growing incidence of battered children that is becoming the leading reason for head injuries.

2. **Infections and toxic conditions.** Meningitis, encephalitis, syphilis, brain abscess, and toxic chemical (e.g., lead poisoning) can cause cerebral palsy.

3. **Brain hemorrhages or clots.** Sudden and spontaneous brain hemorrhages occur in children and most often produce a one-sided limb spastic paralysis. A traveling blood clot or embolus from the heart can lodge in a blood vessel within the brain, resulting in the blood supply being cut off, causing destruction of nerve cells.

4. **Cerebral anoxia (lack of oxygen to the brain).** Carbon monoxide poisoning, drowning, and cardiac arrest are common examples.

5. **Brain tumors.** Due to direct invasion of a tumor or through compression and pressure changes of normal tissues, brain tumors may lead to cerebral palsy.

# DIAGNOSIS

## *The Difficulty of Diagnosis*

The study of normal human development in infants and children has added significant knowledge to the study of individuals who experience abnormal or delayed development. The work of Gesell and others firmly established both uniformity and the concept of variation in the normal developmental sequence of children. Acquaintance with this basic framework is essential to the understanding of the growth process. More importantly, it is the cornerstone upon which identification and understanding of abnormal development rest (Scherzer & Tscharnuter, 1982).

There is a reliable and orderly process from birth which is continuous with in utero development. The basis of this process is the ascending development of brain center control. Newborn infants rely on behavior that is largely reflex, mediated primarily through the brain stem. As the individual acquires maturity, behavior proceeds toward "higher" centers, ultimately reaching independence in full voluntary control. Some degree of voluntary movement is present even in the neonate. Primitive reflexes in the infant give way to more postural reflexes and proceed to full voluntary behavior. Individual responses that come under voluntary control eventually replace all the initial activity based on reflexes. Motor maturation proceeds in an orderly direction: motor control of the head, neck, and trunk precede extension of the trunk, and ultimately full weight bearing and walking occur.

One measure of early human development is that maturation of the normal central nervous system occurs simultaneously at many different levels. There is an orderly sequence in development, yet considerable variation is seen within a given child in achieving stages of motor and intellectual achievement. Motor development is a succession of integrated milestones leading to more complex and independent function.

The challenge for those dealing with developmental problems in children is to accurately assess the significance of delay that falls outside the limits of variability. Knowledge of the normal orderly sequence of developmental achievement and patterns of integration of behavior is the basis upon which one can gauge possible significant deviation in maturation. There is no early pathognomonic sign (pathology predicting), x-ray, or laboratory test, which confirms the condition; it is based on a combination of factors.

A diagnosis of cerebral palsy is not easily made in the immediate postnatal period. Such a diagnosis is usually clinical, made by a physician specializing in pediatrics or a general practitioner with a thorough knowledge of cerebral palsy. The beginning point is often contact by a concerned parent whose child is not progressing in motor milestones of speech. Too often, the concerns shown by the parents toward their child's development may not be given serious consideration unless definite focal motor abnormality is found. A starting point is a sensitivity of the professional to possible neurological deficit in a child with developmental delay or infant behavior problems. The professional needs to conduct information gathering in an orderly and sequential manner including the important factors discussed below.

## Laboratory Testing

Laboratory tests in cerebral palsy rule out the possibility of progressive neurological illnesses or indicate where the brain damage occurred and its extent. The following tests are used selectively and carefully (Bleck, 1975).

1. **Skull x-ray.** This may be used to rule out abnormalities such as toxoplasmosis evidenced, which may be by calcifications (white spots) on the skull.

2. **Electroencephalogram (EEG).** EEG is used in the diagnosis of seizure disorders, or to find focal lesions such as brain tumor or old scars from prior brain injury.

3. **Pneumoencephalogram.** Because of newer and more informative procedures, such as magnetic resonance imaging, this procedure is rarely used. In this procedure, air is injected into the ventricles of the brain. The air shadows show up on x-ray. A displaced ventricle may mean a tumor in the brain. The physician can sometimes diagnose cerebral atrophy (shrinkage of part of the brain).

4. **Brain scan.** Radioactive isotopes are injected into the blood stream. The resultant recording or radiation from brain tissue can often localize brain tumors.

5. **Cerebral arteriogram.** As in pneumoencephalogram, this procedure is less frequently used. A dye that can be seen on x-ray (radiopaque) is injected into the blood stream. The x-ray of the skull will show the blood vessels and pick-up abnormalities of the arteries in the brain (e.g., aneurysm, local dilation of a blood vessel).

6. **Computerized axial tomography (CAT scan).** CAT scan is a procedure wherein the electronic impulses of the x-ray beam are processed by a computer which reconstitutes and displays the cross-section of the part of the brain being studied.

7. **Magnetic resonance imaging (MRI).** MRI is a non x-ray procedure which utilizes the application of an external magnetic field to distinguish hydrogen atoms in different environments of soft tissue. This information is processed by a computer that produces an image.

8. **Blood and urine analyses.** These laboratory tests may show chemical abnormalities related to cerebral palsy.

# TREATMENT

## Early Intervention

The rehabilitation process for a child with cerebral palsy is a complex undertaking, enhanced significantly by beginning early treatment when prompt diagnosis permits. Parent involvement is a key to the overall success of any rehabilitation program.

Despair and denial are common emotions parents frequently feel after the diagnosis of any disability, cerebral palsy being no exception. The power of these emotions can be an asset when redirected toward a more constructive adjustment if therapy is suggested immediately. Parents and siblings receive reassurance when a treatment plan includes intensive training and guidance of the family in techniques of management and proper developmental stimulation designed to suit the functional level of the child.

According to Molnar and Taft (1977), early sensorimotor experiences are crucial for cognitive development at a young age. This becomes even more crucial when the opportunity to learn through exploration is limited from birth by a motor disability with consequent deprivation during development. Currently held practice suggests the sooner early intervention begins, the more possibilities there will be that motor function will occur in a more desirable manner at any developmental stage. The onset of therapy during the first few weeks of life is not too soon to begin such programming with families of children who experience cerebral palsy. Early intervention in knowledge of how to work with their children and what to expect about realistic development are important.

## Treatment Approaches and Programs

**Treatment approaches.** Treatment approaches recommended for the movement disorder of cerebral palsy have been evolving since the first works of Jennie Colby (Molnar & Taft, 1977). The recent trend toward very early diagnosis and intervention has greatly shifted initial emphasis away from orthopedic surgery, and placed major priority on global remediation of the existing developmental deficits (Scherzer & Tscharnuter, 1982). According to Bobath (1967), the aims of early treatment are the following:

1. To develop normal postural reactions and postural tone against gravity for support and control of movement.

2. To counteract the development of abnormal postural reactions and abnormal postural tone.

3. To give the child, by means of handling and play, the functional patterns that will be later used for feeding, dressing, washing, and other self-help activities.

4. To prevent the development of contractures and deformities.

**Treatment program.** When formulating a treatment program, it is necessary to anticipate: (a) whether, in the future, the child will be able to sit, stand, and walk; (b) what degree of bimanual or unilateral hand dexterity one expects the individual to have; (c) in which activities of daily life the person is likely to achieve independence; and (d) whether the individual can accomplish any of these skills, with or without adaptive techniques or assistive devices. The treatment procedures professionals may recommend for the movement disorder of cerebral palsy are orthopedic surgery, medications, physical therapy, occupational therapy, and bracing (orthotics). Early treatment, when the condition is first diagnosed, is aimed at improving function through measures that decrease muscle spasm and improve mobility.

## Physical Therapy Treatment Techniques

**Crothers.** The approach of Crothers, while not a unique treatment procedure, is a basic guide to involving the child in a meaningful program. Crothers stressed the need for a variety of movement and stimulation activities to help prevent contractures and encourage active participation, even in the most severely involved children. Another aspect of his treatment technique is to counsel parents against overprotectiveness to enable the child to be more independent. Crothers' philosophy is considered mainstream thinking today because of its comprehensive approach, which includes individualized assessment that prepares and guides the child in realistic and appropriate activities.

**Phelps.** This method uses an orthopedic approach with conventional techniques from poliomyelitis treatment regimens. Individual muscle therapy is stressed. Emphasis is also placed on training in gross movement patterns and inhibition of abnormal movements. This method also employs deep massage for muscle stimulation. Auditory and kinesthetic treatment activities are used, especially a combination of rhymes and music together with desired movement patterns to develop a conditioned reflex. The training technique theory holds that once an association is established between a musical rhyme and movement, the child can perform the movement upon hearing or reciting the rhyme.

Phelps also encouraged visual stimulation and eye-hand-foot coordination activities in addition to particular emphasis on the use of orthotic devices for regulation of tone and postural adjustment. Additionally, the method uses relaxation techniques for dyskinesias (defects in voluntary movement).

Weights are highly regarded in the treatment of ataxia (defective muscular coordination). Stretching exercises are advocated for spasticity. Ultimately, the goal is to reduce the extent of bracing used for control at a particular joint. The techniques developed by Phelps remain in active use today because they represent the first coherent systematic approach to treatment of the individual with cerebral palsy.

**Deaver.** Deaver's emphasis is on functional ability rather than patterns of movement. Objectives within his treatment model include:

1. Performance of bed and wheelchair activities.

2. Maximum use of hands.

3. Performance of ambulation and stair climbing.

4. Achievement of adequate speech and hearing.

5. Achievement of as near normal appearance as possible.

This method employs extensive bracing designed to restrict all but two movements of an extremity in functional activity. Bracing requirements are reduced as functional control is achieved. Deaver places considerable emphasis on intensive training, as well as activities of daily living (ADL), particularly wheelchair use. These required treatment training periods are prescribed in a residential unit, at frequent intervals, as the child develops or needs to acquire new skills for function.

**Fay-Doman.** Fay, a neurophysiologist, pursued the idea of motor developmental levels of the brain comparable to the evolutionary process. The most primitive levels are related to the lowest evolutionary life forms with development progressing through maturation at each level. This highly controversial concept suggests that first the brain must evolve through the developmental stages of fish and reptile, then evolve toward mammalian species, and ultimately humans. Insult or injury to the central nervous system interrupts this process with fixation at some given lower or immature stage.

Glen Doman and Carl Delacato, who co-founded the Institution for the Achievement of Human Potential, integrated the theory described above into a treatment system, which is based upon the level of neurological organization. The belief is that within this system, the child must become proficient at each neurological level before advancing to the next level.

Expectations for parent involvement in this program is extremely high. Parents are trained, at the institute, to utilize a variety of activities with their child in an effort to enhance the child's neurological organization. Because of the intensity of this program, it is frequently necessary to enlist the services of other family members, neighbors, and volunteers from the community to help in fulfilling this demanding treatment regimen.

**Rood.** Margaret Rood's treatment approach emphasizes both sensory and motor aspects of movement. The basis of this approach is in activating muscles through sensory receptors, and then using a sequence of developmental patterns of movement. Muscles are activated through modalities of heat, cold, and brushing.

**Bobath and Neurodevelopmental Therapy (NDT).** The Bobaths have enjoyed the most recent and perhaps most extensive influence in the therapy field today. Their treatment system is a neurodevelopmental approach to the total underlying deficits that relate to tone, movement, and posture. Theoretically, this method is designed to inhibit abnormal reflex activity and facilitate normal automatic movement. Before actual treatment, the therapist assesses the child's reflexes, the variations in muscle tone, and how the child performs. The test is most often called the "basic motor maturity evaluation." This information is then used in practice of normal movement patterns with the child, consistent with motor development. The Bobath Treatment Method enjoys wide appeal throughout the United States and Europe where NDT therapy has led to extensive training programs for therapists. Certification in NDT has considerable status as a mark of professional expertise in this field.

**Others.** Frequently called the Eclectic Method, many knowledgeable therapists prefer to use a combination of approaches and a variety of modalities as the basis of treatment. Following thorough evaluation of a patient including deficits and needs, professionals develop a management plan, incorporating various approaches. This selective approach offers much flexibility and allows the therapist to individually tailor a program to a child's needs. Lack of uniformity and systematization can create difficulty in evaluating and comparing results. Proper identification and record keeping, including therapy descriptions and progress, can aid in the understanding of a patient's program between therapists and settings.

## Occupational Therapy

This therapy discipline complements the efforts put forth by the physical therapist in treatment of the individual with cerebral palsy. In many settings, physical and occupational therapists work as a team, frequently with other specialties in coordinated efforts to serve the individual and family. Activities of daily living are significant goals for a child who may experience life-long deficits in even the simplest of activities involving eating, dressing, mobility, and other everyday activities. Observation and testing in areas of motor, perceptual, and visual-motor activities can aid in the development of successful strategies for independence. For example, rather than concentrating on handwriting activities, the person receives training and necessary adaptive aids to write successfully with an electric typewriter or computer. Also, activities such as cooking, eating, and toileting might all require adaptation that allows for partial or total independence in these activities.

## Medication

The use of drugs to alter motor deficits and improve movement has been generally unsuccessful, particularly in efforts to control spasticity. Professionals have tried a variety of muscle relaxants with little benefit. The greatest amount of use has been with infants and preschool age children.

Dantrolene sodium, while showing evidence of helping stroke patients recover some use of functional abilities, has not had the same benefits with cerebral palsy. This drug does show some benefit in reducing muscle excitability in the individual by reducing spasticity. It appears the effectiveness of the drug is highly individual. Dantrolene sodium helps manage spastic paralysis and mixed types of spasticity and athetosis.

Prescribed medications play a significant role in the control of various associated disabilities for the individual affected by cerebral palsy. Anticonvulsants are essential in the management of seizure disorders. Medication also has become standard treatment practice for hyperactive behaviors and attention disorders in children, by facilitating their opportunities in education and other life areas. Drug treatment in the older child is especially important as requirements in independence at school, social activities, and transition into adulthood begin to take on importance for the individual and the family.

## Surgery

The medical treatment team and consequent surgical management has priority over any other treatment considerations. Surgical correction of any brain lesion associated with cerebral palsy in an infant may involve treatment of hydrocephalus, vascular abnormalities, cysts, or benign tumors. Intractable seizures may respond to partial resection of brain tissue; recent developments in this arena have been successful.

Recently, implant of an electrical pacemaker in a portion of the cerebellum has been successful in reduction of abnormal tone, extrinsic movements, and increase in functional ability in some adults. This procedure has generally not been used with infants. It remains an area of great interest and hope as technology and engineering help to shape the future of surgical possibilities.

Orthopedic care and management are primary in effective early medical treatment. With other medical specialists and therapy staff, the orthopedic surgeon provides guidance and direction in conservative approaches to limit or prevent abnormality and use of specialized equipment. The developing child receives maximum benefit obtained from therapy, bracing, and what would be considered other conservative measures. Orthopedic surgical procedures often are essential to overcome residual deformity and improve function in the individual. Complicated procedures are performed in stages as need demands.

Corrective eye surgery for strabismus (deviation of the eye) is common practice in helping the child and should be performed as early as appropriate to prevent amblyopia (loss of vision). Repair of cleft lip and palate is similarly essential and should be done while the child is still young. Other types of corrective procedures may be necessary, and, as mentioned earlier, would likely be planned in conjunction with the total treatment program, including therapy team members and the family. The importance of the team approach to treatment cannot be stressed enough in the overall success of any individual's gaining increased independence and functional abilities. Isolated treatment approaches, while common in the past, cannot compare in general effectiveness with the team approach.

# VOCATIONAL POTENTIAL

## Legislation and Accessibility

The vocational potential of people who have cerebral palsy is as broad as the range of disabilities caused by the condition. Some, due to the severe extent of physical and cognitive involvement, may be very unlikely candidates for vocational rehabilitation services. Changes in the types of jobs that are and will be available in the future place greater emphasis on intelligence and creativity, and less emphasis on physical strength (Naisbitt & Aburdene, 1990). The shift from greater physical exertion in the workplace to more intellectual demands, coupled with the development of high-tech assistive devices, will make jobs available for many to whom competitive employment was not previously a realistic goal.

Legislation has played an important role in making employment a more viable goal for many people with cerebral palsy. Section 504 of the Rehabilitation Act of 1973 provides assurances to people with physical disabilities that public buildings and places of business receiving federal funds are fully accessible. In 1990, the Americans with Disabilities Act (ADA) was passed to make most other businesses, workplaces, and public transportation accessible to persons with disabilities. Under the ADA, employers cannot refuse employment based on a person's disability. Laws such as these have helped eliminate limited mobility as a barrier to employment for many people with cerebral palsy and related conditions (Holmes, 1990).

As the workplace becomes more accessible to persons with disabilities, many opportunities for knowledge about people with disabilities should be available for the nondisabled population. It is hoped that such knowledge and familiarity will lead to a decrease in attitudinal barriers imposed upon those with disabilities.

## *Other Factors*

Speed and manual dexterity are requirements on many jobs that may be impediments to some people with cerebral palsy. A goal of the vocational training program should be to evaluate qualities such as speed and manual dexterity and examine the various requirements in any vocation.

A further consideration is the social development of the person in terms of ability to function and interact with others in the workplace. The level of social maturity will directly affect the person's successfully functioning in competitive employment.

## *Integrated Employment*

Integrated employment was described by Turnbull, Turnbull, Bronicki, Summers, and Roeder-Gordon (1989) as a work situation where most of the workers are not disabled. There are two kinds of integrated employment. The first is "supported employment" in which the worker is employed in a paid position but receives some type of training or assistance while on the job. The second type is "competitive employment" in which the employee is hired over others in the work force due to being the best qualified for the job. These jobs are held independently of any type of support (Turnbull et al., 1989).

There are several benefits both for the person with cerebral palsy and for society when these people are engaged in competitive employment. First, when a person is engaged in competitive employment, the opportunities to earn more wages and benefits are greater than for those in sheltered employment situations. The need for public assistance is thus decreased.

A second advantage is that persons with disabilities, who are competitively employed, have opportunities to be integrated into society with nondisabled workers. They have opportunities to interact with nondisabled people, not only in receiving services, but in providing services as well. As integration on the job increases, so do opportunities for friendships to develop between co-workers.

There are other advantages of competitive employment. These include the chance to function in a more normal setting, a greater opportunity for advancement, improved attitudes by family, friends, and employers, and improved perceptions by legislators who provide funds for vocational rehabilitation (Wehman, 1981).

# FUNCTIONAL LIMITATIONS

## *Physical Considerations*

The extent of physical limitations of the person with cerebral palsy is an important consideration when planning prevocational and vocational training strategies. Input from physicians, physical therapists, occupational therapists, speech and language specialists, vocational evaluators, rehabilitation counselors, and psychologists is essential in planning for long-range vocational goals.

Modern treatment for people who have cerebral palsy begins in infancy or sometimes before the child is born, if the mother or her pregnancy is considered "at risk" for having medical complications. Medical personnel, therapists, and educators with special training may be part of these early intervention programs. Parents are taught skills necessary in properly caring for a child with a disability to help the child develop functional independence. Staff members and educators work with the parents and child in developmental assessment and training. This includes pre-speech and feeding endeavors, activities designed to assist in reflex development and integration, functions to stimulate more normal growth and development, and therapeutic exercises to help develop greater mobility.

Children may need orthopedic surgery as they continue to mature. The purpose of surgery is to correct for abnormal brain input to muscles that may leave the child with deformed limbs and severely limited ability for normal movement in the affected limbs. With the help of surgery, corrective bracing of affected limbs, and physical therapy, children with cerebral palsy are often able to gain mobility and greater independence.

## Intellectual Considerations

Distorted physical appearance resulting from motor involvement and accompanying speech problems associated with many individuals with cerebral palsy encourages negative assumptions to be made regarding intellectual abilities. Caution must be exercised by professionals involved with the assessment for training and career exploration for these individuals. The underestimation of an individual's intellectual ability has the potential for denying them training opportunities, ideal residential settings, and vocational and educational opportunities.

As a population, individuals with cerebral palsy are found to have a higher incidence of intellectual deficits than the general population. Studies have indicated that mental retardation accompanies cerebral palsy in approximately half to three-quarters of those studied (Best, 1978; Nelson & Ellenberg, 1978). While mental retardation is noted in higher levels than in the general population, the actual intelligence levels measured within this group also includes many individuals who demonstrate average and above average intellect.

## Emotional Considerations

Management of cerebral palsy is a team process that often subjects the person with the condition to extensive periods of time spent in hospitals and treatment and training programs. The constant demand of these regimens may lead to emotional complications in persons with cerebral palsy and their families. Emotional stress from intensive programs are not the only pressures related to this condition.

Buscaglia (1983) discussed the development of self in persons with disabilities. While these people develop in the same way as those without disabilities, there are many additional negative influences on the development of people with disabilities that may combine to cause lower self-concept. Buscaglia described the forces influencing self-concept development of people with disabilities in the following manner: "These major forces seem to relate mostly to interpersonal relationships, disability-related frustrations, social acceptance and rejection, limitations of experience, physical and emotional suffering, and inferiority and lowered status" (p. 173).

The interactive effects of powerful forces upon the emotional stability of an individual or upon a family unit may be dramatic. Emotional considerations should be an integral part of any cerebral palsy management program.

Persons with cerebral palsy also may experience emotional and other psychological problems. It is advisable for the management team to include a professional with a psychological counseling background who may work with individuals with cerebral palsy and provide guidance to other team members in this important area. Teachers, physicians, nurses, therapists, counselors, and family members may participate in providing emotional support and guidance.

## Social Considerations

A most difficult challenge is to develop acceptable social skills. Social development may range from extreme self-centered behavior to behavior that is normal in all respects.

The family and management team must be aware of social development and assist in developing traits that are acceptable in the home, workplace, and society. If these traits are not present when the person enters vocational training, social skills training should be included in the vocational training program.

# REHABILITATION POTENTIAL

## Legislation

Public Law 94-142, the Education for all Handicapped Children Act of 1975, was enacted to assure children with a broad range of disabilities a free, appropriate public education. To broaden the impact of Public Law 94-142, Congress passed Public Law 99-457, the Education for all Handicapped Act Amendments of 1986. The purposes of the amendments were to extend the impact of Public Law 94-142 into the areas of career development and life skills. Besides reauthorizing the transition program and funding activities for persons with disabilities, the act also provided for grants for demonstration projects and technical assistance for transition programs and programs for early childhood special needs (birth to 5 years) (Berkel & Brown, 1989).

## Education and Functioning in Society

Individuals who may have remained at home or been placed in residential institutions, are now offered the opportunities to enter and complete school in preparation for entering the labor market. Those students and graduates present a problem to all who are concerned with the provision of services for persons who have cerebral palsy. The problem may be expressed through several pertinent questions. What happens after students with cerebral palsy complete public school programs? Can they function successfully in independent living situations? Can they enter vocational training programs? Are they capable of earning a living? Do they have skills that are in demand in the workplace? Have they been given an opportunity to develop skills in leisure-time activities? Have they developed the social skills necessary to interact in a satisfactory manner with the public or with co-workers on the job?

These questions and similar ones need to be answered if we are to succeed in preparing children and adults with disabling conditions to function to their maximum potential in society. Due in part to the availability of new, "high-tech" devices, many people who have cerebral palsy can answer "yes" to most of the questions listed above. Many still continue to be unemployed or underemployed. Roessler (1987) pointed out the staggering rates of unemployment among people with disabilities. He reported that only one-third of men and one-fifth of women with disabilities were employed. To curb this trend, many school systems have instituted transition programs to assist older high school students with meeting the demands of self-sufficiency.

Transition is a term that is used to denote the move from-school to the world of adult life. Many people, representing various fields, may be involved in this transition and the adult working life of people with cerebral palsy.

## Technology

The extraordinary gains in technology during the past two decades have helped provide persons with cerebral palsy and other physically disabling conditions to have much brighter prospects in the vocational area. Computers are used to perform many job functions in the modern workplace. While the physical challenges facing people with cerebral palsy often make it difficult to perform many manual tasks required on some jobs, others are finding they can perform many of these job functions with computers and other electronic equipment.

A person who works in the field of accounting, for example, often uses computers. The computer, through application of the many available adaptive input devices, may be operated equally well by workers who function with a wide range of physical abilities and disabilities. Computers may be operated with one finger, one hand, one foot, the user's head, a puff of breath, voice input, eye input (through eye blinks or eye movement), and other methods (Ridgeway & McKears, 1985). Voice synthesizers are available to help those with unintelligible speech in communicating orally. They may allow a person with a severe form of cerebral palsy to communicate well enough to gain employment which otherwise would be denied.

Computer input devices are available to assist in environmental control. With such a system, a person can control electrical appliances and electrical equipment anywhere in the home or workplace from one centralized control unit.

Products for people with disabilities are now commonly available from many companies. This development of "high-tech" products for use by individuals with disabilities has provided many opportunities for vocational training and education not previously available. While much of this electronic equipment is expensive, there are agencies in government and the private sector which may provide financial aid to the person who needs such devices but is unable to afford the cost.

## Vocational Assessment and Training

People with cerebral palsy have historically presented serious problems to those who provide prevocational and vocational training programs. As Christy Brown shared in the book, **My Left Foot** (1955), others often have difficulty communicating with and assessing the ability of people with cerebral palsy. Often, due to severe physical involvement, others tend to immediately associate the condition with impaired mental ability. Brown represents many authors, artists, and other successful people who have cerebral palsy.

Service providers assist in locating vocational assessment and training, whether it be through vocational rehabilitation or similar agencies. The person with cerebral palsy also may need assistance in matching particular personal strengths and abilities with compatible jobs or training programs.

## Employment

Turnbull et al. (1989) presented an in-depth discussion of the importance of being employed. The authors described employment as a crucial aspect of our lives. Besides financial rewards, work gives us a feeling we are productive citizens and not a burden on society. Our job provides us with friends and social acquaintances with whom we interact daily and gives us a means in which to identify. We often identify ourselves as teachers, carpenters, assemblers, or with the company where we work. Having a job with a regular paycheck also provides a sense of security and independence.

Common to many endeavors in life, a person often faces uncertainty and a host of other obstacles that can, without guidance and confidence in one's abilities, intimidate the individual. The field of rehabilitation counseling requires thoughtful and deliberate methods to make accurate assessments of individuals who are at a distinct disadvantage for enjoying many aspects of daily life. Because of mental, emotional, physical, social, or other conditions that affect their well-being, persons with cerebral palsy may be unable to realize their potential without adequate rehabilitation and proper intervention techniques.

# CASE STUDY

Cynthia Wagner is a 22 year-old student attending a local community college. Currently, in her sophomore year, Ms. Wagner is struggling with the selection of an appropriate major that meets her interests and abilities. She has shown exceptionally high aptitude in the area of computers and computer science and has been encouraged by her advisors and professors to consider a major in computer science at the regional state university. Unsure about those recommendations, Cynthia acknowledges her interest in computers, but also is aware of her strong love for agriculture.

This individual grew up on the family farm that produces table grapes, walnuts, and oranges. She loves farming activities and, in keeping with her childhood development on the farm, has been drawn to potential careers that are related to farming. In reality, however, Cynthia realizes that her physical disabilities, which have limited her in an ability to work on the family farm, will present obstacles which she must overcome.

At an early age, a physician diagnosed Ms. Wagner as having athetoid cerebral palsy. Medical records indicate the degree of involvement to be Class III (moderate to great limitation of activity) evidenced in all four limbs (quadriplegia). For mobility, she uses a wheelchair.

The availability of state services has helped Cynthia and her family, both for her therapeutic and educational training. Therapy intervention by the state children's services began in Cynthia's infancy, followed by educational programming from local public schools. Early education was provided in a specialized facility staffed by a multidisciplinary team of teachers, physical therapists, speech therapists, occupational therapists, nurse, and a school psychologist. All these professionals were trained in providing the specialized services required of children who have physical and health-related impairments.

After passage of the Education for All Handicapped Children Act of 1975, P.L. 94-142, Cynthia was able to benefit by attending a regular educational program with her disabled peers through junior high and high school. Transition was made possible by available school district support services and the emerging availability of technology.

Cynthia was able to compensate for her severe speech impairment by learning to use and communicate with electronic communication devices. Furthermore, curricular adaptations were made possible because of advances in computer technology. Through these available adaptations, Ms. Wagner was able to display her above average intelligence to her teachers and peers, finally gaining their understanding and appreciation for her talents.

Upon completion of high school and having earned a 3.5 grade point average, Cynthia selected a college. A local community college was chosen in part because of the availability of its Enabler Program, which provided supportive services. This program offers services beyond those provided by the regular college program and "enables" students to successfully pursue educational, vocational, and personal goals.

Ms. Wagner voiced her career concerns to the counseling staff of the Enabler Program who referred her to the rehabilitation counselor for advice. After analyzing her aptitudes and interests, the rehabilitation counselor worked with Cynthia to identify professions which would incorporate her aptitude with computers and her love of farming. They examined the occupations described in the *Occupational Outlook Handbook* (U.S. Department of Labor, 1990) and the **Dictionary of Occupational Titles** (U.S. Department of Labor, 1991). Cynthia eventually decided to enter a professional preparation program for agricultural scientists D.O.T.# 040.061-010 (crop scientist), -014 (animal scientist), -018 (dairy scientist), -038 (horticulturist), -042 (poultry scientist), and -058 (soil scientist);

041.061-014 (animal breeder), -018 (apiculturist - the study and breeding of bees), -046 (entomologist - the study of insects), and -082 (plant breeder); and 041.081-010 (food technologist).

Within this broad category, she found a number of professional occupations which fit her aptitudes and interests. After successful completion of her Associate of Science (A.S.) degree, she plans to transfer to a 4-year college or university. With the assistance of her rehabilitation counselor, Ms. Wagner now has additional career choices to make. Will she use her expertise to help her father make the family farm more automated and productive? Will she work in a U.S. Department of Agriculture research laboratory? Will she work in private industry? Will she select a career in higher education and teach others to become agricultural scientists? These options in career direction await Cynthia because of her strong intellect and spirit, the availability of emerging technology, and the dedication and expertise of countless professionals.

## Questions

1. What additional medical needs might Cynthia have that could affect her choice of careers?

2. Are her career goals compatible with her abilities and limitations?

3. Describe additional rehabilitation assessment information which may be required in this case.

4. Should Ms. Wagner be encouraged to explore additional career options? Why?

5. How might this client's educational and career options have differed if she had been born 20 years earlier?

6. What do you believe are Cynthia's greatest obstacles in fulfilling her chosen career? Is she limited more by her disability or by society's perception of her as a "disabled person?" Explain.

# REFERENCES

Berkell, D.E., & Brown, J.M. (1989). **Transition from school to work for persons with disabilities.** New York: Longman.

Best, G.A. (1978). **Individuals with physical disabilities: An introduction for educators.** St. Louis, MO: C.V. Mosby.

Bleck, E.E. (1975). Cerebral palsy. In E.E. Bleck & D.A. Nagel (Eds.), **Physically handicapped children: A medical atlas for teachers** (pp. 37-89). New York: Grune & Stratton.

Bleck, E.E. (1982). Cerebral palsy. In E.E. Bleck & D.A. Nagel (Eds.), **Physically handicapped children: A medical atlas for teachers** (2nd ed., pp. 59-132). New York: Grune & Stratton.

Bobath, B. (1967). The very early treatment of cerebral palsy. **Developmental Medicine and Child Neurology, 9,** 373-390.

Brown, C. (1955). **My left foot.** New York: Simon and Schuster.

Buscaglia, L. (1983). **The disabled and their parents: A counseling challenge.** Thorofare, NJ: Slack.

Cruickshank, W.M., & Raus, G.M. (Eds.). (1955). **Cerebral palsy - Its individual and community problems.** Syracuse, NY: Syracuse University.

Green, W. (1975). Historical notes - The past generation. In R. Samilson (Ed.), **Orthopedic aspects of cerebral palsy** (pp. 1-4). Philadelphia, PA: J.B. Lippincott.

Holmes, S.A. (1990, July 14). Rights bill for disabled is sent to Bush. **The New York Times,** p. 6, L.

Keats, S. (1965). **Cerebral palsy**. Springfield, IL: Charles C Thomas.

Minear, W. L. (1956). A classification of cerebral palsy. **Pediatrics, 18,** 841-852.

Molnar, G.E., & Taft, L.T. (1977). Pediatric rehabilitation, Part I: Cerebral palsy and spinal cord injuries. **Current Problems in Pediatrics, 7,** 3-46.

Naisbitt, J., & Adurdene, P. (1990). **Megatrends 2000: Ten new directions for the 1990s**. New York: William Morrow.

Nelson, K.B., & Ellenberg, J.H. (1978). Epidemiology of cerebral palsy. In B.S. Schoenburg (Ed.), **Advances in Neurology** (Vol. 19, pp. 421-435). New York: Raven Press.

Ridgeway, L., & McKears, S. (1985). **Computer help for disabled people**. London, England: Souvenir Press (E & A).

Roessler, R.T. (1987). Work, disability and the future: Promoting employment for people with disabilities. **Journal of Counseling and Development, 66,** 188-190.

Scherzer, A.L., & Tschamuter, I. (1982). **Early diagnosis and therapy in cerebral palsy**. New York: Marcel Dekker.

Turnbull, H.R., Turnbull, A.P., Bronicki, G.J., Summers, J.A., & Roeder-Gordon, C. (1989). **Disability and the family: A guide to decisions for adulthood**. Baltimore, MD: Paul H. Brookes.

U.S. Department of Labor (1990). **Occupational outlook handbook**. Washington, DC: Author.

U.S. Department of Labor (1991). **Dictionary of occupational titles** (4th ed., revised). Washington, DC: Author.

Wehman, P. (1981). **Competitive employment: New horizons for severely disabled individuals**. Baltimore, MD: Paul H. Brookes.

## About the Authors

Peter Kopriva, Ed.D., is Director and Professor, Programs in Special Education, Graduate School, Fresno Pacific College, Fresno, California. Dr. Kopriva has worked in a variety of teaching and administrative capacities in California and Colorado involving educational programming for individuals that have physical, mental, and other developmental disabilities. Current research interests include teacher preparation and service delivery options that provide lifespan programming, both in urban and rural communities, and include family support.

Joseph R. Taylor, Ed.D., is Professor of Special Education, Graduate School, Fresno Pacific College, Fresno, California. Dr. Taylor has served in various capacities as teacher and administrator in special education and regular programs in Mississippi, Alabama, Louisiana, and California. His current research interests include the provision for special educational services in rural and small school settings.

# INDEX

# INDEX

539